2019 GUIDE TO

MEDICATIONS FOR THE TREATMENT OF DIABETES MELLITUS

Edited by
John R. White, Jr., PA-C, PharmD

American Diabetes Association

Associate Publisher, Books, Abe Ogden; *Director, Book Operations,* Victor Van Beuren; *Managing Editor, Books,* John Clark; *Associate Director, Book Marketing,* Annette Reape; *Acquisitions Editor,* Jaclyn Konich; *Senior Manager, Book Editing,* Lauren Wilson; *Project Manager, Editor, and Composition,* Jeska Horgan-Kobelski; *Editor,* Brian Keating; *Printer,* Lightning Source®.

Printed in the United States of America
1 3 5 7 9 10 8 6 4 2

The suggestions and information contained in this publication are generally consistent with the *Standards of Medical Care in Diabetes* and other policies of the American Diabetes Association, but they do not represent the policy or position of the Association or any of its boards or committees. Reasonable steps have been taken to ensure the accuracy of the information presented. However, the American Diabetes Association cannot ensure the safety or efficacy of any product or service described in this publication. Individuals are advised to consult a physician or other appropriate health care professional before undertaking any diet or exercise program or taking any medication referred to in this publication. Professionals must use and apply their own professional judgment, experience, and training and should not rely solely on the information contained in this publication before prescribing any diet, exercise, or medication. The American Diabetes Association—its officers, directors, employees, volunteers, and members—assumes no responsibility or liability for personal or other injury, loss, or damage that may result from the suggestions or information in this publication.

♾ The paper in this publication meets the requirements of the ANSI Standard Z39.48-1992 (permanence of paper).

American Diabetes Association titles may be purchased for business or promotional use or for special sales. To purchase more than 50 copies of this book at a discount, or for custom editions of this book with your logo, contact the American Diabetes Association at the address below or at booksales@diabetes.org.

American Diabetes Association
2451 Crystal Drive, Suite 900
Arlington, VA 22202

DOI: 10.2337/9781580407007

Library of Congress Cataloging-in-Publication Data

Names: White, John R., Jr., 1958- editor. | American Diabetes Association, issuing body.
Title: 2019 guide to medications for the treatment of diabetes mellitus / John R. White Jr., editor.
Other titles: Guide to medications for the treatment of diabetes mellitus | Medications for the treatment of diabetes mellitus
Description: Arlington : American Diabetes Association, [2019] | Includes bibliographical references.
Identifiers: LCCN 2018056668 | ISBN 9781580407007 (softcover : alk. paper)
Subjects: | MESH: Diabetes Mellitus—drug therapy | Insulins—pharmacology | Hypoglycemic Agents—pharmacology
Classification: LCC RC661.I6 | NLM WK 815 | DDC 616.4/62061--dc23
LC record available at https://lccn.loc.gov/2018056668

This book is dedicated to the memory of R. Keith Campbell.

Keith was a close friend, a mentor, and an inspiration to me as well as to innumerable other healthcare providers, patients, students, and other people. This book was originally his brainchild. He co-edited each of the previous editions/permutations of this book.

Keith was diagnosed with type 1 diabetes when he was 8 years old. He lived with diabetes for more than 68 years, all the while remaining positive and helping myriad others with diabetes. He was always firmly at the forefront of knowledge in the diabetes arena. He published more than 600 manuscripts, 14 books, 55 book chapters, and made over 1,500 professional presentations. His multifaceted career at Washington State University as an academic spanned 45 years and included many roles and titles. He received numerous awards including the American College of Clinical Pharmacy's Paul F. Parker Medal, the National Community Pharmacists Association's Outstanding Pharmacy Administration Professor in the U.S., the American Diabetes Association's Outstanding Health Care Educator in the Field of Diabetes, and the American Association of Diabetes Educator's (AADE's) Distinguished Service Award. He served on the board of directors of the American Diabetes Association, Washington State Pharmacy Association, and AADE. He was beloved by his friends, family, and students, and was known for his outgoing personality. He was a remarkable, one-of-a-kind individual who is greatly missed. He will always be remembered for his indefatigable ability to manage a difficult, complicated, chronic disease with grace, for his larger-than-life personality, and for his ever-present cat-that-caught-the-mouse smile.

—*John R. White, Jr.*

Contents

Contributors   ix

1. **Pharmacologic Therapy for Type 1 Diabetes**   1

2. **Management of Hyperglycemia in Type 1 Diabetes Mellitus**   8
   Joshua J. Neumiller, PharmD, CDE, FASCP

3. **Insulin**   26
   Joshua J. Neumiller, PharmD, CDE, FASCP, and Kimberly C. McKeirnan, PharmD, BCACP

4. **Pharmacologic Therapy for Type 2 Diabetes**   48

5. **Overview of Medications Used to Treat Type 2 Diabetes**   66
   John R. White, Jr., PA-C, PharmD

6. **Biguanides**   80
   Peggy Soule Odegard, BSPharm, PharmD, CDE; Jennifer Danielson, PharmD, CDE; and Kam L. Capoccia, PharmD, BCPS, CDE

7. **Thiazolidinediones**   103
   Kam L. Capoccia, PharmD, BCPS, CDE; Jennifer Danielson, PharmD, CDE; and Peggy Soule Odegard, BSPharm, PharmD, CDE

8. **Sulfonylureas**   124
   Lisa Kroon, PharmD, and Crystal Zhou, PharmD

9. **Glinides**   138
   Lisa Kroon, PharmD, and Crystal Zhou, PharmD

10. SGLT2 Inhibitors   151

John R. White, Jr., PA-C, PharmD

11. α-Glucosidase Inhibitors   168

Kimberly C. McKeirnan, PharmD, BCACP, and Nicole M. Perea, PharmD

12. Dipeptidyl Peptidase-4 (DPP-4) Inhibitors   176

Kimberly C. McKeirnan, PharmD, BCACP, and Joshua J. Neumiller, PharmD, CDE, FASCP

13. Glucagon-Like Peptide-1 Receptor Agonists   190

Jennifer M. Trujillo, PharmD, BCPS, FCCP, CDE, BC-ADM

14. Pramlintide   211

Jennifer M. Trujillo, PharmD, BCPS, FCCP, CDE, BC-ADM

15. Bile Acid Sequestrants   223

Christina R. Buchman, PharmD, BCACP

16. Dopamine-2 Receptor Agonists   233

Christina R. Buchman, PharmD, BCACP

17. Cardiovascular Disease and Risk Management   241

18. Microvascular Complications and Foot Care   286

19. Hypertension   322

Cheyenne Newsome, PharmD, PhC, BCACP

20. Lipids   339

Cheyenne Newsome, PharmD, PhC, BCACP

21. Antiplatelets   355

Megan Willson, PharmD, BCPS, and Kimberly C. McKeirnan, PharmD, BCACP

22. Medications for Smoking Cessation   370
Anne P. Kim, PharmD, MPH, MIT

23. Medications for the Management of Neuropathy   395
Damianne Brand-Eubanks, PharmD, and Anne P. Kim, PharmD, MPH, MIT

24. Medications for the Management of Nephropathy   411
Emmeline Tran, PharmD

25. Medications for the Management of Retinopathy   439
Emmeline Tran, PharmD

26. Medications for the Management of Depression   460
Megan Willson, PharmD, BCPS

27. Medications for the Management of Hypoglycemia   472
Megan Giruzzi, PharmD, BCPS

28. Medications for the Management of Obesity   482
Nicholas R. Giruzzi, PharmD, BCPS

29. Immunizations and Diabetes   503
Kimberly C. McKeirnan, PharmD, BCACP, and Nicole M. Perea, PharmD

Index   509

Contributors

EDITOR

John R. White, Jr., PA-C, PharmD
Professor and Department Chair
Department of Pharmacotherapy
College of Pharmacy and
  Pharmaceutical Sciences
Washington State University
Spokane, WA

CONTRIBUTORS

Damianne Brand-Eubanks, PharmD
Clinical Assistant Professor,
  Pharmacotherapy
College of Pharmacy and
  Pharmaceutical Sciences
Washington State University
Yakima, WA

Christina R. Buchman, PharmD, BCACP
Clinical Assistant Professor,
  Pharmacotherapy
College of Pharmacy and
  Pharmaceutical Sciences
Washington State University
Yakima, WA

Kam L. Capoccia, PharmD, BCPS, CDE
Clinical Professor of Community Care
PGY-1 Community-Based Residency
  Program Director
College of Pharmacy and Health
  Sciences
Western New England University
Springfield, MA

Jennifer Danielson, PharmD, CDE
Associate Professor
Director, Introductory Practice
  Experiential Education
School of Pharmacy
University of Washington
Seattle, WA

Megan Giruzzi, PharmD, BCPS
Clinical Assistant Professor,
  Pharmacotherapy
College of Pharmacy and
  Pharmaceutical Sciences
Washington State University
Yakima, WA

Nicholas R. Giruzzi, PharmD, BCPS
Clinical Assistant Professor,
  Pharmacotherapy
College of Pharmacy and
  Pharmaceutical Sciences
Washington State University
Yakima, WA

Anne P. Kim, PharmD, MPH, MIT
Clinical Assistant Professor,
  Pharmacotherapy
College of Pharmacy and
  Pharmaceutical Sciences
Washington State University
Yakima, WA

Lisa Kroon, PharmD
Chair and Professor
Department of Clinical Pharmacy
School of Pharmacy
University of California, San Francisco
San Francisco, CA

Kimberly C. McKeirnan, PharmD, BCACP
Clinical Assistant Professor
Department of Pharmacotherapy
College of Pharmacy and
  Pharmaceutical Sciences
Washington State University
Spokane, WA

Joshua J. Neumiller, PharmD, CDE, FASCP
Vice Chair and Allen I. White
  Distinguished Associate Professor,
  Pharmacotherapy
Department of Pharmacotherapy
College of Pharmacy and
  Pharmaceutical Sciences
Washington State University
Spokane, WA

Cheyenne Newsome, PharmD, PhC, BCACP
Clinical Assistant Professor,
  Pharmacotherapy
College of Pharmacy and
  Pharmaceutical Sciences
Washington State University
Spokane, WA

Peggy Soule Odegard, BSPharm, PharmD, CDE
Associate Dean, Professional
  Pharmacy Education
Lynn and Geraldine Brady Endowed
  Professor of Pharmacy
School of Pharmacy
University of Washington
Seattle, WA

Nicole M. Perea, PharmD
PGY1 Academic Fellow
Department of Pharmacotherapy
College of Pharmacy and
  Pharmaceutical Sciences
Washington State University
Spokane, WA

Emmeline Tran, PharmD
Assistant Professor
College of Pharmacy
Medical University of South Carolina
Charleston, SC

Jennifer M. Trujillo, PharmD, BCPS, FCCP, CDE, BC-ADM
Associate Professor
Skaggs School of Pharmacy and
  Pharmaceutical Sciences
University of Colorado Anschutz
  Medical Campus
Aurora, CO

Megan Willson, PharmD, BCPS
Clinical Associate Professor,
  Pharmacotherapy
College of Pharmacy and
  Pharmaceutical Sciences
Washington State University
Spokane, WA

Crystal Zhou, PharmD
Assistant Professor
Department of Clinical Pharmacy
School of Pharmacy
University of California, San Francisco
San Francisco, CA

Chapter 1
Pharmacologic Therapy for Type 1 Diabetes

9.1 Most people with type 1 diabetes should be treated with multiple daily injections of prandial and basal insulin, or continuous subcutaneous insulin infusion. **A***

9.2 Most individuals with type 1 diabetes should use rapid-acting insulin analogs to reduce hypoglycemia risk. **A**

9.3 Consider educating individuals with type 1 diabetes on matching prandial insulin doses to carbohydrate intake, premeal blood glucose levels, and anticipated physical activity. **E**

9.4 Individuals with type 1 diabetes who have been successfully using continuous subcutaneous insulin infusion should have continued access to this therapy after they turn 65 years of age. **E**

INSULIN THERAPY

Because the hallmark of type 1 diabetes is absent or near-absent β-cell function, insulin treatment is essential for individuals with type 1 diabetes. Insufficient provision of insulin causes not only hyperglycemia but also systematic metabolic disturbances like hypertriglyceridemia and ketoacidosis, as well as tissue catabolism. Over the past three decades, evidence has accumulated supporting multiple daily injections of insulin or continuous subcutaneous administration through an insulin pump as providing the best combination of effectiveness and safety for people with type 1 diabetes.

Generally, insulin requirements can be estimated based on weight, with typical doses ranging from 0.4–1.0 units/kg/day. Higher amounts are required during puberty, pregnancy, and medical illness. The *American Diabetes Association/JDRF Type 1 Diabetes Sourcebook* notes 0.5 units/kg/day as a typical starting dose in patients with type 1 diabetes who are metabolically stable, with half administered as prandial insulin given to control blood glucose after meals and the other half as

---

Chapter 1 is an excerpt from American Diabetes Association, 9. Pharmacologic Approaches to Glycemic Treatment: *Standards of Medical Care in Diabetes—2019. Diabetes Care* 2019; 42(Suppl. 1):S90–S102. DOI:10.2337/dc19-S009

* See Table 1.1 (p. 4) for an explanation of the American Diabetes Association evidence-grading system for *Standards of Medical Care in Diabetes.*

basal insulin to control glycemia in the periods between meal absorption;[1] this guideline provides detailed information on intensification of therapy to meet individualized needs. In addition, the American Diabetes Association position statement "Type 1 Diabetes Management Through the Life Span" provides a thorough overview of type 1 diabetes treatment.[2]

Physiologic insulin secretion varies with glycemia, meal size, and tissue demands for glucose. To approach this variability in people using insulin treatment, strategies have evolved to adjust prandial doses based on predicted needs. Thus, education of patients on how to adjust prandial insulin to account for carbohydrate intake, premeal glucose levels, and anticipated activity can be effective and should be considered. Newly available information suggests that individuals in whom carbohydrate counting is effective can incorporate estimates of meal fat and protein content into their prandial dosing for added benefit.[3–5]

Most studies comparing multiple daily injections with continuous subcutaneous insulin infusion (CSII) have been relatively small and of short duration. However, a recent systematic review and meta-analysis concluded that pump therapy has modest advantages for lowering A1C (–0.30% [95% CI –0.58 to –0.02]) and for reducing severe hypoglycemia rates in children and adults.[6] There is no consensus to guide choosing which form of insulin administration is best for a given patient, and research to guide this decision making is needed.[7] The arrival of continuous glucose monitors to clinical practice has proven beneficial in specific circumstances. Reduction of nocturnal hypoglycemia in people with type 1 diabetes using insulin pumps with glucose sensors is improved by automatic suspension of insulin delivery at a preset glucose level.[7–9] The U.S. Food and Drug Administration (FDA) has also approved the first hybrid closed-loop pump system. The safety and efficacy of hybrid closed-loop systems has been supported in the literature in adolescents and adults with type 1 diabetes.[10,11] Intensive diabetes management using CSII and continuous glucose monitoring should be considered in selected patients. See Section 7 "Diabetes Technology" for a full discussion of insulin delivery devices.

The Diabetes Control and Complications Trial (DCCT) demonstrated that intensive therapy with multiple daily injections or CSII reduced A1C and was associated with improved long-term outcomes.[12–14] The study was carried out with short-acting and intermediate-acting human insulins. Despite better microvascular, macrovascular, and all-cause mortality outcomes, intensive therapy was associated with a higher rate of severe hypoglycemia (61 episodes per 100 patient-years of therapy). Since the DCCT, rapid-acting and long-acting insulin analogs have been developed. These analogs are associated with less hypoglycemia, less weight gain, and lower A1C than human insulins in people with type 1 diabetes.[15–17] Longer-acting basal analogs (U-300 glargine or degludec) may convey a lower hypoglycemia risk compared with U-100 glargine in patients with type 1 diabetes.[18,19] Rapid-acting inhaled insulin to be used before meals is now available and may reduce rates of hypoglycemia in patients with type 1 diabetes.[20]

Postprandial glucose excursions may be better controlled by adjusting the timing of prandial insulin dose administration. The optimal time to administer prandial insulin varies, based on the type of insulin used (regular, rapid-acting analog, inhaled, etc.), measured blood glucose level, timing of meals, and carbohydrate consumption. Recommendations for prandial insulin dose administration should therefore be individualized.

INSULIN INJECTION TECHNIQUE

Ensuring that patients and/or caregivers understand correct insulin injection technique is important to optimize glucose control and insulin use safety. Thus, it is important that insulin be delivered into the proper tissue in the right way. Recommendations have been published elsewhere outlining best practices for insulin injection.[21] Proper insulin injection technique includes injecting into appropriate body areas, injection site rotation, appropriate care of injection sites to avoid infection or other complications, and avoidance of intramuscular (IM) insulin delivery.

Exogenous-delivered insulin should be injected into subcutaneous tissue, not intramuscularly. Recommended sites for insulin injection include the abdomen, thigh, buttock, and upper arm.[21] Because insulin absorption from IM sites differs according to the activity of the muscle, inadvertent IM injection can lead to unpredictable insulin absorption and variable effects on glucose, with IM injection being associated with frequent and unexplained hypoglycemia in several reports.[21–23] Risk for IM insulin delivery is increased in younger and lean patients when injecting into the limbs rather than truncal sites (abdomen and buttocks) and when using longer needles.[24] Recent evidence supports the use of short needles (e.g., 4-mm pen needles) as effective and well tolerated when compared to longer needles,[25,26] including a study performed in obese adults.[27] Injection site rotation is additionally necessary to avoid lipohypertrophy and lipoatrophy.[21] Lipohypertrophy can contribute to erratic insulin absorption, increased glycemic variability, and unexplained hypoglycemic episodes.[28] Patients and/or caregivers should receive education about proper injection site rotation and to recognize and avoid areas of lipohypertrophy.[21] As noted in Table 4.1 in the *Standards of Medical Care in Diabetes—2019* (DOI:10.2337/dc19-S009), examination of insulin injection sites for the presence of lipohypertrophy, as well as assessment of injection device use and injection technique, are key components of a comprehensive diabetes medical evaluation and treatment plan. As referenced above, there are now numerous evidence-based insulin delivery recommendations that have been published. Proper insulin injection technique may lead to more effective use of this therapy and, as such, holds the potential for improved clinical outcomes.

NONINSULIN TREATMENTS FOR TYPE 1 DIABETES

Injectable and oral glucose-lowering drugs have been studied for their efficacy as adjuncts to insulin treatment of type 1 diabetes. Pramlintide is based on the naturally occurring β-cell peptide amylin and is approved for use in adults with type 1 diabetes. Results from randomized controlled studies show variable reductions of A1C (0–0.3%) and body weight (1–2 kg) with addition of pramlintide to insulin.[29,30] Similarly, results have been reported for several agents currently approved only for the treatment of type 2 diabetes. The addition of metformin to adults with type 1 diabetes caused small reductions in body weight and lipid levels but did not improve A1C.[31,32] The addition of the glucagon-like peptide 1 (GLP-1) receptor agonists liraglutide and exenatide to insulin therapy caused small (0.2%) reductions in A1C compared with insulin alone in people with type 1 diabetes and also reduced body weight by ~3 kg.[33] Similarly, the addition of a sodium–glucose cotransporter 2 (SGLT2) inhibitor to insulin therapy has been associated with improvements in A1C and body weight when compared with insulin alone;[34-36]; however, SGLT2 inhibitor use is also associated with more adverse events including ketoacidosis. The dual SGLT1/2 inhibitor sotagliflozin is currently under consideration by the FDA and, if approved, would be the first adjunctive oral therapy in type 1 diabetes.

The risks and benefits of adjunctive agents beyond pramlintide in type 1 diabetes continue to be evaluated through the regulatory process; however, at this time, these adjunctive agents are not approved in the context of type 1 diabetes.[37]

Table 1.1—American Diabetes Association Evidence-grading System for *Standards of Medical Care in Diabetes*

Level of evidence	Description
A	Clear evidence from well-conducted, generalizable randomized controlled trials that are adequately powered, including ■ Evidence from a well-conducted multicenter trial ■ Evidence from a meta-analysis that incorporated quality ratings in the analysis Compelling nonexperimental evidence, i.e., "all or none" rule developed by the Centre for Evidence-Based Medicine at the University of Oxford Supportive evidence from well-conducted randomized controlled trials that are adequately powered, including ■ Evidence from a well-conducted trial at one or more institutions ■ Evidence from a meta-analysis that incorporated quality ratings in the analysis
B	Supportive evidence from well-conducted cohort studies ■ Evidence from a well-conducted prospective cohort study or registry ■ Evidence from a well-conducted meta-analysis of cohort studies Supportive evidence from a well-conducted case-control study
C	Supportive evidence from poorly controlled or uncontrolled studies ■ Evidence from randomized clinical trials with one or more major or three or more minor methodological flaws that could invalidate the results ■ Evidence from observational studies with high potential for bias (such as case series with comparison with historical controls) ■ Evidence from case series or case reports Conflicting evidence with the weight of evidence supporting the recommendation
E	Expert consensus or clinical experience

REFERENCES

1. Peters A, Laffel L (Eds.). *American Diabetes Association/JDRF Type 1 Diabetes Sourcebook.* Alexandria, VA, American Diabetes Association, 2013

2. Chiang JL, Kirkman MS, Laffel LMB, Peters AL; *Type 1 Diabetes Sourcebook* Authors. Type 1 diabetes through the life span: a position statement of the American Diabetes Association. *Diabetes Care* 2014;37:2034–2054

3. Wolpert HA, Atakov-Castillo A, Smith SA, Steil GM. Dietary fat acutely increases glucose concentrations and insulin requirements in patients with type 1 diabetes: implications for carbohydrate-based bolus dose calculation and intensive diabetes management. *Diabetes Care* 2013;36:810–816

4. Bell KJ, Toschi E, Steil GM, Wolpert HA. Optimized mealtime insulin dosing for fat and protein in type 1 diabetes: application of a model based approach to derive insulin doses for open loop diabetes management. *Diabetes Care* 2016;39:1631–1634

5. Bell KJ, Smart CE, Steil GM, Brand-Miller JC, King B, Wolpert HA. Impact of fat, protein, and glycemic index on postprandial glucose control in type 1 diabetes: implications for intensive diabetes management in the continuous glucose monitoring era. *Diabetes Care* 2015;38:1008–1015

6. Yeh H-C, Brown TT, Maruthur N, et al. Comparative effectiveness and safety of methods of insulin delivery and glucose monitoring for diabetes mellitus: a systematic review and meta-analysis. *Ann Intern Med* 2012;157:336–347

7. Pickup JC. The evidence base for diabetes technology: appropriate and inappropriate meta-analysis. *J Diabetes Sci Technol* 2013;7:1567–1574

8. 8. Bergenstal RM, Klonoff DC, Garg SK, et al.; ASPIRE In-Home Study Group. Threshold-based insulin-pump interruption for reduction of hypoglycemia. *N Engl J Med* 2013;369:224–232

9. Buckingham BA, Raghinaru D, Cameron F, et al.; In Home Closed Loop Study Group. Predictive low-glucose insulin suspension reduces duration of nocturnal hypoglycemia in children without increasing ketosis. *Diabetes Care* 2015;38:1197–1204

10. Bergenstal RM, Garg S, Weinzimer SA, et al. Safety of a hybrid closed-loop insulin delivery system in patients with type 1 diabetes. *JAMA* 2016;316:1407–1408

11. Garg SK, Weinzimer SA, Tamborlane WV, et al. Glucose outcomes with the in-home use of a hybrid closed-loop insulin delivery system in adolescents and adults with type 1 diabetes. *Diabetes Technol Ther* 2017;19:155–163

12. Cleary PA, Orchard TJ, Genuth S, et al.; DCCT/EDIC Research Group. The effect of intensive glycemic treatment on coronary artery calcification in type 1 diabetic participants of the Diabetes Control and Complications Trial/Epidemiology of Diabetes Interventions and Complications (DCCT/EDIC) Study. *Diabetes* 2006;55:3556–3565

13. Nathan DM, Cleary PA, Backlund J-YC, et al.; Diabetes Control and Complications Trial/Epidemiology of Diabetes Interventions and Complications (DCCT/EDIC) Study Research Group. Intensive diabetes treatment and cardiovascular disease in patients with type 1 diabetes. *N Engl J Med* 2005;353:2643–2653

14. Diabetes Control and Complications Trial(DCCT)/Epidemiology of Diabetes Interventions and Complications (EDIC) Study Research Group.

Mortality in type 1 diabetes in the DCCT/EDIC versus the general population. *Diabetes Care* 2016;39:1378–1383

15. Tricco AC, Ashoor HM, Antony J, et al. Safety, effectiveness, and cost effectiveness of long acting versus intermediate acting insulin for patients with type 1 diabetes: systematic review and network meta-analysis. *BMJ* 2014;349:g5459

16. Bartley PC, Bogoev M, Larsen J, Philotheou A. Long-term efficacy and safety of insulin detemir compared to Neutral Protamine Hagedorn insulin in patients with type 1 diabetes using a treat-to-target basal-bolus regimen with insulin aspart at meals: a 2-year, randomized, controlled trial. *Diabet Med* 2008;25:442–449

17. DeWitt DE, Hirsch IB. Outpatient insulin therapy in type 1 and type 2 diabetes mellitus: scientific review. *JAMA* 2003;289:2254–2264

18. Lane W, Bailey TS, Gerety G, et al.; Group Information; SWITCH 1. Effect of insulin degludec vs insulin glargine U100 on hypoglycemia in patients with type 1 diabetes: the SWITCH 1 randomized clinical trial. *JAMA* 2017;318:33–44

19. Home PD, Bergenstal RM, Bolli GB, et al. New insulin glargine 300 units/mL versus glargine 100 units/mL in people with type 1 diabetes: a randomized, phase 3a, open-label clinical trial (EDITION 4). *Diabetes Care* 2015;38:2217–2225

20. Bode BW, McGill JB, Lorber DL, Gross JL, Chang PC, Bregman DB; Affinity 1 Study Group. Inhaled technosphere insulin compared with injected prandial insulin in type 1 diabetes: a randomized 24-week trial. *Diabetes Care* 2015;38:2266–2273

21. Frid AH, Kreugel G, Grassi G, et al. New insulin delivery recommendations. *Mayo Clin Proc* 2016;91:1231–1255

22. Karges B, Boehm BO, Karges W. Early hypoglycaemia after accidental intramuscular injection of insulin glargine. *Diabet Med* 2005;22:1444–1445

23. Frid A, Gunnarsson R, Güntner P, Linde B. Effects of accidental intramuscular injection on insulin absorption in IDDM. *Diabetes Care* 1988;11:41–45

24. Gibney MA, Arce CH, Byron KJ, Hirsch LJ. Skin and subcutaneous adipose layer thickness in adults with diabetes at sites used for insulin injections: implications for needle length recommendations. *Curr Med Res Opin* 2010;26:1519–1530

25. Hirsch LJ, Gibney MA, Albanese J, et al. Comparative glycemic control, safety and patient ratings for a new 4 mm × 32G insulin pen needle in adults with diabetes. *Curr Med Res Opin* 2010;26:1531–1541

26. Miwa T, Itoh R, Kobayashi T, et al. Comparison of the effects of a new 32-gauge × 4-mm pen needle and a 32-gauge × 6-mm pen needle on glycemic control, safety, and patient ratings in Japanese adults with diabetes. *Diabetes Technol Ther* 2012;14:1084–1090

27. Bergenstal RM, Strock ES, Peremislov D, Gibney MA, Parvu V, Hirsch LJ. Safety an efficacy of insulin therapy delivered via a 4mm pen needle in obese patients with diabetes. *Mayo Clin Proc* 2015;90:329–338

28. Famulla S, Hövelmann U, Fischer A, et al. Insulin injection into lipohypertrophic tissue: blunted and more variable insulin absorption and action and impaired postprandial glucose control. *Diabetes Care* 2016;39:1486–1492

29. Ratner RE, Dickey R, Fineman M, et al. Amylin replacement with pramlintide as an adjunct to insulin therapy improves long-term glycaemic and weight control in type 1 diabetes mellitus: a 1-year, randomized controlled trial. *Diabet Med* 2004;21:1204–1212

30. Edelman S, Garg S, Frias J, et al. A double-blind, placebo-controlled trial assessing pramlintide treatment in the setting of intensive insulin therapy in type 1 diabetes. *Diabetes Care* 2006;29:2189–2195

31. Meng H, Zhang A, Liang Y, Hao J, Zhang X, Lu J. Effect of metformin on glycaemic control in patients with type 1 diabetes: a meta-analysis of randomized controlled trials. *Diabetes Metab Res Rev* 2018;34:e2983

32. Petrie JR, Chaturvedi N, Ford I, et al.; REMOVAL Study Group. Cardiovascular and metabolic effects of metformin in patients with type 1 diabetes (REMOVAL): a double-blind, randomised, placebo-controlled trial. *Lancet Diabetes Endocrinol* 2017;5:597–609

33. Wang W, Liu H, Xiao S, Liu S, Li X, Yu P. Effects of insulin plus glucagon-like peptide-1 receptor agonists (GLP-1RAs) in treating type 1 diabetes mellitus: a systematic review and meta-analysis. *Diabetes Ther* 2017;8:727–738

34. Henry RR, Thakkar P, Tong C, Polidori D, Alba M. Efficacy and safety of canagliflozin, a sodium–glucose cotransporter 2 inhibitor, as add-on to insulin in patients with type 1 diabetes. *Diabetes Care* 2015;38:2258–2265

35. Dandona P, Mathieu C, Phillip M, et al.; DEPICT-1 Investigators. Efficacy and safety of dapagliflozin in patients with inadequately controlled type 1 diabetes (DEPICT-1): 24 week results from a multicentre, double-blind, phase 3, randomised controlled trial. *Lancet Diabetes Endocrinol* 2017;5:864–876

36. Patoulias D, Imprialos K, Stavropoulos K, Athyros V, Doumas M. SGLT-2 inhibitors in type 1 diabetes mellitus: a comprehensive review of the literature. *Curr Clin Pharmacol*. 7 August 2018 [Epub ahead of print]. DOI:10.2174/1574884713666180807150509

37. Lexicon Pharmaceuticals. FDA to review Zynquista™ (sotagliflozin) as potential treatment for type 1 diabetes [Internet], 2018. Available from http://www.lexpharma.com/media-center/news/673-fda-to-review-zynquista-sotagliflozinas-potential-treatment-for-type-1-diabetes. Accessed 30 September 2018

Chapter 2
Management of Hyperglycemia in Type 1 Diabetes Mellitus

Joshua J. Neumiller, PharmD, CDE, FASCP

INTRODUCTION

According to the Centers for Disease Control and Prevention (CDC) estimates, 30.3 million people currently live with diabetes in the U.S.[1] It is estimated that 5–10% of those living with diabetes have type 1 diabetes (T1D).[2] T1D is the major form of diabetes seen in youth, with almost all cases of diabetes being T1D in children under the age of 10 years.[2] T1D is classically associated with childhood and adolescents and was formerly known as "juvenile diabetes," but T1D (sometimes referred to as "immune-mediated diabetes") can be diagnosed at any age.[2] For people living with T1D, optimization of glycemic control is one of several key treatment approaches central to avoiding or delaying the microvascular and macrovascular complications of diabetes. Although lifestyle interventions (such as consuming a healthy diet and engaging in regular physical activity) are integral to any T1D management plan, this chapter will focus primarily on the pharmacological management of hyperglycemia in people with T1D.

PATHOPHYSIOLOGY

T1D is classically considered an autoimmune disorder leading to the destruction of pancreatic β-cells and a subsequent lack of endogenous insulin production.[3] While mediated by a complex interplay of environmental and genetic factors,[2] as many as 80–90% of people diagnosed with T1D do not have a positive family history of the disorder.[4] Figure 2.1 provides an overview of a classic model of T1D pathophysiology.[2] The model suggests that autoimmunity ensues when people with a genetic predisposition are exposed to an environmental trigger (such as an infection). Once the process is triggered, autoimmunity and β-cell loss progress at a variable rate, but typically proceed until symptoms of diabetes present.[2] The rate of progression and onset of symptoms can be quite variable from one individual to the next. Some people may present at the time of diagnosis in severe diabetic ketoacidosis (DKA), while others may be diagnosed with relatively mild symptoms and residual β-cell function.[2] Ultimately, the lack of insulin secretion that is associated with T1D results in the classic symptoms of hyperglycemia: polyuria, polydipsia, and polyphagia. Owing to the hallmark autoimmune destruction of pancreatic β-cells that occurs in T1D, supplementation with exogenous insulin therapy is absolutely required to manage hyperglycemia.

GLYCEMIC MANAGEMENT IN PEOPLE WITH T1D

Exogenous insulin therapy is a requirement for people with T1D due to an absolute lack of endogenous insulin secretion from pancreatic β-cells. As such, all people with T1D should be managed with an intensive insulin regimen designed to cover both basal and prandial (mealtime) insulin needs, with the ultimate goal of achieving individualized glycemic goals.[5] Indeed, the Diabetes Control and Complications Trial (DCCT) showed that intensive therapy with multiple daily injections or continuous subcutaneous insulin infusion (CSII) resulted in improved glycemic control and better long-term outcomes in people with T1D.[6–8] The American Diabetes Association makes the following specific recommendations pertaining to insulin therapy in people with T1D:[9]

- Most people with T1D should be treated with multiple daily injections of prandial insulin and basal insulin or CSII.
- Most individuals with T1D should use rapid-acting insulin analogs to reduce hypoglycemia risk.
- Consider educating individuals with T1D on matching prandial insulin doses to carbohydrate intake, premeal blood glucose levels, and anticipated physical activity.

Although there are multiple important interventions to consider in decreasing microvascular and macrovascular risk in people with T1D, the following sections

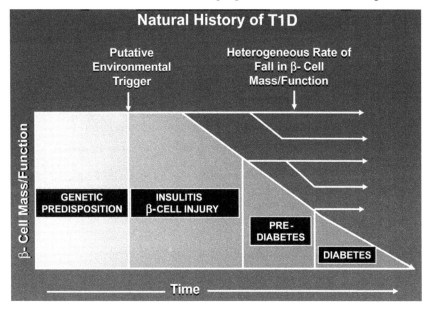

Figure 2.1—Natural history of T1D. *Source:* Reprinted with permission from American Diabetes Association.[2]

Table 2.1 — Glycemic Recommendations for Many Nonpregnant Adults with Diabetes

A1C	<7.0%*
Fasting (Preprandial) Glucose	80–130 mg/dL*
Postprandial Glucose	<180 mg/dL*

*More or less stringent goals may be appropriate for individuals. *Source:* Adapted from American Diabetes Association.[10]

will focus specifically on glycemic goal setting and use of pharmacologic interventions to meet individualized glycemic goals.

GLYCEMIC TREATMENT GOALS IN PEOPLE WITH T1D

As is the case for all people with diabetes, treatment goals and expectations should be individualized for people with T1D. Aside from the importance of individualization, major organizations such as the American Diabetes Association recommend different general treatment targets for children and adolescents when compared to adults with T1D. Table 2.1 provides a summary of general glycemic recommendations for nonpregnant adults with diabetes,[10] and Table 2.2 provides a summary of general glycemic goals for children and adolescents with T1D.[11] It should be noted that while general recommendations for glycated hemoglobin A_{1c} (A1C) and blood glucose levels are provided, all glycemic goals should be individualized based on person-specific considerations.[9] Factors that may inform glycemic goals in an individual may include risk of hypoglycemia and other adverse drug events, diabetes disease duration, life expectancy, comorbidity burden, presence of vascular complications, attitudes and treatment expectations of the individual, and resources and support available to implement a given treatment plan.[9] As pertaining to glycemic goal setting in children and adolescents with T1D, the American Diabetes Association outlines the following key concepts to consider:[11]

- Glycemic goals should be individualized, and lower goals may be reasonable based on a benefit/risk assessment.
- Blood glucose goals should be modified in children with frequent hypoglycemia or hypoglycemia unawareness.
- Postprandial blood glucose values should be measured when there is a discrepancy between preprandial blood glucose values and A1C levels and to assess preprandial insulin doses in those on basal-bolus or CSII regimens.

Ultimately, the American Diabetes Association recommends that treatment decisions and glycemic goal setting should be made in collaboration with the individual, whenever possible, to incorporate his or her needs, preferences, and values.[10]

ANTIHYPERGLYCEMIC DRUG THERAPY IN T1D: INSULIN THERAPY

Insulin both increases glucose uptake by adipose and muscle tissues and suppresses hepatic glucose release. The primary limitation to the usefulness of insulin

Table 2.2—Glycemic Goals for Children and Adolescents with T1D

A1C	<7.5%*
Premeal Glucose	90–130 mg/dL*
Bedtime/Overnight Glucose	90–150 mg/dL*

*More or less stringent goals may be appropriate for individuals.
Source: Adapted from American Diabetes Association.[11]

as an antihyperglycemic agent is the development of hypoglycemia. In addition, insulin use often leads to weight gain. There are many common challenges involved in prescribing insulin as well—from choosing insulin regimens to minimizing the hypoglycemia and weight gain that often accompany improved glycemic control. While all insulin products work via stimulation of insulin receptors, their pharmacokinetic and pharmacodynamic profiles can vary significantly. The insulin primarily in use today is manufactured via recombinant DNA technology as either human insulin or as rapid- or longer-acting human insulin analogs. Analog insulins are structurally modified such that the amino acid sequence is intentionally altered to achieve the desired pharmacokinetic characteristics, as detailed in the following sections.[5]

Pharmacokinetics

Several factors impact the pharmacokinetic properties of insulin, regardless of insulin type. The site of injection, thickness of the subcutaneous tissue, amount of total body adipose tissue, subcutaneous blood flow, and amount of insulin administered can all impact the pharmacokinetics of exogenous insulin.[5,12,13] Temperature variation can also have a major influence on insulin absorption. Elevated skin temperature can lead to increased subcutaneous vasodilation and blood flow to the injection site, thus causing insulin to be more rapidly absorbed.[14,15] Additionally, subcutaneous injections can be administered at multiple anatomical sites, such as the abdominal wall area, thigh, or upper arm. Many practitioners recommend use of the abdomen for consistency of absorption. Although most insulin manufacturers recommend rotating injection sites, changing the anatomical site of injection can affect insulin absorption.[5,16] People using insulin should be educated about factors that may influence insulin absorption when initiating insulin therapy and periodically thereafter.

Table 2.3 provides a summary of individual insulin products currently available in the U.S.[2,17–21] Because U-500 regular human insulin is used primarily in people with significant insulin resistance and rarely in T1D, it will not be discussed in this chapter. The following sections discuss individual insulin products, as grouped by their pharmacokinetic and pharmacodynamic profiles, and their relative effects on glucose control.

Short-Acting Insulin

Regular human insulin (RHI) is generally classified as a short-acting insulin product. RHI is a prandial (mealtime) insulin product used to cover carbohydrate intake with meals.[5] When compared to rapid-acting insulin analogs, RHI has a

Table 2.3—Summary of Insulin Products*

Generic name	Brand name(s)	Time to onset of action (h)	Time to peak action (h)	Duration of action (h)
Regular Human Insulin (U-100)	Humulin R; Novolin R	0.5	1.5–2.5	8
Lispro (U-100, U-200)	Humalog; Admelog	within 0.25	0.5–1.5	4–6
Aspart[†]	Novolog, Fiasp	within 0.25	0.5–1.5	4–6
Glulisine	Apidra	within 0.25	0.5–1.5	4–6
Inhaled Human Insulin Powder	Afrezza	within 0.25	0.5–1	1.5–4.5
NPH Insulin	Humulin N; Novolin N	2–4	4–10	12–18
Detemir	Levemir	2–4	flat	14–24
Glargine (U-100)	Lantus; Basaglar	2–4	flat	20–24
Glargine (U-300)	Toujeo	6	flat	up to 36
Degludec (U-100, U-200)	Tresiba	1	flat	>42
Regular Human Insulin (U-500)	Humulin R U-500	0.5	4–8	13–24

* Person-specific onset, peak, and duration may vary from times listed in table. Peak and duration are dose-dependent with shorter durations of action seen for smaller doses and longer durations of action with larger doses; † Insulin aspart is available as two branded products: Novolog and Fiasp. Fiasp has a relatively fast onset of action and has been shown to provide greater reductions in 1 h PPG levels when compared to Novolog. *Source*: refs. 2,17–25,27.

slower onset and a longer duration of action (see Table 2.3). The glucose-lowering effect of RHI starts approximately 30 min after subcutaneous administration, thus RHI is typically injected 30–45 min before a meal to best match the expected postprandial rise in blood glucose.[5,17,18] Although rapid-acting insulin analogs have possible advantages related to their faster onset and shorter durations of action, RHI costs considerably less and can be used effectively in patients unable to afford newer analog insulin products.

Rapid-Acting Insulin Analogs

Currently available injectable rapid-acting analogs (RAAs) include insulin lispro, insulin aspart, and insulin glulisine.[22–25] As noted previously, RAAs are preferred for use in people with T1D over RHI.[9] Injectable RAAs are structurally engineered to dissociate and be absorbed more rapidly than RHI,[2] resulting in a faster onset and shorter duration of action.[2,26] The faster onset of action allows for RAAs to be administered closer to the time of meal ingestion (typically from 15 min prior to just before a meal), and the shorter duration of action leads to a reduction in postabsorptive hypoglycemic events.[2] Insulin lispro is commercially available in both U-100 and U-200 strengths, with a follow-on U-100 insulin lispro product recently approved by the U.S. Food and Drug Administration (FDA) under the brand name Admelog.[22,27] Insulin aspart is likewise available as two different branded products: Novolog and Fiasp.[23,24] The faster-acting insulin aspart product (Fiasp) is formulated with niacinamide, which is believed to promote formation of insulin monomers after subcutaneous injection, leading to more rapid absorption.[28] Clinical trials comparing Fiasp to Novolog in people with T1D showed a statistically significant improvement in lowering of 1 h postprandial glucose (PPG) levels with Fiasp.[29] It is generally recommended that RAAs be administered no more than 15 min before a meal; however, it is acceptable for people to inject after a meal if carbohydrate intake is difficult to predict or their rate of carbohydrate absorption is variable due to gastroparesis.[5] It is possible that the faster-acting insulin aspart product (Fiasp) may have an advantage in this scenario due to its relatively rapid absorption.[28]

The mechanism of action of inhaled human insulin powder (brand name Afrezza), also classified as an RAA, differs from the injectable rapid-acting insulins. The product is composed of insulin formulated in "microspheres" with a carrier molecule that allows for the insulin to be delivered into the deep lung for rapid absorption following inhalation.[30] Following oral inhalation of 4, 12, and 48 units, the time to maximum serum concentration ranged from 10–20 min in people with T1D.[19]

Intermediate-Acting Insulin

Neutral protamine Hagedorn (NPH) insulin, also known as isophane insulin, is generally classified as "intermediate-acting" in terms of its pharmacokinetic profile. NPH insulin contains an absorption-inhibiting substance called protamine, which prolongs the action and contributes to the cloudy appearance of NPH insulin.[5] For this reason, NPH and NPH-type insulins should be agitated/mixed prior to injection to resuspend the insulin mixture. NPH insulin may be used to cover basal insulin needs, in which case NPH is typically administered twice daily. NPH reaches peak plasma levels anywhere from 4–10 h after subcutaneous administration.[2,31,32] Because of the notable peak with NPH insulin, its use is associated with higher rates of hypoglycemia when compared to long-acting insulin analogs.[2] Although NPH does carry a higher hypoglycemia risk, it is considerably less expensive than long- and ultra-long-acting insulin analogs and can be used effectively in people who have difficulty obtaining more expensive insulin products.

Long-Acting Insulin

Long-acting insulin products are basal insulin analogs that provide basal insulin coverage for up to 24 h. The two medications within this group include insulin glargine (U-100) and insulin detemir. Some people can realize a full 24 h of basal coverage with these insulin products; others can experience end-of-dose "wearing off," as noted by the duration of action ranges presented in Table 2.3.

Insulin Glargine (U-100)

Insulin glargine (U-100) was approved by the FDA in the year 2000, and differs structurally from human insulin by the addition of two arginines after position B30 and the replacement of asparagine with glycine at position A21.[33] Unlike NPH insulin, insulin glargine is soluble at a pH of 4.0.[33,34] Following subcutaneous injection, the acidic insulin solution is neutralized leading to the formation of insulin microprecipitates from which small amounts of insulin are gradually released over time.[33] U-100 insulin glargine exhibits a duration of action generally ranging from 20–24 h, with a relatively flat pharmacokinetic profile.[2] In clinical trials, U-100 insulin glargine demonstrated similar effects on glycemic control when compared to once- or twice-daily NPH, with the advantage of a decreased rate of hypoglycemic events, particularly nocturnal hypoglycemic events.[33] In addition to the product Lantus, a follow-on U-100 insulin glargine product is available in the U.S., marketed as Basaglar.[35] Although some people can realize a full 24 h of basal coverage with a single injection of U-100 insulin glargine, some people require twice-daily administration for a full day of basal coverage. This can be especially true in people with T1D on relatively low doses of basal insulin (e.g., 20 units/day).

Insulin Detemir

Insulin detemir is another long-acting basal insulin analog. Insulin detemir has a prolonged duration of action (14–24 h) due to the insulin's ability to reversibly bind to albumin at the injection site and within the bloodstream.[2,36] Unlike insulin glargine, insulin detemir is soluble at a neutral pH. Structurally, insulin detemir differs from human insulin by the omission of threonine at position B30 and the attachment of myristic acid to lysine at position B29.[36] The presence of myristic acid contributes to delayed dissociation and absorption of insulin detemir hexamers and also facilitates a >98% binding of insulin detemir to albumin molecules in the plasma and interstitial fluid.[36] Because only free, non-albumin-bound insulin can be absorbed and bind to insulin receptors, albumin binding contributes to the prolonged duration of action seen with this insulin product. Since the duration of action of insulin detemir can range from 14–24 h, many people with T1D require twice-daily dosing with insulin detemir.

Insulin Glargine (U-300)

U-300 insulin glargine is a concentrated version of insulin glargine. U-300 insulin glargine is similar to the U-100 product in terms of structure and solubility at an acidic pH of 4.0. The longer duration of action realized with the concentrated U-300 product is attributable to the smaller injection volume, which results in a smaller precipitate surface area.[37] The smaller surface area is associated with a slower dissolution rate and a resultant longer duration of action.[37] Please refer to Table 2.3 for specifics related to the pharmacokinetic properties of U-300 insulin glargine. Due to the long half-life of U-300 insulin glargine, time is needed for this insulin product to accumulate and reach steady-state levels, which are generally achieved after 5 days of once-daily administration.[20] The manufacturer recommends titrating the dose no more frequently than every 3–4 days to minimize the risk of hypoglycemia.[20]

Potential advantages of U-300 insulin glargine over the U-100 insulin glargine product include a longer duration of action, the potential for delivery of large insulin doses in a smaller injection volume, and a lower incidence of nocturnal hypoglycemia. Of note, when converting someone from the U-100 insulin glargine product to the U-300 product, larger doses (on a unit per unit basis) are typically needed to achieve the same glucose-lowering effect.[20] Therefore, it can be expected that higher unit doses of U-300 insulin glargine will be required to maintain glycemic control when compared to the previous U-100 insulin glargine dose.

Insulin Degludec (U-100; U-200)

Insulin degludec is another ultra-long-acting basal insulin analog with a duration of action in excess of 42 h at steady state.[21] Steady-state insulin concentrations are achieved by 3–4 days of once-daily subcutaneous administration.[21] When stored in solution with phenol and zinc, insulin degludec forms small, soluble, and stable dihexamers. Upon injection, the phenol component slowly dissipates allowing for self-association of the insulin molecules into large multihexameric chains consisting of thousands of dihexamers connected to one another.[38] Over time, these chains slowly begin to dissolve as the zinc component diffuses, resulting in the release of insulin from the terminal ends of the chain to be absorbed.[38] Insulin degludec is commercially available in U-100 and U-200 concentrations. Similar to U-300 insulin glargine, the manufacturer recommends titrating the dose no more frequently than every 3–4 days to minimize the risk of hypoglycemia.[21] Potential advantages of insulin degludec include its long duration of action, the potential for delivery of large insulin doses in a smaller injection volume (U-200 product), and a lower incidence of nocturnal hypoglycemia when compared to U-100 insulin glargine.

Insulin Adverse Effects

While insulin therapy has been associated with a variety of adverse effects in clinical trials, the more salient adverse effects and monitoring recommendations for insulin products are provided in this section.

Table 2.4   Symptoms of Hypoglycemia

Shakiness	Blurred/impaired vision
Nervousness or anxiety	Tingling or numbness in the lips or tongue
Sweating, chills, or clamminess	Headache
Irritability or impatience	Anger, stubbornness, or sadness
Confusion	Lack of coordination
Rapid/fast heartbeat	Nightmares
Lightheadedness or dizziness	Seizures
Hunger	Unconsciousness
Sleepiness/fatigue	

Source: Adapted from American Diabetes Association.[5]

Hypoglycemia

Hypoglycemia is the most common and serious adverse event associated with insulin use. Hypoglycemia is defined generally as a blood glucose value ≤70 mg/dL, with lower blood glucose levels associated with worsening hypoglycemic symptoms.[10] Although not an exhaustive list, Table 2.4 provides a list of potential hypoglycemic symptoms.[5] People with hypoglycemia unawareness may not have recognizable symptoms and are at particular risk for severe hypoglycemic events. In people with hypoglycemia unawareness less stringent glycemic targets may be warranted to reduce hypoglycemia risk, especially during the night.[5]

All people who use insulin should be counseled regarding the signs, symptoms, and proper treatment of hypoglycemia. Mild hypoglycemia can be treated by following the "rule of 15": treat with 15 g carbohydrate, wait 15 min, and then check the blood glucose level.[5] If after 15 min blood glucose remains below 70 mg/dL, another 15 g carbohydrate should be consumed. Once the blood glucose is normalized, a snack or meal that includes complex carbohydrates and protein should be consumed to prevent a secondary hypoglycemic episode. When a severe hypoglycemic event occurs and glucose cannot be delivered orally, subcutaneous or intramuscular glucagon use is indicated.[5] The American Diabetes Association *Standards of Medical Care in Diabetes* recommends that glucagon be prescribed to individuals at significant risk of severe hypoglycemia,[10] which would include people who use prandial insulin products, or all people with T1D.

Weight Gain

Weight gain is associated with insulin use and is observed as improvements in glycemic control are achieved. Weight gain can additionally be seen in people with T1D due to increased caloric intake to treat hypoglycemia. As glycemic control improves, glucose is used by the tissues instead of being lost in the urine, thus resulting in weight gain. People starting insulin therapy should be informed of the potential for weight gain and encouraged to implement healthy lifestyle measures to minimize insulin-induced weight gain.[5] In people with T1D, pramlintide can be used as an adjunct therapy with the goal of lowering insulin doses and inducing weight loss.[5] Please see additional information about pramlintide in the section "Other Adjunctive Drug Therapies" presented later in this chapter.

Injection Site Reactions

Long-term use of insulin can lead to lipoatrophy or lipohypertrophy, which can adversely affect insulin absorption. Injection site rotation is important to avoid lipoatrophy and lipohypertrophy. If either occurs, injection into the affected area(s) should be avoided. Lipoatrophy and lipohypertrophy are particularly problematic in people with T1D and can impair long-term glycemic management as the number of viable injection sites decreases over time.

Modes of Insulin Delivery

The method of insulin delivery can include multiple daily injections (with vial and syringe or insulin pens) or use of CSII. The choice of which delivery method to use should be tailored to the individualized needs and preferences of the person with T1D.[5]

Insulin Vials and Syringes

Vials of insulin are typically less expensive than prefilled insulin pens or durable pens that use insulin cartridges. Many people can do quite well with vials and syringes, but use may be difficult for people with vision or dexterity issues. People should be instructed to use a new, clean needle for every dose to prevent injection site infections.

Insulin Pens

Insulin pens provide a mode of delivery that is more convenient, and often more accurate, than insulin administration via vial and syringe. These devices can be very beneficial for people who have vision or dexterity issues that make drawing insulin into a syringe difficult. A new disposable pen needle should be tightened onto the insulin pen before each use to prevent infection. Patients should also be counseled to never share insulin pens. Some of the pens also require priming the pen needle before each use and holding the needle in the injection site for a specific number of seconds (typically 10 seconds), so manufacturer's instructions should be explained to the patient prior to initiation.

Continuous Subcutaneous Insulin Infusion

CSII via an insulin pump or patch allows for precise insulin delivery. CSII requires considerable patient education and support until the individual becomes familiar with the use of the device. Insulin pumps use rapid-acting insulin (insulin lispro, insulin aspart, or insulin glulisine) to cover both basal and bolus insulin needs.[5] Insulin pump and patch technology advances very quickly, with new-generation devices entering the market regularly. Examples of recent technological advancements with insulin pump therapies are the incorporation of threshold suspend features and the introduction of the first hybrid closed-loop system that is able to automatically adjust basal insulin delivery in response to continuous glucose monitoring (CGM) input. The American Diabetes Association's *Diabetes Forecast* publishes consumer guides, inclusive of an insulin pump consumer guide, on an annual basis that are readily accessible via the publication's website (www.diabetesforecast.org).

Insulin Inhalation

As discussed previously, inhaled human insulin is currently available in the U.S. for prandial use in T1D.[19] The product is available in single-use cartridges for use in the corresponding inhalation device. The product is available in 4-unit, 8-unit, and 12-unit single-use cartridges, which are color-coded to prevent medication errors.[19]. Individual cartridges can be used in combination to customize the dose or if higher doses are needed.

INSULIN DOSING IN T1D

Ideally the exogenous insulin regimen used in people with T1D mimics physiologic insulin secretory patterns to the extent possible. Such an approach involves either initiation of an intensive multiple daily injection (MDI) insulin regimen or use of CSII.[5] An intensive basal/bolus regimen in someone with T1D is generally inclusive of a long- or ultra-long-acting insulin that mimics the normal basal insulin release seen in people without diabetes, where approximately 1 unit of insulin is secreted every hour to handle the fasting insulin needs of the liver and muscle. A short- or rapid-acting insulin is also administered in conjunction with the ingestion of carbohydrates at mealtimes, which simulates the rapid release of insulin from the pancreas that typically occurs in the fed state. Similarly, CSII allows for the infusion of rapid-acting insulin to cover both basal and prandial insulin needs.

Insulin Initiation and Titration

When initiating insulin therapy in someone newly diagnosed with T1D, the starting insulin dose is generally calculated based on weight, with starting doses typically ranging from 0.4–1.0 units/kg/day of total insulin.[2] Many clinicians will begin at 0.5 units/kg/day when the person is metabolically stable, with subsequent titration of the insulin per glycemic response. After calculating the total daily insulin dose, approximately half of the calculated total daily dose is administered as basal insulin, with the other half distributed across meals as prandial insulin (for example, 20% of the total daily dose injected at breakfast, 10% at lunch, and 20% at dinner)[2] It is important to note that this weight-based total daily dose calculation and allocation is a starting point only and should be subsequently adjusted according to individualized insulin needs. The following provides an example total daily insulin dose calculation in a person recently diagnosed with T1D:

Example: RJ is a 60-kg female recently diagnosed with T1D. It is decided that a total daily dose of 0.5 units/kg/day is an appropriate starting point.

- Total Daily Dose = 60 kg x 0.5 units/kg/day = 30 units/day
- Basal Dose = 30 units/2 = 15 units of basal insulin daily
- Prandial Insulin = Remaining 15 units/3 meals = 5 units of prandial insulin per meal

Of note, there is no one gold standard method for initiating insulin in people with T1D. While the example provided above provides a starting point for initiating an intensive insulin regimen, the weight-based dose calculation is an estimation of insulin needs only. The basal and prandial insulin doses will inevitably require adjustment to meet individualized glycemic goals. Blood glucose monitoring data and continuous glucose monitoring (CGM) are important tools to evaluate an insulin regimen and inform insulin titration decisions. Ideally, people with T1D will promptly learn to count carbohydrates and adjust insulin doses based on carbohydrate intake, and also use insulin correction doses to account for residual hyperglycemia before meals and at bedtime.

Insulin:Carbohydrate (I:C) Ratios

Ideally, prandial (mealtime) insulin doses are calculated in people with T1D to cover the amount of carbohydrate to be consumed. A typical ballpark insulin-to-carbohydrate ratio (I:C ratio) in someone with T1D is 1:10 (1 unit of prandial insulin to cover 10 g carbohydrate) or 1:15.[5] These are estimates, however, and each individual's needs vary. For people taking rapid-acting analogs to cover meals, the "500 Rule" provides a reasonable initial estimate for determining a person's I:C ratio.[39] To use the 500 Rule, the current total daily dose of insulin is simply divided into 500 to determine an estimated I:C ratio.

Example: SR, a person with T1D, is currently taking 30 units of U-100 insulin glargine once daily and a total of 20 units of insulin aspart divided among breakfast, lunch, and dinner. His total daily insulin dose is 50 units. SR would like to begin adjusting his mealtime insulin doses using an I:C ratio.

- The 500 Rule = 500/total daily insulin dose = 500/50 = 10
- Interpretation: 1 unit of insulin aspart will cover approximately 10 g carbohydrate consumed with meals
- Application: SR is planning to consume 40 g carbohydrate at lunch. Using his estimated I:C ratio, he will inject 4 units of insulin aspart prior to the meal. RJ was advised to check his blood glucose before the meal and 2 h after the meal to assess and reevaluate the appropriateness of his I:C ratio estimate.

Correction Doses

Correction doses are important when blood glucose levels are unexpectedly elevated. A correction factor is ultimately used to correct for a blood glucose reading in the hyperglycemic range before meals or at bedtime, as examples.[39] The "1800 Rule" is another simple estimating calculation that can be used in people using rapid-acting analogs at meals. The calculation estimates how far 1 unit of rapid-acting insulin will drop an individual's blood glucose in mg/dL. To use the 1800 Rule, the number 1800 is divided by the total daily dose of insulin to determine the individual's correction factor. The following is an example of how to use the 1800 Rule to estimate a correction factor:

Example: RJ is currently taking 30 units of U-100 insulin glargine once daily and an average total of 30 units of insulin aspart divided among breakfast, lunch, and dinner after recently implementing an I:C ratio of 1:10. His total daily insulin dose is approximately 60 units. RJ would now like to determine his correction factor to better control his blood glucose throughout the day.

- The 1,800 Rule = 1,800/total daily insulin dose = 1,800/60 = 30
- Interpretation: 1 unit of insulin aspart will drop RJ's blood glucose by an estimated 30 mg/dL
- Application: RJ is about to consume 40 g carbohydrate at lunch. His premeal blood glucose reading is 160 mg/dL (his goal premeal blood glucose is 100 mg/dL). Using his I:C ratio he will administer 4 units to cover carbohydrates, and using his correction factor he will administer an additional 2 units of insulin to account for the 60 mg/dL he is above his target premeal blood glucose. In total, RJ will administer 6 units of insulin aspart prior to lunch.

Ongoing Insulin Adjustment in T1D

Although there are a variety of tools and estimates that can be used to initiate and titrate insulin in people with T1D, the job of optimizing insulin therapy in the individual with T1D is an ongoing and iterative process. Insulin needs can and will change based on numerous factors. Illness, stress, diet, physical activity, and even the changing of the seasons can have drastic effects on glycemic control and insulin needs in people with T1D. Using information obtained from blood glucose monitoring and CGM can be extremely valuable in pinpointing glycemic trends and making adjustments to diet, physical activity, or insulin doses to improve glucose control. People with T1D should be encouraged and empowered to take an active role in identifying trends and factors that impact their blood glucose to improve their glucose control and quality of life. For additional information and recommendations related to the overall management of people with

T1D, please refer to the American Diabetes Association Position Statement "Type 1 Diabetes Through the Life Span."[40]

ADJUNCTIVE DRUG THERAPIES IN T1D

Insulin is the foundation of all pharmacotherapeutic regimens in T1D, but there are several other antihyperglycemic classes of medication that are used on- and off-label for the management of hyperglycemia. A brief discussion of the use of adjunctive antihyperglycemic therapies in T1D follows.

Pramlintide

Amylin is a 37-amino-acid hormone co-secreted with insulin from pancreatic β-cells.[2] Because people with T1D do not have functioning β-cells, they have an absolute deficiency of both insulin and amylin. As a neuroendocrine hormone, amylin acts to slow the appearance of glucose into the bloodstream through three primary mechanisms: suppression of glucagon secretion from pancreatic α-cells, slowing of gastric emptying, and promotion of satiety.[41] Taken together, these actions work in concert with the physiologic actions of insulin to maintain glucose homeostasis.[42]

Pramlintide is an amylinomimetic agent indicated as an adjunctive treatment for people with T1D (and type 2 diabetes [T2D]) receiving mealtime insulin therapy who have failed to achieve desired glucose control despite optimal insulin therapy.[43] Pramlintide is an injectable agent that is administered in addition (as a separate injection) to mealtime insulin prior to meals. In people with T1DM, the starting dose is 15 micrograms (μg) injected subcutaneously before each meal.[43] Because pramlintide slows gastric emptying, some of the most common adverse reactions experienced with use include nausea and vomiting, which are dose related. As such, the dose of pramlintide is gradually increased in 15-μg increments to a target premeal dose of 30 or 60 μg, as tolerated.[43] It is recommended that dose increases not be made any more frequently than every 3 days to minimize nausea.[43] The labeling for pramlintide includes a black box warning for severe hypoglycemia,[43] and mealtime insulin doses should be decreased by approximately 50% upon the initiation of pramlintide to minimize the risk of severe hypoglycemia. The mealtime insulin dose can subsequently be titrated based on individualized response.

The potential advantages of pramlintide use in people with T1D include improved overall glycemic control and potential weight loss. Potential disadvantages, however, include the need for additional injections, severe hypoglycemia risk, and the possible occurrence of common adverse events such as nausea and vomiting.

Other Adjunctive Drug Therapies

Although not approved by the FDA, several other antihyperglycemic classes of medications have been studied and used off-label in people with T1D. Immunotherapies under investigation for the treatment and/or prevention of T1D and β-cell transplant will not be covered in this chapter.

Metformin

The addition of metformin to insulin therapy in people with T1D may have benefits.[9] One report found that the addition of metformin led to reduced insulin requirements and modest reductions in weight and total and LDL cholesterol levels.[44] A randomized clinical trial additionally found that among overweight adolescents with T1D, the addition of metformin to insulin did not improve glycemic control, but did increase the risk for gastrointestinal adverse events when compared to placebo.[45] When studied in adults with T1D and increased risk of cardiovascular disease, the addition of metformin to insulin did not significantly improve glycemic control beyond the initial 3 months of treatment, and the progression of atherosclerosis was not significantly improved.[46] Other cardiovascular risk factors such as weight and LDL cholesterol were, however, improved with metformin treatment.[46]

Incretin-Based Therapies

Interest exists for the use of glucagon-like peptide 1 (GLP-1) receptor agonists and dipeptidyl peptidase-4 (DPP-4) inhibitors in T1D, owing to their potential effects on preservation of β-cell mass and suppression of glucagon release.[9] No GLP-1 receptor agonists or DPP-4 inhibitors are currently approved for use in people with T1D. GLP-1 receptor agonists are currently being investigated (and used off-label) in people with T1D due to their insulin-sparing and weight loss effects.[2] The safety and efficacy of incretin-based therapy in people with T1D remains to be fully defined.

Sodium-Glucose Cotransporter 2 (SGLT2) Inhibitors

SGLT2 inhibitors, via inhibition of glucose reabsorption in the proximal renal tubule, decrease glucose levels in an insulin-independent fashion. Because SGLT2 inhibitors lower glucose independent of β-cell function, there is great interest in the potential adjunctive use of these agents in people with T1D. Limited evidence published to date shows potential glycemic benefits in people with diabetes receiving insulin therapy, inclusive of people with T1D.[47] Despite these potential benefits, SGLT2 inhibitor use has been associated with cases of euglycemic diabetic ketoacidosis (eDKA) in people with both T1D and T2D,[9] thus calling into question the safety of using these agents in people with T1D. That said, an SGLT2 inhibitor is currently under FDA review for a formal indication to treat T1D. Similar to incretin-based therapies, the role of SGLT2 inhibition in people with T1D requires further investigation.

MONOGRAPHS

INSULIN PRODUCTS

Insulin Aspart (Fiasp): https://dailymed.nlm.nih.gov/dailymed/drugInfo. cfm?setid=834e7efc-393f-4c55-9125-628562a8a5cf

Insulin Aspart (Novolog): https://dailymed.nlm.nih.gov/dailymed/drugInfo. cfm?setid=3a1e73a2-3009-40d0-876c-b4cb2be56fc5

Insulin Degludec [U-100, U-200] (Tresiba): https://dailymed.nlm.nih.gov/dailymed/drugInfo.cfm?setid=456c5e87-3dfd-46fa-8ac0-c6128d4c97c6

Insulin Detemir (Levemir): https://dailymed.nlm.nih.gov/dailymed/drugInfo.cfm?setid=d38d65c1-25bf-401d-9c7e-a2c3222da8af

Insulin Glargine [U-100] (Lantus, Basaglar): https://dailymed.nlm.nih.gov/dailymed/drugInfo.cfm?setid=6328c99d-d75f-43ef-b19e-7e71f91e57f6

Insulin Glargine [U-300] (Toujeo): https://dailymed.nlm.nih.gov/dailymed/drugInfo.cfm?setid=c9561d96-124d-48ca-982f-0aa1575bff36

Insulin Glulisine (Apidra): https://dailymed.nlm.nih.gov/dailymed/drugInfo.cfm?setid=e7af6a7a-8046-4fb4-9979-4ec4230b23aa

Inhaled Human Insulin (Afrezza): https://dailymed.nlm.nih.gov/dailymed/drugInfo.cfm?setid=29f4637b-e204-425b-b89c-7238008d8c10

Insulin Lispro [U-100, U-200] (Humalog, Admelog): https://dailymed.nlm.nih.gov/dailymed/drugInfo.cfm?setid=c6b8ff07-d3e2-457f-8a38-b60de60adf75

NPH Insulin (Humulin N, Novolin N): https://dailymed.nlm.nih.gov/dailymed/drugInfo.cfm?setid=f6edd793-440b-40c2-96b5-c16133b7a921

Regular Human Insulin [U-100] (Humulin R, Novolin R): https://dailymed.nlm.nih.gov/dailymed/drugInfo.cfm?setid=b519bd83-038c-4ec5-a231-a51ec5cc291f

NONINSULIN PRODUCTS (FDA APPROVED FOR USE IN T1D)

Pramlintide (Symlin): https://dailymed.nlm.nih.gov/dailymed/drugInfo.cfm?setid=4aea30ff-eb0d-45c1-b114-3127966328ff

---

REFERENCES

1. Centers for Disease Control and Prevention. National Diabetes Statistics Report, 2017. Estimates of Diabetes and Its Burden in the United States. Available from https://www.cdc.gov/diabetes/pdfs/data/statistics/national-diabetes-statistics-report.pdf. Accessed 18 June 2018

2. American Diabetes Association/JDRF. *Type 1 Diabetes Sourcebook*. Peters A, Laffel L, Eds. Alexandria, American Diabetes Association, 2013

3. American Diabetes Association. 14. Classification and diagnosis of diabetes: *Standards of Medical Care in Diabetes—2018*. *Diabetes Care* 2018;41(Suppl. 1):S13–S27

4. Haller MJ, Atkinson MA, Schatz DA. Efforts to prevent and halt autoimmune beta cell destruction. *Endocrinol Metab Clin North Am* 2010;39:527–539

5. American Diabetes Association. *Practical Insulin: A Handbook for Prescribing Providers.* 3rd ed. Alexandria, American Diabetes Association, 2015

6. Nathan DM, Genuth S, Lachin J, et al.; Diabetes Control and Complications Trial Research Group. The effect of intensive treatment of diabetes on the development and progression of long-term complications in insulin-dependent diabetes mellitus. *N Engl J Med* 1993;329:977–986

7. Nathan DM, Cleary PA, Backlund J-YC, et al.; Diabetes Control and Complications Trial/Epidemiology of Diabetes Interventions and Complications (DCCT/EDIC) Study Research Group. Intensive diabetes treatment and cardiovascular disease in patients with type 1 diabetes. *N Engl J Med* 2005;353:2643–2653

8. DCCTEDIC Study Research Group. Mortality in type 1 diabetes in the DCCT/EDIC versus the general population. *Diabetes Care* 2016;39:1378–1383

9. American Diabetes Association. 8. Pharmacologic approaches to glycemic treatment: *Standards of Medical Care in Diabetes—2018. Diabetes Care* 2018;41(Suppl. 1):S73–S85

10. American Diabetes Association. 6. Glycemic targets: *Standards of Medical Care in Diabetes—2018. Diabetes Care* 2018;41(Suppl. 1):S55–S64

11. American Diabetes Association. 12. Children and adolescents: *Standards of Medical Care in Diabetes—2018. Diabetes Care* 2018;41(Suppl. 1):S126–S136

12. Evans M, Schumm-Draeger PM, Vora J, King AB. A review of modern insulin analogue pharmacokinetic and pharmacodynamics profiles in type 2 diabetes: improvements and limitations. *Diabetes Obes Metab* 2011;13:677–684

13. Ryysy L, Häkkinen AM, Goto T, et al. Hepatic fat content and insulin action on free fatty acids and glucose metabolism rather than insulin absorption are associated with insulin requirements during insulin therapy in type 2 diabetic patients. *Diabetes* 2000;49:749–758

14. Koivisto VA. Sauna-induced acceleration in insulin absorption from subcutaneous injection site. *Br Med J* 1980;280:1411–1413

15. Berger M, Cuppers HJ, Hegner H, Jorgens V, Berchtold P. Absorption kinetics and biologic effects of subcutaneously injected insulin preparations. *Diabetes Care* 1982;5:77–91

16. ter Braak EW, Woodworth JR, Bianchi R, et al. Injection site effects on the pharmacokinetics and glucodynamics of insulin lispro and regular insulin. *Diabetes Care* 1996;19:1437–1440

17. Humulin R (insulin human injection) [package insert]. Indianapolis, IN, Lilly USA, LLC, 2015

18. Novolin R (insulin human injection) [package insert]. Plainsboro, NJ, Novo Nordisk Inc., 2018

19. Afrezza (insulin human inhalation powder) [package insert]. Danbury, CT, MannKind Corporation, 2018

20. Toujeo (insulin glargine injection) [package insert]. Bridgewater, NJ, Sanofi-aventis U.S. LLC, 2018

21. Tresiba (insulin degludec injection) [package insert]. Plainsboro, NJ, Novo Nordisk Inc., 2018

22. Humalog (insulin lispro injection) [package insert]. Indianapolis, IN, Lilly USA, LLC, 2017

23. Novolog (insulin aspart injection) [package insert]. Plainsboro, NJ, Novo Nordisk Inc., 2017

24. Fiasp (insulin aspart injection) [package insert]. Plainsboro, NJ, Novo Nordisk Inc., 2017

25. Apidra (insulin glulisine injection) [package insert]. Bridgewater, NJ, Sanofi-aventis U.S. LLC, 2015

26. Tibaldi JM. Evolution of insulin: From human to analog. *Am J Med* 2014;127:S25–S38

27. Admelog (insulin lispro injection) [package insert]. Bridgewater, NJ, Sanofi-aventis U.S. LLC, 2017

28. Mathieu C, Bode BW, Franek E, et al. Efficacy and safety of fast-acting insulin aspart in comparison with insulin aspart in type 1 diabetes (onset 1): a 52-week, randomized, treat-to-target, phase III trial. *Diabetes Obes Metab* 2018;20:1148–1155

29. Russell-Jones D, Bode BW, De Block C, et al. Fast-acting insulin aspart improves glycemic control in basal-bolus treatment for type 1 diabetes: results of a 26-week multicenter, active-controlled, treat-to-target, randomized, parallel-group trial (onset 1). *Diabetes Care* 2017;40:943–950

30. Neumiller JJ, Campbell RK. Technosphere insulin: an inhaled prandial insulin product. *Biodrugs* 2010;24:165–172

31. Humulin N (human insulin isophane suspension) [package insert]. Indianapolis, IN, Lilly USA, LLC, 2017

32. Novolin N (isophane insulin human suspension) [package insert]. Plainsboro, NJ, Novo Nordisk Inc., 2018

33. Campbell RK, White JR, Levien T, Baker D. Insulin glargine. *Clin Ther* 2001;23:1938–1957

34. Lantus (insulin glargine injection) [package insert]. Bridgewater, NJ, Sanofi-aventis U.S. LLC, 2015

35. Basaglar (insulin glargine injection) [package insert]. Indianapolis, IN, Lilly USA, LLC, 2016

36. Soran H, Younis N. Insulin detemir: a new basal insulin analogue. *Diabetes Obes Metab* 2006;8:26–30

37. Blair HA, Keating GM. Insulin glargine 300 U/mL: a review in diabetes mellitus. *Drugs* 2016;76:363–374

38. Robinson JD, Neumiller JJ, Campbell RK. Can a new ultra-long-acting insulin analogue improve patient care? Investigating the potential role of insulin degludec. *Drugs* 2012;72:2319–2325

39. Walsh J, Roberts R, Varma C, Bailey T. *Using Insulin.* San Diego, Torrey Pines Press, 2003

40. Chiang JL, Kirkman MS, Laffel LM, et al. Type 1 diabetes through the life span: a position statement of the American Diabetes Association. *Diabetes Care* 2014;37:2034–2054

41. Younk LM, Mikeladze M, Davis SN. Pramlintide and the treatment of diabetes: a review of the data since its introduction. *Expert Opin Pharmacother* 2011;12:1439–1451

42. Edelman SV, Weyer C. Unresolved challenges with insulin therapy in type 1 and type 2 diabetes: potential benefit of replacing amylin, a second beta-cell hormone. *Diabetes Technol Ther* 2002;4:175–189

43. Symlin (pramlintide acetate) [package insert]. Wilmington, DE, AstraZeneca Pharmaceuticals LP, 2015

44. Vella S, Buetow L, Royle P, et al. The use of metformin in type 1 diabetes: a systematic review of efficacy. *Diabetologia* 2010;53:809–820

45. Libman IM, Miller KM, DiMeglio LA, et al.; T1D Exchange Clinic Network Metformin RCT Study Group. Effect of metformin added to insulin on glycemic control among overweight/obese adolescents with type 1 diabetes: a randomized clinical trial. *JAMA* 2015;314:2241–2250

46. Petrie JR, Chaturvedi N, Ford I, et al.; REMOVAL Study group. Cardiovascular and metabolic effects of metformin in patients with type 1 diabetes (REMOVAL): a double-blind, randomised, placebo-controlled trial. *Lancet Diabetes Endocrinol* 2017;5:597–609

47. Yang Y, Chen S, Pan H, et al. Safety and efficiency of SGLT2 inhibitor combining with insulin in subjects with diabetes: systematic review and meta-analysis of randomized controlled trials. *Medicine (Baltimore)* 2017;96:e6944

Chapter 3
Insulin

Joshua J. Neumiller, PharmD, CDE, FASCP
Kimberly C. McKeirnan, PharmD, BCACP

INTRODUCTION

Since the introduction of commercially available insulin (Iletin) in the U.S. in 1923, insulin has remained a cornerstone of diabetes management.[1] Prior to the availability of exogenous insulin, a diagnosis of T1D was essentially a death sentence. While insulin products and delivery systems have drastically improved since the introduction of Iletin in the 1920s, insulin remains a medical necessity for all people with T1D.[2,3] The use of insulin is not reserved only for those with T1D, however; insulin is often used in people with T2D to meet individualized glycemic goals.[4]

This chapter will provide an overview of insulin products currently available for use in the U.S. Additional topics covered in this chapter include safety considerations when using insulin therapy, general approaches to insulin use in T1D and T2D, and a brief overview of insulin delivery devices.

PHARMACOLOGY

MECHANISM OF ACTION

Insulin action involves a complex series of responses that affect carbohydrate, lipid, and protein metabolism.[5] Insulin carries out its metabolic and growth-promoting effects via binding to insulin receptors on cell plasma membranes.[5] A key metabolic effect of insulin receptor activation is the stimulation of glucose transport and metabolism. In the context of T1D, patients have an absolute insulin deficiency and are unable to effectively transport and metabolize glucose.[2] In T2D, the tissues are resistant to the effects of insulin leading to a relative deficiency in insulin release.[6] Over time, pancreatic β-cells begin to fail as they continually work to produce more insulin to counterbalance the persistent insulin resistance within the tissues. Eventually, β-cell function can decline to a level that requires exogenous insulin administration to adequately control blood glucose.[7] While all insulin products work via stimulation of insulin receptors, their pharmacokinetic and pharmacodynamic profiles can vary significantly. The insulin primarily in use today is manufactured via recombinant DNA technology as either human insulin (Figure 3.1) or as rapid- or longer-acting human analogs. Analog insulins are structurally modified such that the amino acid sequence is intentionally altered to achieve desired pharmacokinetic characteristics, as detailed in the next section.[7]

PHARMACOKINETICS

Several factors impact the pharmacokinetic properties of insulin, regardless of insulin type. The site of injection, thickness of the subcutaneous tissue, amount of total body adipose tissue, subcutaneous blood flow, and amount of insulin administered can all impact the pharmacokinetics of exogenous insulin.[7–9] Factors such as level of endogenous insulin secretion (T1D vs. T2D) and obesity may additionally contribute to pharmacokinetic differences observed among individual patients.[8] Temperature variation can also have a major influence on insulin absorption. Elevated skin temperature can lead to increased subcutaneous vasodilation, increasing blood flow to the injection site, thus causing insulin to be more rapidly absorbed.[10,11] Additionally, subcutaneous injections can be administered at multiple anatomical sites, such as the abdominal wall area, thigh, or upper arm. While most insulin manufacturers recommend rotating injection sites, changing the anatomical site of injection can affect insulin absorption.[7,12] People using insulin should be educated about factors that may influence insulin absorption when initiating insulin therapy and periodically thereafter.

Table 3.1 provides a summary of key pharmacokinetic properties of individual insulin products currently available in the U.S.[2,13–17] The following sections discuss individual insulin products, as grouped by their pharmacokinetic profiles, and their relative effects on glucose control.

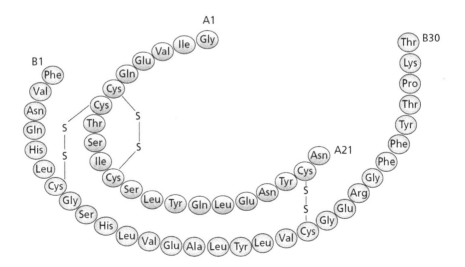

Figure 3.1—Structure of human insulin. Reprinted with permission from American Diabetes Association.[7]

Table 3.1—Summary of Insulin Pharmacokinetics*

Generic name	Brand name(s)	Time to onset of action (h)	Time to peak action (h)	Duration of action (h)
Regular Human Insulin (U-100)	Humulin R; Novolin R	0.5	1.5–2.5	8
Lispro (U-100, U-200)	Humalog; Admelog	within 0.25	0.5–1.5	4–6
Aspart[†]	Novolog; Fiasp	within 0.25	0.5–1.5	4–6
Glulisine	Apidra	within 0.25	0.5–1.5	4–6
Inhaled Human Insulin Powder	Afrezza	within 0.25	0.5–1	1.5–4.5
NPH Insulin	Humulin N; Novolin N	2–4	4–10	12–18
Detemir	Levemir	2–4	flat	14–24
Glargine (U-100)	Lantus; Basaglar	2–4	flat	20–24
Glargine (U-300)	Toujeo	6	flat	up to 36
Degludec (U-100, U-200)	Tresiba	1	flat	>42
Regular Human Insulin (U-500)	Humulin R U-500	0.5	4–8	13–24

* Person-specific onset, peak, and duration may vary from times listed in table. Peak and duration are dose-dependent with shorter durations of action seen for smaller doses and longer durations of action with larger doses. † Insulin aspart is available as two branded products—Novolog and Fiasp. Fiasp has a relatively fast onset of action and has been shown to provide greater reductions in 1 h PPG levels than Novolog. *Source:* refs. 2,13–17,19–22,24,29,30,32,33,40,47.

SHORT-ACTING INSULIN

RHI is generally classified as a short-acting insulin product. RHI is a prandial (mealtime) insulin product used to cover carbohydrate intake with meals.[7] When compared to rapid-acting insulin analogs, RHI has a slower onset and a longer duration of action (see Table 3.1). Following a single subcutaneous injection of 0.1 unit/kg of RHI to healthy subjects, peak insulin concentrations occurred between 1.5–2.5 h post dose, with insulin concentrations returning to baseline after approximately 5 h.[13,14] The glucose-lowering effect of RHI starts approximately 30 min after subcutaneous administration; thus RHI is typically injected 30–45 min before a meal to best match the expected postprandial rise in blood glucose.[7,13,14] RHI administration via continuous intravenous infusion is typically the treatment of choice for managing hyperglycemia in the critical care setting.[18] Although rapid-acting insulin analogs have possible advantages related to their faster onset and shorter durations of action, RHI costs considerably less and can be used effectively in patients unable to afford newer analog insulin products.

RAPID-ACTING INSULIN ANALOGS

Currently available injectable RAAs include insulin lispro, insulin aspart, and insulin glulisine.[19–22] Injectable RAAs are structurally engineered to dissociate and be absorbed more rapidly than RHI,[2] resulting in a faster onset and shorter duration of action.[2,23] The faster onset of action allows for RAAs to be administered closer to the time of meal ingestion (typically from 15 min prior to just before a meal), and the shorter duration of action lends to a reduction in postabsorptive hypoglycemic events.[2] As an example, following subcutaneous administration of insulin lispro at doses ranging from 0.1–0.4 unit/kg, peak serum levels were seen within 30–90 min, compared to 50–120 min with RHI.[19] Similar observations have been noted in studies with insulin aspart and insulin glulisine.[20,22] Insulin lispro is commercially available in both U-100 and U-200 strengths, with a follow-on U-100 insulin lispro product recently approved by the FDA under the brand name Admelog.[19,24] Insulin aspart is likewise available as two different branded products: Novolog and Fiasp.[20,21] The faster-acting insulin aspart product (Fiasp) is formulated with niacinamide, which is believed to promote the formation of insulin monomers after subcutaneous injection leading to more rapid absorption.[25] Clinical trials comparing Fiasp with Novolog in people with T1D and T2D showed a statistically significant improvement in lowering of 1-h PPG levels with Fiasp.[26,27] It is generally recommended that RAAs be administered no more than 15 min before a meal; however, it is acceptable for people to inject after a meal if carbohydrate intake is difficult to predict or their rate of carbohydrate absorption is variable due to gastroparesis.[7] It is possible that the faster-acting insulin aspart product (Fiasp) may have an advantage in this scenario due to its relatively rapid absorption.[25]

The mechanism of action of inhaled human insulin powder (brand name Afrezza), also classified as an RAA, differs from the injectable rapid-acting insulins. The product is composed of insulin formulated in "microspheres" with a carrier molecule that allows for the insulin to be delivered into the deep lung for rapid absorption following inhalation.[28] Following oral inhalation of 4, 12, and 48 units, the time to maximum serum concentration ranged from 10–20 min in people with T1D.[15] Serum concentrations declined to baseline 60–240 min after inhalation, with a half-life of the inhaled insulin product ranging from 120–206 min.[15] Inhaled human insulin is approved for use in T1D and T2D and is a viable option for people who are unwilling to initiate subcutaneous self-injection and can benefit from prandial insulin administration.[28]

INTERMEDIATE-ACTING INSULIN

NPH insulin, also known as isophane insulin, is generally classified as "intermediate-acting" in terms of its pharmacokinetic profile. NPH insulin contains an absorption-inhibiting substance called protamine, which prolongs the action and contributes to the cloudy appearance of NPH insulin.[7] For this reason, NPH and NPH-type insulins should be agitated/mixed prior to injection to resuspend the insulin mixture. NPH insulin may be used to cover basal insulin needs, in which case NPH is typically administered twice daily. NPH reaches peak plasma levels anywhere from 4–10 h after subcutaneous administration.[2,29,30] Because of the notable peak with NPH insulin, its use is associated with higher rates of hypoglycemia than that of long-acting insulin analogs.[2] Although NPH does carry a higher hypoglycemia risk, it is considerably less expensive than long- and ultra-long-acting insulin analogs and can be used effectively in people who have difficulty obtaining more expensive insulin products.

LONG-ACTING INSULIN

Long-acting insulin products are basal insulin analogs that provide basal insulin coverage for up to 24 h. The two medications within this group include insulin glargine (U-100) and insulin detemir. Some people can realize a full 24 h of basal coverage with these insulin products, but others can experience end-of-dose "wearing off," as noted by the duration of action ranges presented in Table 3.1.

Insulin Glargine (U-100)

Insulin glargine (U-100) was approved by the FDA in the year 2000, and differs structurally from human insulin by the addition of two arginines after position B30 and the replacement of asparagine with glycine at position A21.[31] Unlike NPH insulin, insulin glargine is soluble at a pH of 4.0.[31,32] Following subcutaneous injection, the acidic insulin solution is neutralized leading to the formation of insulin microprecipitates from which small amounts of insulin are gradually released over time.[31] As noted in Table 3.1, U-100 insulin glargine exhibits a duration of action generally ranging from 20–24 h with a relatively flat pharmacokinetic profile.[2] In clinical trials, U-100 insulin glargine demonstrated effects on glycemic control similar to once- or twice-daily NPH, with the advantage of a decreased rate of hypoglycemic events, particularly nocturnal hypoglycemic events.[31] In addition to the product Lantus, a follow-on U-100 insulin glargine product is available in the U.S., marketed as Basaglar.[33] Although some people can realize a full 24 h of basal coverage with a single injection of U-100 insulin glargine, some people require twice-daily administration for a full day of basal coverage.

Insulin Detemir

Insulin detemir is another long-acting basal insulin analog. Insulin detemir has a prolonged duration of action (14–24 h) due to the insulin's ability to reversibly bind to albumin at the injection site and within the bloodstream.[2,34] Unlike insulin glargine, insulin detemir is soluble at a neutral pH. Structurally, insulin detemir differs from human insulin by the omission of threonine at position B30 and the attachment of myristic acid to lysine at position B29.[34] The presence of myristic acid contributes to delayed dissociation and absorption of insulin detemir hexamers and also facilitates a >98% binding of insulin detemir to albumin molecules in the plasma and interstitial fluid.[34] Because only free, non-albumin-bound insulin can be absorbed and bind to insulin receptors, albumin binding contributes to the prolonged duration of action seen with this insulin product. Since the duration of action of insulin detemir can range from 14–24 h, not everyone can realize a full 24 h of basal insulin coverage with once-daily administration, and twice-daily administration may be required.

ULTRA-LONG-ACTING INSULIN ANALOGS

"Ultra-long-acting" basal insulin products are those that have a duration of action in excess of 24 h. These insulin products will provide a full 24 h of basal coverage with a single daily injection, and may be beneficial in people who do not realize a full 24 h of coverage with U-100 insulin glargine or insulin detemir.

Insulin Glargine (U-300)

U-300 insulin glargine is a concentrated version of insulin glargine. U-300 insulin glargine is similar to the U-100 product in terms of structure and solubility at an acidic pH of 4.0. The longer duration of action realized with the concentrated U-300 product is attributable to the smaller injection volume, which results in a smaller precipitate surface area.[35] The smaller surface area is associated with a slower dissolution rate and a resultant longer duration of action.[35] In terms of its pharmacokinetic profile, the median time to maximum serum concentration following doses of 0.4, 0.6, and 0.9 U/kg of insulin glargine U-300 was 12 (8–14), 12 (12–18), and 16 (12–20) h, respectively, and the mean concentrations declined to the lower limit of quantitation by 16, 28, and beyond 36 h, respectively.[16] Please refer to Table 3.1 for general pharmacokinetic properties of U-300 insulin glargine. Due to the pharmacokinetic properties of U-300 insulin glargine, time is needed for this insulin product to accumulate and reach steady-state levels, which are generally achieved after 5 days of once-daily administration.[16] The manufacturer recommends titrating the dose no more frequently than every 3–4 days to minimize the risk of hypoglycemia.[16]

Potential advantages of U-300 insulin glargine over the U-100 insulin glargine product include a longer duration of action, the potential for delivery of large insulin doses in a smaller injection volume, and a lower incidence of nocturnal hypoglycemia. Of note, when converting someone from the U-100 insulin glargine product to the U-300 product, larger doses (on a unit per unit basis) are typically needed to achieve the same glucose-lowering effect.[16] Therefore, it can be expected that higher unit doses of U-300 insulin glargine will be required to maintain glycemic control when compared to the previous U-100 insulin glargine dose.

Insulin Degludec (U-100; U-200)

Insulin degludec is another ultra-long-acting basal insulin analog with a duration of action of action in excess of 42 h at steady state.[17] Steady-state insulin concentrations are achieved by 3–4 days of once-daily subcutaneous administration.[17] To achieve this prolonged glycemic effect, insulin degludec is modified such that the amino acid at B30 is deleted and the lysine at position B29 is conjugated to hexadecanoic acid via a γ-L-glutamyl spacer.[36] When stored in solution with phenol and zinc, insulin degludec forms small, soluble and stable dihexamers. Upon injection, the phenol component slowly dissipates, allowing for self-association of the insulin molecules into large multihexameric chains consisting of thousands of dihexamers connected to one another.[36] Over time, these chains slowly begin to dissolve as the zinc component diffuses, resulting in the release of insulin from the terminal ends of the chain to be absorbed.[36] Insulin degludec is commercially available in U-100 and U-200 concentrations. Similar to U-300 insulin glargine, the manufacturer recommends titrating the dose no more frequently than every 3–4 days to minimize the risk of hypoglycemia.[17] Potential advantages of insulin degludec include its long duration of action, the potential for delivery of large insulin doses in a smaller injection volume (U-200 product), and a lower incidence of nocturnal hypoglycemia when compared to U-100 insulin glargine.

U-500 Regular Insulin

U-500 regular insulin was first introduced in the U.S. in 1952 for use in people with extreme insulin resistance caused by antibody formation against animal-derived insulin products.[37] Although it is a 5-times concentrated RHI product, the pharmacokinetics of U-500 insulin are considerably different than U-100 RHI. U-500 insulin peaks around 30 min after subcutaneous injection and has a duration of action that can range widely (see Table 3.1)[38,39] Historically, U-500 insulin use was associated with a high risk of insulin overdose errors due to injection of U-500 with U-100 insulin syringes. In recent years, however, the availability of U-500 insulin pens and dedicated U-500 insulin syringes has improved the safety of this insulin product. Given the unique pharmacokinetics of U-500 insulin, its use is generally reserved for people with T2D and significant insulin resistance who take in excess of 200 units of insulin daily.[40] Following publication of a U-500 clinical trial that used two dosing algorithms for the initiation and titration of U-500 in T2D patients not achieving adequate glycemic control with high-dose U-100 insulin therapy,[41] dosing algorithms are now readily available to help guide clinicians in the use of U-500 insulin in appropriate patients.

TREATMENT ADVANTAGES/DISADVANTAGES

Insulin therapy has the greatest potential for lowering A1C and improving glycemic control among all available glucose-lowering therapies. The degree to which glycemia can be reduced with insulin is limited only by hypoglycemia. Unlike many other antihyperglycemic options that target either fasting plasma glucose (FPG) or PPG, insulin can be used to target FPG, PPG, or both depending on the needs of the individual. Although insulin is unmatched in terms of glucose-lowering potential, its use comes with risks of hypoglycemia, weight gain, and injection site reactions (please see the section below, "Adverse Effects and Monitoring"). In addition, with the exception of inhaled insulin, insulin administration requires subcutaneous self-injection. Initiation of insulin therapy inherently comes with a requirement of more intensive medical oversight and training related to proper insulin use and administration. These considerations can lead to hesitancy to initiate insulin on the part of both people with diabetes and healthcare providers. The following sections provide a general description of the approaches to insulin use in people with T1D and T2D. The information below may be helpful in understanding the generally recommended approaches to insulin use in these patient populations, but the information provided is by no means the only approach to successfully manage people with insulin.

APPROACH TO THE USE OF INSULIN IN T1D

As noted at the beginning of this chapter, exogenous insulin therapy is a requirement for people with T1D due to an absolute lack of endogenous insulin secretion from pancreatic β-cells. As such, all people with T1D should use an intensive insulin regimen designed to cover both basal and prandial (mealtime) insulin needs with the ultimate goal of achieving individualized glycemic targets.[7] Regarding insulin therapy in T1D, the American Diabetes Association *Standards of Medical Care in Diabetes* make the following recommendations:[4]

- Most people with T1D should be treated with multiple daily injections of prandial insulin and basal insulin or CSII.
- Most individuals with T1D should use rapid-acting insulin analogs to reduce hypoglycemia risk.
- Consider educating individuals with T1D on matching prandial insulin doses to carbohydrate intake, premeal blood glucose levels, and anticipated physical activity.

When initiating insulin therapy in someone newly diagnosed with T1D, the starting insulin dose is generally calculated based on weight, with starting doses ranging from 0.4–1.0 units/kg/day of total insulin.[2] Many clinicians will begin at 0.5 units/kg/day when the person is metabolically stable, with titration of the insulin per glycemic response. After calculating the total daily insulin dose, approximately half of the calculated total daily dose is administered as basal insulin, with the other half distributed across meals as prandial insulin (such as 20% of the total daily dose injected at breakfast, 10% at lunch, and 20% at dinner).[2] The insulin is thereafter titrated based on blood glucose monitoring data, with the individual ideally learning to count carbohydrates and dose their prandial insulin based on carbohydrate intake at each meal and snack.

The method of insulin delivery can include multiple daily injections (with vial and syringe or insulin pens) or use of CSII. The choice of which delivery method to use should be tailored to the individualized needs and preferences of the person with T1D. For a more detailed discussion of insulin use and glycemic management in people with T1D please refer to "Chapter 2: Management of Hyperglycemia in Type 1 Diabetes Mellitus."

APPROACH TO THE USE OF INSULIN IN T2D

The approach to insulin use in T2D is quite different than the approach taken in people with T1D. People with T1D initiate an intensive insulin regimen shortly after diagnosis; people with T2D can often be managed with noninsulin therapies for years before the addition of insulin is required to meet individualized glycemic goals. That said, many people with T2D can benefit from early basal insulin initiation, depending on individualized needs and preferences. Once people with T2D reach a point where they are not achieving individualized glycemic goals despite the use of multiple noninsulin therapies, people may need to progress to the use of injectable therapies. Figure 3.2 provides recommendations from the 2018 ADA/EASD consensus report on management of hyperglycemia in T2D regarding treatment intensification to injectable therapies.[42] As noted in Figure 3.2, for people with T2D who have an elevated A1C despite dual or triple therapy, it is recommended that a GLP-1 receptor agonist be considered as the first injectable agent in most patients. Insulin is recommended as the first injectable in those with very high A1C (>11%), those with symptoms or evidence of catabolism (weight loss, polyuria, polydipsia, etc.), or if a diagnosis of T1D is a possibility.[42] The figure provides some guidance on the initiation and titration of basal insulin, inclusive of a recommended starting dose (10 units/day or 0.1–0.2 units/kg/day) and guidance on titration of the basal insulin to achieve an individualized FPG target.[4] If goal A1C is not met following basal insulin optimization and achieving the target FPG level, the addition of prandial insulin is recommended. Prandial insulin is recommended to be started at 4 units/day, or 10% of the basal dose, typically initiated once daily with the largest meal (or meal with the largest PPG excursion). The dose can be up-titrated by 1–2 units or 10–15% twice weekly, with dose reductions of 10–20% recommended in the presence of hypoglycemia. Depending on response, additional injections of prandial insulin can be added until individualized glycemic goals are achieved.[42] While Figure 3.2 provides a framework for insulin initiation and titration in people with T2D, individual patient needs will differ, and strategies should be individualized to meet glycemic goals and minimize hypoglycemia risk.

THERAPEUTIC CONSIDERATIONS

SIGNIFICANT WARNINGS/PRECAUTIONS

The following are warnings and precautions to be considered for use of insulin products.

Hypoglycemia

Hypoglycemia is the most common adverse reaction for all insulin therapies. Extra caution is warranted in people who have recently begun treatment with insulin and those with hypoglycemia unawareness who may not readily recognize hypoglycemic symptoms. Individuals experiencing a hypoglycemic event may experience impaired concentration and/or reaction time, thus hypoglycemia may present risk during activities such as driving or operating machinery.

Hypokalemia

Insulin stimulates potassium movement intracellularly, potentially causing hypokalemia. The risk of hypokalemia is particularly high when administering insulin intravenously.[13,14] Potassium levels should be monitored closely when administering insulin intravenously.

Figure 3.2—Combination injectable therapy for Type 2 diabetes. Reprinted with permission from Davies.[42]

Table 3.2—Symptoms of Hypoglycemia

Shakiness	Tingling or numbness in the lips or tongue
Nervousness or anxiety	Headache
Sweating, chills, or clamminess	Anger, stubbornness, or sadness
Irritability or impatience	Lack of coordination
Confusion	Nightmares
Rapid/fast heartbeat	Seizures
Lightheadedness or dizziness	Unconsciousness
Hunger	
Sleepiness/fatigue	
Blurred/impaired vision	

Source: Adapted from American Diabetes Association.[7]

Hypersensitivity and Allergic Reactions

Severe, life-threatening hypersensitivity and allergic reactions can occur with insulin products. If hypersensitivity reactions occur, the offending insulin product should be discontinued until the person is medically treated and evaluated.

SPECIAL POPULATIONS

Although all people with T1D require insulin therapy, and many people with T2D will eventually require insulin to meet glycemic goals there are some considerations with insulin use in special populations as outlined below.

Pregnancy

According to the American Diabetes Association *Standards of Medical Care in Diabetes*, insulin is the preferred medication for treating hyperglycemia during gestational diabetes as well as during pregnancy in women with T1D or T2D.[43] In people with diabetes or gestational diabetes, insulin requirements may decrease during the first trimester, generally increase during the second and third trimesters, and rapidly decline after delivery.[43]

Renal Impairment

In contrast to endogenously secreted insulin, which undergoes substantial degradation in the liver, exogenous insulin is to a larger degree eliminated by the kidneys.[44] Insulin is filtered by the glomerulus followed by reabsorption in the proximal tubule of the kidney. Insulin clearance decreases in parallel with a decrease in glomerular filtration rate (GFR), leading to an overall decrease in exogenous insulin requirements.[44] Because individual insulin preparations have not been well studied in the context of chronic kidney disease (CKD) and considering individual needs vary considerably, no definitive recommendations exist for insulin dose adjustment based on estimated GFR. Many noninsulin therapies are contraindicated in CKD, so insulin therapy is a mainstay of hyperglycemia management in people with CKD. To mitigate hypoglycemia risk, blood glucose levels should be monitored closely to inform insulin dose adjustments.[44]

Hepatic Impairment

As with renal disease, individual insulin products have not been well studied in people with hepatic impairment. In general, more frequent glucose monitoring and insulin dose adjustment may be warranted to prevent possible hypoglycemia in people with liver disease.

ADVERSE EFFECTS AND MONITORING

Insulin therapy has been associated with a variety of adverse effects in clinical trials, and the more salient adverse effects and monitoring recommendations for insulin products are provided below.

Hypoglycemia

As noted in the "Significant Warnings/Precautions" section above, hypoglycemia is the most common and serious adverse event associated with insulin use. Hypoglycemia is defined generally as a blood glucose value $\leq$70 mg/dL, with lower blood glucose levels associated with worsening hypoglycemic symptoms.[45] Hypoglycemia is much more common with the use of prandial insulin products. Careful and methodical titration of basal insulin products can minimize hypoglycemia risk. As such, people with T1D are generally at greater risk for hypoglycemia, as intensive insulin therapy is required for adequate glycemic control. That said, some people with T2D also receive intensive insulin therapy and should be considered high risk for hypoglycemic events, particularly when used in combination with sulfonylureas or other insulin secretagogue medications. Although not an exhaustive list, Table 3.2 provides a list of potential hypoglycemic symptoms.[7] People with hypoglycemia unawareness may not have recognizable symptoms and are at particular risk for severe hypoglycemic events. In people with hypoglycemia unawareness, less stringent glycemic targets may be warranted to reduce hypoglycemia risk, especially during the night.[7]

All people who use insulin should be counseled regarding the signs, symptoms, and proper treatment of hypoglycemia. Mild hypoglycemia can be treated by following the "rule of 15": treat with 15 g carbohydrate, wait 15 min, and then check the blood glucose level.[7] If after 15 min the blood glucose remains below 70 mg/dL, another 15 g carbohydrate should be consumed. Once the blood glucose is normalized, a snack or meal that includes complex carbohydrates and protein should be consumed to prevent a secondary hypoglycemic episode. When a severe hypoglycemic event occurs and glucose cannot be delivered orally, subcutaneous or intramuscular glucagon use is indicated.[7] The American Diabetes Association *Standards of Medical Care in Diabetes* recommend that glucagon be prescribed to individuals at significant risk of severe hypoglycemia,[45] which would include people who use prandial insulin products.

Weight Gain

Weight gain is associated with insulin use and is observed as improvements in glycemic control are achieved. As glycemic control improves, glucose is used by the tissues instead of being lost in the urine, thus resulting in weight gain. Although weight gain is initially viewed as desirable in people with T1D due to weight loss experienced due to glucosuria and catabolism that is frequently present at the time of diagnosis, intensive insulin therapy can result in undesirable weight gain over time.[46] Indeed, some patients with T1D may even underdose insulin in an effort to avoid weight gain.[46] For those with T2D, who often struggle with overweight and obesity, insulin therapy can further contribute to weight gain. Use of prandial insulin in people with T2D generally contributes to more weight gain than does the use of basal insulin products alone, with both hypoglycemia treatment and possibly increased caloric intake in defense against hypoglycemia.[46] People starting insulin therapy should be informed of the potential for weight gain and encouraged to implement healthy lifestyle measures to minimize insulin-induced weight gain.[7] In people with T2D, adjunctive antihyperglycemic agents such as GLP-1 receptor agonists, SGLT2 inhibitors, and pramlintide can also be used for their insulin-sparing and weight-mitigating effects.[7] Medications approved by the FDA for weight loss can also be considered.

Injection Site Reactions

Long-term use of insulin can lead to lipoatrophy or lipohypertrophy, which can adversely affect insulin absorption. Injection site rotation is important to avoid lipoatrophy and lipohypertrophy. If either occurs, injection into the affected area(s) should be avoided.

Pulmonary Adverse Events (Inhaled Insulin)

Due to its route of administration, inhaled human insulin carries unique adverse-event considerations related to pulmonary function. In clinical trials, the most common reason for discontinuation of inhaled insulin was cough.[15] In addition, participants using the product in clinical trials experienced a greater decline from baseline in forced expiratory volume in 1 second (FEV_1) compared to people treated with other antihyperglycemic therapies.[15] For these reasons, at least in part, inhaled insulin is contraindicated for use in people with chronic lung disease, such as asthma or chronic obstructive pulmonary disease (COPD), due to the risk of acute bronchospasm.[15] For people using the product, pulmonary function testing is recommended at baseline, after the first 6 months of therapy, and annually thereafter, even in the absence of pulmonary symptoms.[15] It is recommended that the product be considered for discontinuation if a $\geq 20\%$ decline in FEV_1 from baseline is observed.

DRUG INTERACTIONS

Drugs affecting glucose metabolism have the potential to interact with insulin and impact overall glycemic control. Some examples of commonly used medications that may lower blood glucose and potentially increase the effect of insulin include oral antihyperglycemic agents, angiotensin converting enzymes inhibitors, angiotensin II receptor blocking agents, disopyramide, pramlintide, fibrates, monoamine oxidase inhibitors, salicylates, sulfonamide antibiotics, and fluoxetine.[13–17,19–22,24,29,30,32,33,40,47] Conversely, examples of medications that may reduce the effect of insulin by increasing blood glucose include corticosteroids, niacin, diuretics, sympathomimetic agents (such as epinephrine or albuterol), isoniazid, thyroid hormones, estrogens, progestin, protease inhibitors, and antipsychotics.[13–17,19–22,24,29,30,32,33,40,47] More specific to the inhaled human insulin product, when coadministered with albuterol, the area under the curve for inhaled human insulin increased by 25%.[15] For patients taking albuterol and inhaled human insulin, dose adjustment of the insulin may be necessary with more frequent blood glucose monitoring recommended.[15] Medications, such as β-blockers, clonidine, lithium salts, and alcohol have been associated with both increasing and decreasing blood glucose levels.[13–17,19–22,24,29,30,32,33,40,47] Signs of hypoglycemia may also be reduced or absent in patients taking antiadrenergic medications, such as β-blockers, clonidine, guanethidine, and reserpine.[13–17,19–22,24,29,30,32,33,40,47] People taking any of these medications in combination with insulin should monitor their blood glucose more closely during use and be counseled on the signs, symptoms, and proper management of hypoglycemic events. Of note, while some antihyperglycemic agents have a low risk of hypoglycemia when used as monotherapy, the risk of hypoglycemia is always increased when additional antihyperglycemic agents are added to background insulin therapy. More diligent blood glucose monitoring with a potential decrease in insulin dose may be warranted when adding additional antihyperglycemic therapies.

DOSAGE AND ADMINISTRATION

The dose of insulin required varies considerably and is dependent on the type of insulin used and the needs of the individual. Although guidelines provide recommendations for insulin initiation and titration for basal and prandial insulin products, these are merely starting points from which to individualize the insulin dose and schedule.

A variety of insulin delivery options are also available, including vials and syringes, pens with disposable cartridges (penfills), prefilled disposable pens with disposable pen needles, and insulin pumps.[7] Table 3.3 provides a summary of individual insulin products available in the U.S., and how the products are supplied, storage recommendations, and pen dosing capabilities (if applicable).[13–17,19–22,24,29,30,32,33,40,47]

Insulin Vials and Syringes

Vials of insulin are typically less expensive than prefilled insulin pens or insulin cartridges. Many people can do quite well with vials and syringes, but use may be difficult for people with vision or dexterity issues. People should be instructed to use a new, clean needle for every dose to prevent injection site infections.

Insulin Pens

Insulin pens provide a mode of delivery that is more convenient, and often more accurate, than insulin administration via vial and syringe. These devices can be beneficial for people who have vision or dexterity issues that make drawing

Table 3.3—Insulin Product Availability and Storage Information

Generic name	Brand name(s)	Product availability	Units per pen (if applicable)	Dose range per injection (pens only)	Recommended pen storage at room temperature (days)
Prandial (Mealtime) Insulin Products					
Regular Human Insulin	Humulin R, Novolin R	Vial	N/A	N/A	N/A
	Humulin R U-500	Vial, Prefilled pen	1,500 units	5–300 units	28
Insulin Lispro	Humalog (U-100)	Vial, Prefilled pen, Pen Cartridges	300 units	1–60 units	28
	Admelog (U-100)	Vial, Prefilled pen	300 units	1–80 units	28
	Humalog (U-200)	Prefilled pen	600 units	1–60 units	28
Insulin Aspart	Novolog	Vial, Prefilled pen, Pen Cartridges	300 units	1–60 units (FlexPen) 1–80 units (FlexTouch)	28
	Fiasp	Vial, Prefilled pen	300 units	1–80 units	28
Insulin Glulisine	Apidra	Vial, Prefilled pen	300 units	1–80 units	28
Inhaled Human Insulin	Afrezza	Inhalation cartridges	N/A	N/A	N/A
Basal Insulin Products					
Human Insulin Isophane (NPH)	Humulin N Novolin N	Vial, Prefilled pen	300 units	1–60 units	14
Insulin Detemir	Levemir	Vial, Prefilled pen	300 units	1–80 units	42

(continued)

Table 3.3 (continued)

Generic name	Brand name(s)	Product availability	Units per pen (if applicable)	Dose range per injection (pens only)	Recommended pen storage at room temperature (days)
Insulin Glargine (U-100)	Lantus	Vial, Prefilled pen	300 units	1–80 units	28
	Basaglar	Prefilled pen	300 units	1–80 units	28
Insulin Glargine (U-300)	Toujeo	Prefilled pen	450 units (SoloStar) 900 units (Max SoloStar)	1–80 units (SoloStar) 2–160 units (Max SoloStar)	42
Insulin Degludec (U-100, U-200)	Tresiba	Prefilled pen	300 units (U-100) 600 units (U-200)	1–80 units (U-100) 2–160 (U-200)	56

N/A, not applicable. *Source:* refs. 13–17,19–22,24,29,30,32,33,40,47.

insulin into a syringe difficult. A new disposable pen needle should be tightened onto the insulin pen before each use to prevent infection. Some of the pens also require priming the pen needle before each use and holding the needle in the injection site for a specific number of seconds, so manufacturer's instructions should be explained to the patient prior to initiation.

Continuous Subcutaneous Insulin Infusion

CSII via use of an insulin pump or patch allows for precise insulin delivery. CSII is largely limited to people with T1D at the current time, due to limitations of insulin volume that can be loaded into an insulin pump. CSII requires considerable patient education and support until the individual becomes familiar with use of the device. Insulin pumps use rapid-acting insulin (insulin lispro, insulin aspart, or insulin glulisine) to cover both basal and bolus insulin needs.[7] Insulin pump and patch technology advances very quickly with new-generation devices entering the market regularly. The American Diabetes Association's *Diabetes Forecast* publishes consumer guides, inclusive of an insulin pump consumer guide, on an annual basis that are readily accessible via the publication's website (www.diabetesforecast.org).

Insulin Inhalation

As discussed previously, inhaled human insulin is currently available in the U.S. for prandial use in T1D and T2D.[15] The product is available in single-use cartridges for use in the corresponding inhalation device. The product is available in 4-unit, 8-unit, and 12-unit single-use cartridges, which are color-coded to prevent medication errors.[15] Individual cartridges can be used in combination to customize the dose or if higher doses are needed.

COMBINATION THERAPY

Insulin combination therapy is commonly needed in people with T1D (unless they use an insulin pump) and in many people with longstanding T2D. Please refer back to the sections "Approach to the Use of Insulin in Type 1 Diabetes" and "Approach to the Use of Insulin in Type 2 Diabetes" for specific information on approaches to insulin use in these patient groups. When using multiple insulin products, they can be injected individually, mixed in a single syringe (if compatible), or purchased in fixed-ratio combination (FRC) insulin pens.

MIXING INSULIN

Some insulin products can be combined, or "mixed," in the same syringe to reduce the number of required daily injections. NPH or NPH-type insulin can be mixed with either regular human insulin or rapid-acting insulin analogs.[7] By mixing NPH-type insulins with regular insulin or a rapid-acting insulin analog, a biphasic action profile is created, providing both basal and prandial coverage with a single injection. When mixing insulins in a single syringe, the rapid- or short-acting insulin should be drawn up first.[7] It should be noted that long-acting insulins such as insulin glargine, insulin detemir, and insulin degludec should not be mixed with other insulin products.

PREMIXED INSULIN PRODUCTS

Commercially available premixed insulin products contain set percentages of two types of insulin in the same solution. These include mixtures of NPH and RHI (70/30), mixtures of protamine suspensions of rapid-acting analogs with the respective rapid-acting analog (75/25 lispro protamine/insulin lispro, 50/50 lispro protamine/insulin lispro, and 70/30 aspart protamine/aspart), and a combination of insulin degludec with insulin aspart (70/30).[48-53] The primary advantages of these insulin products are convenience and accuracy of administration, particularly for people with vision or dexterity limitations for whom mixing insulin would be difficult or unreliable.[7]

In addition to fixed-dose insulin combination products, there are currently two products available that combine a basal insulin analog with a GLP-1 receptor agonist.[54,55] As discussed in the section "Approach to the Use of Insulin in Type 2 Diabetes," combination therapy with basal insulin and a GLP-1 receptor agonist can effectively target both FPG and PPG values and thus improve A1C and overall glycemic control, while also mitigating insulin-associated weight gain. Table 3.4 provides a summary of fixed-dose combination products currently available in the U.S.[48-55]

Table 3.4—Fixed-Dose Combination (FDC) Insulin Products

Generic name	Brand name(s)	Product availability	Units per pen	Dose range per injection (pens only)	Recommended pen storage at room temperature (days)
Fixed-Dose Combination Insulin Products					
Regular/NPH 70/30	Humulin 70/30 Novolin 70/30	Vial, Prefilled pen	300 units	1–60	10
Lispro mix 50/50	Humalog Mix 50/50	Vial, Prefilled pen	300 units	1–60 units	10
Lispro mix 75/25	Humalog Mix 75/25	Vial, Prefilled pen	300 units	1–60 units	10
Aspart mix 70/30	Novolog Mix 70/30	Vial, Prefilled pen	300 units	1–60 units	14
Degludec/ Aspart mix 70/30	Ryzodeg 70/30	Prefilled pen	300 units	1–80 units	28
Fixed-Dose Insulin/GLP-1 Receptor Agonist Products					
Insulin Glargine/ Lixisenatide	Soliqua	Prefilled pen	300 units (insulin glargine)	15–60 units (insulin glargine)	28
Insulin Degludec/ Liraglutide	Xultophy	Prefilled pen	300 units (insulin degludec)	10–50 units (insulin degludec)	21

Source: refs. 48–55.

SINGLE INSULIN PRODUCTS

Insulin Aspart (Fiasp): https://dailymed.nlm.nih.gov/dailymed/drugInfo.cfm?setid=834e7efc-393f-4c55-9125-628562a8a5cf

Insulin Aspart (Novolog): https://dailymed.nlm.nih.gov/dailymed/drugInfo.cfm?setid=3a1e73a2-3009-40d0-876c-b4cb2be56fc5

Insulin Degludec [U-100, U-200] (Tresiba): https://dailymed.nlm.nih.gov/dailymed/drugInfo.cfm?setid=456c5e87-3dfd-46fa-8ac0-c6128d4c97c6

Insulin Detemir (Levemir): https://dailymed.nlm.nih.gov/dailymed/drugInfo.cfm?setid=d38d65c1-25bf-401d-9c7e-a2c3222da8af

Insulin Glargine [U-100] (Lantus, Basaglar): https://dailymed.nlm.nih.gov/dailymed/drugInfo.cfm?setid=6328c99d-d75f-43ef-b19e-7e71f91e57f6

Insulin Glargine [U-300] (Toujeo): https://dailymed.nlm.nih.gov/dailymed/drugInfo.cfm?setid=c9561d96-124d-48ca-982f-0aa1575bff36

Insulin Glulisine (Apidra): https://dailymed.nlm.nih.gov/dailymed/drugInfo.cfm?setid=e7af6a7a-8046-4fb4-9979-4ec4230b23aa

Inhaled Human Insulin (Afrezza): https://dailymed.nlm.nih.gov/dailymed/drugInfo.cfm?setid=29f4637b-e204-425b-b89c-7238008d8c10

Insulin Lispro [U-100, U-200] (Humalog, Admelog): https://dailymed.nlm.nih.gov/dailymed/drugInfo.cfm?setid=c6b8ff07-d3e2-457f-8a38-b60de60adf75

NPH Insulin (Humulin N, Novolin N): https://dailymed.nlm.nih.gov/dailymed/drugInfo.cfm?setid=f6edd793-440b-40c2-96b5-c16133b7a921

Regular Human Insulin [U-100] (Humulin R, Novolin R): https://dailymed.nlm.nih.gov/dailymed/drugInfo.cfm?setid=b519bd83-038c-4ec5-a231-a51ec5cc291f

Regular Human Insulin [U-500] (Humulin R U-500): https://dailymed.nlm.nih.gov/dailymed/drugInfo.cfm?setid=b60e8dd0-1d48-4dc9-87fd-e14675255e8c

---

REFERENCES

1. White JR. A brief history of the development of diabetes medications. *Diabetes Spectr* 2014;27:82–86

2. American Diabetes Association/JDRF. *Type 1 Diabetes Sourcebook*. Peters A, Laffel L, Eds. Alexandria, American Diabetes Association, 2013

3. Chiang JL, Kirkman MS, Laffel LMB, Peters AL. Type 1 diabetes through the life span: a position statement of the American Diabetes Association. *Diabetes Care* 2014;37:2034–2054

4. American Diabetes Association. 8. Pharmacologic approaches to glycemic treatment: *Standards of Medical Care in Diabetes—2018. Diabetes Care* 2018;41(Suppl. 1):S73–S85

5. Kahn CR, Baird KL, Flier JS, et al. Insulin receptors, receptor antibodies and the mechanism of insulin action. *Recent Prog Horm Res* 1981;37:477–538

6. Skyler JS, Bakris GL, Bonifacio E, et al. Differentiation of diabetes by pathophysiology, natural history, and prognosis. *Diabetes* 2017;66:241–255

7. American Diabetes Association. *Practical Insulin: A Handbook for Prescribing Providers*. 3rd ed. Alexandria, American Diabetes Association, 2015

8. Evans M, Schumm-Draeger PM, Vora J, King AB. A review of modern insulin analogue pharmacokinetic and pharmacodynamics profiles in type 2 diabetes: improvements and limitations. *Diabetes Obes Metab* 2011;13:677–684

9. Ryysy L, Häkkinen AM, Goto T, et al. Hepatic fat content and insulin action on free fatty acids and glucose metabolism rather than insulin absorption are associated with insulin requirements during insulin therapy in type 2 diabetic patients. *Diabetes* 2000;49:749–758

10. Koivisto VA. Sauna-induced acceleration in insulin absorption from subcutaneous injection site. *Br Med J* 1980;280:1411–1413

11. Berger M, Cuppers HJ, Hegner H, Jorgens V, Berchtold P. Absorption kinetics and biologic effects of subcutaneously injected insulin preparations. *Diabetes Care* 1982;5:77-91

12. ter Braak EW, Woodworth JR, Bianchi R, et al. Injection site effects on the pharmacokinetics and glucodynamics of insulin lispro and regular insulin. *Diabetes Care* 1996;19:1437–1440

13. Humulin R (insulin human injection) [package insert]. Indianapolis, IN, Lilly USA, LLC, 2015

14. Novolin R (insulin human injection) [package insert]. Plainsboro, NJ, Novo Nordisk Inc., 2018

15. Afrezza (insulin human inhalation powder) [package insert]. Danbury, CT, MannKind Corporation, 2018

16. Toujeo (insulin glargine injection) [package insert]. Bridgewater, NJ, Sanofi-aventis U.S. LLC, 2018

17. Tresiba (insulin degludec injection) [package insert]. Plainsboro, NJ, Novo Nordisk Inc., 2018

18. American Diabetes Association. 14. Diabetes care in the hospital: *Standards of Medical Care in Diabetes—2018*. *Diabetes Care* 2018;41(Suppl. 1):S144–S151

19. Humalog (insulin lispro injection) [package insert]. Indianapolis, IN, Lilly USA, LLC, 2017

20. Novolog (insulin aspart injection) [package insert]. Plainsboro, NJ, Novo Nordisk Inc., 2017

21. Fiasp (insulin aspart injection) [package insert]. Plainsboro, NJ, Novo Nordisk Inc., 2017

22. Apidra (insulin glulisine injection) [package insert]. Bridgewater, NJ, Sanofi-aventis U.S. LLC, 2015

23. Tibaldi JM. Evolution of insulin: from human to analog. *Am J Med* 2014;127:S25–S38

24. Admelog (insulin lispro injection) [package insert]. Bridgewater, NJ, Sanofi-aventis U.S. LLC, 2017

25. Mathieu C, Bode BW, Franek E, et al. Efficacy and safety of fast-acting insulin aspart in comparison with insulin aspart in type 1 diabetes (onset 1): a 52-week, randomized, treat-to-target, phase III trial. *Diabetes Obes Metab* 2018;20:1148–1155

26. Russell-Jones D, Bode BW, De Block C, et al. Fast-acting insulin aspart improves glycemic control in basal-bolus treatment for type 1 diabetes: results of a 26-week multicenter, active-controlled, treat-to-target, randomized, parallel-group trial (onset 1). *Diabetes Care* 2017;40:943–950

27. Bowering K, Case C, Harvey J, et al. Faster aspart versus insulin aspart as part of a basal-bolus regimen in inadequately controlled type 2 diabetes: the onset 2 trial. *Diabetes Care* 2017;40:951–957

28. Neumiller JJ, Campbell RK. Technosphere insulin: an inhaled prandial insulin product. *Biodrugs* 2010;24:165–172

29. Humulin N (human insulin isophane suspension) [package insert]. Indianapolis, IN, Lilly USA, LLC, 2017

30. Novolin N (isophane insulin human suspension) [package insert]. Plainsboro, NJ, Novo Nordisk Inc., 2018

31. Campbell RK, White JR, Levien T, Baker D. Insulin glargine. *Clin Ther* 2001;23:1938–1957

32. Lantus (insulin glargine injection) [package insert]. Bridgewater, NJ, Sanofi-aventis U.S. LLC, 2015

33. Basaglar (insulin glargine injection) [package insert]. Indianapolis, IN, Lilly USA, LLC, 2016

34. Soran H, Younis N. Insulin detemir: a new basal insulin analogue. *Diabetes Obes Metab* 2006;8:26–30

35. Blair HA, Keating GM. Insulin glargine 300 U/mL: a review in diabetes mellitus. *Drugs* 2016;76:363–374

36. Robinson JD, Neumiller JJ, Campbell RK. Can a new ultra-long-acting insulin analogue improve patient care? Investigating the potential role of insulin degludec. *Drugs* 2012;72:2319–2325

37. Kahn CR, Flier JS, Bar RS, et al. The syndromes of insulin resistance and acanthosis nigricans: insulin-receptor disorders in man. *N Engl J Med* 1976;294:739–745

38. Lamos EM, Younk LM, Davis SN. Concentrated insulins: the new basal insulins. *Ther Clin Risk Manag* 2016;12:389–400

39. de la Peña A, Riddle M, Morrow LA, et al. Pharmacokinetics and pharmacodynamics of high-dose human regular U-500 insulin versus human regular U-100 insulin in healthy obese subjects. *Diabetes Care* 2011;34:2496–2501

40. Humulin R U-500 (insulin human injection) [package insert]. Indianapolis, IN, Lilly USA, LLC, 2018

41. Hood RC, Arakaki RF, Wysham C, et al. Two treatment approaches for human regular U-500 insulin in patients with type 2 diabetes not achieving adequate glycemic control on high-dose U-100 insulin therapy with or without oral agents: a randomized, titration-to-target clinical trial. *Endocr Pract* 2015;21:782–793

42. Davies MJ, D'Alessio DA, Fradkin J, et al. Management of hyperglycemia in type 2 diabetes, 2018. A consensus report by the American Diabetes Association (ADA) and the European Association for the Study of Diabetes (EASD). *Diabetes Care* 2018 Oct 4. DOI:10.2337/dci18-0033. [Epub ahead of print]

43. American Diabetes Association. 13. Management of diabetes in pregnancy: *Standards of Medical Care in Diabetes—2018. Diabetes Care* 2018;41 (Suppl. 1):S137–S143

44. Neumiller JJ, Alicic RZ, Tuttle KR. Therapeutic considerations for antihyperglycemic agents in diabetic kidney disease. *J Am Soc Nephrol* 2017;28:2263–2274

45. American Diabetes Association. 6. Glycemic targets: *Standards of Medical Care in Diabetes—2018. Diabetes Care* 2018;41(Suppl. 1):S55–S64

46. Russell-Jones D, Khan R. Insulin-associated weight gain in diabetes—causes, effects and coping strategies. *Diabetes Obes Metab* 2007;9(6):799–812

47. Levemir (insulin detemir injection) [package insert]. Plainsboro, NJ, Novo Nordisk Inc., 2015

48. Humulin 70/30 (insulin human injection) [package insert]. Indianapolis, IN, Lilly USA, LLC, 2017

49. Novolin 70/30 (human insulin isophane suspension and human insulin injection) [package insert]. Plainsboro, NJ, Novo Nordisk Inc., 2018

50. Humalog Mix50/50 (insulin lispro injection, suspension) [package insert]. Indianapolis, IN, Lilly USA, LLC, 2015

51. Humalog Mix75/25 (insulin lispro injection, suspension) [package insert]. Indianapolis, IN, Lilly USA, LLC, 2015

52. Novolog Mix 70/30 (insulin aspart protamine and insulin aspart injectable suspension) [package insert]. Plainsboro, NJ, Novo Nordisk Inc., 2017

53. Ryzodeg 70/30 (insulin degludec and insulin aspart injection) [package insert]. Plainsboro, NJ, Novo Nordisk Inc., 2016

54. Soliqua 100/33 (insulin glargine and lixisenatide injection) [package insert]. Bridgewater, NJ, Sanofi-aventis U.S. LLC, 2017

55. Xultophy 100/3.6 (insulin degludec and liraglutide injection) [package insert]. Plainsboro, NJ, Novo Nordisk Inc., 2016

Chapter 4
Pharmacologic Therapy for Type 2 Diabetes

9.5 Metformin is the preferred initial pharmacologic agent for the treatment of type 2 diabetes. **A**[*]

9.6 Once initiated, metformin should be continued as long as it is tolerated and not contraindicated; other agents, including insulin, should be added to metformin. **A**

9.7 Long-term use of metformin may be associated with biochemical vitamin B_{12} deficiency, and periodic measurement of vitamin B_{12} levels should be considered in metformin-treated patients, especially in those with anemia or peripheral neuropathy. **B**

9.8 The early introduction of insulin should be considered if there is evidence of ongoing catabolism (weight loss), if symptoms of hyperglycemia are present, or when A1C levels (>10% [86 mmol/mol]) or blood glucose levels (≥300 mg/dL [16.7 mmol/L]) are very high. **E**

9.9 Consider initiating dual therapy in patients with newly diagnosed type 2 diabetes who have A1C ≥1.5% (12.5 mmol/mol) above their glycemic target. **E**

9.10 A patient-centered approach should be used to guide the choice of pharmacologic agents. Considerations include comorbidities (atherosclerotic cardiovascular disease, heart failure, chronic kidney disease), hypoglycemia risk, impact on weight, cost, risk for side effects, and patient preferences. **E**

9.11 Among patients with type 2 diabetes who have established atherosclerotic cardiovascular disease, sodium–glucose cotransporter 2 inhibitors, or glucagon-like peptide 1 receptor agonists with demonstrated cardiovascular disease benefit (Table 4.1) are recommended as part of the antihyperglycemic regimen. **A**

9.12 Among patients with atherosclerotic cardiovascular disease at high risk of heart failure or in whom heart failure coexists, sodium–glucose cotransporter 2 inhibitors are preferred. **C**

9.13 For patients with type 2 diabetes and chronic kidney disease, consider use of a sodium–glucose cotransporter 2 inhibitor or glucagon-like peptide 1

Chapter 4 is an excerpt from American Diabetes Association, 9. Pharmacologic Approaches to Glycemic Treatment: *Standards of Medical Care in Diabetes—2019. Diabetes Care* 2019; 42(Suppl. 1):S90–S102. DOI:10.2337/dc19-S009

[*] See Table 1.1 (p. 4) for an explanation of the American Diabetes Association evidence-grading system for *Standards of Medical Care in Diabetes.*

receptor agonist shown to reduce risk of chronic kidney disease progression, cardiovascular events, or both. **C**

9.14 In most patients who need the greater glucose-lowering effect of an injectable medication, glucagon-like peptide 1 receptor agonists are preferred to insulin. **B**

9.15 Intensification of treatment for patients with type 2 diabetes not meeting treatment goals should not be delayed. **B**

9.16 The medication regimen should be reevaluated at regular intervals (every 3–6 months) and adjusted as needed to incorporate new patient factors (Table 4.1). **E**

The American Diabetes Association/European Association for the Study of Diabetes consensus report "Management of Hyperglycemia in Type 2 Diabetes, 2018"[1] recommends a patient-centered approach to choosing appropriate pharmacologic treatment of blood glucose (Fig. 9.1). This includes consideration of efficacy and key patient factors: *1)* important comorbidities such as atherosclerotic cardiovascular disease (ASCVD), chronic kidney disease (CKD), and heart failure (HF), *2)* hypoglycemia risk, *3)* effects on body weight, *4)* side effects, *5)* cost, and *6)* patient preferences. Lifestyle modifications that improve health (see Section 5 "Lifestyle Management") should be emphasized along with any pharmacologic therapy. See Sections 12 and 13 for recommendations specific for older adults and for children and adolescents with type 2 diabetes, respectively.

INITIAL THERAPY

Metformin should be started at the time type 2 diabetes is diagnosed unless there are contraindications; for most patients this will be monotherapy in combination with lifestyle modifications. Metformin is effective and safe, is inexpensive, and may reduce risk of cardiovascular events and death.[2] Metformin is available in an immediate-release form for twice-daily dosing or as an extended-release form that can be given once daily. Compared with sulfonylureas, metformin as first-line therapy has beneficial effects on A1C, weight, and cardiovascular mortality;[3] there is little systematic data available for other oral agents as initial therapy of type 2 diabetes. The principal side effects of metformin are gastrointestinal intolerance due to bloating, abdominal discomfort, and diarrhea. The drug is cleared by renal filtration, and very high circulating levels (e.g., as a result of overdose or acute renal failure) have been associated with lactic acidosis. However, the occurrence of this complication is now known to be very rare, and metformin may be safely used in patients with reduced estimated glomerular filtration rates (eGFR); the FDA has revised the label for metformin to reflect its safety in patients with eGFR $\geq$30 mL/min/1.73 m^2.[4] A recent randomized trial confirmed previous observations that metformin use is associated with vitamin B_{12} deficiency and worsening of symptoms of neuropathy.[5] This is compatible with a recent report from the Diabetes Prevention Program Outcomes Study (DPPOS) suggesting periodic testing of vitamin B_{12}.[6]

In patients with contraindications or intolerance of metformin, initial therapy should be based on patient factors; consider a drug from another class depicted in Fig. 9.1. When A1C is $\geq$1.5% (12.5 mmol/mol) above glycemic target (see Section 6 "Glycemic Targets" for more information on selecting appropriate targets), many patients will require dual combination therapy to achieve their target A1C level.[7] Insulin has the advantage of being effective where other agents are not and should be considered as part of any combination regimen when hyperglycemia is severe, especially if catabolic features (weight loss, hypertriglyceridemia, ketosis) are present. Consider initiating insulin therapy when blood glucose is ≥300 mg/dL (16.7 mmol/L) or A1C is ≥10% (86 mmol/mol) or if the patient has symptoms of hyperglycemia (i.e., polyuria or polydipsia), even at diagnosis or early in the course of treatment (Fig. 9.2). As glucose toxicity resolves, simplifying the regimen and/or changing to oral agents is often possible.

COMBINATION THERAPY

Although there are numerous trials comparing dual therapy with metformin alone, few directly compare drugs as add-on therapy. A comparative effectiveness meta-analysis suggests that each new class of noninsulin agents added to initial therapy generally lowers A1C approximately 0.7–1.0%.[8] If the A1C target is not achieved after approximately 3 months and the patient does not have ASCVD or CKD, consider a combination of metformin and any one of the preferred six treatment options: sulfonylurea, thiazolidinedione, dipeptidyl peptidase 4 (DPP-4) inhibitor, SGLT2 inhibitor, GLP-1 receptor agonist, or basal insulin; the choice of which agent to add is based on drug-specific effects and patient factors (Fig. 9.1 and Table 4.1). For patients in whom ASCVD, HF, or CKD predominates, the best choice for a second agent is a GLP-1 receptor agonist or SGLT2 inhibitor with demonstrated cardiovascular risk reduction, after consideration of drug-specific and patient factors (Table 4.1). For patients without established ASCVD or CKD, the choice of a second agent to add to metformin is not yet guided by empiric evidence. Rather, drug choice is based on avoidance of side effects, particularly hypoglycemia and weight gain, cost, and patient preferences.[9] Similar considerations are applied in patients who require a third agent to achieve glycemic goals; there is also very little trial-based evidence to guide this choice. In all cases, treatment regimens need to be continuously reviewed for efficacy, side effects, and patient burden (Table 4.1). In some instances, patients will require medication reduction or discontinuation. Common reasons for this include ineffectiveness, intolerable side effects, expense, or a change in glycemic goals (e.g., in response to development of comorbidities or changes in treatment goals). See Section 12 "Older Adults" for a full discussion of treatment considerations in older adults.

Even though most patients prefer oral medications to drugs that need to be injected, the eventual need for the greater potency of injectable medications is common, particularly in people with a longer duration of diabetes. The addition of basal insulin, either human NPH or one of the long-acting insulin analogs, to oral agent regimens is a well-established approach that is effective for many patients. In addition, recent evidence supports the utility of GLP-1 receptor agonists in patients not reaching glycemic targets with oral agent regimens. In trials comparing the addition of GLP-1 receptor agonists or insulin in patients needing further glucose lowering, the efficacy of the two treatments was similar.[10–12] However, GLP-1 receptor agonists had a lower risk of hypoglycemia and beneficial effects on body weight compared with insulin, albeit with greater gastrointestinal side effects. Thus, trial results support a GLP-1 receptor agonist as the preferred option for patients requiring the potency of an injectable therapy for glucose control (Fig. 9.2). However, high costs and tolerability issues are important barriers to the use of GLP-1 receptor agonists.

Cost-effectiveness models of the newer agents based on clinical utility and glycemic effect have been reported.[13] Table 4.2 provides cost information for currently approved noninsulin therapies. Of note, prices listed are average wholesale prices (AWP)[14] and National Average Drug Acquisition Costs (NADAC)[15] and do not account for discounts, rebates, or other price adjustments often involved in prescription sales that affect the actual cost incurred by the patient. While there are alternative means to estimate medication prices, AWP and NADAC were utilized to provide two separate measures to allow for a comparison of drug prices with the primary goal of highlighting the importance of cost considerations when prescribing antihyperglycemic treatments.

CARDIOVASCULAR OUTCOMES TRIALS

There are now multiple large randomized controlled trials reporting statistically significant reductions in cardiovascular events in patients with type 2 diabetes treated with an SGLT2 inhibitor (empagliflozin, canagliflozin) or GLP-1 receptor agonist (liraglutide, semaglutide). In people with diabetes with established ASCVD, empagliflozin decreased a composite three-point major cardiovascular event (MACE) outcome and mortality compared with placebo.[16] Similarly, canagliflozin reduced the occurrence of MACE in a group of subjects with, or at high risk for, ASCVD.[17] In both of these trials, SGLT2 inhibitors reduced hospitalization for HF;[16,17] this was a secondary outcome of these studies and will require confirmation in more defined populations. In people with type 2 diabetes with ASCVD or increased risk for ASCVD, the addition of liraglutide decreased MACE and mortality,[18] and the closely related GLP-1 receptor agonist semaglutide also had favorable effects on cardiovascular endpoints in high-risk subjects.[19] In these cardiovascular outcomes trials, empagliflozin, canagliflozin, liraglutide, and semaglutide all had beneficial effects on composite indices of CKD.[16–19] See antihyperglycemic therapies and cardiovascular outcomes in Section 10 "Cardiovascular Disease and Risk Management" and Table 10.4 for a detailed description of these cardiovascular outcomes trials, as well as a discussion of how HF may impact treatment choices. See Section 11 "Microvascular Complications and Foot Care" for a detailed discussion on how CKD may impact treatment choices. Additional large randomized trials of other agents in these classes are ongoing.

The subjects enrolled in the cardiovascular outcomes trials using empagliflozin, canagliflozin, liraglutide, and semaglutide had A1C ≥7%, and more than 70% were taking metformin at baseline. Moreover, the benefit of treatment was less evident in subjects with lower risk for ASCVD. Thus, extension of these results to practice is most appropriate for people with type 2 diabetes and established ASCVD who require additional glucose-lowering treatment beyond metformin and lifestyle management. For these patients, incorporating one of the SGLT2 inhibitors or GLP-1 receptor agonists that have been demonstrated to reduce cardiovascular events is recommended (Table 4.1).

Table 4.1—Drug-Specific and Patient Factors to Consider When Selecting Antihyperglycemic Treatment in Adults With T2D

	Efficacy	Hypo-glycemia	Weight change	CV effects		Cost	Oral/SQ	Renal effects		Additional considerations
				ASCVD	CHF			Progression of DKD	Dosing/use considerations*	
Metformin	High	No	Neutral (potential for modest loss)	Potential benefit	Neutral	Low	Oral	Neutral	■ Contraindicated with eGFR <30	■ Gastrointestinal side effects common (diarrhea, nausea) ■ Potential for B_{12} deficiency
SGLT2 inhibitors	Intermediate	No	Loss	Benefit: empa-gliflozin†, cana-gliflozin	Benefit: empa-gliflozin†, cana-gliflozin	High	Oral	Benefit: cana-gliflozin, empa-gliflozin	■ Renal dose adjustment required (canagliflozin, dapagliflozin, empagliflozin, ertugliflozin)	■ FDA Black Box: Risk of amputation (canagliflozin) ■ Risk of bone fractures (canagliflozin) ■ DKA risk (all agents, rare in T2DM) ■ Genitourinary infections ■ Risk of volume depletion, hypotension ■ ↑LDL cholesterol ■ Risk of Fournier's gangrene
GLP-1 RAs	High	No	Loss	Neutral: lix-isenatide Benefit: liraglutide† > sema-glutide > exenatide extended release	Neutral	High	SQ	Benefit: liraglutide	■ Renal dose adjustment required (exenatide, lix-isenatide) ■ Caution when initiating or increasing dose due to potential risk of acute kidney injury	■ FDA Black Box: Risk of thyroid C-cell tumors (liraglutide, albiglutide, dulaglutide, exenatide extended release) ■ Gastrointestinal side effects common (nausea, vomiting, diarrhea) ■ Injection site reactions ■ ?Acute pancreatitis risk

(continued)

Table 4.1 (continued)

DPP-4 inhibitors	Intermediate	No	Neutral	Neutral	Potential risk: saxagliptin, alogliptin	High	Oral	Neutral	■ Renal dose adjustment required (sitagliptin, saxagliptin, alogliptin); can be used in renal impairment ■ No dose adjustment required for linagliptin	■ Potential risk of acute pancreatitis ■ Joint pain
Thiazolidinediones	High	No	Gain	Potential benefit: pioglitazone	Increased risk	Low	Oral	Neutral	■ No dose adjustment required ■ Generally not recommended in renal impairment due to potential for fluid retention	■ FDA Black Box: Congestive heart failure [pioglitazone, rosiglitazone] ■ Fluid retention (edema; heart failure) ■ Benefit in NASH ■ Risk of bone fractures ■ Bladder cancer (pioglitazone) ■ ↑LDL cholesterol (rosiglitazone)
Sulfonylureas (2nd generation)	High	Yes	Gain	Neutral	Neutral	Low	Oral	Neutral	■ Glyburide: not recommended ■ Glipizide and glimepiride: initiate conservatively to avoid hypoglycemia	■ FDA Special Warning on increased risk of cardiovascular mortality based on studies of an older sulfonylurea (tolbutamide)
Insulin — Human insulin	Highest	Yes	Gain	Neutral	Neutral	Low	SQ	Neutral	■ Lower insulin doses required with a decrease in eGFR; titrate per clinical response	■ Injection site reactions
Insulin — Analogs						High	SQ			■ Higher risk of hypoglycemia with human insulin (NPH or premixed formulations) vs. analogs

*For agent-specific dosing recommendations, please refer to the manufacturers' prescribing information. †FDA approved for CVD benefit. CHF, congestive heart failure; CV, cardiovascular; DPP-4, dipeptidyl peptidase 4; DKA, diabetic ketoacidosis; DKD, diabetic kidney disease; GLP-1 RAs, glucagon-like peptide 1 receptor agonists; NASH, nonalcoholic steatohepatitis; SGLT2, sodium–glucose cotransporter 2; SQ, subcutaneous; T2DM, type 2 diabetes.

INSULIN THERAPY

Many patients with type 2 diabetes eventually require and benefit from insulin therapy (Fig. 9.2). See the section above, INSULIN INJECTION TECHNIQUE, for important guidance on how to administer insulin safely and effectively. The progressive nature of type 2 diabetes should be regularly and objectively explained to patients, and providers should avoid using insulin as a threat or describing it as a sign of personal failure or punishment. Rather, the utility and importance of insulin to maintain glycemic control once progression of the disease overcomes the effect of oral agents should be emphasized. Educating and involving patients in insulin management is beneficial. Instruction of patients in self-titration of insulin doses based on self-monitoring of blood glucose improves glycemic control in patients with type 2 diabetes initiating insulin.[20] Comprehensive education regarding self-monitoring of blood glucose, diet, and the avoidance and appropriate treatment of hypoglycemia are critically important in any patient using insulin.

BASAL INSULIN

Basal insulin alone is the most convenient initial insulin regimen and can be added to metformin and other oral agents. Starting doses can be estimated based on body weight (e.g., 10 units a day or 0.1–0.2 units/kg/day) and the degree of hyperglycemia, with individualized titration over days to weeks as needed. The principal action of basal insulin is to restrain hepatic glucose production, with a goal of maintaining euglycemia overnight and between meals.[21,22] Control of fasting glucose can be achieved with human NPH insulin or with the use of a long-acting insulin analog. In clinical trials, long-acting basal analogs (U-100 glargine or detemir) have been demonstrated to reduce the risk of symptomatic and nocturnal hypoglycemia compared with NPH insulin,[23–28] although these advantages are generally modest and may not persist.[29] Longer-acting basal analogs (U-300 glargine or degludec) may convey a lower hypoglycemia risk compared with U-100 glargine when used in combination with oral agents.[30–36] Despite evidence for reduced hypoglycemia with newer, longer-acting basal insulin analogs in clinical trial settings, in practice they may not affect the development of hypoglycemia compared with NPH insulin.[37]

The cost of insulin has been rising steadily, and at a pace several times that of other medical expenditures, over the past decade.[38] This expense contributes significant burden to the patient as insulin has become a growing "out-of-pocket" cost for people with diabetes, and direct patient costs contribute to treatment nonadherence.[38] Therefore, consideration of cost is an important component of effective management. For many patients with type 2 diabetes (e.g., individuals with relaxed A1C goals, low rates of hypoglycemia, and prominent insulin resistance, as well as those with cost concerns), human insulin (NPH and Regular) may be the appropriate choice of therapy, and clinicians should be familiar with its use.[39] Table 4.3 provides AWP[14] and NADAC[15] information (cost per 1,000 units) for currently available insulin and insulin combination products in the U.S. As stated for Table 4.2, AWP and NADAC prices listed do not account for discounts, rebates, or other price adjustments that may affect the actual cost to the patient. For example, human regular insulin, NPH, and 70/30 NPH/Regular products can

Table 4.2—Median Monthly Cost of Maximum Approved Daily Dose of Noninsulin Glucose-Lowering Agents in the U.S.

Class	Compound(s)	Dosage strength/ product (if applicable)	Median AWP (min, max)†	Median NADAC (min, max)†	Maximum approved daily dose*
Biguanides	• Metformin	500 mg (IR)	$84 ($4, $93)	$2	2,000 mg
		850 mg (IR)	$108 ($6, $109)	$3	2,550 mg
		1,000 mg (IR)	$87 ($4, $88)	$2	2,000 mg
		500 mg (ER)	$89 ($82, $6,671)	$4 ($4, $1,267)	2,000 mg
		750 mg (ER)	$72 ($65, $92)	$4	1,500 mg
		1,000 mg (ER)	$1,028 ($1,028, $7,214)	$311 ($311, $1,321)	2000 mg
Sulfonylureas (2nd generation)	• Glimepiride	4 mg	$71 ($71, $198)	$4	8 mg
	• Glipizide	10 mg (IR)	$75 ($67, $97)	$5	40 mg (IR)
		10 mg (XL)	$48	$15	20 mg (XL)
	• Glyburide	6 mg (micron- ized)	$50 ($48, $71)	$10	12 mg (micronized)
		5 mg	$93 ($63, $103)	$13	20 mg

(continued)

Table 4.2 (continued)

Class	Compound(s)	Dosage strength/ product (if applicable)	Median AWP (min, max)†	Median NADAC (min, max)†	Maximum approved daily dose*
Thiazolidinedio-nes	• Pioglitazone	45 mg	$348 ($283, $349)	$4	45 mg
	• Rosiglitazone	4 mg	$407	$329	8 mg
α-Glucosidase inhibitors	• Acarbose	100 mg	$106 ($104, $106)	$23	300 mg
	• Miglitol	100 mg	$241	$311	300 mg
Meglitinides (glinides)	• Nateglinide	120 mg	$155	$46	360 mg
	• Repaglinide	2 mg	$878 ($162, $898)	$48	16 mg
DPP-4 inhibitors	• Alogliptin	25 mg	$234	$170	25 mg
	• Saxagliptin	5 mg	$490 ($462, $490)	$392	5 mg
	• Linagliptin	5 mg	$494	$395	5 mg
	• Sitagliptin	100 mg	$516	$413	100 mg
SGLT2 inhibitors	• Ertugliflozin	15 mg	$322	$257	15 mg
	• Dapagliflozin	10 mg	$557	$446	10 mg
	• Canagliflozin	300 mg	$558	$446	300 mg
	• Empagliflozin	25 mg	$558	$448	25 mg

(continued)

Table 4.2 (continued)

Class	Compound(s)	Dosage strength/ product (if applicable)	Median AWP (min, max)†	Median NADAC (min, max)†	Maximum approved daily dose*
GLP-1 receptor agonists	• Exenatide (extendedre-lease)	2 mg powder for suspension or pen	$792	$634	2 mg**
	• Exenatide	10 µg pen	$850	$680	20 µg
	• Dulaglutide	1.5/0.5 mL pen	$876	$702	1.5 mg**
	• Semaglutide	1 mg pen	$875	$704	1 mg**
	• Liraglutide	18 mg/3 mL pen	$1,044	$835	1.8 mg
Bile acid seques-trants	• Colesevelam	625 mg tabs	$712 ($674, $712)	$354	3.75 g
		3.75 g suspen-sion	$674	$598	3.75 g
Dopamine-2 agonists	• Bromocriptine	0.8 mg	$855	$685	4.8 mg
Amylin mimetics	• Pramlintide	120 µg pen	$2,547	$2,036	120 µg/injec-tion†††

AWP, average wholesale price; DPP-4, dipeptidyl peptidase 4; ER and XL, extended release; GLP-1, gluca-gon-like peptide 1; IR, immediate release; NADAC, National Average Drug Acquisition Cost; SGLT2, sodium–glucose cotransporter 2. †Calculated for 30-day supply (AWP [44] or NADAC [45] unit price × number of doses required to provide maximum approved daily dose × 30 days); median AWP or NADAC listed alone when only one product and/or price. *Utilized to calculate median AWP and NADAC (min, max); generic prices used, if available commercially. **Administered once weekly. †††AWP and NADAC calculated based on 120 µg three times daily.

be purchased for considerably less than the AWP and NADAC prices listed in Table 4.3 at select pharmacies.

PRANDIAL INSULIN

Individuals with type 2 diabetes may require doses of insulin before meals in addition to basal insulin. The recommended starting dose of mealtime insulin is either 4 units or 10% of the basal dose at each meal. Titration is done based on home glucose monitoring or A1C. With significant additions to the prandial insulin dose, particularly with the evening meal, consideration should be given to decreasing the basal insulin dose. Meta-analyses of trials comparing rapid-acting insulin analogs with human regular insulin in patients with type 2 diabetes have not reported important differences in A1C or hypoglycemia.[40,41]

PREMIXED INSULIN

Premixed insulin products contain both a basal and prandial component, allowing coverage of both basal and prandial needs with a single injection. The NPH/Regular premix is composed of 70% NPH insulin and 30% regular insulin. The use of premixed insulin products has its advantages and disadvantages, as discussed below in combination injectable therapy.

CONCENTRATED INSULIN PRODUCTS

Several concentrated insulin preparations are currently available. U-500 regular insulin is, by definition, five times more concentrated than U-100 regular insulin. Regular U-500 has distinct pharmacokinetics with delayed onset and longer duration of action, characteristics more like an intermediate-acting insulin. U-300 glargine and U-200 degludec are three and two times as concentrated, respectively, as their U-100 formulations and allow higher doses of basal insulin administration per volume used. U-300 glargine has a longer duration of action than U-100 glargine but modestly lower efficacy per unit administered.[42,43] The FDA has also approved a concentrated formulation of rapid-acting insulinlispro, U-200 (200 units/mL). These concentrated preparations may be more convenient and comfortable for patients to inject and may improve adherence in those with insulin resistance who require large doses of insulin. While U-500 regular insulin is available in both prefilled pens and vials (a dedicated syringe was FDA approved in July 2016), other concentrated insulins are available only in prefilled pens to minimize the risk of dosing errors.

INHALED INSULIN

Inhaled insulin is available for prandial use with a limited dosing range; studies in people with type 1 diabetes suggest rapid pharmacokinetics.[44] A pilot study found evidence that compared with injectable rapid-acting insulin, supplemental doses of inhaled insulin taken based on post-prandial glucose levels may improve blood glucose management without additional hypoglycemia or weight gain, although results from a larger study are needed for confirmation.[45]

Table 4.3—Median Cost of Insulin Products in the U.S. Calculated as AWP (44) and NADAC (45) per 1,000 Units of Specified

Insulins	Compounds	Dosage form/product	Median AWP (min, max)*	Median NADAC (min, max)*
Rapid-acting analogs	• Lispro biosimilar	U-100 vial	$280	$226
		U-100 prefilled pen	$361	$289
	• Glulisine	U-100 vial	$324	$260
		U-100 prefilled pen	$417	$334
	• Lispro	U-100 vial	$330	$264
		U-100 3 mL cartridges	$408	$326
		U-100 prefilled pen; U-200 prefilled pen	$424	$340
	• Aspart	U-100 vial	$347	$278
		U-100 3 mL cartridges	$430	$343
		U-100 prefilled pen	$447	$358
	• Inhaled insulin	Inhalation cartridges	$993	$606
Short-acting	• Human Regular	U-100 vial	$165 ($165, $178)	$135 ($135, $146)
Intermediate-acting	• Human NPH	U-100 vial	$165 ($165, $178)	$135 ($135, $144)
		U-100 prefilled pen	$377	$304
Concentrated Human Regular insulin	• U-500 Human Regular insulin	U-500 vial	$178	$142
		U-500 prefilled pen	$230	$184
Basal analogs	• Glargine biosimilar	U-100 prefilled pen	$261	$209
	• Glargine	U-100 vial; U-100 prefilled pen	$323	$259
		U-300 prefilled pen	$331	$266
	• Detemir	U-100 vial; U-100 prefilled pen	$353	$281
	• Degludec	U-100 prefilled pen; U-200 prefilled pen	$388	$310

(continued)

Table 4.3 (continued)

Insulins	Compounds	Dosage form/product	Median AWP (min, max)*	Median NADAC (min, max)*
Premixed insulin products	• NPH/Regular 70/30	U-100 vial	$165 ($165, $178)	$135 ($135, $144)
		U-100 prefilled pen	$377	$306
	• Lispro 50/50	U-100 vial	$342	$274
		U-100 prefilled pen	$424	$340
	• Lispro 75/25	U-100 vial	$342	$273
		U-100 prefilled pen	$424	$340
	• Aspart 70/30	U-100 vial	$360	$288
		U-100 prefilled pen	$447	$358
Premixed insulin/GLP-1 Receptor Agonist products	• Degludec/Liraglutide	100/3.6 prefilled pen	$793	$638
	• Glargine/Lixisenatide	100/33 prefilled pen	$537	$431

AWP, average wholesale price; GLP-1, glucagon-like peptide 1; NADAC, National Average Drug Acquisition Cost. *AWP or NADAC calculated as in Table 4.2; median listed alone when only one product and/or price.

Inhaled insulin is contraindicated in patients with chronic lung disease, such as asthma and chronic obstructive pulmonary disease, and is not recommended in patients who smoke or who recently stopped smoking. All patients require spirometry (FEV_1) testing to identify potential lung disease prior to and after starting inhaled insulin therapy.

COMBINATION INJECTABLE THERAPY

If basal insulin has been titrated to an acceptable fasting blood glucose level (or if the dose is >0.5 units/kg/day) and A1C remains above target, consider advancing to combination injectable therapy (Fig. 9.2). This approach can use a GLP-1 receptor agonist added to basal insulin or multiple doses of insulin. The combination of basal insulin and GLP-1 receptor agonist has potent glucose-lowering actions and less weight gain and hypoglycemia compared with intensified insulin regimens.[46-48] Two different once-daily fixed-dual combination products containing basal insulin plus a GLP-1 receptor agonist are available: insulin glargine plus lixisenatide and insulin degludec plus liraglutide.

Intensification of insulin treatment can be done by adding doses of prandial to basal insulin. Starting with a single prandial dose with the largest meal of the day is simple and effective, and it can be advanced to a regimen with multiple prandial doses if necessary.[49] Alternatively, in a patient on basal insulin in whom additional prandial coverage is desired, the regimen can be converted to two or three doses of a premixed insulin. Each approach has advantages and disadvantages. For example, basal/prandial regimens offer greater flexibility for patients who eat on irregular schedules. On the other hand, two doses of premixed insulin is a simple, convenient means of spreading insulin across the day. Moreover, human insulins, separately or as premixed NPH/Regular (70/30) formulations, are less costly alternatives to insulin analogs. Figure 9.2 outlines these options, as well as recommendations for further intensification, if needed, to achieve glycemic goals. When initiating combination injectable therapy, metformin therapy should be maintained while sulfonylureas and DPP-4 inhibitors are typically discontinued. In patients with suboptimal blood glucose control, especially those requiring large insulin doses, adjunctive use of a thiazolidinedione or an SGLT2 inhibitor may help to improve control and reduce the amount of insulin needed, though potential side effects should be considered. Once a basal/bolus insulin regimen is initiated, dose titration is important, with adjustments made in both mealtime and basal insulins based on the blood glucose levels and an understanding of the pharmacodynamic profile of each formulation (pattern control). As people with type 2 diabetes get older, it may become necessary to simplify complex insulin regimens because of a decline in self-management ability (see Section 12 "Older Adults").

REFERENCES

1. Davies MJ, D'Alessio DA, Fradkin J, et al. Management of hyperglycemia in type 2 diabetes, 2018. A consensus report by the American Diabetes Association (ADA) and the European Association for the Study of Diabetes (EASD). *Diabetes Care* 2018;41:2669–2701

2. Holman RR, Paul SK, Bethel MA, Matthews DR, Neil HAW. 10-year follow-up of intensive glucose control in type 2 diabetes. *N Engl J Med* 2008;359:1577–1589

3. Maruthur NM, Tseng E, Hutfless S, et al. Diabetes medications as monotherapy or metformin-based combination therapy for type 2 diabetes: a systematic review and meta-analysis. *Ann Intern Med* 2016;164:740–751

4. U.S. Food and Drug Administration. FDA Drug Safety Communication: FDA revises warnings regarding use of the diabetes medicine metformin in certain patients with reduced kidney function [Internet]. Available from http://www.fda.gov/Drugs/DrugSafety/ucm493244.htm. Accessed 14 October 2016

5. Out M, Kooy A, Lehert P, Schalkwijk CA, Stehouwer CDA. Long-term treatment with metformin in type 2 diabetes and methylmalonic acid: post hoc analysis of a randomized controlled 4.3 year trial. *J Diabetes Complications* 2018;32:171–178

6. Aroda VR, Edelstein SL, Goldberg RB, et al.; Diabetes Prevention Program Research Group. Long-term metformin use and vitamin B12 deficiency in the Diabetes Prevention Program Outcomes Study. *J Clin Endocrinol Metab* 2016;101:1754–1761

7. Henry RR, Murray AV, Marmolejo MH, Hennicken D, Ptaszynska A, List JF. Dapagliflozin, metformin XR, or both: initial pharmacotherapy for type 2 diabetes, a randomised controlled trial. *Int J Clin Pract* 2012;66:446–456

8. Bennett WL, Maruthur NM, Singh S, et al. Comparative effectiveness and safety of medications for type 2 diabetes: an update including new drugs and 2-drug combinations. *Ann Intern Med* 2011;154:602–613

9. Vijan S, Sussman JB, Yudkin JS, Hayward RA. Effect of patients' risks and preferences on health gains with plasma glucose level lowering in type 2 diabetes mellitus. *JAMA Intern Med* 2014;174:1227–1234

10. Singh S, Wright EE Jr, Kwan AYM, et al. Glucagon-like peptide-1 receptor agonists compared with basal insulins for the treatment of type 2 diabetes mellitus: a systematic review and meta-analysis. *Diabetes Obes Metab* 2017;19:228–238

11. Levin PA, Nguyen H, Wittbrodt ET, Kim SC. Glucagon-like peptide-1 receptor agonists: a systematic review of comparative effectiveness research. *Diabetes Metab Syndr Obes* 2017;10:123–139

12. Abd El Aziz MS, Kahle M, Meier JJ, Nauck MA. A meta-analysis comparing clinical effects of short- or long-acting GLP-1 receptor agonists versus insulin treatment from head-to-head studies in type 2 diabetic patients. *Diabetes Obes Metab* 2017;19:216–227

13. Institute for Clinical and Economic Review. Controversies in the management of patients with type 2 diabetes [Internet], December 2014. Available from https://icer-review.org/wp-content/uploads/2015/03/CEPAC-T2D-Final-Report-December-22.pdf. Accessed 9 November 2018

14. Truven Health Analytics. Micromedex 2.0 Introduction to RED BOOK Online [Internet], 2018. Available from http://www.micromedexsolutions.com/micromedex2/4.34.0/WebHelp/RED_BOOK/Introduction_to_REDB_BOOK_Online.htm. Accessed 5 September 2018

15. Centers for Medicare & Medicaid Services. NADAC (national average drug acquisition cost), drug pricing and payment [Internet], 2018. Available from https://data.medicaid.gov/Drug-Pricing-and-Payment/NADAC-National-Average-Drug-Acquisition-Cost-/a4y5-998d.Accessed5 September 2018

16. Zinman B, Wanner C, Lachin JM, et al.; EMPA-REG OUTCOME Investigators. Empagliflozin, cardiovascular outcomes, and mortality in type 2 diabetes. *N Engl J Med* 2015;373:2117–2128

17. Neal B, Perkovic V, Mahaffey KW, et al.; CANVAS Program Collaborative Group. Canagliflozin and cardiovascular and renal events in type 2 diabetes. *N Engl J Med* 2017;377:644–657

18. Marso SP, Daniels GH, Brown-Frandsen K, et al.; LEADER Steering Committee; LEADER Trial Investigators. Liraglutide and cardiovascular outcomes in type 2 diabetes. *N Engl J Med* 2016;375:311–322

19. Marso SP, Bain SC, Consoli A, et al.; SUSTAIN-6 Investigators. Semaglutide and cardiovascular out comes in patients with type 2 diabetes. *N Engl J Med* 2016;375:1834–1844

20. Blonde L, Merilainen M, Karwe V, Raskin P; TITRATE Study Group. Patient-directed titration for achieving glycaemic goals using a once-daily basal insulin analogue: an assessment of two different fasting plasma glucose targets – the TITRATE study. *Diabetes Obes Metab* 2009;11:623–631

21. Porcellati F, Lucidi P, Cioli P, et al. Pharmacokinetics and pharmacodynamics of insulin glargine given in the evening as compared with in the morning in type 2 diabetes. *Diabetes Care* 2015;38:503–512

22. Wang Z, Hedrington MS, Gogitidze Joy N, et al. Dose-response effects of insulin glargine in type 2 diabetes. *Diabetes Care* 2010;33:1555–1560

23. Singh SR, Ahmad F, Lal A, Yu C, Bai Z, Bennett H. Efficacy and safety of insulin analogues for the management of diabetes mellitus: a meta-analysis. *CMAJ* 2009;180:385–397

24. Horvath K, Jeitler K, Berghold A, et al. Long-acting insulin analogues versus NPH insulin (human isophane insulin) for type 2 diabetes mellitus. *Cochrane Database Syst Rev* 2007;2:CD005613

25. Monami M, Marchionni N, Mannucci E. Long-acting insulin an alogues versus NPH human insulin in type 2 diabetes: a meta-analysis. *Diabetes Res Clin Pract* 2008;81:184–189

26. Owens DR, Traylor L, Mullins P, Landgraf W. Patient-level meta-analysis of efficacy and hypoglycaemia in people with type 2 diabetes initiating insulin glargine 100 U/mL or neutral protamine Hagedorn insulin analysed according to concomitant oral antidiabetes therapy. *Diabetes Res Clin Pract* 2017;124(Suppl. C):57–65

27. Riddle MC, Rosenstock J, Gerich J; Insulin Glargine 4002 Study Investigators. The treat-totarget trial: randomized addition of glargine or human NPH insulin to oral therapy of type 2 diabetic patients. *Diabetes Care* 2003;26:3080–3086

28. Hermansen K, Davies M, Derezinski T, Martinez Ravn G, Clauson P, Home P. A 26-week, randomized, parallel, treat-to-target trial comparing insulin detemir with NPH insulin as add-on therapy to oral glucose-lowering drugs in insulin-naive people with type 2 diabetes. *Diabetes Care* 2006;29:1269–1274

29. Yki-Järvinen H, Kauppinen-Mäkelin R, Tiikkainen M, et al. Insulin glargine or NPH combined with metformin in type 2 diabetes: the LANMET study. *Diabetologia* 2006;49:442–451

30. Bolli GB, Riddle MC, Bergenstal RM, et al.; EDITION 3 study investigators. New insulin glargine 300 U/ml compared with glargine 100 U/ml in insulin-naïve people with type 2 diabetes on oral glucose-lowering drugs: a randomized controlled trial (EDITION 3). *Diabetes Obes Metab* 2015;17:386–394

31. Terauchi Y, Koyama M, Cheng X, et al. New insulin glargine 300 U/ml versus glargine 100 U/ml in Japanese people with type 2 diabetes using

basal insulin and oral antihyperglycaemic drugs: glucose control and hypo-glycaemia in a randomized controlled trial (EDITION JP 2). *Diabetes Obes Metab* 2016;18:366–374

32. Yki-Järvinen H, Bergenstal RM, Bolli GB, et al. Glycaemic control and hypoglycaemia with new insulin glargine 300 U/ml versus insulin glargine 100 U/ml in people with type 2 diabetes using basal insulin and oral antihy-perglycaemic drugs: the EDITION 2 randomized 12-month trial including 6-month extension. *Diabetes Obes Metab* 2015;17:1142–1149

33. Marso SP, McGuire DK, Zinman B, et al.; DEVOTE Study Group. Efficacy and safety of degludec versus glargine in type 2 diabetes. *N Engl J Med* 2017;377:723–732

34. Rodbard HW, Cariou B, Zinman B, et al.; BEGIN Once Long trial investi-gators. Comparison of insulin degludec with insulin glargine in insulin-naive subjects with type 2 diabetes: a 2-year randomized, treat-to-target trial. *Diabet Med* 2013;30:1298–1304

35. Wysham C, Bhargava A, Chaykin L, et al. Effect of insulin degludec vs insu-lin glargine U100 on hypoglycemia in patients with type 2 diabetes: the SWITCH 2 randomized clinical trial. *JAMA* 2017;318:45–56

36. Zinman B, Philis-Tsimikas A, Cariou B, et al.; NN1250-3579 (BEGIN Once Long) Trial Investigators. Insulin degludec versus insulin glargine in insulin-naive patients with type 2 diabetes: a 1-year, randomized, treat-to-target trial (BEGIN Once Long). *Diabetes Care* 2012;35:2464–2471

37. Lipska KJ, Parker MM, Moffet HH, Huang ES, Karter AJ. Association of initiation of basal insulin analogs vs neutral protamine Hagedorn insulin with hypoglycemia-related emergency department visits or hospital admis-sions and with glycemic control in patients with type 2 diabetes. *JAMA* 2018;320:53–62

38. Cefalu WT, Dawes DE, Gavlak G, et al.; Insulin Access and Affordability Working Group. Insulin Access and Affordability Working Group: conclu-sions and recommendations. *Diabetes Care* 2018;41:1299–1311

39. Lipska KJ, Hirsch IB, Riddle MC. Human insulin for type 2 diabetes: an effective, less-expensive option. *JAMA* 2017;318:23–24

40. Mannucci E, Monami M, Marchionni N. Short-acting insulin analogues vs. regular human insulin in type 2 diabetes: a meta-analysis. *Diabetes Obes Metab* 2009;11:53–59

41. Heller S, Bode B, Kozlovski P, Svendsen AL. Meta-analysis of insulin aspart versus regular human insulin used in a basal-bolus regimen for the treat-ment of diabetes mellitus. *J Diabetes* 2013;5:482–491

42. Riddle MC, Yki-Järvinen H, Bolli GB, et al. One-year sustained glycaemic control and less hypoglycaemia with new insulin glargine 300 U/ml com-pared with 100 U/ml in people with type 2 diabetes using basal plus meal-time insulin: the EDITION 1 12-month randomized trial, including 6-month extension. *Diabetes Obes Metab* 2015;17:835–842

43. Yki-Järvinen H, Bergenstal R, Ziemen M, et al.; EDITION 2 Study Investigators. New insulin glargine 300 units/mL versus glargine 100 units/mL in people with type 2 diabetes using oral agents and basal insulin: glucose control and hypoglycemia in a 6-month randomized controlled trial (EDITION 2). *Diabetes Care* 2014;37:3235–3243

44. Bode BW, McGill JB, Lorber DL, Gross JL, Chang PC, Bregman DB; Affinity 1 Study Group. Inhaled technosphere insulin compared with injected prandial insulin in type 1 diabetes: a randomized 24-week trial. *Diabetes Care* 2015;38:2266–2273

45. Akturk HK, Snell-Bergeon JK, Rewers A, et al. Improved postprandial glucose with inhaled technosphere insulin compared with insulin aspart in patients with type 1 diabetes on multiple daily injections: the STAT study. *Diabetes Technol Ther* 2018;20:639–647

46. Diamant M, Nauck MA, Shaginian R, et al.; 4B Study Group. Glucagon-like peptide 1 receptor agonist or bolus insulin with optimized basal insulin in type 2 diabetes. *Diabetes Care* 2014;37:2763–2773

47. Eng C, Kramer CK, Zinman B, Retnakaran R. Glucagon-like peptide-1 receptor agonist and basal insulin combination treatment for the management of type 2 diabetes: a systematic review and meta-analysis. *Lancet* 2014;384:2228–2234

48. Maiorino MI, Chiodini P, Bellastella G, Capuano A, Esposito K, Giugliano D. Insulin and glucagon-like peptide 1 receptor agonist combination therapy in type 2 diabetes: a systematic review and meta-analysis of randomized controlled trials. *Diabetes Care* 2017;40:614–624

49. Rodbard HW, Visco VE, Andersen H, Hiort LC, Shu DHW. Treatment intensification with step-wise addition of prandial insulin aspart boluses compared with full basal-bolus therapy (FullSTEP Study): a randomised, treat-to-target clinical trial. *Lancet Diabetes Endocrinol* 2014;2:30–37

Chapter 5
Overview of Medications Used to Treat Type 2 Diabetes

JOHN R. WHITE, JR., PA-C, PHARMD

INTRODUCTION

The options available to clinicians in the U.S. for the management of hyperglycemia secondary to T2D have changed dramatically in the past three decades. Currently there are a dozen categories of medications that may be used in the management of diabetes. These include insulins, sulfonylureas, thiazolidinediones (TZDs), glinides, biguanides, amylin derivatives, gliptins (DPP-4 inhibitors), α-glucosidase inhibitors, bile-acid sequestrants, GLP-1 receptor agonists (GLP-1 RAs), dopamine-2 agonists, and SGLT2 inhibitors.[1] The dopamine-2 agonists, amylin derivatives, and bile acid sequestrants will not be mentioned in this chapter, as they are rarely used for the management of hyperglycemia in T2D but are covered in later individual chapters. The glinides and the α-glucosidase inhibitors are mentioned in this chapter but are not widely used. Overall, this chapter will provide a brief introduction to the medications used in the management of T2D.

CHOICE OF MEDICATION

The efficacy associated with single-drug therapy and with various permutations of multiple drug combinations continues to be evaluated as newer agents are released. The selection of the best medication or combination of medications for the management of hyperglycemia in patients with T2D, while based in science, remains to a large degree in the realm of "art." Although in some situations the choice of medication is relatively simple, in the majority of situations the decision-making process is complex and does not necessarily lead to a clear-cut choice. Algorithms can sometimes provide an overall framework through which decisions can be made, but they often ignore pertinent patient-specific characteristics and are not powerful enough to provide specific recommendations for the best medications in the multitude of complex situations often encountered in clinical practice. However, the new approach proffered by the American Diabetes Association and the European Association for the Study of Diabetes (EASD) provides us with a circumspect perspective and a solid roadmap to the management of hyperglycemia in patients with T2D. This new approach includes consideration of the major factors that are pertinent to choice of medication.[1]

Several factors should be considered when choosing a medication, including degree of glycemic lowering needed to get the patient into target goal ranges, renal effects, cardiovascular effects, ease of compliance, effect of the medication on weight and lipids, contraindications, side effects, cost and patient insurance coverage, and the need for dose adjustment with renal and/or hepatic impairment. This chapter will provide a cursory and abbreviated review of the use of the above-mentioned categories of medications. More detailed information regarding specific medications is provided in subsequent chapters and linked monographs.

Using the American Diabetes Association/EASD schema, patients presenting with T2D should first be treated with metformin and comprehensive lifestyle interventions (Figure 5.1). If metformin monotherapy has been instituted and the patient's glycemic indices are not appropriately controlled, the patient should next be categorized as: *1)* having established atherosclerotic cardiovascular disease (ASCVD) or chronic kidney disease (CKD), or *2)* not having established ASCVD or CKD. In patients with predominately ASCVD, either a GLP-1 RA or an SGLT2i that has been shown to provide cardiovascular disease (CVD) benefit should be used. In patients with predominately CKD or HF, an SGLT2i with evidence of the ability to reduce CKD or HF (empagliflozin or canagliflozin) should be used (unless contraindicated). In patients without established ASCVD or CKD, either a DPP-4 inhibitor, GLP-1 RA, SGLT2 inhibitor, TZD, or sulfonylurea should be used. The decision regarding specific agent should be made with consideration to level of hyperglycemia, need for weight loss, cost, and other issues. Additional antihyperglycemic medications may be added as needed to achieve the appropriate level of glycemic control. If the patient's initial A1C is >10% and/or is 2 percentage points above target, the consensus statement recommends considering injectable combination therapy (basal insulin plus GLP-1 RA). Also, in patients who are not at their A1C target despite dual or triple therapy, insulin and/or GLP-1 RA should be considered. The considerations involved in this decision are articulated in Figure 5.2.[1]

The number of medications available for the management of hyperglycemia has grown consistently since the first use of exogenous insulin in the 1920s. However, the rate of growth of the introduction of new medications and new categories of medications has burgeoned over the past 30 years (Figure 5.3).

ORAL THERAPY

BIGUANIDES

The biguanide metformin (Glucophage) was first introduced in 1959 as an antihyperglycemic agent for use in patients with T2D but was not approved for use in the U.S. until the 1990s.

Metformin is the usual first choice in the management of hyperglycemia in patients with T2D if it is not contraindicated, is tolerated, and if the patient does not have a presenting initial A1C of >10%.[1]

The physiologic effects of this compound on carbohydrate metabolism and disposition occur primarily in the liver via inhibition of hepatic glucose production.[2] Additionally, it may also cause a reduction in the intestinal absorption of glucose.[3] At a molecular level, metformin probably elicits its glycemic effects by activation of AMP kinase although other mechanisms may be in play as well.[1]

Figure 5.1—Glucose-lowering medication in type 2 diabetes: overall approach. Reprinted with permission from Davies.[1]

While it is difficult to assign an expected drop in A1C with any medications because of the myriad confounding factors, generally metformin therapy can be expected to cause about a 1–1.5 percentage point reduction in A1C.[4,5]

Metformin does not typically cause hypoglycemia when used as monotherapy and may be associated with weigh loss.[2] In a medication review carried out by the Agency for Healthcare Research and Quality (AHRQ), metformin was superior to TZDs and sulfonylureas in terms of effect on weight (mean 2.6 kg).[6] It is potentially beneficial in ASCVD and is neutral in its impact on congestive heart failure (CHF).[1] Additionally, metformin was associated with a reduction in LDL compared to pioglitazone, sulfonylureas, and DPP-4 inhibitors.[6]

Conversely, metformin is also associated with gastrointestinal side effects. Patients treated with metformin may experience a 30% higher incidence of abdominal bloating, nausea, cramping, feeling of fullness, and diarrhea.[5] These side effects can be a particular problem during the initiation phases of therapy. However, these side effects are usually self-limiting and transient and can be mitigated by starting with a low dose, titrating up slowly, and taking the medication with food.

Less common side effects include a reduction in cyanocobalamin levels (vitamin B_{12}) and a metallic taste in the mouth. Periodic testing of B_{12} should be con-

DECISION CYCLE FOR PATIENT-CENTERED GLYCEMIC MANAGEMENT IN TYPE 2 DIABETES

Figure 5.2—Decision cycle for patient-centered glycemic management in type 2 diabetes. Reprinted with permission from Davies.[1]

sidered in patients treated with metformin, particularly those with peripheral neuropathy or anemia.[1] Lactic acidosis can occur with the administration of metformin, but it is extremely rare (0.03 cases per 1,000 patient-years) and has occurred primarily in patients with significant renal dysfunction.[5]

Metformin is contraindicated in patients with an estimated glomerular filtration rate (eGFR) of ≤ 30 mL/min/1.73 m^2. Metformin should not be initiated in patients with an eGFR of 30–45 mL/min/1.73 m^2 and its use should be evaluated in any patient with these renal parameters who is already being treated with the drug. Other warnings and contraindications are detailed in chapter 6.

Metformin is available generically and is relatively inexpensive.

SULFONYLUREAS

Sulfonylureas have been widely used in the management of T2D since their introduction in the late 1950s. In the past, it was estimated that 40% of all T2D patients were treated with sulfonylureas. However, since the introduction of newer antihyperglycemic medications, the fraction of patients with T2D treated with sulfonylureas has probably dropped.

Sulfonylureas exhibit both pancreatic and extrapancreatic effects and are clinically useful only in patients with viable β-cells. The primary effect of sulfonylureas is due to direct stimulation of insulin release.[7] In-vivo studies of sulfonylureas show that they sensitize β-cells to glucose, increasing insulin secretion indirectly.

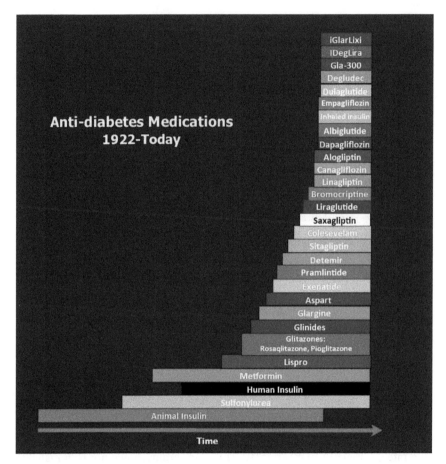

Figure 5.3—Adapted by Dawn Scartozzi from a figure created by Dr. Sam Dagogo-Jack. Reprinted with permission.

Therefore, under the influence of sulfonylureas, more insulin is secreted at all glucose levels than would be expected in the absence of sulfonylureas. Sulfonylureas may also affect glucose metabolism via several extrapancreatic mechanisms, such as increasing insulin's effect by a postreceptor action, decreasing hepatic insulin extraction, and increasing insulin receptor number and receptor binding affinity; however, the relative clinical relevance of each of these mechanisms of action is still subject to research and debate.

In terms of glycemic lowering, sulfonylureas can be expected to reduce A1C values between 1 and 2%.[5]

The sulfonylureas have also been associated with weight gain. Lastly, sulfonylureas are true hypoglycemic agents and can cause significant hypoglycemia. There remains a question regarding cardiovascular risk/outcomes with the use of sulfonylureas. This is well outlined in chapter 8. Generally speaking, validated randomized controlled trials do not demonstrate added cardiovascular risk, but meta-analyses suggest added risk. However, their long track record of relative safety, efficacy in reducing hypoglycemia, and very low cost probably make them a reasonable choice early on in the treatment of some patients with T2D. While there is not a clear drug of choice in this category, the two that are generally preferred are glipizide and glimepiride.

GLINIDES

Repaglinide and nateglinide are nonsulfonylurea insulinotropic agents whose biochemical mechanism of action—closure of ATP-sensitive potassium channels in β-cells—is similar to that of sulfonylureas. Closure of ATP-sensitive potassium channels causes an influx of calcium by way of voltage-dependent calcium channels. Insulin release is stimulated after intercellular calcium concentrations reach a threshold.[8] Therefore, similar to sulfonylureas, the glinides reduce blood glucose levels by stimulating insulin release from the pancreas.

The glycemic lowering afforded by the glinides is generally less than that of the sulfonylureas. Typically, A1C lowering of about 1–1.5% can be expected in a secretagogue-naïve patient.[5] These agents do not work in patients who do not respond to sulfonylureas. The glinides are associated with a lower incidence of hypoglycemia than are sulfonylureas. The major disadvantages of the glinides are the need for multiple daily doses and less A1C-lowering capacity than the sulfonylureas. More information about these agents can be found in chapter 9.

α-GLUCOSIDASE INHIBITORS (AGIs)

Two drugs in the α-glucosidase inhibitor category have been approved for use in the U.S.: acarbose and miglitol. These drugs exhibit mild antihyperglycemic activity. They may be used as monotherapy in newly onset T2D if the hyperglycemia is low grade and metformin was contraindicated—although other agents would likely be preferable. They may also be useful in combination with other antihyperglycemic medications.

The primary mechanism of action of α-glucosidase inhibitors is competitive inhibition of the α-glucosidase enzymes in the brush border of the small intestine.[9] Inhibition of these enzyme systems effectively reduces the rate of absorption of carbohydrates without altering the absolute absorption. The result is reduced PPG levels. There is also a modest effect on fasting glucose.

The most common side effects of the α-glucosidase inhibitors are dose-related gastrointestinal complaints, abdominal pain, flatulence, and diarrhea.[10] In many cases these side effects may be mitigated with continued administration of the drug and with slow stepwise titration.

Elevated hepatic enzymes have been reported at higher doses of acarbose (200 and 300 mg t.i.d.); however, the occurrence of hepatic dysfunction with doses of ≤100 mg t.i.d. is rare.[11] In fact, elevated serum transaminase levels are no more frequent than those observed with placebo when doses of ≤100mg t.i.d. were used.

Contraindications for the use of α-glucosidase inhibitors primarily revolve around gastrointestinal side effects. Acarbose should be avoided in patients with inflammatory bowel disease, colonic ulceration, or obstructive bowel disorders.[7] Relative contraindications include medical conditions that might deteriorate with increased intestinal gas formation and chronic intestinal disorders of digestion or absorption.

Both AGIs should be avoided in patients with significant renal dysfunction: Acarbose, avoid if eGFR <30 mL/min/1.73 m²; miglitol, avoid if eGFR <25 mL/min/1.73 m².[1]

Typically an A1C reduction of about 0.5–1% can be expected with AGIs.[10] However, they must be dosed three times daily and are sometimes avoided due to their gastrointestinal side effects.

More information about these agents can be found in chapter 11.

THIAZOLIDINEDIONES

Currently two TZDs are available for use in the U.S.: pioglitazone and rosiglitazone. These medications appear to work by affecting insulin action without affecting insulin secretion. They are sometimes referred to as insulin sensitizers. Although several mechanisms of action may contribute to their antihyperglycemic properties, it is known that these compounds stimulate receptors on the nuclear surface, PPAR-γ (peroxisome-proliferator-activated receptor γ). Therefore, the TZDs are also referred to as PPAR activators. Stimulation of PPAR-γ leads to increased glucose uptake by upregulation of the genes responsible for the production of GLUT1 and GLUT2.

Several studies have suggested a link between the use of TZDs and reduced bone density and fractures. Because of this, TZDs should be avoided in patients who are at risk for fracture. TZDs have also been associated with mild to moderate weight gain (1–5 kg) in some patients. Initially, this weight gain was thought to be due primarily to edema but has since been shown to be nonedema weight gain.

Rosiglitazone and pioglitazone have different effects on lipid profiles. This difference may be related to relative effect of these agents on the nuclear receptor. Pioglitazone has a higher affinity for PPAR-α and is associated with mild improvements in lipid profiles (reduction of TG and increases in HDL). Both agents may cause an increase in LDL. Indirect comparisons of pioglitazone and rosiglitazone suggest that rosiglitazone probably causes more LDL elevation than pioglitazone.[5]

Both agents can cause edema. This may in turn increase the incidence of exacerbations of CHF in patients who have underlying disease. This effect seems to be more pronounced in patients who are also treated with insulin. Edema, if it occurs, can sometimes be mitigated through the use of diuretics. However, TZDs are contraindicated in patients with New York Heart Association (NYHA) class III or IV failure.

The published conclusions regarding the impact of TZDs on overall cardiovascular mortality are conflicting. A handful of contradictory manuscripts and a plethora of opposing opinions and editorials on this subject have been published. While it is clear that untreated hyperglycemia is a major risk factor for cardiovascular mortality, it is not clear that treating hyperglycemia in patients with TZDs results in significantly more cardiovascular mortality than is encountered in patients treated with other modalities.

A1C lowering can be expected somewhere between 0.5 and 1.5% in most patients. Significant differences between the two available agents, in terms of glycemic lowering, are not obvious. However the TZDs are less effective than insulin and slightly less effective than metformin or sulfonylureas. In most cases, the latter agents should probably be used initially.

More information about these agents can be found in chapter 7.

DPP-4 INHIBITORS

GLP-1 and glucose-dependent insulinotropic polypeptide (GIP) hormone, under normal physiologic conditions, have very short half-lives and short durations of action. These small half-lives are due to degradation of GLP by a dipeptidyl peptidase-4 (DPP-4).[12] Pharmacologic inhibition of this system results in prolonged activity of the incretin hormones, which in turn are associated with enhanced insulin secretion and a reduction in glucagon secretion. Currently, four DPP-4 inhibitors are available in the U.S.: sitagliptin, saxagliptin, alogliptin, and linagliptin.

The four DPP-4 inhibitors differ in terms or pharmacokinetics and drug interactions. For example, linagliptin does not require dosage adjustment with renal dysfunction while the others three agents in this class do.[13] There are other nuances among the four agents with regard to drug interactions. These differences are reviewed in chapter 12.

Therapeutic use of DPP-4 inhibitors generally results in a modest A1C reduction. A reduction in A1C of about 0.4–0.9% can be expected in most cases.[13] These medications, however, do tend to be weight neutral, are taken once daily, and are generally well tolerated. Cardiovascular outcome trials (CVOT) have to date demonstrated no particular cardiovascular benefit, and there has been some concern that DPP-4 inhibitors may be linked to a slight increase in HF.[14,15,16] Considering their high cost and mild glucose-lowering effect, DPP-4 inhibitors are probably considered by most to be a third- or fourth-line agent.

More information about these agents can be found in chapter 12.

SGLT2 INHIBITORS

Currently, there are four SGLT2 inhibitors on the market in the U.S. (canagliflozin, dapagliflozin, empagliflozin, and ertugliflozin) and others are in development. These compounds are analogs to the natural compound phlorizin, which is found in the bark of apple trees.[17] The first SGLT2 inhibitor (canagliflozin) was approved for use in the U.S. in 2013.[18]

The mechanism of action of the SGLT2 inhibitors is through inhibition of the transporter SGLT2, which in turn results in an increase in urine glucose excretion (UGE). These medications essentially lower the renal threshold for glucose excretion. The SGLT2 inhibitors prevent the reabsorption of between 30 and 50% of filtered glucose. The result of this inhibition is renal loss of glucose and a concomitant reduction in blood glucose. It should be noted that a mixed SGLT1 and SGLT2 inhibitor, sotagliflozin, is currently under development. This medication will modulate glucose transport in both the gastrointestinal tract and kidneys.[19]

The SGLT2 inhibitors are generally associated with an A1C reduction (difference from placebo) of approximately 0.8% when used as monotherapy and

0.6% when used as add-on therapy.[20] Individual response will vary, of course, depending on the agent used and patient characteristics.

The SGLT2 inhibitors have grown in popularity for several reasons. They are associated with weight loss, and may have positive cardiovascular and renal effects. Additionally, they are in and of themselves associated with low rates of hypoglycemia. The SGLT2 inhibitors have been consistently associated with weight loss. The level of weight loss varies but may in some cases be as high as 4.7 kg.[21] Although the magnitude of weight loss varies depending on conditions of the study and population evaluated, a positive effect on weight (i.e., loss) has been consistently observed. One of the more exciting and salient findings with the SGLT2 inhibitors has been the correlation between their use (canagliflozin and empagliflozin) and positive cardiovascular outcomes. SGLT2 inhibition has shown promise in several studies evaluating the impact of these agents on renal disease. The cardiovascular and renal findings are detailed in chapter 10.

The SGLT2 inhibitors are associated with the potential for acute kidney injury (probably secondary to volume depletion) and an increase in urogenital infections; they are relatively expensive.

The use of or the need for dose adjustment with these agents in cases of renal or hepatic impairment varies from agent to agent.

Generally speaking, these agents have been widely accepted and used. They offer a unique mechanism of action, are effective in lowering glycemic indices, have low rates of hypoglycemia, and may have positive cardiovascular and renal effects.

More information about these agents can be found in chapter 10.

INJECTABLES

GLP-1 AGONISTS

GLP-1 7–37, is a naturally occurring peptide that stimulates insulin secretion. It, along with GIP, is secreted under the influence of glucose in the L-cells of the small intestine.[22] These compounds both have very short half-lives, rendering them ineffective, or at least not practical, as pharmacologic agents. A compound isolated from the Gila monster, exendin-4, was found to have homology with the human GLP-1 sequence but with a longer circulating half-life. This finding circumvented the issue of short half-life encountered with native GLP-1 and led to the development of the first pharmacologically viable GLP-1 receptor agonist (GLP-1 RA), exenatide (Byetta), a synthetic version of exendin-4. It was approved for use in the U.S. in 2005. Since that time, multiple other GLP-1 RAs have been approved: liraglutide (Victoza, approved 2010), exenatide XR (Bydureon, approved 2012; BCise pen, approved 2017), albiglutide (Tanzeum, approved 2014), dulaglutide (Trulicity, approved 2014), lixisenatide (Adlyxin, approved 2016), and semaglutide (Ozempic, approved 2017). Albiglutide was discontinued in 2017.

The mechanism of action of the GLP-1 RAs is complex and multifaceted. First, they stimulate insulin secretion from functional β-cells. Second, they suppress glucagon secretion and slow gastric motility. They also have a central effect on satiety and are associated with reduced food intake and weight loss.[22]

GLP-1 RAs are associated with significant reductions in A1C. Placebo-subtracted changes from baseline generally range from 0.5–2%, depending on the particular medication and the population being evaluated.[13] Additionally, GLP-1 RAs are associated with weight loss that has been reported to be as high as 6.5 kg (mean).[23] However, across other studies, weight loss ranged from 0.3–4.7 kg (mean).[13] In fact, these agents are now being used for weight loss in individuals without diabetes. GLP-1 RAs are associated with very low rates of hypoglycemia. This is due primarily to their glucose-lowering actions being linked to ambient glucose concentrations.[24] Two of these agents (liraglutide and semaglutide) have demonstrated cardiovascular benefits. Additionally, liraglutide has been shown to be beneficial in terms of slowing the progression of chronic kidney disease.[1]

GLP-1 RAs are associated with a relatively high frequency of gastrointestinal side effects. These gastrointestinal events are generally mild to moderate in intensity, transient, self-limiting, and do not usually result in the need for discontinuation of the medication.[24] Early in the evolution of GLP-1 RAs, there was concern about a potential correlation with these medications and acute pancreatitis. However, retrospective observational evaluations have concluded that there is essentially no increase in the incidence of pancreatitis with these agents.[25] No prospective trials have conclusively addressed the potential correlation between this category of medication and pancreatitis; it is recommended that they be used cautiously in patients with a history of pancreatitis, and be discontinued in those who develop it. These agents also carry a black box warning for risk of thyroid C-cell tumors. This concern arose from rodent studies, and no cases of tumors caused by GLP-1 RAs have been reported, but these agents are contraindicated in patients with a family or personal history of medullary thyroid cancer or multiple endocrine neoplasia type 2 (MEN2).[25] Other possible adverse event issues include acute kidney injury, hypersensitivity, and injection site reactions.[1,25]

The currently available GLP-1 RAs differ by duration of action, other elements of their pharmacokinetic profiles, A1C-lowering potency, level of weight loss, and potential cardiovascular benefits. All of these characteristics should be considered when choosing a particular agent.

More information about these agents can be found in chapter 13.

INSULIN

Insulin has been used widely for monotherapy since its introduction in 1922 and has been used in combination with oral agents since the late 1950s.[5] It is difficult to estimate the fraction of patients with T2D who are treated with insulin, but one study estimated that about 24% of Medicare beneficiaries with T2D were treated with insulin.[26] Although one could argue about the absolute fraction or number of those with T2D treated with insulin, insulin is probably underutilized in this population. It is the one type of therapy that, with appropriate titration, can consistently bring a patient's blood glucose levels into the target range.

Insulin binds to the α-subunit of the insulin receptor, activating tyrosine kinase activity of the α-subunit. Activation of tyrosine kinase initiates a cascade of reactions, resulting in several physiological events, including inhibition of hepatic glucose production, stimulation of hepatic glucose uptake, stimulation of glucose uptake by muscle, and mild stimulation of glucose uptake by adipose tissue. Insulin therapy has been associated with as much as a 44% reduction in hepatic glucose production and between a 17 and 80% increase in peripheral glucose uptake.[5]

The most significant side effects of insulin in patients with T2D include hypoglycemia and weight gain. Severe hypoglycemia, while a major concern in patients with T2D, probably occurs much less frequently than in patients with T1D. In clinical trials where patients were treated toward an A1C of <7%, rates of severe hypoglycemia occurred at about 1/50th (1–3 episodes per 100 patient-years) of the rate encountered in T1D during the Diabetes Control and Complications Trial (DCCT). Insulin has also been associated with significant weight gain. Studies in patients treated with insulin for between 6 and 12 months have reported weight gain of up to 6 kg but are more commonly on the order of 2–4 kg.

The hyperglycemic-lowering capacity of insulin therapy in patients with T2D is limited only by dose and eventual development of hypoglycemia if too much insulin is used. It is very effective in combination with other pharmacologic modalities. Its titration can be simplified, in many instances, to a point that allows the patient to continue to titrate dose between visits to the provider.

The use of insulin is reviewed in detail in chapter 3.

CONCLUSION

At present, the development of a meaningful, clinically effective, and relevant medication treatment regimen for T2D is complex, and providers do not find it easy to decide which medication to prescribe. The prescriber must consider the patient's weight, diabetes duration, cardiovascular risk, dexterity, and liver and kidney function, as well as the medications that have been tried previously. Fasting plasma glucose, A1C levels, PPG levels, allergies, insurance coverage, cost of therapy, dosing complexity, and the time it takes to titrate to effective doses, degree of insulin resistance, and whether or not the β-cell is still capable of producing and releasing insulin are all additional considerations. For these reasons, an exact step-by-step treatment algorithm is difficult to develop and various clinics follow different guidelines.

As mentioned above, the hyperglycemia encountered in patients with T2D is often accompanied by other metabolic abnormalities, such as hyperlipidemia, hyperinsulinemia, hypertension, and weight gain. In the past several years, many new medications have been introduced that address not only glycemic abnormalities but also other metabolic abnormalities in patients with T2D. Although the cost of medication should be considered, the most effective method of achieving cost savings in the management of T2D is via strict glycemic control with medications that do not adversely affect the patient's metabolic profile and do not carry contraindications to the patient's specific situation. Clinicians presently have an expanded medication tool chest from which to select that will allow achievement of metabolic objectives and still allow patients a flexible and near-normal lifestyle.

Table 5.1—Summary of Antidiabetic Medication Attributes in a Typical Patient

Interventions	Expected decrease in A1C (%)	Advantages	Disadvantages
Metformin	1.5	Weight neutral, inexpensive	GI side effects, rare to questionable lactic acidosis
Insulin	Dose dependent	No dose limit, inexpensive→expensive	Injections, monitoring, hypoglycemia, weight gain
Sulfonylureas	1–2	Inexpensive	Weight gain, hypoglycemia
TZDs	0.5–1.5	Low rates of hypoglycemia	Fluid retention, weight gain, may worsen or facilitate CHF, expensive, fractures
GLP-1 RAs	0.5–2.0	Weight loss, low rates of hypoglycemia, cardiovascular benefits (liraglutide)	Injections, frequent GI side effects, expensive
DPP-4 inhibitors	0.4–0.9	Once-daily oral dosing	Moderate glycemic lowering, expensive
SGLT2 inhibitors	0.8	Weight loss, cardiovascular benefits (empagliflozin)	Genitourinary infections, expensive

GI, gastrointestinal.

REFERENCES

1. Davies MJK, D'Alessio DA, Fradkin J, et al. Management of hyperglycemia in type 2 diabetes, 2018: a consensus report by the American Diabetes Association (ADA) and the European Association for the Study of Diabetes (EASD). *Diabetes Care* 2018 Sep; dci180033. https://doi.org/10.2337/dci18-0033

2. Bailey CJ, Turner RC. Metformin. *N Engl J Med* 1996;334:574–579 DOI: 10.1056/NEJM199602293340906

3. Chung JW, Hartzler ML, Smith A, Hatton J, Kelley K. Pharmacological agents utilized in patients with type-2 diabetes: beyond lowering A1C. *P T* 2018;43;4:214–227

4. Metformin [package insert]. https://dailymed.nlm.nih.gov/dailymed/drugInfo.cfm?setid=2d98aea3-35ba-447a-b88f-a5a20b612b2f&audience=consumer

5. White JR. Biguanides. In *ADA/PDR Medications for the Treatment of Diabetes.* White JR, Campbell RK, Eds. Alexandria, American Diabetes Association, 2008

6. Bennett WL, Wilson LM, Bolen S, et al. Oral diabetes medications for adults with type 2 diabetes: an update. *AHRQ Comparative Effectiveness Reviews* 2011;27:Report No.:11-EHC038-EF

7. Inzucchi SE. Oral antihyperglycemic therapy for type 2 diabetes: scientific review. *JAMA* 2002;287:360–372

8. Guardado-Mendoza R, Prioletta A, Jiménez-Ceja LM, Sosale A, Folli F. The role of nateglinide and repaglinide, derivatives of meglitinide, in the treatment of type 2 diabetes mellitus. *Arch Med Sci* 2013;9;5:936–943

9. Trevor AJ, Katzung BG, Knuidering-Hall M. Pancreatic hormones, antidiabetic agents and glucagon. In *Katzung and Trevor's Pharmacology: Examination and Board Review*, 11th ed. New York, McGraw Hill Education, 2015

10. Krentz AJ, Bailey CJ. Oral antidiabetic agents: current role in type 2 diabetes mellitus. *Drugs* 2005;65:385–411

11. Chiasson JL, Josse RG, Hunt JA, et al. The efficacy of acarbose in the treatment of patients with non-insulin-dependent diabetes mellitus: a multicenter controlled clinical trial. *Ann Intern Med* 1994;121:928–935

12. Neumiller JJ. Incretin pharmacology: a review of the incretin effect and current incretin-based therapies. *Cardiovasc Hematol Agents Med Chem* 2012;10(4):276–288

13. Neumiller JJ. Incretin-based therapies. *Med Clin North Am* 2015;99:107–130

14. White WB, Cannon CP, Heller SR, et al.; EXAMINE Investigators. Alogliptin after acute coronary syndrome in patients with type 2 diabetes. *N Engl J Med* 2013;369:1327–1335

15. Scirica BM, Bhatt DL, Braunwald E. et al.; SAVOR-TIMI 53 Steering Committee and Investigators. Saxagliptin and cardiovascular outcomes in patients with type 2 diabetes mellitus. *N Engl J Med* 2013;369:1317–1326

16. Green JB, Bethel MA, Armstrong PW, et al.; TECOS Study Group. Effect of sitagliptin on cardiovascular outcomes in type 2 diabetes. *N Engl J Med* 2015;373:232–242

17. White J. Apple trees to sodium glucose co-transporter inhibitors: a review of SGLT2 inhibition. *Clin Diabetes* 2010;28(1):5–10

18. Vasilakou D, Karagiannis T, Athanasiadou E, et al. Sodium-glucose cotransporter 2 inhibitors for type 2 diabetes: a systematic review and meta-analysis. *Ann Intern Med.* 2013;159:262–274

19. Garg SK, Henry RR, Banks P, et al. Effects of sotagliflozin added to insulin in patients with type 1 diabetes. *N Engl J Med* 2017;377:2337–2348

20. White JR. Sodium glucose cotransporter 2 inhibitors. *Med Clin North Am* 2015;99:131–144

21. Chao EC. SGLT-2 inhibitors: a new mechanism for glycemic control. *Clin Diabetes* 2014;32(1):4–11

22. Mudaliar S, Henry RR. The incretin hormones: from scientific discovery to practical therapeutics. *Diabetologia* 2012;55:1865–1868

23. Pratley RE, Aroda VR, Lingvay I, Lüdemann J, Andreassen C, Navarria A, Viljoen A; SUSTAIN 7 Investigators. Semaglutide versus dulaglutide once weekly in patients with type 2 diabetes (SUSTAIN 7): a randomised, open-label, phase 3b trial. *Lancet* 2018;6(4):275–286

24. Leiter LA, Nauck MA. Efficacy and safety of GLP-1 receptor agonists across the spectrum of type 2 diabetes mellitus. *Exp Clin Endocrinol Diabetes* 2017;125:419–435

25. Prasad-Reddy L, Isaacs D. A clinical review of GLP-1 receptor agonists: efficacy and safety in diabetes and beyond. *Drugs Context* 2015;4:212283. DOI:10.7573/dic.212283

26. Sargen MR, Hoffstad OJ, Wiebe DJ, Margolis DJ. Geographic variation in pharmacotherapy decisions for U.S. Medicare enrollees with diabetes. *J Diabetes Complications* 2012;26(4):301–307

Chapter 6
Biguanides

PEGGY SOULE ODEGARD, BSPHARM, PHARMD, CDE
JENNIFER DANIELSON, PHARMD, CDE
KAM L. CAPOCCIA, PHARMD, BCPS, CDE

INTRODUCTION

Biguanides[1] in some form have been used since medieval times. French lilac, or goat's rue (*galega officinalis*), was used as a folk treatment for diabetes in southern and eastern Europe. Later, *galega officinalis* was found to be rich in the compound guanidine. In 1918, the hypoglycemic activity of guanidine was confirmed. Unfortunately, guanidine was too toxic for human clinical use, but its chemical congeners, such as the alkyldiguanide synthalin A, were introduced in the early 1920s. Further analysis continued with the biguanide group in the 1920s; however, clinical use of these compounds was not pursued. The compounds fell into disfavor because of the discovery and availability of insulin products.

With the advent of sulfonylureas in the 1950s, biguanides were reinvestigated for possible use in the treatment of diabetes. Metformin and phenformin were introduced in 1957, followed by buformin in 1958. No other active compounds in the biguanide category have been discovered, even though significant work on the structure-activity relationship has taken place. Clinical use of buformin was limited, but phenformin was used widely in the 1960s and 1970s. An association between phenformin and lactic acidosis resulted in the withdrawal of this compound from use in many countries. Metformin was introduced in 1995 and has been the only drug in the biguanide category in the U.S. ever since. Metformin is now the most widely used oral antihyperglycemic agent.

Metformin hydrochloride is indicated for management of T2D as an adjunct to nutrition and exercise. It is used as monotherapy and in combination with other oral agents, GLP-1 RAs, and insulin. It is also used in prevention of diabetes.

PHARMACOLOGY

MECHANISM OF ACTION

Metformin causes a plethora of metabolic effects, including changes in carbohydrate, lipid, and lipoprotein metabolism. The effects of metformin on carbohydrate metabolism occur primarily in the liver and, to a lesser extent, in peripheral muscle tissue. Metformin's main effect is associated with a reduction in basal hepatic glucose production in patients with T2D. Metformin has been shown to enhance insulin-stimulated glucose transport in skeletal muscle, thereby increasing glucose uptake and insulin sensitivity, although this effect is not as significant as that of hepatic glucose production. Metformin also has beneficial effects on lipids in that it decreases plasma triglycerides and low-density lipoprotein cholesterol (LDL-C) and increases high-density lipoprotein cholesterol (HDL-C).

PHARMACOKINETICS

The bioavailability of the immediate-release formulation of metformin ranges from 50–60% when fasting, which is slightly decreased when taken with food. Food increases the absorption of the extended-release formulation. The clinical significance of the increased and decreased absorption caused by food intake is questionable, however. The compound is absorbed mainly through the small intestine. For conventional tablets, peak plasma concentration of 0.4–3 μg/mL is reached ~2–4 h after an oral dose of between 500 and 1,000 mg. For extended-release tablets, peak plasma concentration of 0.6–1.8 μg/mL is reached in 4–8 h. The drug undergoes negligible binding to plasma proteins. The average half-life of metformin in individuals with normal renal function is 6 h. No measurable metabolism of metformin occurs.

In terms of elimination, ~90% of the compound is excreted via the urine within 17–24 h of administration. Elimination occurs via glomerular filtration and tubular secretion. Tubular secretion is thought to be a major route of metformin elimination because the renal clearance of this compound is ~3.5 times greater than creatinine clearance. The drug is widely distributed into most tissues in concentrations similar to those found in peripheral plasma. However, the highest concentrations are found in the salivary glands and in the intestinal wall. Relatively high concentrations are found in the liver and the kidney.

TREATMENT ADVANTAGES/DISADVANTAGES

Metformin has gained position as the primary oral pharmacologic treatment for T2D because of its ability to reduce A1C and fasting glucose, beneficial effect on weight, and relatively low cost compared to other glucose-lowering therapies. In addition to these improved effects on glucose control, data continue to emerge highlighting other potential health benefits of metformin. Specifically, its impact on polycystic ovary syndrome (PCOS), prevention or slowing progression to T2D in those at high risk, reduction of certain cancer risks and improvement in survival rates, reduction in CV disease, and favorable impact on aging-related conditions. There is limited data evaluating the impact of metformin initiation in subjects without diabetes on risk reduction or treatment benefits for these conditions; however, initial studies are underway to explore the use of metformin as an adjunct therapy in certain cancers.

POLYCYSTIC OVARY SYNDROME

Metformin has demonstrated efficacy in the treatment of PCOS, with effects on fertility.[2] The primary actions of metformin in PCOS include resumption of menses, improvement in menses cyclic frequency, and hormonal and metabolic parameters. In one study of 119 women with PCOS, 24 months of metformin treatment was correlated with improved hormonal profiles for testosterone and luteinizing hormone, increased menstrual frequency, and decreased body mass in both overweight and normal weight women.[3]

PREVENTION OF T2D

The Diabetes Prevention Program, a 3-year multicenter trial (n = 3,234) aimed to prevent T2D, compared intensive lifestyle support intervention to metformin and placebo in people at high risk for diabetes. The results substantially favored the lifestyle intervention (7% weight loss and 150 min moderate level physical activity weekly) with a 58% reduction in the incidence of diabetes at 3 years; however, metformin (850 mg twice daily) demonstrated significant benefits on risk reduction as well, with 31% reduced incidence of diabetes as compared to placebo.[4] These findings were reinforced by the 10-year follow-up to the Diabetes Prevention Program study of 924 subjects initially in the metformin group, with an 18% reduction in diabetes incidence for those taking metformin.[5] The American Diabetes Association, in its *Standards of Medical Care in Diabetes*, currently recommends metformin as a pharmacotherapeutic approach for those with prediabetes, especially if BMI is greater than or equal to 35 kg/m[2], in women with a history of gestational diabetes, and for those who are less than 60 years old.[6]

USE IN PREGNANCY

Metformin is not approved by the FDA for the treatment of diabetes during pregnancy. However, it has demonstrated safety in patients who are pregnant, even though it does cross the placenta.[7-11] As it is associated with a lower risk of neonatal hypoglycemia and less maternal weight gain, metformin is used in gestational diabetes and pregnant women with T2D as an alternative to insulin, which is usually considered first-line choice of therapy.[11-15]

CARDIOVASCULAR RISKS

A positive effect of metformin on cardiovascular health has been reported by multiple studies, although the explicit CV benefit—often attributed to its effects on weight, blood pressure, endothelial function, and lipids—has yet to be specifically confirmed. In the United Kingdom Prospective Diabetes Study (UKPDS) and subsequent follow-up study, metformin treatment was associated with reduced all-cause mortality, including reduction in myocardial infarction.[16,17] In a meta-analysis of 40 trials, metformin reduced risk of CV mortality compared to the other oral diabetes agents studied and placebo.[18,19] More recently, the contraindication regarding the use of metformin in patients with advanced HF has been removed from the product labeling in light of several studies demonstrating the safety and benefit of metformin use in people with diabetes and HF, including reduction in HF readmissions and mortality.[20] It is still, however, prudent to consider holding metformin therapy in acute HF exacerbations involving substantial reduction in renal function, until stabilized, to mitigate risk.

IMPACT ON CANCER RISKS AND OUTCOMES

The impact of metformin on cancer risk and survival has been reported in several studies, although current findings are based primarily on studies using a retrospective design. A review of the most recent evidence is reflected in the subsequent sections. Additional prospective, controlled investigations are needed to confirm any potential benefit of metformin in prevention of specific cancers and to more specifically characterize metformin's effects on cancer treatment outcomes. Initial data exploring these effects of metformin is summarized below for certain cancers. Readers are encouraged to conduct updated medical literature searches to confirm the most recent findings to guide therapeutic decision-making.

Endometrial Cancer Risk and Outcomes

In a subset of five pooled studies of a meta-analysis of 11 studies involving more than 766,000 subjects conducted by Tang et al., metformin use in individuals with T2D who had endometrial cancer was associated with a reduction of endometrial cancer risk among patients with diabetes (RR 0.87 [95% CI 0.80–0.95]; $P = 0.006$). Additionally, pooled analysis of six retrospective studies identified survival in patients with endometrial cancer using metformin that was significantly improved compared to nonusers (HR 0.63 [95% CI 0.45–0.87]; $P = 0.006$).[21]

Pancreatic Cancer Risk and Outcomes

Four recent studies have identified a positive impact on survival in people with T2D and pancreatic cancer who were taking metformin. In a systematic review and meta-analysis of nine studies comprising 9,265 subjects taking metformin, Zhou et al. identified a relative survival benefit (overall survival HR 0.84 [95% CI 0.73–0.96]) associated with metformin use compared to no metformin use.[22] In a similar systematic review of 14 studies (12 cohort studies and 2 randomized controlled trials) of over 94,000 patients with pancreatic cancer, metformin use was associated with improved overall survival (adjusted HR 0.77 [95% CI 0.68–0.87]).[23] In the cohort studies, however, no improvement in progression-free survival or overall survival was identified. Separate meta-analyses conducted by Li et al. and Jian-Yu et al. have confirmed these findings with some subanalyses pointing to potential differential effects of this benefit, based on tumor stage.[24,25]

Colorectal Cancer Risk and Outcomes

The risk of colorectal cancer (CRC) in patients with T2D taking metformin has been evaluated in a number of studies with evidence pointing to a reduced incidence of CRC and a survival benefit in those using metformin. In a meta-analysis conducted of 20 studies published prior to 2016, including 12 cohort, 7 case-control, and 1 randomized controlled trial, metformin use was associated with reduced incidence of colorectal adenomas (OR 0.80 [95% CI 0.71–0.90]; $P = 0.0002$).[26] In a similar analysis, Du et al. identified improved overall survival in metformin users with diabetes and CRC as compared to non-metformin users (HR 0.69 [95% CI 0.61–0.77]), with benefit noted in particular for patients with stage II and III CRC disease.[27] Furthering this observation of the positive impact of metformin on CRC, Tian and colleagues conducted a meta-analysis of 81 studies, representing 6,908 cases of CRC patients using metformin and 4,954 CRC patients with T2D not using metformin. This analysis found a significantly improved overall survival (HR 0.82 [95% CI 0.77–0.87]; $P = 0.000$) in patients using metformin, although this benefit was not significant for CRC-specific survival (HR 0.84 [95% CI 0.69–1.02]; $P = 0.079$).[28]

Prostate Cancer Risk and Outcomes

The impact of metformin use on risk reduction for prostate cancer has been reported; however, studies have largely been focused in Asian populations, limiting the ability to generalize findings. With this in mind, Chen and colleagues used a meta-analysis design to investigate this impact further with attention to ethnicity. Of 482 studies identified, 26 were chosen for inclusion (23 Western-based, 3 Asian-based, representing almost 2 million patients). No significant association between metformin use and prostate cancer was identified for Western- or Asian-based studies collectively (RR 1.01 [95% CI 0.86–1.18]). The removal of one large study in an Asian population resulted in similar findings for the Asian-based studies. The authors concluded there is likely no association between metformin and risk of prostate cancer based on the current evidence.[29]

Gastric Cancer Risk and Outcomes

The potential effect of metformin use on the risk of gastric cancer in patients with T2D has been evaluated in limited studies. In a meta-analysis of 7 cohort studies ($n = 591,077$ patients), metformin therapy was associated with a lower incidence of gastric cancer in Asian patients with T2D than that of other therapies for diabetes (HR 0.763 [95% CI 0.642–0.905]). Given these findings were limited to observations in a sample with Asian ethnicity, additional study is needed to clarify the effect and potential benefit of metformin on reducing the risk of gastric cancer in more generalized populations.[30]

Lung Cancer Risk and Outcomes

Several investigations have explored the effect of metformin on overall survival (OS) and progression-free survival (PFS) in patients with lung cancer. This stems from the experimental observation that cancer proliferation rate and tumor progression occur more quickly in patients with diabetes, theoretically due to the influence of hyperinsulinemia, inflammatory cytokines, and hyperglycemia.[31] Cao and colleagues conducted a recent meta-analysis of studies published prior to April 2017. In this analysis of people with T2D and lung cancer, both OS (HR 0.77 [95% CI 0.66–0.9]; $P = 0.001$) and PFS (HR 0.53 [95% CI 0.41–0.68]; $P < 0.001$) improved (23 and 47% reductions, respectively) with metformin use compared to no metformin use. Histological analysis revealed this beneficial effect for both non-small cell lung cancer and small cell lung cancer with statistically significant improvements in OS and PFS.[32]

AGING-RELATED CONDITIONS

Recently, reports in the popular press hinted at the aging benefits of metformin, suggesting far-reaching benefits of age extension. There is not current evidence to support this suggested benefit; however, some research is underway to characterize this potential, but unproven, benefit.[33,34]

SIGNIFICANT WARNINGS/PRECAUTIONS

Metformin is contraindicated in patients with

- Acute or chronic metabolic acidosis, including diabetic ketoacidosis.
- Known hypersensitivity to metformin hydrochloride.
- Severe renal impairment (GFR below 30 mL/min).

Metformin should be discontinued temporarily in patients requiring radiological studies using iodinated contrast medias, because these agents are known to cause renal dysfunction in some individuals.

Monitoring Renal Function

Metformin is excreted via the kidneys; thus, the risk of accumulation of the medication is greater in patients with reduced renal function. The risk of lactic acidosis is increased in these patients as well. Calculation of GFR is recommended for renal monitoring in patients taking metformin. Metformin use in patients with renal impairment should be monitored closely.[35] When the GFR for a patient taking metformin falls below 45 mL/min, assessing risk versus benefit of continued use is recommended. Normally, the annual assessment of renal function is appropriate. In patients with a GFR of less than 60 mL/min, renal function should be assessed every 3–6 months; in those with a GFR of 30–45 mL/min, the dose should be reduced and they should have more frequent renal monitoring. Patients 65 years of age or older can have reduced renal function, so more frequent assessment of renal function in these patients when taking metformin is recommended.

Radiological Studies

Radiological studies involving the use of iodinated contrast media should be undertaken only after metformin has been discontinued. The drug should be withheld on the day of the procedure, and for at least 2–3 days after, until normal renal function has been documented.

Hypoxic States

Lactic acidosis is associated with cardiovascular collapse, acute congestive heart failure, acute myocardial infarction, and other conditions such as septicemia and dehydration that cause hypoxemia. Therefore, metformin should be discontinued in patients with these acute medical conditions and may be reinstituted once the acute illness has resolved and renal function is normal.

Surgical Procedures

Metformin therapy should be discontinued temporarily for any major surgical procedure and should be restarted only after the patient's oral intake has been resumed and renal function has shown to be normal.

Alcohol Intake

Metformin should be used cautiously in patients who are known to consume excessive alcohol, since this may be a precipitating factor increasing risk for lactic acidosis.

Impaired Hepatic Function

Impaired hepatic function has been associated with some cases of lactic acidosis; therefore, it is recommended that metformin not be used in patients with impaired hepatic function. Recently, metformin, along with other medications used for T2D, has been evaluated for effects on reducing nonalcoholic fatty liver disease (NAFLD), with modest effects on steatosis demonstrated when combined with weight loss; however, no appreciable effect on fibrosis was demonstrated.[36]

Vitamin B_{12} Levels

Among patients treated with metformin, 7–9% experience a reduction in vitamin B_{12} to subnormal levels with long-term use.[37] However, this is rarely associated with anemia and appears to be rapidly reversible with discontinuation of the medication or with vitamin B_{12} supplementation. Patients treated with metformin should therefore undergo measurement of hematological parameters annually. Hematological evaluation is also advised in any patient with apparent abnormalities. Routine serum vitamin B_{12} measurements approximately every 2–3 years may be useful in individuals with inadequate B_{12} or calcium intake and/or absorption.

Hypoglycemia

Hypoglycemia does not occur with metformin monotherapy under normal conditions. However, it may occur in patients in whom caloric intake is deficient, in patients who undertake strenuous exercise, in patients who are treated with other glucose-lowering agents, such as sulfonylureas, or in patients who consume ethanol. Patients taking combination products containing metformin along with other agents, especially sulfonylureas and meglitinides, can experience hypoglycemia.

SPECIAL POPULATIONS

Hepatic Impairment

Patients with hepatic impairment have developed lactic acidosis while taking metformin, perhaps not due to metformin itself but because of reduced hepatic lactate clearance. Nevertheless, metformin should be avoided in patients with hepatic impairment.

Pediatrics

The safety and efficacy of metformin in pediatric patients between the ages of 10 and 16 years has been established. Extended-release metformin has been evaluated in this population. Even though combination products are sometimes used for greater medication adherence, the safety and efficacy of combination products containing metformin have not been established in this population except for one (metformin with glyburide).[38]

Geriatrics

Limited published data on the use of metformin in geriatric patients indicates a potential for changes in its pharmacokinetic profile, primarily due to renal function decline. Yet no overall difference in the safety or efficacy of metformin has been found in geriatric patients compared to younger patients. Since metformin is excreted renally and renal function declines with age, elderly patients have an increased likelihood of metformin-associated lactic acidosis. Monitoring renal function more frequently is recommended for this patient population.

Sex

No pharmacokinetic differences have been reported based on sex. Clinically, in controlled trials in patients with T2D, no differences have been observed between males and female patients.

Ethnicity

Although no controlled clinical trials have been conducted evaluating differences in the pharmacokinetics or pharmacodynamics of metformin use among ethnic groups, the effects of metformin have been shown to be comparable in non-Hispanic white, black, and Hispanic subjects.

ADVERSE EFFECTS AND MONITORING

Lactic Acidosis

Lactic acidosis is a very rare but extremely serious condition that can occur secondary to the accumulation of metformin. Lactic acidosis is fatal in ~50% of cases. Currently, the reported incidence of lactic acidosis in patients receiving metformin is extremely low. The majority of these cases have occurred in patients with significant renal insufficiency. The risk of lactic acidosis can be reduced by observing the aforementioned contraindications and precautions. Recent studies have demonstrated that if contraindications are followed, the rates of lactic acidosis in patients treated with metformin are no greater than background rates observed in similar patients not treated with metformin.[39-41]

Gastrointestinal Reactions

Gastrointestinal symptoms, such as abdominal bloating, flatulence, anorexia, diarrhea, nausea, and vomiting, are the most common side effects observed in patients treated with metformin. Importantly, these symptoms may be mitigated by taking with food (e.g., start the dose with the major meal), gradual dose escalation as tolerated against gastrointestinal symptoms, and by using the extended-release (i.e., XR) formulation of the drug. Gastrointestinal complaints are ~30% more frequent in patients on metformin monotherapy than in patients treated with placebo, particularly during the initial phases of therapy. These complaints are generally transient and may resolve with continued treatment and attention to the dosing strategies mentioned above. In some cases, however, temporary dose reduction may be prudent. If significant diarrhea and/or vomiting occur, metformin should be temporarily discontinued or a trial of the extended-release formulation be considered, if not yet attempted.

Dysgeusia

Approximately 1–5% of patients treated with metformin will complain of an unpleasant or metallic taste in their mouths. This usually resolves spontaneously; if not, some clinicians find it helpful for the patient to try taking metformin with saltine crackers or a lemon hard candy (sugar free) to help reduce the unpleasant taste.

Dermatological Reactions

In controlled trials, the incidence of rash or dermatitis in patients treated with metformin monotherapy was comparable to that of placebo.

Hematological Reactions

As mentioned above, metformin therapy may result in a small reduction in vitamin B_{12} levels; however, reports of megaloblastic anemia secondary to metformin are exceedingly rare. Annual monitoring of hematologic parameters is suggested. In patients at risk for low vitamin B_{12} levels (such as those with inadequate B_{12} or calcium intake), such levels should be checked every 2–3 years. Some recommend vitamin B_{12} supplementation in those with excessive use of alcohol, which may result in depletion of vitamin B_{12} stores.

DRUG INTERACTIONS

Antihyperglycemic Agents

Although metformin alone does not cause hypoglycemia, concomitant therapy with other antihyperglycemic agents can result in hypoglycemia, especially when changes in diet and physical activity occur. In a single-dose study of subjects with T2D, administration of metformin with glyburide did not result in changes in metformin pharmacokinetics or pharmacodynamics but did result in reductions in glyburide area under the curve (AUC) and C_{max}.[1] The clinical significance of this interaction is uncertain. In a single-dose study, administration of metformin with an α-glucosidase inhibitor resulted in a decrease in the bioavailability of metformin.[42] The clinical significance of this interaction is uncertain.

Other Drugs

Corticosteroids, such as prednisone, can cause hyperglycemia and lead to loss of glucose control in patients with diabetes. Concurrent use of these agents or agents with a similar impact on glucose may in effect lower the efficacy of metformin; the discontinuation of such agents could lead to hypoglycemia if metformin use is continued. Other drugs with the potential for causing hyperglycemia include: thiazide diuretics, estrogens, thyroid products, oral contraceptives, phenytoin, phenothiazines, niacin, sympathomimetics, β-blockers, calcium channel blockers, and isoniazid.

Metformin/furosemide interaction was studied in healthy subjects in a single-dose trial where both medications were affected. Furosemide caused an increase in metformin's C_{max} and AUC (22 and 15%, respectively) without altering metformin's renal clearance. Furosemide's C_{max} and AUC were reduced by 31 and 12%, respectively. The terminal half-life of furosemide was reduced by 32%, without any significant alteration in renal clearance.

Agents that Enhance Effects of Metformin

The following drugs have the potential to enhance the glucose-lowering effects of metformin. Patients taking these agents with metformin should perform close monitoring of blood glucose to avoid hypoglycemia.

- Alpha-lipoic acid
- Androgens
- Guanethidine
- Mono-amine oxidase inhibitors
- Nifedipine
- Prothionamide
- Pegvisomant
- Salicylates
- Selective serotonin reuptake inhibitors (SSRIs)

Quinolones

Quinolone antibiotics taken with metformin can have a transient impact on metformin effectiveness, with both increases and decreases in effectiveness reported. Patients taking quinolones while taking metformin should monitor their blood glucose more closely to avoid hyper- or hypoglycemia, and to assure ongoing glucose control during antibiotic therapy.

Trospium

A study in healthy volunteers showed that taking metformin with trospium can decrease absorption of trospium. Patients taking both of these agents should be monitored closely for evidence of reduced trospium efficacy.

Cationic Drugs

An interaction between metformin and cimetidine has been observed in normal healthy subjects, with a 60% increase in peak metformin concentrations and a 40% increase in metformin AUC. However, in one single-dose study, the elimination half-life of metformin was unchanged. Metformin apparently has no effect on cimetidine kinetics.

Other compounds that are eliminated via renal tubular secretion have the potential for causing an interaction with metformin by competing for renal tubular transport systems; therefore, these drugs should be used cautiously. Examples include abemaciclib, amiloride, bictegravir, bupropion, cephalexin, dalfampridine, digoxin, dofetilide, dolutegravir, isavuconazonium, lamotrigine, morphine, ondansetron, procainamide, quinidine, quinine, ranitidine, ranolazine, topiramate, triamterene, trimethoprim, and vancomycin.

Agents with Increased Risk of Lactic Acidosis

The following drugs have potential to increase risk of lactic acidosis alone. When taken with metformin, caution should be taken to monitor for signs and symptoms of lactic acidosis as patients may be at increased risk for it.

- Carbonic anhydrase inhibitors
- Glycopyrrolate
- Topiramate
- Ombitasvir, paritaprevir, and ritonavir

Agents that Decrease Effects of Metformin

The following drugs have been found in small studies to significantly decrease the glucose-lowering effect of metformin. Increased self-monitoring of blood glucose should be performed when starting, stopping, or adjusting any of these agents.

- Patiromer
- Ritodrine
- Vandetanib
- Verapamil

β-Blockers

In a single-dose study of metformin taken with propranolol in healthy patients, neither drug was affected in its pharmacokinetic profile. However, β-adrenergic blocking agents as a class have potential for effects on blood glucose. β-Blockers can impair glucose tolerance, increase frequency and severity of hypoglycemia, alter the hemodynamic response to hypoglycemia, and delay the recovery of blood glucose following hypoglycemia. And, because nonselective β-blockers inhibit some of the typical response to hypoglycemia like tachycardia, the only sign of hypoglycemia patients may recognize is sweating.

Angiotensin-Converting Enzyme Inhibitors

Angiotensin-converting enzyme (ACE) inhibitors have been associated with unexplained hypoglycemia and increased insulin sensitivity. The risk of this effect is low, but patients taking metformin who are newly started on ACE inhibitors or who are adjusting doses or discontinuing them should monitor blood glucose for this potential effect.

Clomiphene

Metformin and other antihyperglycemic agents have been known to cause resumption of ovulation in premenopausal women with PCOS. Patients with this syndrome taking metformin, especially if taking clomiphene, should be aware that fertility and chance of pregnancy may improve.

DOSAGE AND ADMINISTRATION

The usual starting dose of 500-mg metformin tablets is once a day, given with the largest meal of the day. In those with anticipated poor gastrointestinal tolerance, a dose of 250 mg may be useful as a starting point. The importance of initiating metformin dosing with a regular-sized meal, especially when the first meal of the day is scant, should be reinforced to minimize gastrointestinal distress. Doses may be titrated in increments of one tablet every week up to a maximum effective dose of 2,000 mg per day, although the total maximum dose is 2,500 mg per day. Metformin is often administered at a dose of 1,000 mg twice a day with the morning and evening meals. If a dose of 2,500 mg is required, the patient may have improved tolerance if it is given three times a day with meals.

The usual starting dose of 850-mg metformin tablets is once daily, given with the largest meal of the day. Dosage increases are usually made in increments of one tablet every other week given in divided doses up to a maximum of 2,550 mg per day. The most common maintenance dose is 850 mg given twice a day with the morning and evening meals. However, if necessary, patients may be given 850 mg three times a day with meals.

The usual starting dose of the extended-release form is 500 mg once a day, given with the largest meal of the day. This formulation may be useful in individuals experiencing ongoing gastrointestinal side effects to improve tolerance. Doses may be titrated in increments of one tablet every week up to a maximum of 2,000 mg given with the evening meal. Patients previously treated with conventional metformin may be safely switched to the extended-release form at the same total daily dose (up to 2,000 mg) given as one daily dose of the extended-release form.

COMBINATION PRODUCTS

The use of combination products containing metformin and other antihyperglycemic medications may be especially helpful for individuals with adherence challenges due to the complexity of taking multiple drug regimens and who may benefit from the dual action of two agents. When using a combination product, it is prudent to approach the decision with consideration to the benefit of each individual product on the health of the patient. An initial titration using metformin as a single agent is ideal to assess its efficacy (e.g., A1c reduction of 1–2%) and to reduce the risk of gastrointestinal toxicity that might occur with a fixed-dose combination without the flexibility to titrate the metformin to gastrointestinal tolerance. If efficacy is demonstrated and additional efficacy with a second agent is desired, a combination product can be useful to keep the dosing regimen simplified to one physical product while gaining the treatment advantages of two medications. In choosing a metformin combination product, the mechanism of action of the second product in the combination should be matched to the perceived therapeutic need for the patient. For example, if the patient appears to need enhanced insulin as well as the effects of metformin on hepatic glucose production and insulin sensitivity, the addition of a sulfonylurea to augment physiologic insulin release through a dual-drug product like glipizide/metformin combination

Table 6.1—Antihyperglycemic Medications Containing Metformin

Metformin formulations	Available strengths	Extended or immediate release	Can be cut?	Dosing interval	Maximum therapeutic effect (time)	Maximum daily dose (MDD)	Renal dose adjustments (mL/min/1.73 m²)	Hepatic dose adjustments	Contraindications	Pregnancy category
					Extended Release (XR)					
Fortamet; Glucophage XR; Glumetza; Generics	Fortamet: 500 mg, 1,000 mg; Glucophage XR: 500 mg, 750 mg; Glumetza: 500 mg, 1000 mg; Generic: 500 mg, 750 mg, 1,000 mg	Extended release	Do not chew, cut, or crush	Once daily–b.i.d.	May take 4–6 weeks to see full effect	2,000 mg/d	eGFR 30–45: Do not initiate; if eGFR falls to <45, consider benefits/risks of continuing therapy eGFR <30: Do not use	Avoid use of metformin in patients with clinical or laboratory evidence of hepatic disease due to risk of lactic acidosis	Hypersensitivity to metformin; eGFR <30; acute or chronic metabolic acidosis, including diabetic ketoacidosis; use cautiously in patients at risk for lactic acidosis	B
					Immediate Release (IR)					
Glucophage; Generic	500 mg, 850 mg, 1,000 mg (scored)	Immediate release	Yes	b.i.d.	May take 4–6 weeks to see full effect	2,000 mg/d	See metformin above	See metformin above	See metformin above	B
					Liquid					
Riomet; Generic	500 mg/5 mL	Immediate release	N/A	Once daily–t.i.d.	May take 4–6 weeks to see full effect	2,000 mg/d	See metformin above	See metformin above	See metformin above	B

(continued)

Table 6.1 (continued)

Metformin formulations	Available strengths	Extended or immediate release	Can be cut?	Dosing interval	Maximum therapeutic effect (time)	Maximum daily dose (MDD)	Renal dose adjustments (mL/min/1.73 m²)	Hepatic dose adjustments	Contraindications	Pregnancy category
Metformin & DPP-4 Inhibitors										
Metformin & Alogliptan (Kazano)	500 mg/12.5 mg; 1,000 mg/12.5 mg	Immediate release	Do not chew, cut, or crush	b.i.d.	Metformin: 4–6 weeks; Alogliptin: 2–4 weeks	Metformin 2,000 mg/d; Alogliptin 12.5 mg/d	See metformin above	See metformin above	See metformin above; Hypersensitivity to alogliptan	B
Metformin & Linagliptan (Jentadueto)	500 mg/2.5 mg; 850 mg/2.5 mg; 1,000 mg/2.5 mg	Immediate release	Yes	b.i.d.	Metformin: 4–6 weeks; Linagliptin: 2–4 weeks	Metformin 2,000 mg/d; Linagliptin 5 mg/d	See metformin above	See metformin above	See metformin above; Hypersensitivity to linagliptin	B
Metformin Extended Release & Linagliptin (Jentadueto XR)	1,000 mg XR/2.5 mg; 1000 mg XR/5 mg	Extended release	Do not crush, cut, or chew	Once daily	Metformin: 4–6 weeks; Linagliptin: 2–4 weeks	Metformin 2,000 mg/d; Linagliptin 5 mg/d	See metformin above	See metformin above	See metformin above; Hypersensitivity to linagliptin	B
Metformin Extended Release & Saxagliptin (Kombiglyze XR)	500 mg XR/5 mg; 1,000 mg XR/2.5 mg; 1,000 mg XR/5 mg	Extended release	Do not crush, cut, or chew	Once daily	Metformin: 4–6 weeks; Saxagliptin: 2–4 weeks	Metformin 2,000 mg/d; Saxagliptin 5 mg/d	See metformin above; Limit saxagliptin dose to 2.5 mg/d	See metformin above	See metformin above; Hypersensitivity to saxagliptin	B
Metformin & Sitagliptin (Janumet)	500 mg/50 mg; 1,000 mg/50 mg	Immediate release	Do not chew, cut, or crush	b.i.d.	Metformin: 4–6 weeks; Saxagliptin: 2–4 weeks	Metformin 2,000 mg/d; Sitagliptin 100 mg/d	See metformin above; Limit sitagliptin dose to 50 mg/day	See metformin above	See metformin above; Hypersensitivity to sitagliptin	B

(continued)

Table 6.1 (continued)

Metformin formulations	Available strengths	Extended or immediate release	Can be cut?	Dosing interval	Maximum therapeutic effect (time)	Maximum daily dose (MDD)	Renal dose adjustments (mL/min/1.73 m²)	Hepatic dose adjustments	Contraindications	Pregnancy category
Metformin Extended Release & Sitagliptin (Janumet XR)	500 mg XR/50 mg, 1,000 mg XR/50 mg, 1,000 mg XR/100 mg	Extended release	Do not chew, cut, or crush	Once daily	Metformin: 4–6 weeks; Sitagliptin: 2–4 weeks	Metformin 2,000 mg/d; Sitagliptin 100 mg/d	See metformin above	See metformin above	See metformin above; Hypersensitivity to sitagliptin	B
Metformin & Meglitinide										
Metformin & Repaglinide (PrandiMet)	500 mg/1 mg, 500 mg/2 mg	Immediate release	Yes	b.i.d.–t.i.d.	Metformin: 4–6 weeks; Repaglinide: 2 weeks	Metformin 2,000 mg/d; Repaglinide 10 mg/d; Do not exceed 1,000 mg metformin/4 mg repaglinide per meal	See metformin above	See metformin above	See metformin above; Hypersensitivity to repaglinide; Concomitant administration of gemfibrozil	C
Metformin & SGLT2 Inhibitors										
Metformin & Canagliflozin (Invokamet)	500 mg/50 mg, 500 mg/150 mg, 1,000 mg/50 mg, 1,000 mg/150 mg	Immediate release	Yes	b.i.d.	Metformin: 4–6 weeks; Canagliflozin: 2 weeks	Metformin 2,000 mg/d; Canagliflozin 300 mg/d	See metformin above; eGFR 45 to <60: Limit the dose of canagliflozin to 100 mg/day; eGFR <45: Do not use	See metformin above	See metformin above; Hypersensitivity to canagliflozin; eGFR <45, end-stage renal disease or patients on dialysis	C

(continued)

Table 6.1 (continued)

Metformin formulations	Available strengths	Extended or immediate release	Can be cut?	Dosing interval	Maximum therapeutic effect (time)	Maximum daily dose (MDD)	Renal dose adjustments (mL/min/1.73 m²)	Hepatic dose adjustments	Contraindications	Pregnancy category
Metformin Extended Release & Canagliflozin (Invokamet XR)	500 mg XR/50 mg 500 mg XR/150 mg 1,000 mg XR/50 mg 1,000 mg XR/150 mg	Extended release	Do not crush, cut, or chew	Once daily	Metformin: 4–6 weeks Canagliflozin: 2 weeks	Metformin 2,000 mg/d Canagliflozin 300mg/d	See metformin above eGFR 45 to <60: Limit the dose of canagliflozin to 100 mg/day eGFR <45: Do not use	See metformin above	See metformin above Hypersensitivity to canagliflozin eGFR <45, end-stage renal disease or patients on dialysis	C
Metformin Extended Release & Dapagliflozin (Xigduo XR)	500 mg XR/5 mg 500 mg XR/10 mg 1,000 mg XR/5 mg 1,000 mg XR/10 mg	Extended release	Do not crush, cut, or chew	Once daily	Metformin: 4–6 weeks Dapagliflozin: 2 weeks	Metformin 2,000 mg/d Dapagliflozin 10 mg/d	See metformin above Dapagliflozin: eGFR <60: Do not initiate; eGFR that declines persistently in the range of 30 to <60 use is not recommended; eGFR <30 Do not use	See metformin above	See metformin above Hypersensitivity to dapagliflozin Moderate to severe renal impairment (eGFR <60), end-stage renal disease or patients on dialysis	C

(continued)

Table 6.1 (continued)

Metformin formulations	Available strengths	Extended or immediate release	Can be cut?	Dosing interval	Maximum therapeutic effect (time)	Maximum daily dose (MDD)	Renal dose adjustments (mL/min/1.73 m²)	Hepatic dose adjustments	Contraindications	Pregnancy category
Metformin & Empagliflozin (Synjardy)	500 mg/5 mg 1000 mg/5 mg 500 mg/12.5 mg 1,000 mg/12.5 mg	Immediate release	Yes	b.i.d.	Metformin: 4–6 weeks Empagliflozin: 2 weeks	Metformin 2,000 mg/d Empagliflozin 25mg/d	See metformin above Empagliflozin: eGFR ≥45: No dosage adjustment necessary. Monitor renal function at least annually eGFR <45: Do not use	See metformin above	See metformin above Hypersensitivity to empagliflozin eGFR <45, end-stage renal disease or patients on dialysis	C
Metformin Extended Release & Empagliflozin (Synjardy XR)	1,000 mg XR/5 mg 1,000 mg XR/10 mg 1,000 mg XR/12.5 mg 1,000 mg XR/25 mg	Extended release	Do not crush, cut, or chew	Once daily	Metformin: 4–6 weeks Empagliflozin: 2 weeks	Metformin 2,000 mg/d Empagliflozin 25 mg/d	See metformin above Empagliflozin: eGFR ≥45: No dosage adjustment necessary. Monitor renal function at least annually eGFR <45: Do not use	See metformin above	See metformin above Hypersensitivity to empagliflozin eGFR <45, end-stage renal disease or patients on dialysis	C

(continued)

Table 6.1 (continued)

Metformin formulations	Available strengths	Extended or immediate release	Can be cut?	Dosing interval	Maximum therapeutic effect (time)	Maximum daily dose (MDD)	Renal dose adjustments (mL/min/1.73 m²)	Hepatic dose adjustments	Contraindications	Pregnancy category
Metformin & Sulfonylurea										
Metformin & Glipizide (Metaglip) Generics	250 mg/2.5 mg 500 mg/2.5 mg 500 mg/5 mg	Immediate release	Yes	b.i.d.	Metformin: 4–6 weeks Glipizide: 2 weeks	Metformin 2,000 mg/d Glipizide 10 mg/d	See metformin above Glipizide: ERSD start with 2.5mg and titrate accordingly	See metformin above	See metformin above Hypersensitivity to glipizide eGFR <30	C
Metformin & Glyburide (Glucovance) Generic	500 mg/2.5 mg 500 mg/5 mg	Immediate release	Yes	b.i.d.	Metformin: 4–6 weeks Glyburide: 2 weeks	Metformin 2,000 mg/d Glyburide 10 mg/d	See metformin above Do not use glyburide in chronic kidney disease	See metformin above	See metformin above Hypersensitivity to glyburide eGFR <30 Concomitant administration of bosentan	C
Metformin & Thiazolidinediones										
Metformin & Pioglitazone (Actoplus Met)	500 mg/15 mg 850 mg/15 mg	Immediate release	Yes	Once daily or b.i.d.	Metformin: 4–6 weeks Pioglitazone: 3–6 months	Metformin 2,000 mg/d Pioglitazone 45 mg/d	See metformin above	See metformin above Do not initiate if ALT > 2.5 times the ULN at baseline; If ALT levels persist above three times the ULN during therapy, discontinue use	See metformin above Hypersensitivity to pioglitazone NYHA Class III or IV heart failure	C Pioglitazone may cause ovulation in anovulatory premenopausal women, increasing the risk of unintended pregnancy

(continued)

Table 6.1 (continued)

Metformin formulations	Available strengths	Extended or immediate release	Can be cut?	Dosing interval	Maximum therapeutic effect (time)	Maximum daily dose (MDD)	Renal dose adjustments (mL/min/1.73 m²)	Hepatic dose adjustments	Contraindications	Pregnancy category
Metformin Extended Release & Pioglitazone (Actoplus Met XR)	1,000 mg XR/15 mg 1,000 mg XR/30 mg	Extended release	Do not crush, cut, or chew	Once daily	Metformin: 4–6 weeks Pioglitazone: 3–6 months	Metformin 2,000 mg/d Pioglitazone 45mg/d	See metformin above	See metformin above Do not initiate if ALT > 2.5 times the ULN at baseline; if ALT levels persist above three times the ULN during therapy, discontinue use	See metformin above Hypersensitivity to pioglitazone NYHA Class III or IV heart failure	C Pioglitazone may cause ovulation in anovulatory premenopausal women, increasing the risk of unintended pregnancy

ALT, alanine aminotransferase; ULN, upper limit of normal; NYHA, New York Heart Association.

may be useful. Table 6.1 provides a list of the currently available combination antihyperglycemic medications containing metformin, their current brand name information, and selected dose or formulation information.

BIGUANIDES

Metformin (Glucophage) and Metformin XR (Glucophage XR): https://dailymed. nlm.nih.gov/dailymed/drugInfo.cfm?setid=4a0166c7-7097-4e4a-9036-6c9a60d08fc6

REFERENCES

1. Glucophage—4079189 [package insert]. Princeton, NJ, Bristol-Myers Squibb Company, 2018, https://packageinserts.bms.com/pi/pi_glucophage.pdf

2. Morley LC, Tang T, Yasmin E, et al. Insulin sensitising drugs (metformin, rosiglitazone, pioglitzaone, D-chiro-inositol) for women with polycystic ovary syndrome, oligo amenorrhoea and subfertility. *Cochrane Database Syst Rev* 2017;11:CDO03053. DOI:10.1002/14651858.CD003053.pub6

3. Yang PK, Hsu CY, Chen MJ, et al. The efficacy of 24-month metformin for improving menses, hormones, and metabolic profiles in polycystic ovary syndrome. *J Clin Endocrinol Metab* 2018;103:890–899

4. Knowler WC, Barrett-Connor E, Fowler SE, et al. Reduction in the incidence of type 2 diabetes with lifestyle intervention or metformin. *N Engl J Med* 2002;346(6):393–403

5. Diabetes Prevention Program Research Group, Knowler WC. 10-year follow-up of diabetes incidence and weight loss in the Diabetes Prevention Program Outcomes Study. *Lancet* 2009;374(9702):1677–1686

6. American Diabetes Association. 5. Prevention or delay of type 2 diabetes: *Standards of Medical Care in Diabetes—2018*. *Diabetes Care* 2018;41(Suppl. 1): S51–S54

7. Rowan JA, Hague WM, Gao W, et al. Metformin versus insulin for the treatment of gestational diabetes. *N Engl J Med* 2008;358:2003–2015

8. Nicholson W, Bolen S, Witkop CT, et al. Benefits and risks of oral diabetes agents compared with insulin in women with gestational diabetes: a systematic review. *Obstet Gynecol* 2009;113:193–205

9. Dhulkotia JS, Ola B, Fraser R, Farrell T. Oral hypoglycemic agents vs insulin in management of gestational diabetes: a systematic review and meta-analysis. *Am J Obstet Gynecol* 2010;203(5):457.e1–9

10. Balsells M, García-Patterson A, Solà I, et al. Glibenclamide, metformin, and insulin for the treatment of gestational diabetes: a systematic review and meta-analysis. *BMJ* 2015;350:h102

11. Jiang YF, Chen XY, Ding T, et al. Comparative efficacy and safety of OADs in management of GDM: network meta-analysis of randomized controlled trials. *J Clin Endocrinol Metab* 2015;100:2017–2080

12. Finneran MM, Landon MB. Oral agents for the treatment of gestational diabetes. *Curr Diab Rep* 2018;18(11):119

13. Patti AM, Giglio RV, Pafili K, Rizzo M, Papanas N. Pharmacotherapy for gestational diabetes. *Expert Opin Pharmacother* 2018;19(13):1407–1414.

14. Martis R, Crowther CA, Shepherd E, Alsweiler J, Downie MR, Brown J. Treatments for women with gestational diabetes mellitus: an overview of Cochrane systematic reviews. *Cochrane Database Syst Rev* 2018;8:CD012327

15. Priya G, Kaira S. Metformin in the managements of diabetes during pregnancy and lactation. *Drugs Context* 2018;7:212523

16. UK Prospective Diabetes Study (UKPDS) Group. Effect of intensive blood-glucose control with metformin on complications in overweight patients with type 2 diabetes (UKPDS 34). *Lancet* 1998;352(9131):854–865

17. Holman RR, Paul SK, Bethel A, Matthews DR, Neil HA. 10-year follow-up of intensive glucose control in type 2 diabetes. *N Engl J Med* 2008;359(15):1577–1589

18. Rojas LB, Gomez MB. Metformin: an old but still the best treatment for type 2 diabetes. *Diabetol Metab Syndr* 2013;5:6

19. Selvin E, Bolen S, Yeh HC, et al. Cardiovascular outcomes in trials of oral diabetes medications: a systematic review. *Arch Int Med* 2008;168:2070–2080

20. MacDonald MR, Eurich DT, Majumdar S, et al. Treatment of type 2 diabetes and outcomes in patients with heart failure: a nested case–control study from the UK General Practice Research Database. *Diabetes Care* 2010;33:1213–1218

21. Tang YL, Zhu LH, Li Y, et al. Metformin use is associated with reduced incidence and improved survival of endometrial cancer: a meta-analysis. *BioMed Res Int* 2017;2017:5905384

22. Zhou PT, Li B, Liu FR, et al. Metformin is associated with survival benefit in pancreatic cancer patients with diabetes: a systematic review and meta-analysis. *Oncotarget* 2017;8(15):25422–25250

23. Zhou DC, Gong H, Chong-Qing T, et al. Prognostic significance of anti-diabetic medications in pancreatic cancer: a meta-analysis. *Oncotarget* 2017;8(37):62349–62357

24. Li X, Li T, Liu Z, et al. The effect of metformin on survival of patients with pancreatic cancer: a meta-analysis. *Sci Rep* 2017;7(1):5825

25. Jian-Yu E, Graber JM, Lu SE, et al. Effect of metformin and statin use on survival in pancreatic cancer patients: a systematic literature review and meta-analysis. *Curr Med Chem* 2018;25(22):2595–2607

26. Liu F, Yan L, Wang Z, et al. Metformin therapy and risk of colorectal adenomas and colorectal cancer in type 2 diabetes mellitus patients: a systematic review and meta-analysis. *Oncotarget* 2017;8(9):16017–16026

27. Du L, Wang M, Kang Y, et al. Prognostic role of metformin intake in diabetic patients with colorectal cancer: an updated qualitative evidence of cohort studies. *Oncotarget* 2017;8(16):26448–26459

28. Tian S, Lei HB, Liu YL, et al. The association between metformin use and colorectal cancer survival among patients with diabetes mellitus: an updated meta-analysis. *Chronic Dis Trans Med* 2017;3(3):169–175

29. Chen CB, Eskin M, Eurich DT, et al. Metformin, Asian ethnicity and risk of prostate cancer in type 2 diabetes: a systematic review and meta-analysis. *BMC Cancer* 2018;18(1):65

30. Zhou XL, Xue WH, Ding XF, et al. Association between metformin and the risk of gastric cancer in patients with type 2 diabetes mellitus: a meta-analysis of cohort studies. *Oncotarget* 2017;8(33):55622–55631

31. Giovannucci E, Harlan DM, Archer MC, et al. Diabetes and cancer: a consensus report. *CA Cancer J Clin* 2010;60:207–221

32. Cao X, Wen ZS, Wang XD, et al. The clinical effect of metformin on the survival of lung cancer patients with diabetes: a comprehensive systematic review and meta-analysis of retrospective studies. *J Cancer* 2017;8(13):2532–2541

33. Metformin in Longevity Study (MILES) [Internet], 2018. Available from https://clinicaltrials.gov/ct2/show/study/NCT02432287

34. Targeting Aging with Metformin (TAME) [Internet]. Available from American Federation for Aging Research, https://www.afar.org/natgeo/

35. FDA Drug Safety Communication: FDA revises warnings regarding use of the diabetes medicine metformin in certain patients with reduced kidney function. U.S. Food and Drug Administration, April 2017. Available from https://www.fda.gov/Drugs/DrugSafety/ucm493244.htm

36. Mills EP, Brown KPD, Smith JD, et al. Treating nonalcoholic fatty liver disease in patients with type 2 diabetes mellitus: a review of efficacy and safety. *Ther Adv Endocrinol Metab* 2018;9(1):15–28. Published online 2017 Dec 7. DOI:10.1177/2042018817741852

37. de Jager J, Kooy A, Lehert P, et al. Long term treatment with metformin in patients with type 2 diabetes and risk of vitamin B-12 deficiency: randomised placebo controlled trial. *BMJ* 2010;340:c2181

38. Glucovance [package insert]. Princeton, NJ, Bristol-Myers Squibb Company, 2017. Available from https://packageinserts.bms.com/pi/pi_glucovance.pdf

39. Salpeter SR, Greyber E, Pasternak GA, Salpeter EE. Risk of fatal and non-fatal lactic acidosis with metformin use in type 2 diabetes mellitus. *Arch Intern Med* 2003;163:2594–2602

40. Salpeter SR, Greyber E, Pasternak GA, Salpeter EE. Risk of fatal and non-fatal lactic acidosis with metformin use in type 2 diabetes mellitus. *Cochrane Database Syst Rev* 2010(4):CD002967. DOI:10.1002/14651858.CD002967.pub4

41. Bodmer M, Meier C, Krähenbühl S, et al. Metformin, sulfonylureas, or other antidiabetes drugs and the risk of lactic acidosis or hypoglyemia. *Diabetes Care* 2008;31:2086–2091

42. Scheen AJ, Ferreira Alves de Magalhaes AC, Salvatore T, et al. Reduction of the acute bioavailability of metformin by the alpha-glucosidase inhibitor acarbose in normal man. *Eur J Clin Invest* 1993;23(1):A43

Chapter 7
Thiazolidinediones

KAM L. CAPOCCIA, PHARMD, BCPS, CDE
JENNIFER DANIELSON, PHARMD, CDE
PEGGY SOULE ODEGARD, BSPHARM, PHARMD, CDE

INTRODUCTION

The first thiazolidinedione (TZD), ciglitazone, was synthesized in 1982. It was soon thereafter discovered that ciglitazone reduced insulin resistance in obese and diabetic animals. Because of their effects on insulin resistance, TZDs have been developed as pharmacological agents for the management of T2D, although they were initially synthesized as potential lipid-reducing agents. Since their discovery, three TZDs have been introduced to the market in the U.S.: troglitazone (Rezulin), rosiglitazone (Avandia), and pioglitazone (Actos). In 2013, the FDA removed the Risk Evaluation and Mitigation Strategy (REMS) program and lifted restrictions on prescribing and dispensing rosiglitazone after concluding that data did not show a higher risk of heart attack with rosiglitazone compared with the standard T2D drugs of metformin and sulfonylurea. Currently, pioglitazone and rosiglitazone are available.

These compounds are taken orally and are unrelated to the other oral antihyperglycemic agents either chemically or by mechanism of action. A thiazolidine-2-4-dione structure is common to these drugs, with differences in potency, receptor binding, metabolic effects, pharmacokinetics, and side effects, governed by modifications in the side chain.[1,2]

Figure 7.1—Thiazolidine-2-4-dione structure.

TZDs have been used in the management of T2D as monotherapeutic agents and in combination with insulin, GLP-1 RAs, and other oral antihyperglycemic agents (metformin, DPP-4 inhibitors, SGLT2 inhibitors, meglitinides, and sulfonylureas). Additionally, they have been studied and found to be effective in treating insulin-resistant women with PCOS, nonalcoholic fatty liver disease, as well as having beneficial effects in some cardiovascular conditions. TZDs are sometimes referred to as "insulin sensitizers."

PHARMACOLOGY

MECHANISM OF ACTION

The relative importance of the mechanisms of action of TZDs are related to their effects on gene regulation. The primary mechanism of action appears to be the direct stimulation of a family of receptors on the nuclear surface of cells that are responsible for the modulation of lipid homeostasis, adipocyte differentiation, and insulin action. TZDs are potent and highly selective agonists for one of the isoforms in this family of receptors, known as peroxisome proliferator-activated receptor γ (PPARγ), which is predominantly expressed in white adipose tissue but also found in brown adipose tissue, muscle, kidney, liver, pancreatic β-cells, vascular endothelium, and macrophages. The TZDs also display some cross-reactivity with other isoforms in the PPAR family; PPARα (alpha), which is found in the liver, cardiac, and skeletal muscle, and PPARβ/δ (beta/delta), which is found in the liver, skeletal muscle, kidney, intestines, and esophagus. The effects of TZDs on PPARα and PPAR β/δ on human tissues remain unclear. Different relative affinities of pioglitazone and rosiglitazone for these three receptor types may explain the different effects that these two agents have on lipid profiles and other organ systems in the body.

These drugs improve glycemic control by increasing insulin sensitivity. PPARγ is the most important of these three receptors in terms of the antihyperglycemic action of TZDs. A relationship between the ability to stimulate PPARγ and antihyperglycemic activity is well understood. TZDs stimulate the expression of genes responsible for the production of glucose transporters (GLUT1 and GLUT4). PPARγ stimulation reduces TNF-α (tumor necrosis factor alpha), resulting in an anti-inflammatory effect and reducing hepatic glucokinase expression, which improves glucose homeostasis.

TZDs cause a reduction in the number of large adipocytes and an increase in the number of small adipocytes, leading to lower free fatty acid and triglyceride levels. PPARγ in the muscle and liver accounts for improved insulin sensitivity and glucose metabolism. The pleiotropic effects and implications of the TZDs have been described in the literature. Pioglitazone has been shown to improve endothelial dysfunction and improve dyslipidemia. Notably, there is a difference on cardiovascular outcomes favoring pioglitazone over rosiglitazone.[3] The cardiovascular data describing these differences is discussed further in this chapter.

PHARMACOKINETICS

Pioglitazone

Following the administration of pioglitazone, C_{max} occurs within approximately 2 h. Food may delay the absorption rate and time to C_{max} but not the extent of absorption. Pioglitazone may be taken without regard to meals. It is extensively bound, primarily to albumin (>99%), and its metabolites M-III and M-IV are >98% bound. The apparent mean volume of distribution (Vd) is 0.63 ±0.41 L/kg. Pioglitazone is extensively metabolized via oxidation and hydroxylation, with metabolites being partially converted to glucuronide or sulfate conjugates. Metabolites M-III (keto derivatives) and M-IV (hydroxy derivatives), along with parent pioglitazone, are the predominant species found in human serum at steady state. Approximately 15–30% of pioglitazone can be recovered in the urine and feces following oral administration. The mean serum half-lives of pioglitazone and pioglitazone metabolites are 3–7 h and 16–24 h, respectively. Pioglitazone clearance is 5–7 L/h.[1]

Rosiglitazone

Following the administration of rosiglitazone, C_{max} occurs within 1 h. Food may delay the absorption rate and time to C_{max}, but the extent of absorption is not clinically significantly changed. Rosiglitazone may be taken without regard to meals. It is extensively bound to serum protein (>99.8%), primarily albumin. The apparent mean volume of distribution (Vd) was 17.6 L/kg. Rosiglitazone is extensively metabolized via N-demethylation and hydroxylation, followed by conjugation with glucuronic acid or sulfate. No unchanged drug is found in the urine. The metabolites of rosiglitazone are less potent than the parent compound and are not thought to contribute to the insulin-sensitizing effects of the drug. After administration of labeled rosiglitazone, ~64% is eliminated via the urine and 23% is eliminated via the feces. The serum half-life for rosiglitazone is 3–4 h, which is prolonged by approximately 2 h in patients with moderate-to-severe hepatic impairment. Rosiglitazone clearance is ~3 L/h.[2]

While the serum half-lives of pioglitazone and rosiglitazone are several hours, the onset of action and duration of effect is delayed due to their mechanism of action. The initial effect on glucose may be seen within a few weeks but it could take upward of a few months to see the maximum effect of these drugs, due to the time intensive mechanism of altering gene expression. Similarly, when these drugs are discontinued, there is a delayed effect on the subsequent rise in glucose.

TREATMENT ADVANTAGES/DISADVANTAGES

As a class, the TZDs are effective in reducing hyperglycemia in patients with T2D. Reductions in hyperglycemia vary significantly between patients. Some researchers have even suggested the terms "responders" and "non-responders" in the population of patients treated with TZDs. A1C lowering can be expected to fall somewhere between 0.5 and 1.5% in most patients. There is no difference between pioglitazone and rosiglitazone in their glucose-lowering effects.

The advantage of the TZDs is predominantly the durability of their insulin-sensitizing effects. Regardless of the amount of insulin secretion in the body, the TZDs still work to decrease peripheral insulin resistance, while other oral antihyperglycemic agents (sulfonylureas, meglitinides) are dependent on insulin secretion and therefore ineffective when the pancreas is no longer secreting insulin. TZDs enhance insulin sensitivity through a variety of mechanisms in multiple tissues (adipose, liver, muscle). As a result, they are valuable agents in the management of metabolic syndrome, due to the underlying cause of insulin resistance.

TZDs have positive effects on the pancreatic β-cell through increased insulin capacity and protection from oxidative stress. They have been shown to improve or preserve β-cell function. The Diabetes Reduction Assessment With Ramipril and Rosiglitazone Medication (DREAM) study showed a 62% reduction in the development of T2D followed for a median of 3 years, while the Actos Now for the Prevention of Diabetes (ACT NOW) study showed a 72% reduction in the development of diabetes with a median follow-up of 2.4 years.[4,5] These studies demonstrated the preservation of β-cell function as well as the insulin-sensitizing effects of TZDs. This class of drugs is useful if metformin is contraindicated or cannot be used and an insulin-sensitizing agent is needed. TZDs are also beneficial if trying to reduce the risk of hypoglycemia or in those occupations that preclude the use of insulin.

The expression of PPARγ in the kidneys may account for the renal benefits seen with TZDs. Pioglitazone and rosiglitazone have shown reductions in albuminuria in people with T2D.[6,7] In hemodialysis patients, those treated with TZDs and/or insulin experienced a reduction in all-cause mortality compared to those treated with other oral agents.[8]

The expression of PPAR in the liver likely accounts for the benefits seen with TZDs in people with T2D and nonalcoholic fatty liver disease (NAFLD). Improvements in fibrosis and resolution of nonalcoholic steatohepatitis (NASH) have been shown with both rosiglitazone and pioglitazone. Continued use of these agents is necessary to sustain these results.[9]

Rosiglitazone and pioglitazone have different effects on lipid profiles. This difference may be related to the relative effect of these agents on the PPARγ nuclear receptor. Pioglitazone has a higher affinity for PPARγ and is associated with improvements in the lipid profile (reduction of triglycerides, increase in HDL-C, and neutral effect on LDL-C). On the other hand, rosiglitazone raises LDL-C levels and the reduction in triglycerides and increase in HDL-C is less than that seen with pioglitazone.

There have been numerous publications with conflicting results suggesting that rosiglitazone is associated with an increased risk of myocardial infarction (MI) and other cardiovascular events. However, several studies have shown that rosiglitazone does not increase cardiovascular mortality or all-cause mortality. In the Rosiglitazone Evaluated for Cardiovascular Outcomes in Oral Agents Combination Therapy for Type 2 Diabetes (RECORD) trial, the primary study endpoint was hospitalization for acute MI, CHF, stroke, unstable angina, transient ischemic attack, unplanned revascularization, amputation of extremities, or any other definitive cardiovascular reason, or cardiovascular mortality. In 4,447 patients with T2D, rosiglitazone was added to metformin or sulfonylurea and compared to a control group of metformin plus sulfonylurea with dose titration to a target A1C of ≤7%. The incidence of HF was greater with rosiglitazone (2.7% compared to control 1.3%, HR 2.10 [CI 1.35–3.27]), but there were no statistically significant differences between rosiglitazone and control groups for MI, stroke, or death.[10] According to a meta-analysis by Mannucci and colleagues, there was no increase in all-cause or cardiovascular mortality observed with rosiglitazone. However, when rosiglitazone was combined with insulin, there was an increased risk of CHF (OR 2.20 [CI 1.28–3.78]).[11] Postmarketing studies indicate the risk of CHF is higher in patients taking TZDs, even with no previously known heart disease. Although change in mortality has not been found to be significant, patients with history of cardiovascular disease, especially those aged 65 years and over, were found to have higher incidence of serious HF requiring hospitalization when taking TZDs.[12–14]

Pioglitazone has been shown to reduce cardiovascular event rates in the PROspective pioglitAzone Clinical Trial In macroVascular Events (PROactive) trial, a large, prospective, randomized, placebo-controlled outcome trial. The study enrolled 5,238 patients with T2D who had a history of a previous cardiovascular event or multiple risk factors for cardiovascular disease. The primary outcome was a composite of seven different cardiovascular endpoints; a 10% reduction was observed but it did not reach statistical significance ($P = 0.09$). However, there was a statistically significant 16% decrease in the secondary endpoint of all-cause mortality, myocardial infarction, and stroke. Pioglitazone was titrated from 15 mg to 45 mg in more than 90% of the patients, compared with at least 95% of those on placebo who reached the maximum dose. Since its original publication in 2005, there have been 19 additional publications from the PROactive investigators describing various subanalyses. Of note, PROactive 04 described a 47% reduction in the incidence of recurrent stroke (HR 0.53 [95% CI 0.34–0.85]; $P = 0.008$).[15,16]

In the Insulin Resistance Intervention After Stroke (IRIS) trial, pioglitazone demonstrated a decreased risk of recurring stroke or transient ischemic attack in people with insulin resistance who did not have diabetes.[17] A meta-analysis by Lee and colleagues describes three randomized trials of pioglitazone use in stroke patients with insulin resistance, prediabetes, and diabetes.[18] Although there was no evidence of an effect on all-cause mortality, pioglitazone was associated with lower risk of recurrent stroke (HR 0.68 [CI 0.50–0.92]; $P = 0.01$) and a lower risk of future vascular events (HR 0.75 [CI 0.64–0.87]; $P = 0.0001$).[17,18] In the RECORD trial, there was a nonsignificant reduction in stroke events when rosiglitazone was added to either metformin or sulfonylurea compared to the metformin-sulfonylurea combination group.[19]

The disadvantages of TZDs are related to the side-effect profile of this class of drugs and likely outweigh the benefits for the majority of patients. This class of drugs is contraindicated in patients with NYHA class III or IV HF. Fluid retention leading to weight gain and peripheral edema may cause or exacerbate CHF. TZDs should not be used in anyone with a history of or active bladder cancer. They also increase the risk of fractures in postmenopausal women and elderly men and therefore should be avoided in these populations. These side effects are further described below in the "Significant Warnings/Precautions" section.

Generally speaking, the use of pioglitazone is favored over rosiglitazone due to its beneficial effects on the lipid profile, in NAFLD, at lower doses, as well as its cardiovascular benefit and decreasing the risk of recurring stroke or TIA. Due to its pleiotropic effects that improve endothelial dysfunction, improve pancreatic β-cell function, reduce blood pressure, improve dyslipidemia, reduce proteinuria, and reduce circulating levels of inflammatory cytokines, pioglitazone is the preferred TZD.[20] Lower doses (7.5–15 mg) have demonstrated fewer side effects with significant improvements in A1C reduction, fasting plasma glucose, PPG, lipid profiles, pancreatic β-cell function, and insulin resistance.[21-24] The addition of low-dose pioglitazone could be incredibly helpful to an obese person who has diabetes and a significant degree of insulin resistance. The low dose may avoid the unwanted side effects of weight gain and fluid retention, while potentially decreasing negative cardiovascular outcomes and the amount of or need for insulin or other medicines for T2D, while improving glucose homeostasis and reducing A1C.

THERAPEUTIC CONSIDERATIONS

SIGNIFICANT WARNINGS/PRECAUTIONS

T1D

These agents should not be used to treat people with T1D or to manage patients in diabetic ketoacidosis.

Hypoglycemia

The risk of hypoglycemia is increased when a TZD is combined with another agent known to cause hypoglycemia such as insulin or sulfonylureas. A decrease in dose of insulin and/or sulfonylurea will likely be necessary to reduce the risk of hypoglycemia.

Ovulation

TZDs may cause resumption of ovulation in premenopausal women with anovulation secondary to insulin resistance. These patients may be at risk for unintended pregnancy. Contraception is recommended in these premenopausal women. TZDs have been studied as a treatment for anovulation in women with PCOS and have been shown to be effective. However, they are no longer recommended as first-line agents due to weight gain and increased risk of fractures.

Hematology

Dose-related reductions in hemoglobin and hematocrit have been observed in patients treated with pioglitazone and rosiglitazone. Reductions in hemoglobin and hematocrit with the TZDs are ≤4% and ≤1 g/dL, respectively. These changes are possibly due to volume expansion and have not been associated with significant hematological effects. The changes occur within the first 4–8 weeks of therapy and remain unchanged thereafter.

Weight Gain and Edema

Dose-related weight gain is the most common side effect of the TZDs. Pioglitazone and rosiglitazone typically cause weight gain of 1–5 kg when used as monotherapy, in combination with oral antihyperglycemic agents, or in combination with insulin. The mechanism of weight gain is not entirely clear but is likely related to the activation of the PPARγ receptors in adipose tissue, resulting in an increase of deposition, and in the kidney, resulting in the retention of salt and water. Edema, fluid retention, and weight gain are problematic in coexisting CHF and require increased patient monitoring. Of note, there is a favorable shift of fat accumulation from visceral to subcutaneous.

Cardiac

The prescribing information for rosiglitazone and pioglitazone includes a black box warning regarding CHF. TZDs are contraindicated in patients with NYHA class III or IV failure. Use of TZDs is not recommended in patients with symptomatic HF. Fluid retention may lead to or exacerbate CHF. Patients should be observed for signs and symptoms of CHF. If CHF develops, it should be managed according to current standards of care and discontinuation or dose reduction of TZDs must be considered.

Hepatic

No evidence of hepatotoxicity has been observed with either rosiglitazone or pioglitazone. In the phase 3 trials of rosiglitazone, 0.2% of patients treated with rosiglitazone had reversible elevations in alanine transaminase (ALT) greater than three times the upper limit of normal (ULN), compared with 0.2% of patients treated with placebo. In the phase 3 trials of pioglitazone, 0.26% of patients treated with pioglitazone had reversible elevations in ALT greater than three times the ULN, compared with 0.25% of patients treated with placebo. Because of the association between the first-marketed TZD (troglitazone) and fulminate hepatic failure, patients treated with TZDs should have their liver function tested prior to initiation of therapy and periodically thereafter. Troglitazone was removed from the market, leaving behind the concern that the hepatotoxic reaction might be a class effect. Although this concern has not been supported by data from the legions of patients treated with pioglitazone and rosiglitazone, testing is still recommended. Current recommendations state to test liver enzymes prior to initiation and periodically thereafter. Evaluate patients with ALT ≥2.5 times ULN at baseline or during therapy for cause of enzyme elevation. If ALT levels remain greater than three times ULN, therapy should be discontinued.

Bladder Cancer

Pioglitazone should not be used in patients with active or a history of bladder cancer. Associations between cumulative dose or cumulative duration of exposure to pioglitazone and bladder cancer have been unfounded. In the 10-year observational follow-up of patients completing PROactive, bladder cancer was reported in 0.8% of patients ($n = 14$) in the pioglitazone versus 1.2% ($n = 21$) in the placebo group [RR 0.65 [95% CI 0.33–1.28]).[25] Inconsistent findings and limitations inherent in these and other studies preclude conclusive interpretations of the observational data.[1]

Fractures

TZDs have demonstrated an increased incidence of bone fractures, especially peripheral factures in women. In the ADOPT and RECORD trials, rosiglitazone demonstrated an increased risk of limb fractures in the first year of treatment that persisted for the length of the trials.[2] In the PROactive trial, pioglitazone demonstrated an increased incidence of bone fracture in women of 5.1% (44/870) vs. 2.5% (23/905) for the placebo group. Fracture risk in men did not differ between the two groups.[15] Although the majority of data has demonstrated an increased risk of fracture in older women, men and younger patients may be susceptible as well. The mechanism is not entirely clear but studies have shown a change in bone mineral density and changes in biochemical markers of bone turnover.[26] Overall, TZDs should not be used in patients who are at an increased risk of fracture.

Pregnancy and Nursing

Pioglitazone and rosiglitazone cross the placenta and are classified as pregnancy category C in all trimesters. It is unknown if TZDs are excreted in breast milk. Therefore, breast-feeding women should not take TZDs as the current evidence is inconclusive.

SPECIAL POPULATIONS

TZDs are not recommended as first-line agents in the treatment of T2D. However, they are used as dual- or triple-combination therapy for the management of T2D and continue to be studied for new applications and potential effectiveness in the treatment of other conditions and diseases.[27] The various cellular effects of TZDs have led to the evaluation in acromegaly, Alzheimer's, Cushing syndrome, mental health disorders, erectile dysfunction (ED), Huntington's, NASH, Parkinson's, PCOS, polycystic kidney disease, and psoriasis. The following information includes human, clinical trials involving pioglitazone or rosiglitazone and is not intended to be all-inclusive. Pioglitazone and rosiglitazone are not FDA approved for any of the following conditions discussed below.[28]

NAFLD

NAFLD is a frequent comorbidity in patients with T2D and obesity. These patients are at an even higher risk of the aggressive liver disease NASH, end-stage liver disease, cirrhosis, hepatocellular carcinoma, and death. The treatment of NAFLD/NASH focuses on the underlying pathology of insulin resistance and dysfunctional adipose tissue that leads to hepatocyte toxicity. The insulin-sensitizing properties of the TZDs are responsible for the beneficial effects seen with this class of drugs. A recent review by Mills and colleagues evaluated the literature on the safety and efficacy of treatment for NAFLD in T2D. They evaluated 23 studies involving metformin, TZDs, statins, and GLP-1 RAs for the treatment of NAFLD. All of the treatment options were safe. TZDs had positive results on fibrosis and resolution of NASH, while the GLP-1 RAs and metformin did not improve fibrosis.[9] Authors Davidson and Pan are calling for the resurrection of the use of pioglitazone due to the small number needed to treat for benefit (2–12) of histological improvement and radiological resolution of NASH based on their findings in the meta-analysis of epidemiological studies.[29] In the clinical practice guidelines for the management of NAFLD by the American Association for the Study of Liver Disease (AASLD), and in the guidelines by the European Associations for the Study of the Liver, Diabetes, and Obesity (EASL, EASD, EASO), pioglitazone is considered an option for treatment of NAFLD.[30,31]

PCOS

Rosiglitazone and pioglitazone have been studied in PCOS because of their insulin-sensitizing properties. Despite positive results, these agents are not commonly used or recommended due to adverse effects, concerns of weight gain, and increased risk of fractures in women.[32]

Secondary Stroke Prevention

The IRIS trial reported that treatment of insulin resistance with pioglitazone (median daily dose each year ranged 29–40 mg) significantly reduced recurrent stroke or MI by 24% compared to placebo (pioglitazone 9.0% vs. placebo 11.8%; HR 0.76 [95% CI 0.62–0.93]; P = 0.007) in 3,876 patients who had a recent (<6 months) history of ischemic stroke or transient ischemic attack and insulin resistance without diabetes, HF, or bladder cancer. There was no difference in all-cause mortality between the pioglitazone and placebo groups. Pioglitazone was associated with greater frequency of weight gain (52.2% vs. 33.7%, P < 0.001), edema (35.6% vs. 24.9%, P < 0.001), and bone fracture requiring surgery or hospitalization (5.1% vs. 3.2%, P = 0.003) compared to placebo, respectively. The pioglitazone group was also associated with a lower risk of diabetes (3.8% vs. 7.7%; HR 0.48 [95% CI 0.33–0.69]; P < 0.001).[17] This study demonstrates the vascular benefits of pioglitazone in a specific subset of patients without diabetes who have insulin resistance. It also demonstrated a lower risk of T2D. The potential impact of pioglitazone in this trial on reducing the burden of stroke and reducing the burden of diabetes could have a global impact.

Bone Health

TZDs have demonstrated an increased incidence of bone fractures, especially peripheral factures in women. Rosiglitazone demonstrated an increased risk of limb fractures in the first year of treatment in the ADOPT and RECORD trials that persisted for the length of the trials.[2] In the PROactive trial, pioglitazone demonstrated an increased incidence of bone fracture in women of 5.1% (44/870) vs. 2.5% (23/905) for the placebo group.[15] Fracture risk in men did not differ between the two groups. Although the majority of data has demonstrated an increased risk of fracture in older women, men and younger patients may be susceptible as well. The mechanism is not entirely clear, but studies have shown a change in bone mineral density, inhibition of bone formation by PPAR-mediated diversion of mesenchymal progenitor cells into the adipocytes rather than osteoblasts, and changes in biochemical markers of bone turnover.[26] Overall, the TZDs should not be used in patients who are at an increased risk of fracture or have had a fracture.

Renal Impairment

Dose adjustments for rosiglitazone or pioglitazone are not required in patients with renal dysfunction or renal failure.

Hepatic Impairment

Patients with impaired hepatic function (Child-Pugh grade B/C) have a 45% reduction in pioglitazone and total pioglitazone mean peak concentrations, but no change in mean AUC when compared with normal subjects. In patients with impaired hepatic function (Child-Pugh grade B/C), C_{max} and AUC values for rosiglitazone were increased two- and threefold, respectively, and elimination half-life was increased by 2 h. Rosiglitazone and pioglitazone should not be used in patients with clinical evidence of active liver disease or with serum ALT concentrations greater than three times the ULN.

Pediatrics

Current use of TZDs in pediatrics is not recommended. No pharmacokinetic, safety, or efficacy data for TZDs is available in children.

Geriatrics

Age does not result in clinically significant changes in the effects or pharmacokinetics of rosiglitazone or pioglitazone. No dosage adjustment is needed in this population.

Sex

Rosiglitazone clearance was reported to be 6% lower in males than females of comparable body weight. In monotherapeutic trials with rosiglitazone, a slightly greater therapeutic response (quantitative differences were not reported) was observed in female patients, while no such difference was reported in metformin/rosiglitazone combination trials. Interestingly, sex-related differences were less marked in more obese patients. Women tend to have a greater fat mass than men for a given BMI. The sex-related differences in effect may be due to this difference in fat mass where the molecular target PPARγ is highly expressed in lipid tissue. Although there are slight differences in the effects of both rosiglitazone and pioglitazone in women, no dose adjustment is recommended. Treatment should be individualized for men and women.

Ethnicity

No differences in the effects of these agents have been observed in any ethnic group.

ADVERSE EFFECTS AND MONITORING

Weight Gain and Edema

Dose-related weight gain is the most common side effect of the TZDs. Pioglitazone and rosiglitazone typically cause weight gain of 1–5 kg when used as monotherapy, in combination with oral antihyperglycemic agents, and in combination with insulin. The mechanism of weight gain is not entirely clear but is likely related to the activation of the PPARγ receptors, resulting in an increase of adipose tissue deposition.

Dose-related edema can be seen with monotherapy, in combination with oral antihyperglycemic agents, and in combination with insulin. Although the mechanism of edema is not clearly understood, it may be due to the activation of the PPARγ receptors in the kidney, which results in the retention of salt and water. Edema, fluid retention, and weight gain are problematic in coexisting CHF and require increased patient monitoring. Rosiglitazone and pioglitazone are contraindicated in NHYA class III or IV HF and should be not be used in patients with symptomatic HF.

Anemia

Dose-related reductions in hemoglobin and hematocrit ($\leq 4\%$ and ≤ 1 g, respectively) have been observed in patients treated with pioglitazone or rosiglitazone. These changes are possibly due to volume expansion and have not been associated with significant hematological effects. The changes occur within the first 4–8 weeks of therapy and remain unchanged thereafter. These effects are usually mild and no routine monitoring for anemia is recommended.

Liver Function Abnormalities

Currently, it is recommended that patients treated with rosiglitazone or pioglitazone undergo serum transaminase monitoring at the initiation of therapy and periodically thereafter, based on the judgment of the clinician. Patients treated with rosiglitazone or pioglitazone who present with ALT levels greater than or equal to 2.5 times the ULN should have their ALT levels assessed with some frequency. Patients treated with rosiglitazone or pioglitazone who present with ALT levels greater than or equal to three times the ULN should have the level repeated and should discontinue the drug if the elevation persists.

Fractures

The risk of fracture should be considered in the care of patients treated with pioglitazone and rosiglitazone, and attention given to assessing and maintaining bone health according to current standards of care. The majority of the observed fractures in the trials were nonvertebral fractures including upper distal limb and lower limb.

Bladder Cancer Risk

Pioglitazone should not be used in patients with active or a history of bladder cancer. Associations between cumulative dose or cumulative duration of exposure to pioglitazone and bladder cancer were not detected in some studies, including the 10-year observational study in the U.S.[25] During the 13 years of both PROactive and observational follow-up, the occurrence of bladder cancer did not differ between patients randomized to pioglitazone or placebo (HR 1.00 [95% CI 0.59–1.72]). Inconsistent findings and limitations inherent in these and other studies preclude conclusive interpretations of the observational data.[1]

Ocular Effects

Rare cases of macular edema have been reported with the use of TZDs, frequently during concurrent peripheral edema. Patients should report any vision changes such as blurred vision or decreased visual acuity. Routine ophthalmological exams should be recommended to all patients with diabetes according to current guidelines.

DRUG INTERACTIONS

Cytochrome P450 enzymes play a role in the metabolism of the TZDs. Rosiglitazone is metabolized predominantly by CYP2C8 and to a lesser degree by CYP2C9. Pioglitazone is metabolized predominantly by CYP2C8 and to a lesser extent by CYP3A4. Inhibitors of CYP2C8 will decrease metabolism of rosiglitazone and pioglitazone and increase serum concentrations. Monitoring for increased hypoglycemia and dose reductions are often needed. CYP2C8 inhibitors include: abiraterone, clopidogrel, deferasirox, gemfibrozil, mifepristone, leflunomide, and teriflunomide. Inducers of CYP2C8 will increase metabolism of rosiglitazone and pioglitazone and thus decrease their effectiveness. Some of the CYP2C8 inducers include: lumacaftor, dabrafenib, ritodrine, and salicylates. In the case of salicylates, this interaction is more likely to occur at doses of 3 g per day or more. Clinical response to TZDs should be monitored when taken in combination with these other agents.

When taken with other antihyperglycemic agents, TZDs can enhance hypoglycemic effects. Risk of hypoglycemia is increased when taken in combination with other antihyperglycemic agents. Doses of the offending drugs may need to be reduced to avoid hypoglycemia.

When taken in combination with other drugs that have been associated with hyperglycemic effects (such as aripiprazole, atazanavir, bumetanide, cortisone, chlorthalidone, clozapine, dexamethasone, epinephrine, estradiol, estrogens, fosamprenavir, furosemide, methylprednisolone, olanzapine, prednisolone, prednisone, quetiapine, risperidone, ritonavir, saquinavir, tacrolimus, thiazide diuretics, torsemide, triamcinolone, ziprasidone), the effectiveness of TZDs can be reduced. The dose of rosiglitazone or pioglitazone may need to be increased to achieve desired effectiveness when taken in combination with these other agents.

When taken in combination with other drugs that have been associated with hypoglycemic effects (such as linezolid, selegiline, monoamine oxidase inhibitors like mebanazine or phenelzine, and serotonin reuptake inhibitors like citalopram, escitalopram, fluoxetine, paroxetine, or sertraline), the effectiveness of TZDs can be enhanced. Increased blood glucose testing should be performed, and the dose of rosiglitazone or pioglitazone may need to be decreased to avoid hypoglycemic effects.

ACE Inhibitors

ACE inhibitors may or may not enhance the hypoglycemic effects of TZDs. Case reports describe episodes of hypoglycemia after taking ACE inhibitors along with antihyperglycemic agents. However, published results are inconsistent and most often reported with sulfonylureas. No action is recommended to manage this potential interaction at this time.

Alpha-Lipoic Acid

Alpha-lipoic acid may enhance the effects of antihyperglycemic agents, including pioglitazone and rosiglitazone. Patients should be monitored closely for signs of hypoglycemia if taking α-lipoic acid with these agents. Intravenous formulations have a greater impact than oral formulations. The dose of rosiglitazone or pioglitazone may need to be reduced to avoid hypoglycemia.

Androgens

Androgen hormones such as fluoxymesterone, mesterolone, methyltestosterone, nandrolone, oxandrolone, oxymetholone, and testosterone may increase the hypoglycemia effect of antihyperglycemic agents like rosiglitazone and pioglitazone. Monitor patients closely for signs of hypoglycemia and reduce the dose of rosiglitazone or pioglitazone if such effects are seen.

Antifungals

Although the AUC of pioglitazone was increased by 34% in a single-dose study administered with ketoconazole, the kinetics of pioglitazone were unaffected when taken with itraconazole in another study.

Clopidogrel

In a study of healthy subjects, clopidogrel was found to significantly increase the AUC and half-life of pioglitazone. Monitor patients closely for increased pioglitazone effects such as hypoglycemia, edema, or hepatotoxicity.

Dabrafenib

Dabrafenib is a strong inducer of CYP2C8, which can decrease serum concentrations of pioglitazone and rosiglitazone. Product labeling recommends finding an alternative to these agents for glucose control in patients taking dabrafenib.

Digoxin

Rosiglitazone and pioglitazone do not alter the pharmacokinetics of digoxin.

Gemfibrozil

Three studies have shown that gemfibrozil increases serum concentrations of pioglitazone when taken together. The dose of pioglitazone should be limited to 15 mg per day when taken with gemfibrozil. Although specific dose limits are not listed, prescribing information for rosiglitazone recommends considering dose reductions when taken with gemfibrozil as well.

Guanethidine

Guanethidine may increase the hypoglycemia effect of antihyperglycemic agents like rosiglitazone and pioglitazone. Monitor patients closely for signs of hypoglycemia and reduce the dose of rosiglitazone or pioglitazone if such effects are seen.

Ethanol

No significant effect has been found between moderate amounts of ethanol and pioglitazone or rosiglitazone.

Leukotriene Receptor Antagonists

In vitro results suggest that leukotriene receptor antagonists may inhibit CYP2C8; however, no change in the kinetics of pioglitazone were seen in a study of 12 healthy subjects.

Oral Contraceptives

When pioglitazone was coadministered with a combination oral contraceptive (ethinyl estradiol/norethindrone) for 21 days, an 11% reduction in ethinyl estradiol AUC and an 11–14% reduction in ethinyl estradiol C_{max} values were reported. The clinical significance of this is unknown. Rosiglitazone has been shown to have no clinically significant effect on the pharmacokinetics of ethinyl estradiol or norethindrone.

Pregabalin

Pregabalin may enhance the fluid-retaining effect of TZDs. Patients taking pregabalin with either rosiglitazone or pioglitazone should be monitored closely for weight gain and edema. Take extra caution in using these agents together in patients at risk for HF.

Quinolones

Quinolone antibiotics may enhance or diminish the effects of blood glucose–lowering agents, such as TZDs. Monitor patients for hypo- or hyperglycemia when initiating a quinolone antibiotic in patients taking rosiglitazone or pioglitazone. Hypoglycemic effects are more likely to occur in the first few days of therapy, while hyperglycemia is at most risk after several days of therapy.

Rifampin

Rifampin has been shown in studies to decrease serum concentrations of both rosiglitazone and pioglitazone. Rifampin likely induces metabolism of these agents, and patients taking them should be monitored for reduced efficacy if therapy with rifampin is initiated.

Topiramate

Concomitant administration with topiramate was found in one study to decrease the serum concentration of pioglitazone. Hypokalemia also occurred when topiramate was added to pioglitazone therapy. Clinical significance of this interaction is uncertain, but glycemic control should be monitored in patients taking pioglitazone when topiramate is initiated.

Trimethoprim

The AUC of rosiglitazone was increased in a study of normal subjects after taking a single dose of rosiglitazone during day 3–4 of a course of trimethoprim therapy. This interaction is thought to be caused by inhibition of CYP2C8, and thus is possible to occur with pioglitazone as well. Monitor for increased effects of TZDs when initiating or discontinuing trimethoprim.

Warfarin

No significant effect has been found between warfarin and pioglitazone or rosiglitazone.

DOSAGE AND ADMINISTRATION

Maximum therapeutic results may not be fully observed for several weeks to months following initiation or change in dose of pioglitazone or rosiglitazone due to the time-intensive mechanism of altering gene expression.

Pioglitazone is available in 15-, 30-, and 45-mg tablets. Pioglitazone is given once daily in doses of 15, 30, or 45 mg. Usual initial doses are either 15 or 30 mg; maximum dose is 45 mg daily. Dose escalation is based on re-evaluation of A1C after 3 months of therapy at a given dose, unless rapid deterioration of glycemic control dictates otherwise. Pioglitazone may be given without regard to meals.

Rosiglitazone is given either once or twice daily, and is available in 2-, 4-, or 8-mg tablets. The typical starting dose is 4 mg daily as a single or divided dose. Dose escalations should be made at 8–12-week intervals. In phase 3 trials, the greatest response was observed in patients treated with 4 mg twice daily. The maximum daily dose is 8 mg.

Table 7.1—Thiazolidinediones

Thiazolidinediones	Available strengths	Can be cut?	Dosing interval	Maximum daily dose (MDD)	Maximum therapeutic effect (time)	Renal dose adjustments (mL/min/1.73 m²)	Hepatic dose adjustments	Contraindications	Pregnancy category
Rosiglitazone									
Avandia	2 mg, 4 mg, 8 mg	Yes	1 or 2 divided doses	8 mg/day	May take 3–6 months to see full effect	No dosage adjustment necessary	Do not initiate if ALT > 2.5 times the ULN at baseline; If ALT levels persist above three times the ULN during therapy, discontinue use	Hypersensitivity to rosiglitazone NYHA Class III or IV heart failure	C TZDs may cause ovulation in anovulatory premenopausal women, increasng the risk of unintended pregnancy
Pioglitazone									
Actos	15 mg, 30 mg, 45 mg	Yes	Once daily	45 mg/day	May take 3–6 months to see full effect	No dosage adjustment necessary	Do not initiate if ALT > 2.5 times the ULN at baseline; If ALT levels persist above three times the ULN during therapy, discontinue use	Hypersensitivity to pioglitazone NYHA Class III or IV heart failure	C TZDs may cause ovulation in anovulatory premenopausal women, increasing the risk of unintended pregnancy
Pioglitazone Combinations									
Pioglitazone & Alogliptan (Oseni)	15 mg/12.5 mg 15 mg/25 mg 30 mg/12.5 mg 30 mg/25 mg 45 mg/12.5 mg 45 mg/25 mg	Do not split tablets	Once daily	Pioglitazone 45 mg/day Alogliptan 25 mg/day	Pioglitazone: 3–6 months alogliptin: 2–4 weeks	eGFR >30 to <50: alogliptin 12.5 mg/day eGFR <30 do not use	Do not initiate if ALT > 2.5 times the ULN at baseline; If ALT levels persist above three times the ULN during therapy, discontinue use	Hypersensitivity to alogliptin or pioglitazone: NYHA Class III or IV heart failure	C TZDs may cause ovulation in anovulatory premenopausal women, increasing the risk of unintended pregnancy

(continued)

Table 7.1 (continued)

Thiazolidinediones	Available strengths	Can be cut?	Dosing interval	Maximum daily dose (MDD)	Maximum therapeutic effect (time)	Renal dose adjustments (mL/min/1.73 m²)	Hepatic dose adjustments	Contraindications	Pregnancy category
Pioglitazone & Glimerpiride (Duetact)	30 mg/2 mg 30 mg/4 mg	Yes	Once daily	Pio-glitazone 45 mg/day Glimepiride 8 mg/day	Pioglitazone: 3–6 months glimerpiride: 2 weeks	Starting dose of glimepiride in renal insufficiency is 1 mg p.o. daily. Do not use combination product unless dose has been titrated	Do not initiate if ALT > 2.5 times the ULN at baseline; If ALT levels persist above three times the ULN during therapy, discontinue use	Hypersensitivity to pioglitazone or glimepiride; history of allergic reaction to sulfonamide derivatives NYHA Class III or IV heart failure	C TZDs may cause ovulation in anovulatory premenopausal women, increasing the risk of unintended pregnancy
Pioglitazone & Metformin (Actoplus Met, Actoplus Met XR)	15 mg/500 mg 15 mg/850 mg XR: 15 mg/1,000 mg XR: 30 mg/1,000 mg	Do not crush, split, or chew XR formulation	Once daily or b.i.d.	Pio-glitazone 45 mg/day Metformin 2,000 mg/day	Pioglitazone: 3–6 months metformin: 4–6 weeks	eGFR 30–45: Do not initiate; if eGFR falls to <45, consider benefits/risks of continuing therapy eGFR <30: Do not use	Do not initiate if ALT > 2.5 times the ULN at baseline; If ALT levels persist above three times the ULN during therapy, discontinue use	Hypersensitivity to pioglitazone or metformin; NYHA Class III or IV heart failure; Lactic acidosis	C TZDs may cause ovulation in anovulatory premenopausal women, increasing the risk of unintended pregnancy

ALT, alanine aminotransferase; ULN, upper limit of normal; NYHA, New York Heart Association.

MONOGRAPHS

THIAZOLIDINEDIONES

Pioglitazone (Actos): https://dailymed.nlm.nih.gov/dailymed/drugInfo.cfm?setid=d2ddc491-88a9-4063-9150-443b4fa4330c

Rosiglitazone (Avandia): https://dailymed.nlm.nih.gov/dailymed/drugInfo.cfm?setid=ec682aec-e98f-41a1-9d21-eb7580ea3a8a

REFERENCES

1. Actos (pioglitazone) [package insert]. Deerfield, IL, Takeda Pharmaceuticals America, Inc., 2011. Available from https://www.accessdata.fda.gov/drugsatfda_docs/label/2011/021073s043s044lbl.pdf. Accessed 12 May 2018

2. Avandia (rosiglitazone) [package insert]. Research Triangle Park, NC, GlaxoSmithKline, 2016. Available from https://www.gsksource.com/pharma/content/dam/GlaxoSmithKline/US/en/Prescribing_Information/Avandia/pdf/AVANDIA-PI-MG.PDF. Accessed 12 May 2018

3. DeFronzo RA, Mehta RJ, Schnure JJ. Pleiotropic effects of thiazolidinediones: implications for the treatment of patients with type 2 diabetes mellitus. *Hosp Pract* 1995;41(2):132–147

4. The DREAM (Diabetes REduction Assessment with ramipril and rosiglitazone Medication) Trial Investigators. Effect of rosiglitazone on the frequency of diabetes in patients with impaired glucose tolerance or impaired fasting glucose: a randomized controlled trial. *Lancet* 2006;368:1096–1105

5. DeFronzo RA, Tripathy D, Schwenke DC, Banerji M, Bray GA, Buchanan TA, Clement SC, Henry RR, Hodis HN, Kitabchi AE, Mack WJ, Mudaliar S, Ratner RE, Williams K, Stentz FB, Musi N, Reaven PD; ACT NOW Study. Pioglitazone for diabetes prevention in impaired glucose tolerance. *N Engl J Med* 2011;364(12):1104–1115

6. Sarafidis PA, Stafylas PC, Georgianos PI, Saratzis AN, Lasaridis AN. Effect of thiazolidinediones on albuminuria and proteinuria in diabetes: a meta-analysis. *Am J Kidney Dis* 2010;55(5):835–847

7. Miyazaki Y, Cersosimo E, Triplitt C, DeFronzo RA. Rosiglitazone decreases albuminuria in type 2 diabetic patients. *Kidney Int* 2007;72(11):1367–1373

8. Brunelli SM, Thadhani R, Ikizler TA, Feldman HI. Thiazolidinedione use is associated with better survival in hemodialysis patients with non-insulin dependent diabetes. *Kidney Int* 2009;75(9):961–968

9. Mills EP, Brown KPD, Smith JD, Vang PW, Trotta K. Treating nonalcoholic fatty liver disease in patients with type 2 diabetes mellitus: a review of efficacy and safety. *Ther Adv Endocrinol Metab* 2018;9(1):15–28

10. Home PD, Pocock SJ, Beck-Nielsen H, Curtis PS, Gomis R, Hanefeld M, Jones NP, Komajda M, McMurray JJ; RECORD Study Team. Rosiglitazone evaluated for cardiovascular outcomes in oral agent combination therapy for type 2 diabetes (RECORD): a multicentre, randomised, open-label trial. *Lancet* 2009;373(9681):2125–2135

11. Mannucci E, Monami M, Di Bari M, Lamanna C, Gori F, Gensini GF, Marchionni N. Cardiac safety profile of rosiglitazone: a comprehensive meta-analysis of randomized clinical trials. *Int J Cardiology* 2010;143:135–140

12. Erdmann E, Charbonnel B, Wilcox RG, et al.; PROactive Investigators. Pioglitazone use and heart failure in patients with type 2 diabetes and pre-existing cardiovascular disease: data from the PROactive study (PROactive 08). *Diabetes Care* 2007;30:2773–2778

13. Nesto RW, Bell D, Bonow RO, et al. Thiazolidinedione use, fluid retention, and congestive heart failure: a consensus statement from the American Heart Association and the American Diabetes Association. *Circulation* 2003;108:2941–2948

14. Lago RM, Singh PP, Nesto RW. Congestive heart failure and cardiovascular death in patients with prediabetes and type 2 diabetes given thiazolidinediones: a meta-analysis of randomised clinical trials. *Lancet* 2007;370:1129–1136

15. Dormandy JA, Charbonnel B, Eckland DJ, Erdmann E, Massi-Benedetti M, Moules IK, Skene AM, Tan MH, Lefèbvre PJ, Murray GD, Standl E, Wilcox RG, Wilhelmsen L, Betteridge J, Birkeland K, Golay A, Heine RJ, Korányi L, Laakso M, Mokán M, Norkus A, Pirags V, Podar T, Scheen A, Scherbaum W, Schernthaner G, Schmitz O, Skrha J, Smith U, Taton J; PROactive Investigators. Secondary prevention of macrovascular events in patients with type 2 diabetes in the PROactive Study (PROspective pioglitAzone Clinical Trial In macroVascular Events): a randomised controlled trial. *Lancet* 2005;366(9493):1279–1289

16. Wilcox R, Bousser MG, Betteridge DJ, Schernthaner G, Pirags V, Kupfer S, Dormandy J; PROactive Investigators. Effects of pioglitazone in patients with type 2 diabetes with or without previous stroke: results from PROactive (PROspective pioglitAzone Clinical Trial In macroVascular Events 04). *Stroke* 2007;38:865–873

17. Kernan WN, Viscoli CM, Furie KL, Young LH, Inzucchi SE, Gorman M, Guarino PD, Lovejoy AM, Peduzzi PN, Conwit R, Brass LM, Schwartz GG, Adams HP Jr., Berger L, Carolei A, Clark W, Coull B, Ford GA, Kleindorfer D, O'Leary JR, Parsons MW, Ringleb P, Sen S, Spence JD, Tanne D, Wang D, Winder TR; IRIS Trial Investigators. Pioglitazone after ischemic stroke or transient ischemic attack. *N Engl J Med* 2016;374(14):1321–1331

18. Lee M, Saver JL, Liao HW, Lin CH, Ovbiagele B. Pioglitazone for secondary stroke prevention: a systematic review and meta-analysis. *Stroke* 2017;48:388–393

19. Bonnet F, Scheen AJ. Impact of glucose-lowering therapies on risk of stroke in type 2 diabetes. *Diabetes Metab* 2017;43:299–313

20. DeFronzo RA. Insulin resistance, lipotoxicity, type 2 diabetes and atherosclerosis: the missing links. *Diabetologia* 2010;53(7):1270–1287

21. Rajagopalan S, Dutta P, Hota D, Bhansali A, Srinivasan A, Chakrabar A. Effect of low dose pioglitazone on glycemic control and insulin resistance in type 2 diabetes: a randomized, double blind, clinical trial. *Diabetes Res Clin Pract* 2015;109(3):e32–e35

22. Kurisu S, Iwasaki T, Ishibashi K, Mitsuba N, Dohi Y, Nishioka K, Kihara Y. Effects of low-dose pioglitazone on glucose control, lipid profiles, renin-angiotensin-aldosterone system and natriuretic peptides in diabetic patients with coronary artery disease. *J Renin Angiotensin Aldosterone Syst* 2013;14(1):51–55

23. Tripathy D, Daniele G, Fiorentino TV, Perez-Cadena Z, Chavez-Velasquez A, Kamath S, Fanti P, Jenkinson C, Andreozzi F, Federici M, Gastaldelli A, DeFronzo RA, Folli F. Pioglitazone improves glucose metabolism and modulates skeletal muscle TIMP-3-TACE dyad in type 2 diabetes mellitus: a randomised, double-blind, placebo-controlled, mechanistic study. *Diabetologia* 2013;56(10):2153–2163

24. Yanai H, Adachi H. The low-dose (7.5 mg/day) pioglitazone therapy. *J Clin Med Res* 2017;9(10):821–825

25. Erdmann E, Harding S, Lam H, Perez A. Ten-year observational follow-up of PROactive: a randomized cardiovascular outcomes trial evaluating pioglitazone in type 2 diabetes. *Diabetes Obes Metab* 2016;18(3):266–273

26. Billington EO, Grey A, Bolland MJ. The effect of thiazolidinediones on bone mineral density and bone turnover: systematic review and meta-analysis. *Diabetologia* 2015;58:2238–2246

27. American Diabetes Association. 5. Prevention or delay of type 2 diabetes: *Standards of Medical Care in Diabetes—2018. Diabetes Care* 2018;41(Suppl. 1):S51–S54

28. Davidson MA, Mattison DR, Azoulay L, Krewski D. Thiazolidinedione drugs in the treatment of type 2 diabetes mellitus: past, present and future. *Crit Rev Toxicol* 2018;48(1):52–108

29. Davidson MB, Pan D. An updated meta-analysis of pioglitazone exposure and bladder cancer and comparison to the drug's effect on cardiovascular disease and non-alcoholic steatohepatitis. *Diabetes Res Clin Pract* 2018;135:102–110.

30. Chalasani N, Younossi Z, Lavine JE, Charlton M, Cusi K, Rinella M, Harrison SA, Brunt EM, Sanyal AJ. The diagnosis and management of nonalcoholic fatty liver disease: practice guideline from the American Association for the Study of Liver Diseases. *Hepatology* 2018;76(1):328–357

31. European Association for the Study of the Liver (EASL), European Association for the Study of Diabetes (EASD), European Association for the Study of Obesity (EASO). EASL-EASD-EASO clinical practice guidelines for the management of non-alcoholic fatty liver disease. *J Hepatol* 2016;64:1388–1402

32. Legro RS, Arslanian SA, Ehrmann DA, Hoeger KM, Murad H, Pasquali R, Welt CK; Endocrine Society. Diagnosis and treatment of polycystic ovary syndrome: an Endocrine Society clinical practice guideline. *J Clin Endocrinol Metab* 2013;89(12):4565–4592

Chapter 8
Sulfonylureas

LISA KROON, PHARMD
CRYSTAL ZHOU, PHARMD

INTRODUCTION

Sulfonylureas have been a mainstay in the pharmacologic treatment of T2D for over 60 years. Three first-generation sulfonylureas (chlorpropamide, tolbutamide, and tolazamide) are rarely used in the United States. The three second-generation sulfonylureas (glyburide, glipizide, and glimepiride) are the most frequently used, so this chapter will focus on these agents. With the availability of many noninsulin classes of medications for T2D, sulfonylurea usage is on the decline.[1] However, they remain some of the most commonly used and effective agents in A1C lowering, are cost effective, and, when dosed appropriately, are well tolerated and easily taken.[2,3]

The American Diabetes Association's pharmacologic treatment approach for glycemic control place insulin secretagogues (sulfonylureas and meglitinides) as an option for a second agent after a patient is on metformin.[4] In clinical practice, sulfonylureas are often initiated as a second or third noninsulin agent. T2D is a progressive disease in which most patients at some point require multiple medications to achieve good glycemic control.[5] As a patient progresses to needing additional pharmacologic therapy, a sulfonylurea is generally discontinued when a patient is advanced to requiring mealtime insulin. At this point, the pancreatic function has declined to a point where the insulin secretagogues likely have no appreciable effect on insulin secretion. In patients with maturity-onset diabetes of the young (MODY), type HNF1A or HNF4A, low-dose sulfonylureas are considered first-line therapy.[6]

PHARMACOLOGY

MECHANISM OF ACTION

Sulfonylureas exert their antihyperglycemic effect by stimulating insulin secretion in the pancreas. Sulfonylureas bind to a high-affinity sulfonylurea receptor on the pancreatic β-cell and increase both basal and meal-stimulated insulin secretion.[7] The second-generation sulfonylureas have greater intrinsic potency than the first-generation agents. Insulin secretion is regulated by ATP-dependent potassium ion channels in the plasma membrane of the β-cell.[7] The ATP-dependent potassium channel consists of two subunits, one containing a sulfonylurea receptor and the other containing the channel. Upon the sulfonylurea binding to its receptor, the ATP-dependent potassium channel closes, blocking the efflux of potassium. As potassium accumulates within the β-cell membrane, the membrane potential lowers, causing depolarization, which opens the voltage-dependent calcium channels; this calcium influx results in increased intracellular calcium, which, in turn, causes insulin granules to migrate to the cell surface, where the granules rupture and release the insulin.[7] Patients with T2D characteristically have defects in both insulin secretion and insulin action. Therefore, sulfonylureas' primary action in improving glycemic control is by affecting the β-cell defect.

With long-term use, sulfonylureas are thought to also exert extrapancreatic effects, including normalizing hepatic glucose production, reducing glucagon levels, enhancing peripheral glucose uptake, enhancing β-cell sensitivity to glucose, and closure of potassium channels in other tissues (e.g., cardiac tissue).[7] These effects are likely due to the improved glycemic control, which then reduces glucose toxicity.[8] The reduction of glucagon levels may be due to the enhanced insulin release, which inhibits α-cell secretion of glucagon. The significance of extrapancreatic potassium channel effects are likely minimal. However, in the heart, the closure of potassium channels on cardiac myocytes can affect ischemic preconditioning, in which vasodilation occurs during an ischemic episode.[9,10]

PHARMACOKINETICS

The sulfonylureas possess differences in their pharmacokinetic profiles. All sulfonylureas are nearly completely absorbed; however, the onset and duration of action are determined by the unique pharmacokinetic features of each agent and its specific formulation.[11] Most sulfonylureas have a relatively short plasma half-life, usually in the range of 4–10 h; only chlorpropamide has a half-life longer than 24 h. All sulfonylureas are highly protein-bound (90–100%), mainly to albumin; however, binding characteristics vary by individual sulfonylurea.[11] Most sulfonylureas effectively maintain glucose control with once- or twice-daily dosing. The longer duration of action seen than would be expected based on plasma half-life is thought to be due to a longer tissue half-life on the β-cell receptor and also the action of any active metabolites.[12] All sulfonylureas are metabolized in the liver, some to weakly active or inactive metabolites.[11] The first-generation sulfonylureas are excreted exclusively by the kidney, whereas the second-generation agents and their metabolites are excreted in differing proportions in the urine and feces. The pharmacokinetic properties of the sulfonylureas are summarized in Table 8.1.

Glyburide (also called glibenclamide) is longer acting compared to glipizide and can be taken once a day. It is metabolized completely by the liver to active metabolites, half of which are excreted in the urine and the rest in the biliary tract. A micronized formulation is available that is not bioequivalent to the conventional tablets. When patients are switched from formulations, they should be carefully monitored for possible dose adjustments.

Glipizide is an intermediate-acting agent, with a duration of action between 12 and 24 h. When taking doses of 20 mg/day or less, patients often can take glipizide once daily. Glipizide is metabolized completely by the liver to inactive metabolites, which are primarily excreted by the kidney. An extended-release formulation is available; the clinical significance on its duration of effect is minimal. Although the FDA-approved maximum dose is 40 mg/day, there is likely little additional glucose-lowering benefit to titrating over 20 mg/day.[13,14] While some clinicians recommend taking sulfonylureas, glipizide in particular, 30 min before the meal, the clinical significance of this on overall glycemic control has not been established and taking at the start of the meal is just as effective.[15]

Glimepiride is a long-acting agent with a duration of action of 24 h, allowing for daily dosing. It is metabolized by the liver to a principle metabolite that has 30% of the activity of glimepiride; metabolites are excreted in the urine and feces. Glimepiride is unique in its selectivity to β-cells. It may be advantageous for use in patients with coronary heart disease, due to the theoretical benefit of not affecting cardiac tissue.

From a pharmacodynamic perspective, sulfonylureas have a rapid onset of effect compared to other noninsulin agents. The full glycemic-lowering effect at a particular dose is seen within 1–2 weeks. Therefore, while most sulfonylureas could be dose adjusted before 1 week, dose titrations are usually done every 1–2 weeks.

TREATMENT ADVANTAGES/DISADVANTAGES

ADVANTAGES

As initial treatment in patients with T2D, sulfonylureas can induce a mean decrease in A1C of 1–2% and can reduce fasting plasma glucose by 60–70 mg/dL (3.3–3.8 mmol/L). However, in most cases, sulfonylureas will be started as an add-on agent to metformin or as a third agent. The ideal candidates for treatment with sulfonylureas are patients with T2D who have significant insulin deficiency (e.g., insulinopenic) but sufficient residual β-cell function to respond to stimulation. Patients are likely to demonstrate a good glycemic response to sulfonylureas if they have a shorter duration of T2D and are not in a state of glucose toxicity (in which insulin therapy may be preferable for short-term use). In the less common condition where a patient with T2D has a thinner phenotype, indicating more insulin secretion defect rather than insulin resistance, a sulfonylurea should be considered.

DISADVANTAGES

The main disadvantages of the sulfonylureas are the side effects of weight gain and hypoglycemia. These are discussed in the "Adverse Effects and Monitoring" section. In addition, with the natural progressive decline in β-cell function associated with T2D over time, the response to sulfonylurea treatment likewise will diminish, and changes to the treatment regimen may be necessary. The ADOPT study assessed the time to monotherapy failure for glyburide, metformin, and rosiglitazone. At 5 years, 34% of patients on a sulfonylurea failed monotherapy, compared to 15 and 21% with rosiglitazone and metformin, respectively.[16] One hypothesis for the lower durability of the sulfonylureas is that the continuous stimulation of β-cells can cause them to fail sooner. This has been studied mainly in animal models and more clinical data is needed to prove this theory.[17] The Glycemia Reduction Approaches in Diabetes: A Comparative Effectiveness Study (GRADE) is assessing the long-term efficacy of a sulfonylurea (glimepiride), insulin glargine, a GLP-1 RA (liraglutide), and a DPP-4 inhibitor (sitagliptin) in patients already on metformin.[18] The primary metabolic outcome is time to primary failure (i.e., A1C ≥7%). This study, funded by the National Institute of Diabetes and Digestive and Kidney Diseases (NIDDK), hopes to provide important information about optimal combinations of antidiabetics.

The progressive decrease in β-cell function is not the only possible cause of the reduced effectiveness of an antidiabetic medication regimen. Patient-specific factors, including poor adherence to the medication or factors that can increase the insulin-resistance component of hyperglycemia such as weight gain, physical inactivity, stress, or intercurrent illness can also reduce the effectiveness of the medication regimen. Medication-related factors are another possible reason for lack of (or diminished) response, such as not uptitrating the dose or initiation of a diabetogenic drug (e.g., glucocorticoids or certain antipsychotics).

THERAPEUTIC CONSIDERATIONS

SIGNIFICANT WARNINGS/PRECAUTIONS

The sulfonylureas are contraindicated in patients with a known hypersensitivity to the drug and in those with DKA, with or without coma. DKA should be treated with insulin. Sulfonylureas should not be used in patients with T1D.

The product information for sulfonylureas contains a special warning that the administration of oral antidiabetic agents has been reported to be associated with increased risk of cardiovascular mortality compared with treatment with nutrition therapy alone or nutrition therapy plus insulin. This warning is based on the results of the long-term, prospective clinical trial, the University Group Diabetes Program that was published in 1970.[19] Although only tolbutamide was included in this study, this warning has been applied to all sulfonylureas. The validity of this finding has been questioned due to design flaws and more recent long-term, randomized, controlled trials, such as the UKPDS and ADVANCE studies, which found no increased cardiovascular mortality in patients on sulfonylureas and provide reassuring evidence.[20,21] However, meta-analyses continue to be published that show an association of sulfonylureas and cardiovascular risk (see "Special Populations").

Hypoglycemia

The most serious acute complication of sulfonylurea therapy is hypoglycemia, and all sulfonylureas are capable of producing severe hypoglycemia. Appropriate patient selection, dosage, and patient education are important to avoid hypoglycemic episodes. Debilitated or malnourished patients and those with adrenal, pituitary, or hepatic insufficiency are particularly susceptible to the hypoglycemic action of insulin secretagogues. Hypoglycemia may be difficult to recognize in the elderly and in people taking β-blockers or other sympatholytic drugs. For patients taking a β-blocker, particularly a nonselective one such as propranolol, hypoglycemic symptoms of tachycardia and shakiness can be blunted, resulting in sweating being the most pronounced symptom. Hypoglycemia is more likely to occur when caloric intake is deficient, after severe or prolonged exercise, when alcohol is ingested, or when more than one glucose-lowering drug is used.

SPECIAL POPULATIONS

Hypoglycemia

Hypoglycemia is the most significant risk of the use of sulfonylureas and other antidiabetic agents in elderly patients and those with multiple comorbidities. Both renal and hepatic insufficiency are substantial risk factors for the development of severe hypoglycemia during sulfonylurea treatment in the elderly. Sulfonylureas should be initiated at lower doses and titrated slowly in elderly patients. See "Adverse Effects and Monitoring" for in-depth discussion.

Pregnancy and Lactation

The sulfonylureas are categorized as pregnancy category C. Glipizide and glimepiride have been found to be fetotoxic in rats at doses that produced maternal hypoglycemia. In some studies in rats, nonteratogenic skeletal deformities were observed after exposure during gestation and lactation. Because a higher incidence of congenital abnormalities is associated with abnormal maternal blood glucose levels during pregnancy, insulin therapy is most often the recommended choice of therapy during pregnancy to maintain blood glucose levels as close to normal as possible.

Pediatrics

The safety and effectiveness of sulfonylureas in pediatric patients has not been established.

Hepatic or Renal Impairment

Because sulfonylureas are major CYP2C9 substrates, caution should be exercised when using this class of medications in patients with hepatic impairment. Due to chlorpropamide and glyburide's longer elimination half-life, they should be avoided in patients with impaired renal function due to the increased risk for hypoglycemia. Glipizide and glimepiride can be initiated at lower doses to avoid hypoglycemia in renal impairment and are the preferred second-generation agents.

Food Insecurity and Homelessness

Patients who are homeless or do not have a reliable source of food may experience more frequent hypoglycemia if taking a longer-acting sulfonylurea. Therefore, in patients with food insecurities who may benefit from sulfonylureas, it is recommended to use glipizide due to its relatively short half-life. In order to prevent hypoglycemia, patients can take glipizide only prior to a meal, as they may not have to plan for future meals. Providers should also help these patients seek local resources to assist them in obtaining regularly distributed food.[22]

Cardiovascular Disease and Increased Cardiovascular Risk

Meta-analyses comparing sulfonylureas to other antidiabetic medications show conflicting results with regard to cardiovascular risk. Two meta-analyses found an increased cardiovascular-related mortality associated with sulfonylureas, with a Mantel-Haenszel odds ratio of 1.22 for patients on glyburide (glibenclamide) specifically in one study and a hazard ratio of 1.46 in another study.[23,24] A network meta-analysis found that sulfonylureas were associated with greater cardiovascular risk, which was partly attributable to a concomitant increased risk of severe hypoglycemia.[25] In another meta-analysis that assessed 47 trials in which patients were on sulfonylureas or other classes of antidiabetic medications for at least 52 weeks, no increase in cardiovascular mortality was found.[26] Therefore, data are inconclusive, and until additional RCT evidence is available, it is reasonable to weigh the benefits (e.g., improved glycemic control) and possible risks when using a sulfonylurea in a patient with known cardiovascular disease.

ADVERSE EFFECTS AND MONITORING

Sulfonylureas are usually well tolerated and the frequency of side effects, other than hypoglycemia, is low. The most common adverse events associated with sulfonylurea treatment, other than hypoglycemia, are dizziness, headache, and nausea. In comparative clinical trials, common adverse events occurred at similar rates with glimepiride and glipizide but were less likely to occur with glimepiride than glyburide.[27] Hematological complications, including thrombocytopenia, agranulocytosis, and hemolytic anemia, have been described with tolbutamide and chlorpropamide but appear to be very rare with the second-generation sulfonylureas. Other rare adverse effects include allergic skin reactions (e.g., rash, urticarial, pruritus), photosensitivity, abnormal liver function tests, and icterus.[12] In the rare event that a patient develops a severe rash or reports a sulfa allergy (although the risk of cross-reactivity is likely extremely low), a meglitinide can be safely used as an alternative.

Certain side effects are unique to the specific agents because of their individual chemical structures. For example, chlorpropamide can increase the secretion of antidiuretic hormone leading to water retention and hyponatremia.[12] A rare, disulfiram-like reaction can occur when patients take chlorpropamide and drink ethanol.[28]

The two adverse effects that are the primary disadvantages of sulfonylureas are weight gain and hypoglycemia.[2,29] Weight gain associated with sulfonylurea use is approximately 2 kg.[12] The weight gain can be attributed to two factors: improved glycemic control and hypoglycemia. Inherent in improving glycemic control is weight gain, as fewer calories are spilling into the urine. Also, a patient consumes additional calories when treating hypoglycemia. Therefore, it is important not only to reduce the risk of hypoglycemia from a safety perspective, but also to limit weight gain associated with sulfonylureas. Data from several studies have suggested that the second-generation sulfonylurea glimepiride may be associated with a lower incidence of hypoglycemia and less weight gain, and may improve insulin sensitivity compared to other sulfonylureas.

In the UKPDS 6-year follow-up, the proportion of patients on sulfonylurea monotherapy reporting at least one episode per year of hypoglycemia (defined as temporarily incapacitated but a patient is able to control symptoms without help, incapacitated and required assistance to control symptoms, or required medical attention) was 1.2% compared to 0.3% with metformin.[30] In a retrospective analysis of a large, national cohort of T2D, use of a sulfonylurea or meglitinide increased the risk of severe hypoglycemia about twofold.[31] This analysis also found that patients with high complexity (i.e., age 75 years and older or multiple comorbidities) on intensive treatment also had nearly double the risk of severe hypoglycemia. A comparable analysis determined that the rate of severe hypoglycemia (defined as requiring an emergency department visit or hospitalization) was between 1.8 and 2.1 events per 100 person-years; again, rates were highest in older patients and those with multiple comorbidities.[1] Chlorpropamide and glyburide are identified in the Beers Criteria as potentially inappropriate medications in patients 65 and older.[32] Sulfonylureas should be used with caution in the elderly and those with multiple comorbidities.

Patients on sulfonylureas should be educated on how to self-monitor their blood glucose (and to monitor regularly), on hypoglycemic symptoms and values, and on how to self-treat for a hypoglycemic episode. A quick-acting source of glucose should be used. Glucagon, while effective for hypoglycemia cause by exogenous insulin, can cause a paradoxical lowering of blood glucose when used with a sulfonylurea, as it stimulates insulin secretion.[33,34] Patients should also be educated to not skip meals, as this, along with irregular eating patterns, will increase the risk of hypoglycemia. Patients who are purposefully trying to eat less, increase physical activity, or lose weight may need their sulfonylurea dose reduced.

Although the sulfonylureas have important side effects to consider, the newer noninsulin agents also have significant side effects (i.e., newer doesn't necessarily mean better or safer). When developing a T2D medication regimen, it is important to tailor the medication selection(s) to the patient, taking into account the unique side effects of the various classes of medications and patient factors (e.g., concurrent medication conditions, ability to adhere, and ability to pay for the medication).

DRUG INTERACTIONS

The hypoglycemic action of sulfonylureas may be enhanced by certain drugs, including nonsteroidal anti-inflammatory drugs (NSAIDs) and other drugs that are highly bound to protein, such as salicylates, sulfonamides, chloramphenicol, warfarin, probenecid, monoamine oxidase inhibitors, and β-blockers (see "Hypoglycemia"). Although the risk is greater with the first-generation sulfonylureas, patients given these drugs concomitantly with any sulfonylurea should be monitored closely for hypoglycemia. Similarly, when these drugs are discontinued, patients on sulfonylurea therapy should be observed closely for worsening of glycemic control.

Pharmacodynamic interactions with all antidiabetics include drugs that can cause hyperglycemia, and when taken may lead to worsening of glycemic control. Examples of these drugs include thiazide diuretics, statins, glucocorticoids, phenothiazines, certain antipsychotics (e.g., chlorpromazine, olanzapine, clozapine), HIV protease inhibitors, estrogens and hormonal contraceptives, phenytoin, immunosuppressive therapies, sympathomimetics, and isoniazid.

DOSAGE AND ADMINISTRATION

A sulfonylurea is typically started at a low dose and then titrated until the glycemic response is achieved. The dose should generally be increased at no shorter than weekly intervals. Most patients will achieve the maximum therapeutic benefit with one-half of the FDA-approved maximum dose. Typical dosing and administration regimens are shown in Table 2.

A number of factors influence the choice of a sulfonylurea, including the duration of action and frequency of administration, patterns of metabolism and excretion, and the side effect profiles. The duration of action of a sulfonylurea is an important consideration. Of the first-generation agents, tolbutamide has a very short duration of action and needs to be taken two or three times a day. Most of the second-generation agents, which have a duration of 16–24 h, can be administered once daily at the usual therapeutic doses, but maximal doses may need to be divided into two daily doses. Glipizide is typically dosed twice daily with breakfast and dinner. Glyburide and glimepiride are usually dosed daily with breakfast, or the first meal of the day. It is important to educate patients to not take a sulfonylurea at bedtime as this can increase the risk of hypoglycemia.

The patterns of metabolism and excretion are also important to the risk of hypoglycemia. Because sulfonylureas are metabolized by and inactivated in the liver, the risk of hypoglycemia is significantly increased in patients with hepatic impairment. Sulfonylureas that are metabolized to active metabolites, such as glyburide, should be avoided in renal dysfunction, as the active metabolites can accumulate, increasing the hypoglycemia risk. Glipizide is preferred for use in renal dysfunction due to its shorter duration of action compared to glyburide and glimepiride, and is metabolized to inactive metabolites.

If a patient is experiencing hypoglycemia on a particular sulfonylurea, their eating pattern should be assessed. Hypoglycemia could occur due to one skipped meal, and thus is explainable. If the hypoglycemia is consistent, the dose should be reduced. If hypoglycemia persists, a meglitinide, a shorter-acting insulin secretagogue, can be used instead of a sulfonylurea.

Sulfonylurea therapy is used most in patients already on metformin, as second- or third-line treatment. Sulfonylureas can be combined with other antidiabetic medications that have different or complementary mechanisms of action. They should not be used in combination with the meglitinides, as these are also insulin secretagogues. When used with a GLP-1 RA or DPP-4 inhibitor, it is recommended to reduce the dose of the sulfonylurea (e.g., by half) when adding either of these agents to reduce the risk of hypoglycemia. When using combination therapy with noninsulin agents, if a patient experiences hypoglycemia, the sulfonylurea should be the first consideration in dosage reduction versus other agents, as it is the sulfonylurea's insulin secretory effect that causes hypoglycemia.

Sulfonylureas and insulin have been used extensively in combination therapy. Based on the American Diabetes Association's treatment algorithm, basal insulin is usually initiated first and used in combination with other noninsulin medications.[4]

At this point in treatment, a sulfonylurea is usually continued, as it still may have some therapeutic benefit. In fact, an older term for this therapy was BIDS: bedtime insulin (with a basal insulin), daytime sulfonylurea. As a patient progresses to needing mealtime insulin, then the sulfonylurea is typically discontinued.

Table 8.1 Sulfonylurea Pharmacokinetic Properties

Sulfonylurea	Peak effect (h)	Approximate duration of action (h)	Protein binding	Metabolism	Half-life (h)	Excretion
Chlorpropamide	3 to 6	36	90%	Hepatic via CYP2C9 (~80%) to metabolites (inactive and active)	~36	Urine (unchanged drug and metabolites)
Glimepiride	2 to 3	24	>99.5%	Hepatic oxidation via CYP2C9 to M1 metabolite (one-third activity compared to parent); further oxidative metabolism to M2 metabolite (inactive)	5 to 9	Urine (60%; 80%–90% as M1 and M2 metabolites); feces (40%; 70% as M1 and M2 metabolites)
Glipizide	IR: 1 to 3 ER: 6 to 12	12 to 24	98% to 99%, primarily to albumin	Hepatic via CYP2C9 to inactive metabolites	IR: 2 to 4 ER: 4–13	Urine (<10% unchanged drug; 80% as metabolites); feces (10%)
Glyburide	2 to 4	≤24	Extensive, primarily to albumin	Hepatic via CYP2C to metabolites (weakly active)	~10; Glynase PresTab: ~4	Urine (50%, as metabolites); feces (50%, as metabolites)
Tolazamide	3 to 4	10 to 24	94%	Extensively hepatic to 5 major metabolites (some active)	7	Urine (85%); feces (7%)
Tolbutamide	3 to 4	6 to 24	~95% (concentration dependent)	Hepatic via CYP2C9 to 2 inactive metabolites	4.5 to 6.5	Urine (75% to 85%, primarily as metabolites); feces

Source: Individual drug monographs on DAILYMED

Table 8.2 Sulfonylurea Dosage Information

Sulfonylurea	Available strengths	Usual starting dose	Dose titration	Dosage range
Chlorpropamide	100 mg, 250 mg	100–250 mg daily	50–125 mg every 1–2 weeks	100–500 mg daily
Tolazamide	250 mg, 500 mg	100–250 mg daily*	100–250 mg every 1–2 weeks	250–1,000 mg daily (if >500 mg, take twice daily)
Tolbutamide	500 mg	250–500 mg twice daily	250 mg every 1–2 weeks	0.25–3 g daily (taken with meals two to three times daily; usual maintenance dose is up to 2 g)
Glimepiride	1 mg, 2 mg, 4 mg	1–2 mg daily*	2 mg every 1–2 weeks	1–8 mg daily (usual maintenance dose is up to 4 mg)
Glipizide	IR: 5 mg, 10 mg ER: 2.5 mg, 5 mg, 10 mg	IR: 5 mg daily* ER: 2.5–10 daily*	IR: 2.5–5 mg at intervals of at least several days ER: 2.5 mg at intervals of at least a week	IR: 10–40 mg once daily (if >15 mg, take twice daily) ER: 2.5–20 mg daily
Glyburide (Glibenclamide)	1.25 mg, 2.5 mg, 5 mg Micronized: 1.5 mg, 3 mg, 6 mg	2.5–5 mg daily* Micronized: 1.5–3 mg daily	2.5 mg every 1–2 weeks Micronized: 1.5 mg every 1–2 weeks	1.25–20 mg daily (or twice daily) Micronized: 1.5–12 mg daily (if >6 mg, take twice daily)

* Daily is usually at breakfast or with first main meal. *Source*: Individual drug monographs at DAILYMED.

COMBINATION PILLS CONTAINING A SULFONYLUREA

Available combination tablets with sulfonylureas are listed below. They can be considered for patients on stable doses of each medication, which can assist with adherence and possibly lower costs. However, if the dose of either agent is being dose adjusted, it is best to for a patient to take each medication as a separate pill. This will avoid any confusion on how much of each medication to take and even medication errors.

Glyburide/metformin (Glucovance; generics)

- 1.25 mg/250 mg: Glyburide 1.25 mg and metformin hydrochloride 250 mg
- 2.5 mg/500 mg: Glyburide 2.5 mg and metformin hydrochloride 500 mg
- 5 mg/500 mg: Glyburide 5 mg and metformin hydrochloride 500 mg
- Glipizide/metformin (Metaglip; generics)
- Glipizide 2.5 mg and metformin hydrochloride 250 mg
- Glipizide 2.5 mg and metformin hydrochloride 500 mg
- Glipizide 5 mg and metformin hydrochloride 500 mg
- Pioglitazone/glimepiride (Duetact; generics)
- Pioglitazone 30 mg and glimepiride 2 mg
- Pioglitazone 30 mg and glimepiride 4 mg

MONOGRAPHS

Chlorpropamide: https://dailymed.nlm.nih.gov/dailymed/drugInfo.cfm?setid=baa54287-8065-da1a-f19e-ce8daf61bd01

Glimepiride (Amaryl): https://dailymed.nlm.nih.gov/dailymed/drugInfo.cfm?setid=222b630b-7e09-43b4-9894-3d87f10add91

Glipizide (Glucotrol): https://dailymed.nlm.nih.gov/dailymed/drugInfo.cfm?setid=504567d2-e4f1-428d-b524-f29db76e6dfb

Glipizide extended-release (Glucotrol XL): https://dailymed.nlm.nih.gov/dailymed/drugInfo.cfm?setid=8438b406-9259-46d1-b26a-90fdcb5cbc50

Glyburide: https://dailymed.nlm.nih.gov/dailymed/drugInfo.cfm?setid=5d0e406f-285d-4716-8971-82f665345517

Glyburide-micronized (Glynase PresTab): https://dailymed.nlm.nih.gov/dailymed/drugInfo.cfm?setid=a7fce80a-2f13-43cc-8e1c-561f7d3ec3d5

Tolbutamide: https://dailymed.nlm.nih.gov/dailymed/drugInfo.cfm?setid=3995eed8-39ec-ce5e-8cc2-062f93445c8d

Tolazamide: https://dailymed.nlm.nih.gov/dailymed/drugInfo.cfm?setid=f82dcff5-4afa-45d8-bc8c-f0f7c0c96272

REFERENCES

1. Lipska KJ, Yao X, Herrin J, et al. Trends in drug utilization, glycemic control, and rates of severe hypoglycemia, 2006–2013. *Diabetes Care* 2017;40:468–475

2. Bennett WL, Maruthur NM, Singh S, et al. Comparative effectiveness and safety of medications for type 2 diabetes: an update including new drugs and 2-drug combinations. *Ann Intern Med* 2011;154:602–613

3. UK Prospective Diabetes Study (UKPDS) Group. Intensive blood glucose control with sulfonylureas or insulin compared with conventional treatment and risk of complications in patients with type 2 diabetes (UKPDS 33). *Lancet* 1998;352:837–853

4. American Diabetes Association. 8. Pharmacologic approaches to glycemic treatment: *Standards of Medical Care in Diabetes—2018*. *Diabetes Care* 2018;41(Suppl. 1):S73–S85

5. Turner RC, Cull CA, Frighi V, Holman RR;UKPDS Group. Glycemic control with diet, sulfonylurea, metformin, or insulin in patients with type 2 diabetes mellitus: progressive requirement for multiple therapies (UKPDS 49). *JAMA* 1999;281:2005–2012

6. American Diabetes Association. 2. Classification and diagnosis of diabetes: *Standards of Medical Care in Diabetes—2018*. *Diabetes Care* 2018;41(Suppl. 1):S13–S27

7. Kennedy M, Masharani U. Pancreatic hormones and antidiabetic drugs. In *Basic & Clinical Pharmacology*, 13th ed. Katzung BG, Trevor AJ, Eds. New York, McGraw-Hill, 2015. Available from http://accessmedicine.mhmedical.com/content.aspx?bookid=1193&sectionid=69110459. Accessed 13 August 2018

8. Inzucchi SE. Oral antihyperglycemic therapy for type 2 diabetes: scientific review. *JAMA* 2002;287:360–372

9. Klepzig H, Kober G, Matter C, et al. Sulfonylureas and ischaemic preconditioning: a double-blind, placebo-controlled evaluation of glimepiride and glibenclamide. *Eur Heart J* 1999;20:439–436

10. Quast U, Stephan D, Bieger S, Russ U. The impact of ATP-sensitive K+ channel subtype selectivity of insulin secretagogues for the coronary vasculature and the myocardium. *Diabetes* 2004;53(Suppl. 3): S156–164

11. Groop LC. Sulfonylureas in NIDDM. *Diabetes Care* 1992;15:737

12. Sola D, Rossi L, Schianca GPC, et al. Sulfonylureas and their use in clinical practice. *Arch Med Sci* 2015;11:840–848

13. Groop LC, Barzilai N, Ratheiser K, et al. Dose-dependent effects of glyburide in insulin secretion and glucose uptake in humans. *Diabetes Care* 1991;14:724–727

14. Stenman S, Melander A, Groop PH, Groop LC. What is the benefit of increasing the sulfonylurea dose? *Ann Intern Med* 1993;118:169–172

15. Faber OK, Beck-Nielsen H, Binder C, et al. Acute actions of sulfonylurea drugs during long-term treatment of NIDDM. *Diabetes Care* 1990;13(Suppl. 3):26–31

16. Kahn SE, Haffner SM, Heise MA, et al.; ADOPT Study Group. Glycemic durability of rosiglitazone, metformin, or glyburide monotherapy. *N Engl J Med* 2006;355:2427–2443

17. van Raalte DH, Verchere CB. Improving glycemic control in type 2 diabetes: stimulate insulin secretion or provide beta-cell rest? *Diabetes Obes Metab* 2017;19:1205–1213

18. Nathan DM, Buse JB, Kahn SE, et al.; GRADE Study Research Group. Rationale and design of the glycemia reduction approaches in diabetes: a comparative effectiveness study (GRADE). *Diabetes Care* 2013;36:2254–2261

19. The University Group Diabetes Program. A study of the effects of hypoglycemic agents on vascular complications in patients with adult-onset diabetes I. Design, methods, and baseline results. *Diabetes* 1970;19(Suppl. 2):747–830

20. ADVANCE Collaborative Group. Intensive blood glucose control and vascular outcomes in patients with type 2 diabetes. *N Engl J Med* 2008;358:2560–2572

21. Holman RR, Paul SK, Bethel MA, et al. 10-year follow-up of intensive glucose control in type 2 diabetes. *N Engl J Med* 2008;359:1577–1589

22. Seligman HK, Schillinger D. Hunger and socioeconomic disparities in chronic disease. *N Engl J Med* 2010;363:6–9

23. Monami M, Genovese S, Mannucci E. Cardiovascular safety of sulfonylureas: a meta-analysis of randomized clinical trials. *Diabetes Obes Metab* 2013;15:938–953

24. Bain S, Druyts E, Balijepalli C, et al. Cardiovascular events and all-cause mortality associated with sulphonylureas compared with other antihyperglycaemic drugs: a Bayesian meta-analysis of survival data. *Diabetes Obes Metab* 2017;19:329–335

25. Zhuang XD, He X, Yang DY, et al. Comparative cardiovascular outcomes in the era of novel anti-diabetic agents: a comprehensive network meta-analysis of 166,371 participants from 170 randomized controlled trials. *Cardiovasc Diabetol* 2018;17:79. DOI:10.1186/s12933-018-0722-z

26. Rados DV, Pinto LC, Remonti LR, et al. The association between sulfonylurea use and all-cause and cardiovascular mortality: A meta-analysis with trial sequential analysis of randomized clinical trials. *PLoS Med* 2016;13(4): e1001992. DOI:10.1371/journal.pmed.1001992

27. Korytkowski MT. Sulfonylurea treatment of type 2 diabetes: focus on glimepiride. *Pharmacotherapy* 2004;24:606–620

28. Towell J, Garthwaite T, Wang R. Erythrocyte aldehyde dehydrogenase and disulfiram-like side effects of hypoglycemics and antianginals. *Alcohol Clin Exp Res* 1985;9:438–442

29. Maruthur NM, Tseng E, Hutfless S, et al. Diabetes medications as monotherapy or metformin-based combination therapy for type 2 diabetes: a systematic review and meta-analysis. *Ann Intern Med* 2016;164:740–751

30. Wright AD, Cull CA, Macleod KM, Holman RR; UKPDS Group. Hypoglycemia in type 2 diabetic patients randomized to and maintained on monotherapy with diet, sulfonylurea, metformin, or insulin for 6 years from diagnosis: UKPDS73. *J Diabetes Complications* 2006;20:395–401

31. McCoy RD, Lipska KJ, Yao X, et al. Intensive treatment and severe hypoglycemia among adults with type 2 diabetes. *JAMA Intern Med* 2016;176(7):969–978

32. American Geriatrics Society 2015 Beers Criteria Update Expert Panel. American Geriatrics Society 2015 updated Beers Criteria for potentially inappropriate medication use in older adults. *J Am Geriatr Soc* 2015;63:2227–2246

33. Graudins A, Linden CH, Ferm RP. Diagnosis and treatment of sulfonylurea-induced hyperinsulinemic hypoglycemia. *Am J Emerg Med* 1997;15:95–96

34. Cryer PE, Davis SN, Shamoon H. Hypoglycemia in diabetes. *Diabetes Care* 2003;26:1902–1912

Chapter 9
Glinides

Lisa Kroon, PharmD
Crystal Zhou, PharmD

INTRODUCTION

The meglitinides are insulin secretagogues that are structurally different from the sulfonylureas and have different pharmacokinetics. The meglitinides (or "glinides," as they will be referred to in this chapter) have a similar mechanism of action as the sulfonylureas, causing an increase in insulin release from the β-cells in the pancreas. They are taken at the time of a meal, and thus require multiple daily dosing for patients, but also allow for more flexibility in dose administration with the timing of their meals. Because of their short half-life, they have a reduced risk of hypoglycemia. Although glinides are some of the less frequently used antidiabetic medications, they do offer a niche in T2D therapy that will be reviewed.[1,2] Two compounds are available in this class of antidiabetics: nateglinide and repaglinide, which are analogs of meglitinide. The glinides are FDA approved to improve glycemic control in adults with T2D as an adjunct to diet and exercise.

The American Diabetes Association's pharmacologic treatment approach for glycemic control places insulin secretagogues (sulfonylureas and glinides) as an option for a second agent after a patient is on metformin.[3] In clinical practice, the glinides are often used after a patient is not able to tolerate a sulfonylurea (usually due to hypoglycemia), where the sulfonylurea is discontinued and switched to a glinide. Thus, their place in therapy is generally as a second or third noninsulin agent. T2D is a progressive disease in which most patients at some point require multiple medications to achieve good glycemic control.[4] As a patient progresses to needing additional pharmacologic therapy, a glinide is generally discontinued when a patient is advanced to requiring mealtime insulin. At this point, the pancreatic function has declined to a point where the insulin secretagogues likely have no appreciable effect on insulin secretion. In patients with MODY, type HNF1A or HNF4A, while low-dose sulfonylureas are considered first-line therapy, meglitinides could be considered as well.[5,6]

PHARMACOLOGY

MECHANISM OF ACTION

The glinides are structurally different from the sulfonylureas; however, similar to that class, they lower blood glucose levels by stimulating insulin release from the pancreas.[7,8] As with the sulfonylureas, release of insulin is dependent on functioning β-cells in the pancreatic islets. Repaglinide is a derivative of benzoic acid, and nateglinide is a derivative of the amino acid D-phenylalanine.

The glinides' effect on the β-cell is glucose-dependent and diminishes at lower glucose concentrations.[8] Glinides bind to the sulfonylurea receptor on the β-cell but in a different configuration than the sulfonylureas and at a separate distinct binding site on the β-cell.[7–9] As with the sulfonylureas, the glinides close ATP-dependent potassium channels in the β-cell membrane, blocking the efflux of potassium.[7] As potassium accumulates within the β-cell membrane, the membrane potential lowers causing depolarization, which opens the voltage-dependent calcium channels; the calcium influx results in increased intracellular calcium. The increased concentration of calcium causes insulin granules to migrate to the cell surface, where the granules rupture and release the insulin.[7]

Patients with T2D characteristically have defects in both insulin secretion and insulin action. Glinides' primary action in improving glycemic control is by affecting the β-cell defect, enhancing (and restoring) early-phase insulin release.[8] Glinides thus reduce postprandial glucose excursions.[10] Since they have a more rapid onset and a shorter duration of action than the sulfonylureas, glinides' niche in therapy is to improve glycemic control postprandially while reducing the risk of late hypoglycemia.

PHARMACOKINETICS

Both repaglinide and nateglinide have a rapid onset and short duration of action. They are extensively metabolized to primarily inactive metabolites. The pharmacokinetic properties of glinides are summarized in Table 9.1.

Peak plasma concentrations of repaglinide are reached within 1 h following oral administration.[11] Repaglinide has an absolute bioavailability of 56–63%.[11] Administration with food does not affect the time to peak level, but it reduces the mean peak concentration by 20% and the area under the plasma time concentration curve by 12.4%. Repaglinide should be taken within 30 min before a meal. The volume of distribution of repaglinide is 31 L, and it is highly protein-bound (>98%).[11]

Repaglinide is rapidly and completely metabolized via oxidative biotransformation and direct conjugation with glucuronic acid. CYP2C8 and CYP3A4 isoenzymes are involved in its metabolism to the M1 and M2 metabolites, which are both inactive. Repaglinide's elimination half-life is about 1 h, and its duration of action is 4–7 h.[7,9] The majority of the drug is excreted in the feces (90%) with 8% excreted in urine. Less than 2% of repaglinide is excreted unchanged in the feces.[11]

Nateglinide is rapidly and almost completely absorbed (about 90%) with a peak plasma concentration within 1 h.[12] Peak levels of nateglinide are lower when it is taken after a meal than when taken shortly before a meal. Nateglinide's absolute bioavailability is about 73%, and its volume of distribution is approximately 10.5 L.[12] It should be taken within 30 min before a meal. Similar to repaglinide and the sulfonylureas, nateglinide is highly bound (98%), mainly to albumin.[12]

Table 9.1 — Glinide Pharmacokinetic Properties

Glinide	Peak effect (h)	Approximate duration of action (h)	Protein binding	Metabolism	Half-life (h)	Excretion
Nateglinide	~1	4	98%	Hepatic via CYP2C9 (70%) and CYP3A4 (30%) to metabolites (inactive and 1 active with similar activity to parent)	~1.5	Urine (83%, 16% unchanged drug); feces (10%)
Repaglinide	~1	4–7	>98%	Hepatic via CYP3A4 and CYP2C8 to metabolite (inactive)	~1	Urine (~8%; 0.1% unchanged drug); feces (90%; <2% unchanged drug)

Source: Individual drug monographs on DAILYMED.

Nateglinide is extensively metabolized by hydroxylation and then glucuronide conjugation. The CYP enzymes, CYP3A4 (30%) and CYP2C9 (70%), convert nateglinide to several inactive metabolites, with only one metabolite (M1) having similar pharmacologic activity to nateglinide. However, the overall exposure to the M1 metabolite is less than 5% compared to nateglinide.[12] The metabolites are primarily excreted in the urine (84–87%) with 8–10% excreted in the feces. Approximately 16% of nateglinide is excreted unchanged in the urine. Nateglinide's elimination half-life is about 1.5 h, and its duration of action is 4 h.[7,12]

TREATMENT ADVANTAGES/DISADVANTAGES

ADVANTAGES

As monotherapy in patients with T2D, glinides can induce a mean decrease in A1C of 0.5–1.5% from baseline, with nateglinide typically having a lesser effect on A1C. The expected A1C lowering of the glinides is generally less than that of the sulfonylureas. A Cochrane review found that repaglinide and nateglinide (specifically the 120-mg dose in three studies) reduced A1C by 0.5–2.1% and 0.5%, respectively, compared to placebo.[13] In a head-to-head, open-label, 16-week study, the mean reduction in A1C was significantly greater with repaglinide monotherapy compared to nateglinide (–1.57 vs. –1.04%).[14] The mean change in fasting blood glucose was also significantly greater with repaglinide (–57 vs. –18 mg/dL). Their effects on postprandial glucose AUC were similar.

Given their rapid onset of action and effect on first-phase insulin release, glinides are effective in lowering postprandial glucose excursions. Repaglinide has been shown to reduce postprandial glucose levels by approximately 100 mg/dL and nateglinide by 85 mg/dL.[15–17] In a study comparing nateglinide and glyburide, nateglinide had a greater effect on mealtime glucose excursions, whereas glyburide was more effective in reducing fasting plasma glucose.[18]

Postprandial hyperglycemia has been shown to contribute to cardiovascular risk in patients with T2D. The Diabetes Epidemiology: Collaborative analysis of Diagnostic criteria in Europe (DECODE) and Diabetes Epidemiology: Collaborative analysis of Diagnostic criteria in Asia (DECODA) studies showed that high 2-h postprandial glucose following an oral-glucose tolerance test was an independent risk factor for all-cause mortality and cardiovascular death in patients with T2D.[19,20] Therefore, postprandial blood glucose control and postprandial glucose monitoring can be an important component of T2D management.[21,22] Glinides can play a unique role in this strategy, given their primary effect in lowering postprandial glucose excursions.

Glinides have a relatively low incidence of hypoglycemia and may be preferable over a sulfonylurea in patients who are predisposed to hypoglycemia, such as the elderly. In patients for whom sulfonylureas are effective, but they are experiencing hypoglycemia, glinides can be used in place of sulfonylureas, which are longer-acting insulin secretagogues. It is important to note that glinides will have little, if any, effect when substituted for a sulfonylurea in a patient who is not responding adequately to a sulfonylurea, due to their same mechanism of action. Glinides and sulfonylureas should not be used in combination for the same reason.

Since glinides do not contain a sulfa moiety, they can be used instead of a sulfonylurea in patients with a history of sulfa allergy or patients who experience an allergic reaction to a sulfonylurea.

From a pharmacodynamics perspective, glinides have a rapid onset of effect compared to other noninsulin agents. While general dose titrations are usually made every 1–2 weeks, in practice, the dose is sometimes adjusted daily or at a particular meal.

DISADVANTAGES

The main disadvantages of glinides are the need for multiple daily doses, which can affect adherence, and less A1C efficacy compared to other antidiabetic medications. In addition, with the natural progressive decline in β-cell function associated with T2D over time, the response to glinide treatment likewise will diminish, and changes to the treatment regimen may be necessary. Please see the "Sulfonylureas" chapter for further discussion.

THERAPEUTIC CONSIDERATIONS

SIGNIFICANT WARNINGS/PRECAUTIONS

Glinides are contraindicated in patients with DKA, T1D, or known hypersensitivity to either nateglinide or repaglinide. Unlike the sulfonylureas, glinides do not carry a special warning about an associated increased risk of cardiovascular mortality. Repaglinide has a specific warning about an increased risk of MI with the concurrent use with NPH insulin, based on older literature. Clinical studies have since been published demonstrating safety and efficacy when repaglinide is used with this particular insulin.[9]

Hypoglycemia

Due to their mechanism of action of stimulating insulin release, glinides can cause hypoglycemia. The frequency of hypoglycemia is less with the glinides than with the sulfonylureas primarily due to their pharmacokinetics (e.g., shorter duration of action and conversion to inactive metabolites).[2,10] See further discussion below in "Patients at Risk for Hypoglycemia."

SPECIAL POPULATIONS

Hypoglycemia

The most serious complication of glinide therapy is hypoglycemia. Appropriate patient selection, dosage, and patient education are important to avoid hypoglycemic episodes. Debilitated or malnourished patients and those with adrenal, pituitary, or hepatic insufficiency are particularly susceptible to the hypoglycemic action of insulin secretagogues. Hypoglycemia may be difficult to recognize in the elderly and in people taking β-blockers, particularly nonselective ones. Hypoglycemia is more likely to occur when caloric intake is reduced, meals are skipped (and the glinide still taken), after severe or prolonged exercise, when alcohol is ingested, or when more than one glucose-lowering drug is used. Elderly patients and those with multiple comorbidities are at greater risk of hypoglycemia (see "Adverse Effects and Monitoring" for in-depth discussion on hypoglycemia).

Irregular Eating Patterns

Due to the rapid onset and shorter duration of action, glinides are ideal for patients who eat meals at differing times day to day. For these patients, glinides should be taken just before the meal (0–30 min prior) regardless of the time of the meal. The ability to change the dose timing of these insulin secretagogues to when a patient eats is a niche for glinides in antidiabetic medication options.

Pregnancy and Lactation

Repaglinide is categorized as pregnancy category C. Repaglinide has not been found to be teratogenic in animal studies; however, nonteratogenic skeletal deformities were observed following exposure during gestation and lactation. Nateglinide is also categorized as pregnancy category C. Adverse effects have been observed in some animal reproduction studies. As the studies on the effects of glinides on pregnancy outcomes is limited, it is not recommended to use them during pregnancy.

Although it is not known whether or not the glinides are excreted in human milk, some animal studies do suggest secretion into the milk of lactating animals. It is recommended that neither glinide be used in nursing women, due to the possible risk of hypoglycemia in nursing infants.

Hepatic or Renal Impairment

Because glinides are metabolized by CYP isoenzymes, caution should be exercised when using this class of medications in patients with hepatic impairment. Patients with moderate to severe impairment of liver function will have higher serum concentrations and more unbound repaglinide and metabolites than will patients with normal hepatic function. However, the altered serum concentrations and unbound fraction have not been shown to alter the response to repaglinide. Since some patients with hepatic dysfunction could respond differently, it is reasonable to start with lower doses of repaglinide. Peak concentration and overall drug exposure to nateglinide were increased by about 30% in nondiabetic subjects with mild hepatic dysfunction when compared to healthy volunteers. No dosage adjustment is recommended in patients with mild to moderate hepatic dysfunction; nateglinide should be used with caution in patients with severe hepatic failure.

In patients for whom insulin secretagogue therapy is effective, glinides can be useful for those with renal dysfunction, due to their short duration of action and their reduced risk of hypoglycemia. No adjustment in the initial dose of repaglinide is required in patients with mild to moderate renal dysfunction. In those with severe renal dysfunction, it is recommended to start with the 0.5-mg dose. Although no dosage adjustment is needed for nateglinide in patients with renal dysfunction, patients with severe renal impairment could be more susceptible to hypoglycemia, due to accumulation of the M1 active metabolite. Therefore, it would be reasonable to start with the 60-mg dose in this population.

Pediatrics

The safety and effectiveness of repaglinide and nateglinide has not been established in children.

Geriatrics

The pharmacokinetics of either glinide are not significantly affected by age, and no dose adjustment is recommended in elderly patients.

Patients with Food Insecurities and Homelessness

Patients who are homeless or who do not have a reliable source of food may experience more frequent hypoglycemia if taking a sulfonylurea, particularly a longer-acting one. Therefore, in patients with food insecurities who may benefit from an insulin secretagogue, the glinides may be advantageous, as they are only taken if a meal is available. Use of glinides can therefore help to prevent hypoglycemia in patients who may not have a plan for future meals, whereas use of a sulfonylurea could put these patients at risk for hypoglycemia. Providers should also help these patients seek local resources to assist them in obtaining regularly distributed food.[23]

Patients with Cardiovascular Disease and Increased Cardiovascular Risk

Neither glinide has been shown to be associated with an increased risk of cardiovascular morbidity or mortality compared to other antidiabetic medications.[24-26] In the Nateglinide And Valsartan in Impaired Glucose Tolerance Outcomes Research (NAVIGATOR) study, nateglinide was evaluated in patients with impaired glucose tolerance to see if its use could reduce the risk of cardiovascular outcomes; nateglinide was not found to reduce the risk of cardiovascular events.[27]

ADVERSE EFFECTS AND MONITORING

Glinides are usually well tolerated, and the frequency of side effects, including hypoglycemia, is low. The most common adverse effects associated with glinide treatment other than hypoglycemia are upper respiratory infections, sinusitis, nausea, diarrhea, constipation, arthralgia, weight gain, and headache.[11] Rare side effects include hypersensitivity reactions and hepatic enzyme elevations.[11,28]

The two adverse effects that are the primary disadvantages of glinides are weight gain and hypoglycemia.[2] In a retrospective analysis of a large, national cohort of T2D, use of a sulfonylurea or glinide increased the risk of severe hypoglycemia about twofold.[29] This analysis also found that patients with high complexity (i.e., age 75 years and older or multiple comorbidities) on intensive treatment also had nearly double the risk of severe hypoglycemia. Monitoring blood glucose levels and only taking a glinide when eating a meal can help to reduce the risk of hypoglycemia. Unlike some of the sulfonylureas, glinides do not appear in the Beers Criteria as potentially inappropriate medications in patients 65 years and older.[30]

Glinides can cause a weight gain of 1–3 kg compared to baseline. In a pooled analysis of studies, sulfonylureas and glinides increased weight similarly.[2] The weight gain can be attributed to two factors: improved glycemic control and hypoglycemia. Inherent in improving glycemic control is weight gain, as fewer calories are spilling into the urine. Also, a patient consumes additional calories when treating hypoglycemia. Therefore, it is important not only to reduce the risk of hypoglycemia from a safety perspective, but also to limit weight gain associated with glinides.

Patients on glinides should be educated on how to self-monitor their blood glucose (and to monitor regularly), hypoglycemic symptoms and values, and how to self-treat for a hypoglycemic episode. A quick-acting source of glucose should be used. Patients should also be educated to only take a glinide with the meal; if the meal is skipped, the glinide dose is also skipped. Patients who are purposefully trying to eat less, increase physical activity, or lose weight may need their glinide dose reduced.

DRUG INTERACTIONS

Repaglinide's metabolism can be inhibited by CYP3A4 inhibitors, such as ketoconazole, itraconazole, cyclosporine, and erythromycin.[31,32] When used with cyclosporine, the maximum daily dose of repaglinide is 6 mg. Agents that induce CYP3A4 metabolism, such as rifampin, barbiturates, and carbamazepine, may reduce repaglinide levels. The combination of repaglinide and atazanavir should be avoided, as atazanavir is a CYP2C8 substrate.

Coadministration of repaglinide with the CYP450 inhibitor clarithromycin resulted in significantly higher concentrations of repaglinide.[33,34] This increase may necessitate a dosage reduction of repaglinide in cases when these drugs are used together. Gemfibrozil causes a significant increase in repaglinide serum levels, and their concomitant use is considered a contraindication.[35,36] Itraconazole has been shown to augment the interaction with gemfibrozil and repaglinide.[32]

Clopidogrel can inhibit CYP2C8 and thus increase repaglinide levels.[37] It is recommended to avoid their concomitant use; if it is necessary to use together, the starting dose of repaglinide is 0.5 mg with each meal, and the total daily dose should be limited to 4 mg or less.

The hypoglycemic action of repaglinide may be enhanced by certain drugs, including NSAIDs and other agents that are highly bound to protein, such as salicylates, sulfonamides, chloramphenicol, warfarin, probenecid, monoamine oxidase inhibitors, and β-blockers. Therefore, if using repaglinide with any of the aforementioned drugs, blood glucose should be monitored and the dose adjusted accordingly.

Even though nateglinide is metabolized by CYP2C9 (major) and CYP3A4 (minor), few clinically significant drug-drug interactions exist with nateglinide. Nateglinide's metabolism can be inhibited by CYP2C9 inhibitors, such as amiodarone, fluconazole, and voriconazole; therefore, the dose of nateglinide may need to be reduced. Although nateglinide is highly protein-bound, in vitro displacement studies have found that nateglinide does not have a significant effect on other highly bound drugs.[12]

Pharmacodynamic interactions with all antidiabetics include drugs that can cause hyperglycemia, and when taken may lead to worsening of glycemic control. Examples of these drugs include thiazide diuretics, statins, glucocorticoids, phenothiazines, certain antipsychotics (e.g., chlorpromazine, olanzapine, clozapine), HIV protease inhibitors, estrogens and hormonal contraceptives, phenytoin, immunosuppressive therapies, sympathomimetics, and isoniazid.

DOSAGE AND ADMINISTRATION

For patients whose A1C is <8%, the starting dose of repaglinide is 0.5 mg before each meal. For patients whose A1C is ≥8%, the initial dose is 1 or 2 mg before each meal. Dosage adjustments are determined by blood glucose response. The preprandial dose should be increased (typically doubled) until glycemic control is achieved or until a maximum dose of 4 mg per meal or 16 mg daily is reached. The usual starting dose of nateglinide is 120 mg before each meal. For patients who are close to their target A1C goal, nateglinide can be initiated at the lower 60-mg dose and then titrated up to 120 mg or until the glycemic response is achieved.

Doses should be taken 0–30 min before a meal. Patients who skip a meal or add an extra meal should be instructed to skip or add a dose for that meal, respectively. Most glinide dosage adjustments are typically done at weekly intervals or longer. Monitoring the preprandial and postprandial (e.g., 2 h after the start of the meal) glucose is particularly effective in assessing the dose response to a glinide. Typical dosing and administration regimens are shown in Table 9.2. In practice, depending on a patient's blood glucose profile, a different dose of a glinide may be taken at particular mealtimes, taking into account different types of meals (e.g., the amount of carbohydrates in the meal) and/or the premeal blood glucose.

When switching from a sulfonylurea to a glinide, the first glinide dose may be administered on the day after the final dose of the sulfonylurea. After changing to a glinide, patients should closely monitor their blood glucose, watching for any hypoglycemia, in case there is a residual effect of the sulfonylurea or an enhanced response to the glinide.

Table 9.2—Glinide Dosage Information

Glinide	Available strengths	Usual starting dose	Dose titration	Dosage range
Nateglinide	60 mg, 120 mg	120 mg three times daily before meals 60 mg three times daily before meals if close to A1C goal	Weekly, if started on 60 mg dose	180–360 mg daily
Repaglinide	0.5 mg, 1 mg, 2 mg	A1C <8%: 0.5 mg three times daily before meals A1C ≥8%: 1 or 2 mg three times daily before meals	0.5–2 mg each meal on a weekly basis (mealtime dose is typically doubled)	0.5–4 mg before meals or up to 16 mg daily

Source: Individual drug monographs at DAILYMED.

COMBINATION PILLS CONTAINING A GLINIDE

Currently there are no combination tablets with glinides available.

MONOGRAPHS

Nateglinide: https://dailymed.nlm.nih.gov/dailymed/drugInfo.cfm?setid =a7e9f62e-32f8-4a89-8588-74d029c8f6a2

Repaglinide: https://dailymed.nlm.nih.gov/dailymed/drugInfo.cfm?setid =68064989-47ea-4ed5-a20e-43c4ef6ec271

REFERENCES

1. Lipska KJ, Yao X, Herrin J, et al. Trends in drug utilization, glycemic control, and rates of severe hypoglycemia, 2006–2013. *Diabetes Care* 2017;40:468–75

2. Bennett WL, Maruthur NM, Singh S, et al. Comparative effectiveness and safety of medications for type 2 diabetes: an update including new drugs and 2-drug combinations. *Ann Intern Med* 2011;154:602–613

3. American Diabetes Association. 8. Pharmacologic approaches to glycemic treatment: *Standards of Medical Care in Diabetes—2018. Diabetes Care* 2018;41(Suppl. 1):S73–S85

4. Turner RC, Cull CA, Frighi V, Holman RR; UKPDS Group. Glycemic control with diet, sulfonylurea, metformin, or insulin in patients with type 2 diabetes mellitus: progressive requirement for multiple therapies (UKPDS 49). *JAMA* 1999;281:2005–2012

5. American Diabetes Association. 2. Classification and diagnosis of diabetes: *Standards of Medical Care in Diabetes—2018. Diabetes Care* 2018; 41(Suppl. 1):S13–S27

6. Tuomi T, Honkanen EH, Isomaa B, Sarelin L, Groop LC. Improved prandial glucose control with lower risk of hypoglycemia with nateglinide than with glibenclamide in patients with maturity-onset diabetes of the young type 3. *Diabetes Care* 2006;29:189–194

7. Kennedy M, Masharani U. Pancreatic hormones and antidiabetic drugs. In *Basic and Clinical Pharmacology*, 13th ed. Katzung BG, Trevor AJ, Eds. New York, McGraw-Hill, 2015. Available from http://accessmedicine.mhmedical.com/content.aspx?bookid=1193&sectionid=69110459. Accessed 13 August 2018

8. Dornhorst A. Insulinotropic meglitinide analogues. *Lancet* 2001;358: 1709–1716

9. Guardado-Mendoza R, Prioletta A, Jiménez-Ceja LM, Sosale A, Folli F. The role of nateglinide and repaglinide, derivatives of meglitinide, in the treatment of type 2 diabetes mellitus. *Arch Med Sci* 2013;9:936–943

10. Inzucchi SE. Oral antihyperglycemic therapy for type 2 diabetes: scientific review. *JAMA* 2002;287:360–372

11. Scott LJ. Repaglinide: a review of its use in type 2 diabetes mellitus. *Drugs* 2012;72:249–272

12. McLeod JF. Clinical pharmacokinetics of nateglinide: a rapidly-absorbed, short-acting insulinotropic agent. *Clin Pharmacokinet* 2004;43:97–120

13. Black C, Donnelly P, McIntyre L, Royle PL, Shepherd JP, Thomas S. Meglitinide analogues for type 2 diabetes mellitus. *Cochrane Database Syst Rev* 2007;(2):CD004654

14. Rosenstock J, Hassman DR, Madder RD, et al.; Repaglinide Versus Nateglinide Comparison Study Group. Repaglinide versus nateglinide monotherapy: a randomized, multicenter study. *Diabetes Care* 2004;27:1265–1270

15. Van Gaal LF, Van Acker KL, De Leeuw IH. Repaglinide improves blood glucose control in sulphonylurea-naive type 2 diabetes. *Diabetes Res Clin Pract* 2001;53:141–148

16. Hezarkhani S, Bonakdaran S, Rajabian R, Shahini N, Marjani A. Comparison of glycemic excursion in patients with new onset type 2 diabetes mellitus before and after treatment with repaglinide. *Open Biochem J* 2013;7:19–23

17. Islas-Andrade S, Revilla-Monsalve MC, Martínez de Hurtado E, et al.; Latin American Study Group. Evaluation of the effects of nateglinide on postprandial glycemia in patients with type 2 diabetes mellitus: a multicenter, multinational, non-randomized, non-controlled Latin American study. *Pharmacology* 2003;68:89–95

18. Hollander PA, Schwartz SL, Gatlin MR, Haas SJ, et al. Importance of early insulin secretion: comparison of nateglinide and glyburide in previously diet-treated patients with type 2 diabetes. *Diabetes Care* 2001;26:983–988

19. The DECODE Study Group on behalf of the European Diabetes Epidemiology Group. Glucose tolerance and mortality: comparison of WHO and American Diabetes Association diagnostic criteria. *Lancet* 1999;354:617–621

20. Nakagami T; DECODA Study Group. Hyperglycaemia and mortality from all causes and from cardiovascular disease in five populations of Asian origin. *Diabetologia* 2004;47:385–394

21. Fonseca V. Clinical significance of targeting postprandial and fasting hyperglycemia in managing type 2 diabetes mellitus. *Curr Med Res Opin* 2003;19:635–641

22. Aronoff SL. Rationale for treatment options for mealtime glucose control in patients with type 2 diabetes. *Postgrad Med* 2017;129:231–241

23. Seligman HK, Schillinger D. Hunger and socioeconomic disparities in chronic disease. *N Engl J Med* 2010;363:6–9

24. Mogensen UM, Andersson C, Fosbøl EL, et al. Metformin in combination with various insulin secretagogues in type 2 diabetes and associated risk of cardiovascular morbidity and mortality—a retrospective nationwide study. *Diabetes Res Clin Pract* 2015;107:104–112

25. Schramm TK, Gislason GH, Vaag A, et al. Mortality and cardiovascular risk associated with different insulin secretagogues compared with metformin in type 2 diabetes, with or without a previous myocardial infarction: a nationwide study. *Eur Heart J* 2011;32:1900–1908

26. Huang Y, Abdelmoneim AS, Light P, Qiu W, Simpson SH. Comparative cardiovascular safety of insulin secretagogues following hospitalization for ischemic heart disease among type 2 diabetes patients: a cohort study. *J Diabetes Complications* 2015;29:196–202

27. Derosa G. Nateglinide does not reduce the incidence of diabetes or cardiovascular outcomes in people with impaired glucose tolerance and cardiovascular disease or risk factors. *BMJ Evid Based Med* 2011;16:7–8

28. Nan DN, Hernández JL, Fernández-Ayala M, Carrascosa M. Acute hepatotoxicity caused by repaglinide. *Ann Intern Med* 2004;141:823

29. McCoy RD, Lipska KJ, Yao X, et al. Intensive treatment and severe hypoglycemia among adults with type 2 diabetes. *JAMA Intern Med* 2016; 176:969–978

30. American Geriatrics Society 2015 Beers Criteria Update Expert Panel. American Geriatrics Society 2015 updated Beers Criteria for potentially inappropriate medication use in older adults. *J Am Geriatr Soc* 2015;63: 2227–2246

31. Scheen AJ. Drug-drug and food-drug pharmacokinetic interactions with new insulinotropic agents repaglinide and nateglinide. *Clin Pharmacokinet* 2007;46:93–108

32. Kudo T, Hisaka A, Sugiyama Y, Ito K. Analysis of the repaglinide concentration increase produced by gemfibrozil and itraconazole based on the inhibition of the hepatic uptake transporter and metabolic enzymes. *Drug Metab Dispos* 2013;41:362–371

33. Khamaisi M, Leitersdorf E. Severe hypoglycemia from clarithromycin-repaglinide drug interaction. *Pharmacotherapy* 2008;28:682–684

34. Niemi M, Neuvonen PJ, Kivistö KT. The cytochrome P4503A4 inhibitor clarithromycin increases the plasma concentrations and effects of repaglinide. *Clin Pharmacol Ther* 2001;70:58–65

35. Gan J, Chen W, Shen H, et al. Repaglinide-gemfibrozil drug interaction: inhibition of repaglinide glucuronidation as a potential additional contributing mechanism. *Br J Clin Pharmacol* 2010;70:870–880

36. Honkalammi J, Niemi M, Neuvonen PJ, Backman JT. Dose-dependent interaction between gemfibrozil and repaglinide in humans: strong inhibition of CYP2C8 with subtherapeutic gemfibrozil doses. *Drug Metab Dispos* 2011;39:1977–1986

37. Tornio A, Filppula AM, Kailari O, et al. Glucuronidation converts clopidogrel to a strong time-dependent inhibitor of CYP2C8: a phase II metabolite as a perpetrator of drug-drug interactions. *Clin Pharmacol Ther* 2014;96: 498–507

Chapter 10
SGLT2 Inhibitors
JOHN R. WHITE, JR., PA-C, PHARMD

INTRODUCTION

The kidney has been considered primarily an organ of elimination for several hundred years, as well as a modulator of salt and ion balance. Our construct of the kidney has evolved significantly over the past 2 decades. At one time, it was considered to be the structural cause of diabetes. Later, its role in glucose homeostasis, while recognized, was all but ignored. Today, however, it is recognized for its salient role in the regulation of glucose homeostasis. As the elucidation of the physiology of glucose transport via specific carriers such as the SGLTs developed, the idea that the natural compound phlorizin (which was isolated in the early 1800s) or its analogs could possibly be used pharmacologically began to be investigated.[1] This work led to the development of several SGLT2 inhibitors. Currently, there are four FDA-approved SGLT2 inhibitors on the market in the U.S.: canagliflozin, dapagliflozin, empagliflozin, and ertugliflozin.

PHARMACOLOGY

MECHANISM OF ACTION

The mechanism of action of these agents is novel and unique. The kidney is involved in glucose homeostasis via several mechanisms, including gluconeogenesis, glucose utilization, glomerular filtration, and reabsorption of glucose in the proximal convoluted tubules.[2] However, the primary effect of the kidney on glucose homeostasis is by glomerular filtration, reabsorption, and urine glucose excretion (UGE). UGE can simply be calculated by subtracting the amount of glucose that is reabsorbed from the amount filtered. Under typical conditions, normal healthy adults filter approximately 180 g of glucose daily. In nondiabetic individuals under euglycemic conditions, the majority of glucose (99%) is reabsorbed with only a small fraction being excreted in the urine.

The reabsorption of glucose from the urine begins with the transport of glucose from the tubule (lumen) into the tubular epithelial cells by way of SGLTs. These SGLTs include a number of membrane proteins that transport many compounds across the lumen membrane of renal tubules as well as from the lumen of the intestine across the intestinal epithelium. The two most well-characterized members of this family are SGLT1 and SGLT2. The first of these, SGLT1, is a low-capacity, high-affinity Na+/glucose transporter, located primarily in the gastrointestinal tract and also found in the S3 segment of the proximal tubule. Although the role of SGLT1s in the kidney is relatively small—accounting for only about 10% of glucose reabsorption there—it is the most important transport mechanism for glucose absorption in the gastrointestinal tract. Conversely, SGLT2 is a high-capacity, low-affinity transporter found primarily in the kidney. It accounts for approximately 90% of glucose reabsorption in the kidney. This transporter is found at a relatively high density on the lumen (brush-border) membrane of the S1 segment of the proximal convoluted tubule. This transporter binds with glucose and Na+ in the tubular filtrate and actively transports glucose across the membrane through Na+ coupling. This process is fueled by the Na+ gradient established between the tubular filtrate and the cell (secondary active transport).[2]

After glucose is transported via SGLT2 into the luminal epithelium, it is transported by GLUTs (glucose transporter proteins) through the basolateral membrane along with Na+ back into the peritubular capillary. This basolateral membrane–peritubular capillary transfer uses both GLUT1 transporters in the late proximal tubule and GLUT2 transporters in the early proximal tubule (see Figure 10.1).[2]

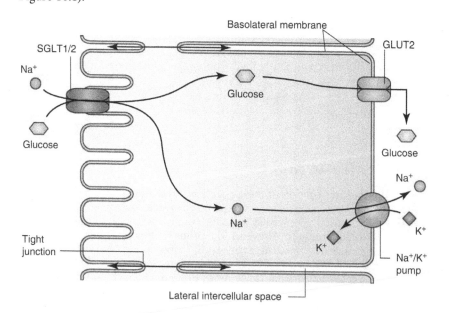

Figure 10.1—Glucose reabsorption from glomerular filtrate through the proximal tubule epithelial cell into the blood. Abbreviations: GLUT, glucose transporter protein. *Source*: Bakris.[3]

The mechanism of action of the SGLT2 inhibitors is through inhibition of SGLT2, which in turn results in an increase in UGE. These medications essentially lower the renal threshold for glucose excretion. The SGLT2 inhibitors prevent the reabsorption of between 30 and 50% of filtered glucose.[4] The result of this inhibition is renal loss of glucose and a concomitant reduction in blood glucose. Also, it should be noted that a mixed SGLT1 and SGLT2 inhibitor, sotagliflozin, is currently under development.[5] This medication will modulate glucose transport in both the gastrointestinal tract and the kidney.

PHARMACOKINETICS

Canagliflozin

Canagliflozin has a mean oral bioavailability of 65%. Although it can probably be taken with or without food, it is recommended that it be taken before the first meal of the day. The mean volume of distribution is approximately 83.5 L, and the drug is 99% bound to plasma proteins. The metabolism of canagliflozin is primarily via uridine diphosphate glucuronosyltransferase (UGT) (1A2 and 2B4) to inactive metabolites, but about 7% is metabolized by CYP3A4. The metabolites are excreted primarily by the fecal route, with about one-third being excreted through the urine. Mean systemic clearance of canagliflozin is 192 mL/min in healthy subjects. The mean terminal half-life ranges from approximately 10–13 h.[6]

Dapagliflozin

The mean bioavailability of dapagliflozin following a 10-mg dose is 78%.[7] Some alterations in C_{max} and T_{max} are observed when the medication is administered with a high-fat meal, but the AUC is unchanged. The observed changes are not considered to be clinically relevant, and this medication can be administered with or without food. Dapagliflozin is extensively metabolized via UGT to an inactive metabolite (~61%). The parent compound and related metabolites are excreted via the kidneys (75%) and the feces (21%). Approximately 2% of the dose is excreted unchanged in the urine, and approximately 15% is excreted in the feces. The mean terminal half-life following a single oral dose of 10 mg is 12.9 h.

Empagliflozin

Administration of empagliflozin with a meal resulted in a slightly reduced AUC (16%) and C_{max} (37%) compared to administration in the fasting state. This difference was deemed not clinically significant, and this medication may be administered with or without food. The apparent mean volume of distribution is estimated to be 73.8 L. Empagliflozin is metabolized via UGT and is also partially excreted unchanged in the urine (11–19%) and feces.[8,9] The mean terminal half-life is estimated to be 12.4 h, and the oral clearance is estimated to be 10.6 L/h (based on population kinetics).

Ertugliflozin

The mean bioavailability of ertugliflozin following a 15-mg dose was 100%.[10] Some alterations in C_{max} and T_{max} are observed when the medication is administered with a high-fat meal, but the AUC is unchanged. The observed changes are not considered to be clinically relevant, and this medication can be administered with or without food. The mean steady-state volume of distribution of ertugliflozin after the administration of an intravenous dose is 85.5 L. Ertugliflozin is primarily metabolized via UGT to two inactive glucuronide metabolites. Approximately 12% of ertugliflozin is metabolized by CYP enzymes. Approximately 1.5% of the parent compound is excreted through the urine, and approximately 33.8% is excreted unchanged in the feces. It is thought that this "unchanged" fecal fraction may actually be secondary to the biliary excretion of the glucuronide metabolite, which is then hydrolyzed back to the parent compound. The mean clearance following an intravenous dose of 100 µg was 11.2 L/h. The mean terminal half-life in patients with T2D was 16.6 h (based on population kinetics).

TREATMENT ADVANTAGES/DISADVANTAGES

ADVANTAGES

There are several characteristics of the SGLT2 inhibitors that could be considered advantageous. These include cardiovascular effects, potential renal protective effects, low rates of hypoglycemia, and weight loss.

Cardiovascular and Renal Outcomes

One of the more exciting and salient findings with the SGLT2 inhibitors has been the correlation between their use (canagliflozin and empagliflozin) and positive cardiovascular outcomes.[11,12] Two landmark trials have suggested cardiovascular benefit with the use of the two SGLT2 medications studied. The first trial, Empagliflozin, Cardiovascular Outcomes, and Mortality in Type 2 Diabetes (EMPA-REG), was a large, multicenter, randomized, double-blind, placebo-controlled trial that evaluated over 7,000 patients with T2D who were at high risk for cardiovascular events. These patients were randomized to either 10 or 25 mg of empagliflozin or placebo against a background of standard diabetes care. The primary composite outcome of the study was cardiovascular death, nonfatal MI, and stroke. The pooled empagliflozin group realized a significant reduction in the composite outcome (14% risk reduction), in the risk of death from cardiovascular causes (38% relative risk reduction), hospitalization for HF (35% relative risk reduction), and death from any cause (32% relative risk reduction). There was no significant difference in the rates of MI or stroke when analyzed singularly.[11] The findings of this study led the American Diabetes Association to recommend that empagliflozin (and also liraglutide) be considered after lifestyle management and metformin in order to reduce cardiovascular events and mortality.[13] The second trial, Canagliflozin Cardiovascular Assessment Study (CANVAS), evaluated more than 10,000 patients with T2D who were at high risk for cardiovascular events.

Patients were randomized to receive canagliflozin or placebo. Patients were treated with either 100 or 300 mg of canagliflozin. The primary outcome of this trial was the same as with EMPA-REG (composite of death from cardiovascular causes, nonfatal MI, stroke). The patients receiving canagliflozin compared to those receiving placebo had a hazard ratio of 0.86 for the composite outcome. The study also demonstrated a possible renal benefit related to canagliflozin, with a hazard ratio of 0.73 for progression of albuminuria and a hazard ratio of 0.6 for the composite renal outcome of 40% reduction in glomerular filtration rate, the need for renal replacement therapy, and death due to renal causes. Unfortunately, the study also reported an almost twofold increase in the risk of lower limb amputation in the patients receiving canagliflozin.

Renal Protection

SGLT2 inhibition has shown promise in several studies evaluating the impact of these agents on renal disease. One recent review stated that the two studies cited above demonstrated overall cardiovascular benefit and "suggest the possibility of dramatic kidney protection in DM2."[14] At least four major trials evaluating this question are currently underway (Dapagliflozin Effect on Cardiovascular Events [DECLARE], Cardiovascular Outcomes Following Ertugliflozin Treatment in Type 2 Diabetes Mellitus Participants With Vascular Disease [VERTIS], Canagliflozin and Renal Outcomes in Type 2 Diabetes and Nephropathy [CREDENCE], A Study to Evaluate the Effect of Dapagliflozin on Renal Outcomes and Cardiovascular Mortality in Patients With Chronic Kidney Disease [DAPA-CKD]) with anticipated completion in 2019–2020.

Low Rates of Hypoglycemia

SGLT2 inhibitors are not associated with high rates of hypoglycemia, in part because they do not completely block renal glucose reabsorption. They inhibit reabsorption of 30–50% of filtered glucose.[4] The reason for this has not been elucidated but may be due to a saturation in the transport mechanism that delivers the medication to the active site. Generally speaking, low rates of hypoglycemia have been consistently reported in clinical trials with SGLT2 inhibitors, except in patients receiving background insulin or sulfonylureas. A meta-analysis of 58 clinical trials reported an odds ratio of 0.44 for hypoglycemia in patients treated with SGLT2 inhibitors when compared to other antihyperglycemic medications.[15]

Weight Loss

The SGLT2 inhibitors have been consistently associated with weight loss. The level of weight loss varies but may in some cases be as high as 4.7 kg.[4] Although the magnitude of weight loss varies depending on conditions of the study and population evaluated, a positive effect on weight (i.e., loss) has been consistently observed in multiple studies. The SGLT2 inhibitors may in some cases be effective in mitigating the increase in weight caused by other medications. In one trial that included the TZD pioglitazone (which is linked to weight gain), dapagliflozin attenuated the TZD-associated weight gain.[16] Another study evaluating weight loss secondary to SGLT2 inhibitors reported that 66% of the weight loss linked to the SGLT2 inhibitor dapagliflozin was due to loss of both visceral and subcutaneous fat.[17]

DISADVANTAGES

There are also several characteristics that could be considered to be disadvantages, including cost, a potential greater risk of lower limb amputation, and other well-recognized adverse events.

Cost

Although the cost of the SGLT2 inhibitors is less than that of GLP-1 RAs, they are higher than most of the other commonly utilized oral antihyperglycemic agents.[13] The average wholesale price for a 1-month supply of canagliflozin, dapagliflozin, or empagliflozin ranges from $512 to $517. The national average acquisition cost ranges from $411 to $415.

Black Box Warning (Lower Limb Amputation)—Canagliflozin

One of the findings of the CANVAS and Canagliflozin Cardiovascular Assessment Study-Renal (CANVAS-R) trials was a twofold increased risk of lower limb amputations in patients with T2D who had established cardiovascular disease. The most frequent types of amputations involved the toe or the midfoot. However, some patients had multiple amputations, in some cases involving both limbs. Prior to initiation of therapy, it is suggested that multiple factors be considered, including history of prior amputation, peripheral vascular disease (PVD), neuropathy, and diabetes-related foot ulcers. Additionally, patients taking this agent should be provided with appropriate caution regarding the early reportage of any signs or symptoms that might be associated with lower limb problems.[6,12]

THERAPEUTIC CONSIDERATIONS

SIGNIFICANT WARNINGS/PRECAUTIONS

Lower Limb Amputations

This warning is described in the section above. The numbers of cases per 1,000 patients per year treated with canagliflozin and placebo in the CANVAS study were 5.9 and 2.8, respectively. The numbers of cases per 1,000 patients per year treated with canagliflozin and placebo in the CANVAS-R study were 7.5 and 4.2, respectively. Appropriate cautions as mentioned above should be instituted.[6,12]

Hypotension/Acute Kidney Injury and Impairment in Renal Function

These agents cause intravascular volume contraction by virtue of their mechanism of action and the diuresis that occurs when they are used. This volume depletion may lead to hypotension and a temporary or transient reduction in glomerular filtration. The package inserts from the currently marketed SGLT2 inhibitors all contain warnings about this potential adverse event and suggest care with patients at high risk for side effects related to intravascular volume contraction.[6-8,10] The greatest increase in incidence of volume contraction–related events has occurred in the elderly, patients with reduced GFRs, patients treated with loop diuretics or renin-angiotensin-aldosterone system modulators, and patients with low systolic blood pressure. Volume status should be addressed and corrected prior to initiation of therapy.

Ketoacidosis

DKA has been observed in both T1D and T2D patients treated with SGLT2 inhibition. The increased risk seems to be greater in patients treated with exogenous insulin. Also, the increased risk is more clearly defined in patients with T1D. As many as 9.4% of patients with T1D enrolled in trials evaluating SGLT2 inhibition developed ketosis while 6% developed DKA.[18] The relationship between ketoacidosis and SGLT2 inhibitors in patients with T2D is less clear. Still, appropriate vigilance should be exercised in patients with T2D being treated with SGLT2 inhibition. SGLT2 inhibition in patients with T1D is being evaluated in well-controlled studies and should probably not be used in the general practice setting until more is known about the risk/benefit ratio of these medications in patients with T1D.

Urogenital Infections

Glucosuria has historically been recognized as a risk factor for urinary tract and other genital infections. Thus, these potential adverse events were anticipated with the SGLT2 inhibitors and have been well documented. Multiple studies have demonstrated that urogenital infections typically occur at a higher rate in patients treated with SGLT2 inhibitors than in those treated with placebo or other medications.[2] However, the incidence of infections in patients treated with SGLT2s varied greatly across those published studies and was even similar to placebo in some.

A meta-analysis of SGLT2 studies reported an odds ratio of 1.34 for the development of urinary tract infections (UTIs) in patients treated with SGLT2 inhibitors when compared to placebo. The study reported an odds ratio of 1.42 in patients treated with SGLT2 inhibitors versus other antihyperglycemic agents.[15] Another study evaluated the rates of UTIs from 12 randomized placebo-controlled trials involving the SGLT2 inhibitor dapagliflozin. The overall rates of UTIs in 3,152 patients treated with dapagliflozin 2.5, 5, 10 mg, or placebo in these trials were 3.6%, 5.7%, 4.3%, and 3.7%, respectively.[19] The overall rates of UTIs in patients treated with empagliflozin 10, 25 mg, or placebo in the phase 3 trials (2,971 patients) were 9.3%, 7.6%, and 7.6%, respectively.[8] The overall rates of UTIs in 2,313 patients treated with canagliflozin 100, 300 mg, or placebo were 5.9%, 4.3%, and 4.0%, respectively.[6] The overall rates of UTIs in 1,544 patients treated with ertugliflozin 5, 15 mg, or placebo in the phase 3 trials were 4.0%, 4.1%, and 3.9% respectively.[10] Females are linked to a higher incidence of UTIs than are males with all of the SGLT2 inhibitors currently on the market.

Genital infections (vulvovaginitis, balanitis, and others) also occur at a higher rate in patients treated with SGLT2 inhibitors than in those treated with placebo.[2]

A meta-analysis of pertinent studies reported an odds ratio of 3.5 for the development of genital infections in patients treated with SGLT2 inhibitors versus placebo and an odds ratio of 5.06 for the development of genital infections in patients treated with SGLT2 inhibitors versus active comparators.[15]

Generally speaking, both UTIs and genital infections that are associated with SGLT2 inhibition are mild and rarely result in discontinuation of the medication. However, there have been occasional reports of urosepsis and pyelonephritis in patients treated with SGLT2 inhibitors.

SPECIAL POPULATIONS

Canagliflozin[6]

Pregnancy
Not recommended during second or third trimesters. There are insufficient data to determine drug-associated risk of major birth defects or miscarriage.

Lactation
No information is available regarding the presence of canagliflozin in human milk, the breast-fed infant, or the effects on milk production.

Pediatrics
Safety and effectiveness in patients under 18 years old has not been established.

Geriatrics
This drug has been studied in the geriatric population in multiple clinical trials. These patients experienced a higher incidence of intravascular volume–related adverse events (particularly at a higher dose of 300 mg/day) and experienced smaller reductions in A1C than were observed in their younger counterparts.

Renal Impairment
Patients with moderate renal dysfunction (eGFR 45–60 mL/min/1.73 m^2) experienced reduced glycemic efficacy, a higher incidence of intravascular volume–related adverse events, and a higher rate of hyperkalemia. The dose should be limited to 100 mg/day in these patients. Canagliflozin has not been studied and is not recommended in patients with an eGFR of <45 mL/min/1.73 m^2.

Hepatic Impairment
No dosage adjustment is required in patients with mild to moderate hepatic impairment. This drug has not been studied and is not recommended in patients with severe hepatic impairment.

Dapagliflozin[7]

Pregnancy
Not recommended during second or third trimesters. There are insufficient data to determine drug-associated risk of major birth defects or miscarriage.

Lactation
No information is available regarding the presence of dapagliflozin in human milk, the breast-fed infant, or the effects on milk production.

Pediatrics

Safety and effectiveness in patients under 18 years old has not been established.

Geriatrics

This drug has been studied in the geriatric population in multiple clinical trials. These patients experienced a higher incidence of intravascular volume and renal-related adverse events. After controlling for changes in eGFR, elderly patients treated with dapagliflozin experienced similar reductions in A1C as were observed in their younger counterparts.

Renal Impairment

Patients with moderate renal dysfunction (eGFR 30–60 mL/min/1.73 m^2) treated with dapagliflozin did not experience an improvement in glycemic control when compared to placebo. They did, however, experience a higher incidence of renal-related adverse events and more bone fractures. Initiation of this drug is not recommended in patients with an eGFR of <60 mL/min/1.73 m^2.

Hepatic Impairment

No dosage adjustment is required in patients with mild, moderate, or severe hepatic impairment. However, this drug has not been studied in patients with severe hepatic impairment and therefore the benefit/risk ratio of its use in this population should be individually assessed.

Empagliflozin[8]

Pregnancy

Not recommended during second or third trimesters. There are insufficient data to determine drug-associated risk of major birth defects or miscarriage.

Lactation

No information is available regarding the presence of empagliflozin in human milk, the breast-fed infant, or the effects on milk production.

Pediatrics

Safety and effectiveness in patients under 18 years old has not been established.

Geriatrics

This drug has been studied in the geriatric population in multiple clinical trials. It is expected that these patients will realize less glycemic impact with renal impairment. No adjustment of dose is recommended for empagliflozin in this population. A subgroup of these patients (>75 years old) experienced a dose-related (2.3%—10 mg daily; 4.4%—25 mg daily) higher incidence of intravascular volume–adverse events.

Renal Impairment

Empagliflozin was studied in patients with mild to moderate renal dysfunction (eGFR 30–90 mL/min/1.73 m^2). The glycemic-lowering effect of this drug was diminished with worsening renal function. These patients experienced a higher incidence of renal- and volume-related adverse events and UTIs as renal function declined. The efficacy and safety of empagliflozin has not been established in patients with severe renal impairment, end-stage renal disease (ESRD), or in those receiving dialysis.

Hepatic Impairment
Empagliflozin may be used in patients with hepatic impairment.

Ertugliflozin[10]

Pregnancy
Not recommended during second or third trimesters. There are insufficient data to determine drug-associated risk of major birth defects or miscarriage.

Lactation
No information is available regarding the presence of ertugliflozin in human milk, the breast-fed infant, or the effects on milk production.

Pediatrics
Safety and effectiveness in patients under 18 years old has not been established.

Geriatrics
This drug has been studied in the geriatric population in clinical trials. It is expected that these patients will realize less glycemic impact from ertugliflozin with renal impairment. No adjustment of dose is recommended for ertugliflozin in this population. These patients (>65 years old) experienced a higher incidence of volume depletion–related adverse events than was reported for younger patients.

Renal Impairment
In patients with T2D and moderate renal impairment, those treated with ertugliflozin did not have an improvement in their glycemic control and had a greater risk of renal impairment, renal-related adverse events, and intravascular volume–related adverse events. Therefore, ertugliflozin is not recommended in patients with moderate renal impairment. Ertugliflozin is contraindicated in patients with severe renal impairment, ESRD, or in those receiving dialysis. No dose adjustment or increased monitoring is needed in patients with mild renal impairment.

Hepatic Impairment
Dose adjustment of ertugliflozin is not needed in patients with mild to moderate hepatic dysfunction. It has not been studied and should not be used in those with severe hepatic impairment.

PHARMACOGENOMICS

There are several potential areas of interest with regard to the intersection of pharmacogenomics and the clinical use of SGLT2 inhibitors. First, genetic variations in UGTs and/or in their expression could potentially be related to clinically significant differences in SGLT2 inhibition response. Second, the SGLT2 gene (SLC5) and many mutations have been identified and mapped. One or more of these SLC5 variants could be related to level of observed response to SGLT2 inhibition. However, at this point there are no studies that have demonstrated a clinically significant relationship between SGLT2 inhibition response and genetic variants.[20]

ADVERSE EFFECTS AND MONITORING[6-8,10]

HYPOTENSION

This adverse effect is possible with all four of the currently approved SGLT2 inhibitors. Greater risk of hypotension is seen in elderly, in patients with renal impairment, and in patients treated with diuretics. Monitor for signs and symptoms of hypotension during initiation and dose escalation.

KETOACIDOSIS

Please see "Significant Warnings/Precautions" above.

LOWER LIMB AMPUTATION

Canagliflozin and ertugliflozin only—please see "Significant Warnings/Precautions" above.

ACUTE KIDNEY INJURY AND IMPAIRMENT

Please see "Significant Warnings/Precautions" above.

HYPERKALEMIA

Canagliflozin only—Use of this medication can lead to hyperkalemia. Those who are at increased risk for this adverse effect are patients with moderate renal impairment who are also taking medications that interfere with potassium excretion (K^+-sparing diuretics) or medications that modulate the renin-angiotensin-aldosterone system. Serum monitoring of potassium is indicated in patients with the risk of developing hyperkalemia. Also, please consider that hyperkalemia in the settings described above could be theoretically possible with any of the SGLT2 inhibitors.

UROSEPSIS AND PYELONEPHRITIS

Please see "Significant Warnings/Precautions: Urogenital Infections" above.

HYPOGLYCEMIA WITH CONCOMITANT USE OF INSULIN AND INSULIN SECRETAGOGUES

Use of any of the SGLT2 inhibitors in the setting of concomitant insulin and/or secretagogue therapy results in an increased risk of hypoglycemia. A lower dose of insulin or secretagogue may be appropriate when used with an SGLT2 inhibitor.

GENITAL MYCOTIC INFECTIONS

Please see "Significant Warnings/Precautions: Urogenital Infections" above.

HYPERSENSITIVITY REACTIONS

Severe hypersensitivity reactions have been reported with canagliflozin and empagliflozin. When this occurs, the medication should be discontinued, and the patient should be treated promptly per standards of care. Also, please note that hypersensitivity reactions are possible with any medication.

BONE FRACTURE

Canagliflozin only—An increased risk of fracture has been observed with the administration of canagliflozin. This effect can occur as early as 12 weeks after initiation of therapy.

BLADDER CANCER

Dapagliflozin only—A slight increase in the incidence of bladder cancer was seen across 22 studies that evaluated dapagliflozin versus placebo (0.17% vs. 0.03%, respectively). The association between bladder cancer and this medication is unclear because there were so few cases. Currently it is recommended that patients with active bladder cancer not be treated with dapagliflozin. The benefit/risk ratio should be considered for those with a prior history of bladder cancer.

INCREASES IN LDL-C

Slight increases in LDL-C have been observed with the four currently marketed SGLT2 inhibitors.

DRUG INTERACTIONS

PHARMACODYNAMICS

One should consider the potential for two types of pharmacodynamic interactions with all four of the currently available SGLT2 inhibitors on the market. First, these medications can potentially interact in a pharmacodynamic manner with diuretics, ACE inhibitors, angiotensin II receptor blockers (ARBs), or aldosterone antagonists to facilitate or cause the worsening of volume depletion–related adverse events. Second, although these medications are associated with a very low risk of hypoglycemia when used as monotherapy, the potential for a pharmacodynamic interaction resulting in an increase in the incidence and level of hypoglycemia exists with insulin and secretagogues.

PHARMACOKINETICS

The primary metabolic pathway for all four SGLT2 inhibitors is via UGT.[6-8,10,21] These drugs are therefore not likely to be involved in the typical

CYP450-mediated interactions that are commonly encountered. Still, SGLT2 inhibitors are likely to be frequently used with multiple other medications; thus, the potential for drug-drug interactions, as with all medications, is present to some degree. The four SGLT2 inhibitors have been evaluated with varying rigor for potential interactions with multiple medications in myriad studies. A review of the interactions related to canagliflozin, dapagliflozin, and empagliflozin has been published elsewhere and provides a more detailed evaluation than is found here.[21] The pharmacokinetic studies were, in most cases, carried out on healthy volunteers and evaluated the potential impact of interactions after the administration of a single dose of an SGLT2 inhibitor. The exposure to SGLT2 inhibitors (as measured by C_{max} and AUC) was not clinically significantly altered by the concomitant administration of cardiovascular agents or antihyperglycemic medications commonly encountered in patients with T2D (metformin, glimepiride, pioglitazone, sitagliptin, linagliptin, voglibose, simvastatin, valsartan, ramipril, hydrochlorothiazide, torasemide, verapamil, warfarin—note that not all of these medications have been evaluated with all four SGLT2 inhibitors). Also, the SGLT2 inhibitors studied did not significantly affect the pharmacokinetic parameters of the second drug studied (those listed above). One exception to this is digoxin and canagliflozin. Canagliflozin has been shown to increase the AUC (20%) and the C_{max} (36%) of digoxin when the two are coadministered.[6]

Additionally, the SGLT2 inhibitors have been evaluated in the context of UGT modulators. Dapagliflozin is primarily metabolized through the UGT1A9 pathway. Dapagliflozin kinetics have been shown to be altered by two UGT1A9 pathway modulators (rifampicin [an inducer] and mefenamic acid [an inhibitor]). Rifampin coadministration with dapagliflozin resulted in a significant reduction in dapagliflozin exposure (AUC reduction of 22%).[7] When mefenamic acid was coadministered with dapagliflozin, a significant increase in dapagliflozin exposure (AUC increase of 51%) was observed. Canagliflozin has been evaluated in combination with rifampicin (600 mg/day × 8 days). In this setting, canagliflozin exposure was significantly reduced (AUC reduction—51%, C_{max} reduction—28%). Empagliflozin is metabolized via multiple UGTs (1A3, 1A8, 1A9, and 2B7). A slight increase in empagliflozin AUC and C_{max} was observed when it was administered with rifampin.[8] The change was deemed to be non-clinically relevant. Ertugliflozin is primarily metabolized via UGT1A9 and 2B7. When evaluated in combination with rifampin, a reduction in AUC (39%) and C_{max} (15%) was observed.[10] These changes were deemed to be non-clinically relevant.

Generally, the SGLT2 inhibitors appear to be relatively free of clinically significant interactions with commonly used medications. This is likely due to the nonexistent to relatively small impact of CYP metabolism on the disposition of these drugs. Still, care should always be taken, particularly when coadministering these agents with modulators of UGT.

Table 10.1—Dosage and Administration[6-8,10]

Medication	Available doses	Initial dose and range	Renal impairment	Hepatic impairment
Canagliflozin	Tablets: 100 mg, 300 mg	Initial Dose: 100 mg daily Range: 100–300 mg daily	eGFR ≥60 mL/min/1.73 m²: No dosage adjustment needed eGFR 45–59 mL/min/1.73 m²: Do not exceed 100 mg/day by mouth eGFR <45 mL/min/1.73 m²: Do not initiate; discontinue in patients currently receiving drug	No adjustment needed for mild or moderate impairment, not recommended with severe impairment
Dapagliflozin	Tablets: 2.5 mg, 5 mg, 10 mg	Initial Dose: 5 mg daily Range: 5–10 mg daily	eGFR <60 mL/min/1.73 m²: Initiation is not recommended eGFR 30–60 mL/min/1.73 m²: Not recommended Contraindicated in those with severe renal impairment, ESRD, or dialysis	No dose adjustment recommended for mild, moderate, or severe impairment. Efficacy and safety has not been studied in severe impairment
Empagliflozin	Tablets: 10 mg, 25 mg	Initial Dose: 10 mg daily Range: 10–25 mg daily	eGFR ≥45 mL/min/1.73 m²: No dosage adjustment needed eGFR <45 mL/min/1.73 m²: Do not initiate; discontinue in patients currently receiving drug	May be used in patients with hepatic impairment
Ertugliflozin	Tablets: 5 mg, 15 mg	Initial Dose: 5 mg daily Range: 5–15 mg daily	eGFR 30–60 mL/min/1.73 m²: Initiation and use is not recommended Contraindicated in those with severe renal impairment, ESRD, or dialysis	No dose adjustment recommended for mild or moderate impairment. Efficacy and safety has not been studied in severe impairment and is not recommended in this population

Source: Invokana [prescribing information],[6] Farxiga [prescribing information],[7] Jardiance [prescribing information],[8] and Steglatro [prescribing information].[10]

COMBINATION PRODUCTS

- Canagliflozin
  - Canagliflozin plus metformin hydrochloride
- Dapagliflozin
  - Dapagliflozin plus metformin hydrochloride
  - Dapagliflozin plus saxagliptin
- Empagliflozin
  - Empagliflozin plus metformin hydrochloride
  - Empagliflozin plus linagliptin
- Ertugliflozin
  - Ertugliflozin plus metformin hydrochloride
  - Ertugliflozin plus sitagliptin

MONOGRAPHS

Canagliflozin: https://dailymed.nlm.nih.gov/dailymed/drugInfo.cfm?setid=b9057d3b-b104-4f09-8a61-c61ef9d4a3f3&audience=consumer

Dapagliflozin: https://dailymed.nlm.nih.gov/dailymed/drugInfo.cfm?setid=72ad22ae-efe6-4cd6-a302-98aaee423d69&audience=consumer

Empagliflozin: https://dailymed.nlm.nih.gov/dailymed/drugInfo.cfm?setid=5777b8a8-ada6-4950-8548-43a1de11f075&audience=consumer

Ertugliflozin: https://dailymed.nlm.nih.gov/dailymed/drugInfo.cfm?setid=e6f3e718-bb99-48f1-ab94-b9f0af05fed6&audience=consumer

REFERENCES

1. White J. Apple trees to sodium glucose co-transporter inhibitors: a review of SGLT2 inhibition. *Clin Diabetes* 2010;28(1):5–10

2. White J. Sodium glucose cotransporter 2 inhibitors. *Med Clin North America* 2015;99:131–143

3. Bakris GL, Fonseca VA, Sharma K, Wright EM. Renal sodium-glucose transport: role in diabetes mellitus and potential clinical implications. *Kidney Int* 2009;75:1272–1277

4. Chao E. SGLT-2 inhibitors: a new mechanism for glycemic control. *Clin Diabetes* 2014;32(1):4–11

5. Garg S, Henry R, Banks P, et al. Effects of sotagliflozin added to insulin in patients with type 1 diabetes. *N Engl J Med* 2017;377:2337–2348

6. Invokana (canagliflozin tablet, film coated) [prescribing information]. Raritan, NJ, Janssen Pharmaceuticals, Inc. Available from https://dailymed.nlm. nih.gov/dailymed/drugInfo.cfm?setid=b9057d3b-b104-4f09-8a61-c61ef9d4a3f3&audience=consumer. Accessed June 2018

7. Farxiga (dapagliflozin propanediol tablet, film coated) [prescribing information]. Princeton, NJ, E. R. Squibb & Sons, LLC. Available from https://dailymed.nlm.nih.gov/dailymed/drugInfo.cfm?setid=72ad22ae-efe6-4cd6-a302-98aaee423d69&audience=consumer. Accessed June 2018

8. Jardiance (empagliflozin tablets, for oral use) [prescribing information]. Ridgefield, CT, Boehringer Ingelheim Pharmaceuticals, Inc. Available from https://dailymed.nlm.nih.gov/dailymed/drugInfo.cfm?setid=faf3dd6a-9cd0-39c2-0d2e-232cb3f67565&audience=consumer. Accessed June 2018

9. Macha S, Mattheus M, Halabi A, et al. Pharmacokinetics, pharmacodynamics and safety of empagliflozin, a sodium glucose cotransporter 2 (SGLT2) inhibitor, in subjects with renal impairment. *Diabetes Obes Metab* 2014;16:215–222

10. Steglatro (ertugliflozin) [prescribing information]. Kenilworth, NJ, Merck Sharp & Dohme Corp. Available from https://dailymed.nlm.nih.gov/dailymed/drugInfo.cfm?setid=e6f3e718-bb99-48f1-ab94-b9f0af05fed6&audience=consumer. Accessed June 2018

11. Zinman B, Wanner C, Lachin JM, et al. Empagliflozin, cardiovascular outcomes, and mortality in type 2 diabetes. *New Engl J Med* 2015;373(22):2117–2128

12. Neal B, Perkovic V, Mahaffey KW, et al. Canagliflozin and cardiovascular and renal events in type 2 diabetes. *New Engl J Med* 2017;377(7):644–657

13. American Diabetes Association. 8. Pharmacologic Approaches to Glycemic Treatment: *Standards of Medical Care in Diabetes—2018. Diabetes Care* 2018;41(Suppl. 1):S73–S85

14. Pecoits-Filho R, Perkovic V. Are SGLT2 inhibitors ready for prime time in CKD? *CJASN*. September 2017 [Epub ahead of print]. DOI:10.2215/CJN.07680717

15. Vasilakou D, Karagiannis T, Athanasiadou E, et al. Sodium-glucose cotransporter 2 inhibitors for type 2 diabetes: a systematic review and meta-analysis. *Ann Intern Med* 2013;159:262–274

16. Rosenstock J, Vico M, Wei L, et al. Effects of dapagliflozin, an SGLT2 inhibitor, on HbA1c, body weight, and hypoglycemia risk in patients with type 2 diabetes inadequately controlled on pioglitazone monotherapy. *Diabetes Care* 2012;35:1473–1478

17. Bolinder J, Ljunggren Ö, Kullberg J, et al. Effects of dapagliflozin on body weight, total fat mass, and regional adipose tissue distribution in patients

with type 2 diabetes mellitus with inadequate glycemic control on metformin. *J Clin Endocrinol Metab* 2012;97:1020–1031

18. Handelsman Y, Henry R, Bloomgarden Z, Dagogo-Jack S, et al. American Association of Clinical Endocrinologists and American College of Endocrinology Position Statement on the association of SGLT-2 inhibitors and diabetic ketoacidosis. *Endocrine Pract* 2016;22(6):753–762

19. Johnsson KM, Ptaszynska A, Schmitz B, et al. Urinary tract infections in patients with diabetes treated with dapagliflozin. *J Diabetes Complications* 2013;27:473–478

20. Scheen AJ. Precision medicine: the future in diabetes care? *Diabetes Res Clin Pract* 2016;117:12–21

21. Scheen AJ. Drug-drug interactions with sodium-glucose cotransporters type 2 (SGLT2) inhibitors, new oral glucose-lowering agents for the management of type 2 diabetes mellitus. *Clin Pharmacokinet* 2014;53:295–304

Chapter 11

α-Glucosidase Inhibitors

Kimberly C. McKeirnan, PharmD, BCACP
Nicole M. Perea, PharmD

INTRODUCTION

α-Glucosidase inhibitors are a versatile class of medications that have been used in a variety of treatment settings since they were first approved by the FDA in 1995 for patients with T1D. α-Glucosidase inhibitors have a unique mechanism of action that allows the drug to alter the rate at which the body absorbs carbohydrates. This allows for the medication to be applied across several spectrums. Of note, α-glucosidase inhibitors are traditionally used in the management of T2D. They can, however, be used in the management of T1D as well. There are two medications available in the U.S. within this class: acarbose (Precose, Bayer) and miglitol (Glyset, Pfizer Inc.). Voglibose (Volix, Ranbaxy Laboratories Limited) is a third medication in this class available outside the U.S.

Several large clinical trials with acarbose, including the large postmarketing PROTECT (Precose Resolution of Optimal Titration to Enhance Current Therapies) trial, have shown a decrease in A1C values of ~0.5–0.7%, or ~0.6–1.1% from baseline when compared to placebo.[1] In the PROTECT trial, which enrolled over 6,000 patients, postprandial glucose levels decreased 40–50 mg/dL (2.2–2.8 mmol/L), and fasting plasma glucose levels decreased 25–30 mg/dL (1.4–1.7 mmol/L).[1] On average, these medications have been shown to reduce A1C by about 0.5–1%.[2] α-Glucosidase inhibitors have the biggest impact on postprandial blood glucose, creating a niche for this class within the many options used to treat diabetes mellitus.

PHARMACOLOGY

MECHANISM OF ACTION

α-Glucosidase inhibitors are named for their ability to competitively inhibit the α-glucosidase enzyme in the brush borders of the intestines through reversible binding.[3] α-Glucosidase enzymes maltase, isomaltase, sucrase, and glucoamylase break down complex carbohydrates into monosaccharides that can then be absorbed.[4] Inhibition of α-glucosidase enzymes leads to the delayed breakdown of oligosaccharides and disaccharides into monosaccharides suitable for absorption.[3] The delayed absorption of carbohydrates from the small intestine results in reduction of the postprandial hyperglycemia that occurs during digestion of a meal.[3]

This slower rise in postprandial blood glucose concentrations is beneficial to patients with T1D or T2D.

PHARMACOKINETICS

Following oral administration, acarbose has very low bioavailability. Minimal absorption by the small intestine leads to <2% of the acarbose being systemically active.[5] Acarbose peak plasma concentration occurs 1 h after administration, while miglitol peak concentrations are reached in 2–3 h.[5,6] Miglitol absorption is also saturable at high doses because miglitol is absorbed via an active transport mechanism, a rate-limiting step, which impacts both the bioavailability and onset of action. A dose of 25 mg, for example, is completely absorbed, but a dose of 100 mg only achieves 50–70% absorption.[6] At higher doses, absorption is also delayed and may take up to 7 h. However, the absorption rate of miglitol does not influence clinical efficacy, since the site of action is the brush border of the intestines.

Acarbose is metabolized exclusively by the intestines. Natural intestinal bacteria and digestive enzymes break acarbose into 13 different metabolites, although only one metabolite inhibits α-glucosidase.[5] Miglitol is not metabolized in humans or any of the animals studied. Miglitol metabolites have not been detected in plasma, urine, or feces, demonstrating the lack of metabolization.[6] Protein binding of miglitol is very low (<4%), and the volume of distribution is 0.18 L/kg, consistent with distribution largely into extracellular fluid.[6] Miglitol also has very low permeability of the blood-brain barrier.

Most of the acarbose dose—approximately 51%—is excreted in the feces, while 34% of the metabolized drug is absorbed systemically and is eliminated in the urine as sulfate, methyl, and glucuronide conjugates.[5] The active metabolite accounts for only 2% of the administered dose and is completely excreted via the kidney. Miglitol is eliminated through renal excretion, and the small amount of miglitol absorbed systemically in the small intestine is excreted in feces. Following a dose of 25 mg, >95% of the dose is recovered in the urine within 24 h.[6] After a 100-mg dose, the amount of drug recovered after 24 h is lower due to the incomplete bioavailability.[6] The elimination half-life for both miglitol and acarbose is approximately 2 h.[5,6]

TREATMENT ADVANTAGES/DISADVANTAGES

Acarbose and miglitol appear to be similar in terms of efficacy. However, there are no head-to-head clinical trials comparing the two drugs, so it is difficult to judge whether there is any advantage for one product over the other. Patients typically do not experience weight gain or hypoglycemia unless α-glucosidase inhibitors are taken in combination with other glucose-lowering medications. α-Glucosidase inhibitors may also have a positive impact on prevention of negative cardiovascular outcomes due to the weight loss seen while on the medication. This impact was seen more in populations in the Eastern Hemisphere. Further research is needed to confirm this theory.[7]

Some studies show patients taking α-glucosidase inhibitors may experience weight loss. A 2014 meta-analysis showed acarbose had a small but statistically significant incidence of weight loss (0.5 kg on average) compared with placebo.[8] The weight loss effect from acarbose was superior to both nateglinide and metformin. Additionally, a significantly greater weight loss (0.92 kg) was seen in Eastern populations compared to Western populations.[8]

α-Glucosidase inhibitors may be used as monotherapy or in combination with other agents. When used in combination, α-glucosidase inhibitors can enhance glycemic control because they have a different mechanism of action than other agents. A study by Wang published in 2013 showed treatment with a combination of acarbose and metformin brought proportionally more patients to goal A1C, had superior effects in lowering blood glucose, and reduced body weight when compared to acarbose alone.[9] Acarbose may be used with insulin, metformin, or sulfonylureas, and miglitol has been approved for use with sulfonylureas.

α-Glucosidase inhibitors are effective at lowering A1C levels by 0.5–1%, which can play a significant role in the treatment of T2D.[10] However, gastrointestinal side effects make these medications challenging to tolerate and unsuitable for patients with chronic intestinal disorders.[11] Slow titration over 10–12 weeks may reduce the likelihood of side effects, but many patients still choose to discontinue use due to these issues. Other classes of medication reduce A1C levels more substantially and have fewer gastrointestinal side effects, relegating α-glucosidase inhibitors to one of the less commonly used classes of medications for diabetes in the U.S.[12]

THERAPEUTIC CONSIDERATIONS

SIGNIFICANT WARNINGS/PRECAUTIONS

Both miglitol and acarbose are contraindicated for patients with inflammatory bowel disease, colonic ulceration, partial intestinal obstruction, predisposition to intestinal obstruction, or chronic intestinal diseases involving digestion or absorption.[5,6] α-Glucosidase inhibitors should not be used for patients with DKA or with any known hypersensitivity to a medication in this class. Acarbose is also contraindicated for patients with liver cirrhosis.

α-Glucosidase inhibitors do not cause hypoglycemia. However, when used in combination with oral sulfonylureas or insulin, hypoglycemia may result. Because α-glucosidase inhibitors block the absorption of dietary carbohydrates, patients experiencing hypoglycemia must use glucose tablets or gels instead of foods containing complex carbohydrates to raise blood glucose levels.[5,6] In the case of severe hypoglycemia, a glucagon injection or intravenous glucose may be necessary. Patients must remember to monitor blood glucose levels, particularly in stressful situations such as illness, trauma, or surgery, all of which can impact blood glucose levels.

SPECIAL POPULATIONS

No significant differences in pharmacokinetics have been observed in either pediatric or geriatric patients or by sex. However, appropriate studies have not been conducted on a pediatric population, so safe and effective use in children has not been established.[13] Following administration of acarbose, the mean steady-state AUC and maximum concentrations were approximately 1.5 times higher in the elderly population, but this difference was not statistically significant.[5]

In controlled clinical studies of acarbose in patients with T2D in the U.S., reductions in A1C were similar between Caucasians ($n = 478$) and African-Americans ($n = 167$), with better responses in Latin Americans ($n = 132$).[5] A 2014 review of 10 large studies of acarbose use in 21 countries around the world (total $n = 30,730$) showed acarbose was effective across all ethnicities and regions examined.[14] However, the most pronounced effects were seen in Southeast and East Asians and those patients with a higher baseline A1C.[14]

Both medications should be used with caution in patients with renal impairment. Participants with severe renal impairment (CrCl <25 mL/min) who took acarbose exhibited a peak plasma concentration five times higher and an AUC six times higher than participants with normal renal function. Subjects with CrCl <25 mL/min taking 25 mg of miglitol three times daily attained a greater than twofold increase in plasma levels compared to subjects with CrCl >60 mL/min.[5,6]

Both medications are pregnancy category B. Studies in rats given miglitol at doses corresponding to 1.5, 4, and 12 times the maximum recommended human dose, and rabbits given doses corresponding to 0.5, 3, and 10 times the maximum recommended human dose, showed no evidence of fetal malformations attributed to miglitol.[6] However, there are no adequate and well-controlled studies in humans. In 2000, a case report in Mexico showed that six pregnant women successfully took acarbose without issue through the pregnancy, delivering what were considered "normal newborns," while a 1998 case report in England showed that out of five women who took acarbose early in pregnancy, two miscarried.[15,16] Both medications should be used in pregnancy only after weighing the risks and benefits of this and other medication options. Miglitol is excreted in human milk, with 0.02% of a 100-mg maternal dose detected. Use of both miglitol and acarbose is not recommended for nursing mothers, even though the amount of drug found in milk is very small.

ADVERSE EFFECTS AND MONITORING

The most common adverse effects from α-glucosidase inhibitors are gastrointestinal symptoms, including flatulence (acarbose 74%, miglitol 41.5%), diarrhea (acarbose 31%, miglitol 28.7%), and abdominal pain (acarbose 19%, miglitol 11.7%).[5,6] These symptoms occur because of intestinal gas from the formation of short-chain fatty acids resulting from undigested carbohydrates in the colon.[3] Both acarbose and miglitol exert their action locally in the small intestine, blocking the breakdown and absorption of complex carbohydrates. The delayed absorption results in the complex sugars moving to the large intestine. The natural flora of the large intestine ferment the carbohydrates, resulting in the production of gas. These drugs are less popular among patients as a result of these gastrointestinal side effects. However, these side effects can be minimized by slowly titrating doses and encouraging patients to eat meals containing complex, rather than simple, carbohydrates.[11]

α-Glucosidase inhibitors may also impact serum iron. Small reductions in serum iron were found in 9.2% of patients taking miglitol versus 4.2% taking placebo.[6] Changes were not associated with reductions in hemoglobin or other hematologic indices. Similar results were seen with acarbose.[6] Patients with known iron deficiency anemia should be monitored when starting an α-glucosidase inhibitor.

Elevated liver function tests have also been observed in patients taking doses above the manufacturer's recommendations. Increased serum transaminases were detected in 4% of patients taking acarbose at doses of 600–900 mg per day. Patients were asymptomatic, and elevated transaminases were reversible with discontinuation of therapy.[12]

A dermatologic rash was reported in 4.3% of patients taking miglitol compared with 2.4% taking placebo. Rashes were found by physician investigators to be transient and likely unrelated to taking the medication, but are included within the package insert along with a recommendation to monitor liver function tests every 3 months during the first year taking acarbose.[6]

DRUG INTERACTIONS

As described previously in the "Significant Warnings/Precautions" section, an additive hypoglycemic effect may occur when α-glucosidase inhibitors are used in combination with sulfonylureas or insulin. A study of combination therapy with α-glucosidase inhibitors and insulin demonstrated a decreased need for insulin, sometimes requiring a reduction in insulin dosage to avoid a hypoglycemic event.[6,17] Patients taking both an α-glucosidase inhibitor and insulin should be closely monitored to prevent a hypoglycemic event.[13]

Medications that elevate glucose levels may also reduce the efficacy of α-glucosidase inhibitors. These may include thiazide diuretics, corticosteroids, estrogen, and calcium channel blockers, among others.

Miglitol taken in combination with glyburide has been shown to reduce the AUC and peak concentrations of glyburide, but the clinical significance of this interaction is unknown. A similar interaction occurs with metformin, but the reduction was minimal.[13] Acarbose has no effect on the absorption and distribution of glyburide but does cause a significant reduction in the acute bioavailability of metformin. However, after a 24 h urine collection, it was found that overall bioavailability of metformin is not affected by this interaction, so it is not clinically significant.[18]

Results from administering the combination of miglitol and digoxin have been contradictory, showing a reduction of digoxin levels by 19–28% in healthy volunteers but not in patients with diabetes.[19] The reason for this discrepancy is unknown, but providers may wish to consider monitoring digoxin levels periodically in patients taking these two drugs concomitantly. Miglitol also significantly reduces the bioavailability of propranolol by 40% and ranitidine by 60%, but has no drug interactions with nifedipine, antacids, or warfarin.[6,19] Acarbose does not interact with digoxin, nifedipine, or propranolol, so it may be the better choice in patients with a heart condition.

DOSAGE AND ADMINISTRATION

There is no fixed dosage regimen for treatment of diabetes mellitus with either α-glucosidase inhibitor. Treatment must be individualized for each patient based on effectiveness and tolerance to assure maximal clinical efficacy with minimal adverse effects. Both medications should be given with the first bite of each meal, since α-glucosidase inhibitors work in the small intestine when dietary carbohydrates are present. The gastrointestinal side effects can be reduced by starting with a low initial daily dose and titrating slowly to the appropriate maintenance dose.

Initial treatment with acarbose is suggested at a dose of 25 mg orally three times daily with a gradual increase if needed to achieve glycemic control up to the maximum dose of 100 mg three times a day. However, some patients may benefit from a slower titration, starting with 25 mg once per day and titrating up to 25 mg three times a day to reduce gastrointestinal adverse events. The usual maintenance dose is 50 mg three times a day, but some patients may need up to 100 mg three times a day.[3] Patients with body weight below 60 kg should not be considered for doses above 50 mg three times a day because of higher risk for elevated serum transaminases.[5] Once the effective and tolerable dose has been established, it should be maintained.

Miglitol should be started at 25 mg orally three times a day and gradually increased until the minimum dose needed to achieve adequate glycemic control is identified. This titration may also reduce the gastrointestinal adverse effects. During this initiation phase, 1 h postprandial plasma glucose can be used to determine response to the medication. A1C should be measured after 3 months to confirm efficacy and appropriateness. The maximum recommended dose of 100 mg three times a day should not be exceeded.[6] Available products and recommended dosing is described in Table 11.1.

Table 11.1—Product Strengths and Dosing Recommendations for α-Glucosidase Inhibitors

Drug name	How supplied	Initial dose*	Usual maintenance dose	Maximum dose
Acarbose (Precose)	25-mg, 50-mg, 100-mg tablets	25 mg t.i.d.	50 mg t.i.d.	For patients ≤60 kg: 50 mg t.i.d.; for patients >60 kg: 100 mg t.i.d.
Miglitol (Glyset)	25-mg, 50-mg, 100-mg tablets	25 mg t.i.d.	50 mg t.i.d.	100 mg t.i.d.

* Some patients may need to begin with once-daily dosing to decrease potential for adverse effects. *Source:* Precose [prescribing information][5] and Glycet [prescribing information].[6]

MONOGRAPHS

Acarbose: https://dailymed.nlm.nih.gov/dailymed/drugInfo.cfm?setid=e4148493-e3bd-4530-8fb6-cdb5197c010e

Miglitol: https://dailymed.nlm.nih.gov/dailymed/drugInfo.cfm?setid=75711d16-2d27-476e-a312-d5af448a0e25

REFERENCES

1. Buse J, Hart K, Minasi L. The PROTECT Study: final results of a large multicenter postmarketing study in patients with type 2 diabetes. Precose Resolution of Optimal Titration to Enhance Current Therapies. *Clin Ther* 1998;20(2):257–269

2. Drent ML, Tollefsen AT, van Heusden FH, Hoenderdos EB, et al. Dose-dependent efficacy of miglitol, an alpha-glucosidase inhibitor, in type 2 diabetic patients on diet alone: results of a 24-week double-blind placebo-controlled study. *Diabetes Nutr Metab* 2002;15:152–159

3. Trevor AJ, Katzung BG, Knuidering-Hall M. Pancreatic hormones, antidiabetic agents and glucagon. In *Katzung and Trevor's Pharmacology: Examination and Board Review*, 11th ed. New York, McGraw Hill Education, 2015

4. Triplitt CL, Repas T, Alvarez C. Diabetes mellitus. In *Pharmacotherapy: A Pathophysiologic Approach*, 10th ed. DiPiro JT, Talbert RL, Yee GC, et al., Eds. New York, McGraw-Hill, 2017, p. 1173

5. Precose (acarbose) [prescribing information]. Whippany, NJ, Bayer Health-Care Pharmaceuticals, March 2015

6. Glycet (miglitol) [prescribing information]. Whippany, NJ, Bayer Health-Care Pharmaceuticals, August 2016

7. Standl E, Theodorakis MJ, Erbach M, Schnell O, Tuomilehto J. On the potential of acarbose to reduce cardiovascular disease. *Cardiovasc Diabetol* 2014;13:81

8. Li Y, Tong Y, Zhang Y, Huang L, et al. Acarbose monotherapy and weight loss in Eastern and Western populations with hyperglycaemia: an ethnicity-specific meta-analysis. *Int J Clin Pract* 2014;68(11):1318–1332

9. Wang JS, Huang CN, Hung YJ, Kwok CF, et al.; acarbose/metformin fixed-dose combination study investigators. Acarbose plus metformin fixed-dose combination outperforms acarbose monotherapy for type 2 diabetes. *Diabetes Res Clin Pract* 2013;102(1):16–24

10. Krentz AJ, Bailey CJ. Oral antidiabetic agents: current role in type 2 diabetes mellitus. *Drugs* 2005;65:385–411

11. Linn WD. Diabetes Mellitus Management. In *Pharmacotherapy in Primary Care*. Linn WD, Wofford MR, O'Keefe ME, Posey LM, Eds. New York, McGraw-Hill Education, 2009

12. Chiasson JL, Josse RG, Hunt JA, et al. The efficacy of acarbose in the treatment of patients with non-insulin-dependent diabetes mellitus: a multicenter controlled clinical trial. *Ann Intern Med* 1994;121:928

13. Campbell LK, Baker DE, Campbell RK. Miglitol: assessment of its role in the treatment of patients with diabetes mellitus. *Ann Pharmacother* 2000;34:1291–1301

14. Weng J, Soegondo S, Schnell O, Sheu W, et al. Efficacy of acarbose in different geographical regions of the world: analysis of a real-life database. *Diabetes Metab Res Rev* 2015;31:155–167

15. Zárate A, Ochoa R, Hernández M, Basurto L. Effectiveness of acarbose in the control of glucose tolerance worsening in pregnancy. *Ginecol Obstet Mex* 2000;68:42–45

16. Wilton LV, Pearce GL, Martin RM, Mackay FJ, Mann RD. The outcomes of pregnancy in women exposed to newly marketed drugs in general practices in England. *Br J Obstet Gynaecol* 1998;105:882–889

17. Dimitriadis G, Hatziagellaki E, Alexopoulos E, Kordonouri O, et al. Effects of α-glucosidae inhibition on meal glucose tolerance and timing of insulin administration in patients with type I diabetes mellitus. *Diabetes Care* 1991;14:393–398

18. Scheen AJ, de Magalhaes AC, Salvatore T, Lefebvre PJ. Reduction of the acute bioavailability of metformin by the alpha-glucosidase inhibitor acarbose in normal man. *Eur J Clin Invest* 1994;24(Suppl. 3):50–54

19. Schall R, Müller FO, Hundt HK, Duursema L, et al. Study of the effect of miglitol on the pharmacokinetics and pharmacodynamics of warfarin in healthy males. *Arzneimittelforschung* 1996;46:41–46

Chapter 12

Dipeptidyl Peptidase-4 (DPP-4) Inhibitors

Kimberly C. McKeirnan, PharmD, BCACP
Joshua J. Neumiller, PharmD, CDE, FASCP

INTRODUCTION

D PP-4 inhibitors improve glycemic control by preventing the proteolytic degradation of endogenous incretin hormones. Enhancement of the effects of these hormones leads to increased glucose-dependent insulin secretion by pancreatic β-cells, reduction in glucagon secretion from pancreatic α-cells, and the slowing of gastric emptying.[1] This class of medication is effective at reducing A1C and plays an important role as an antihyperglycemic treatment option in the management of people with T2D.[2] DPP-4 inhibitors are generally used in combination with other antihyperglycemic medications, such as metformin, TZDs, sulfonylureas, SGLT2 inhibitors, and insulin.

DPP-4 inhibitors are approved as adjunct to diet and exercise to improve glycemic control in adults with T2D.[3-6] Sitagliptin was the first DPP-4 inhibitor approved by the FDA in October 2006. Since the approval of sitagliptin, several more agents have followed within the class. There are currently four DPP-4 inhibitors approved for use in the U.S.: sitagliptin (Januvia, Merck & Co.), which was FDA approved in 2006; saxagliptin (Onglyza, AstraZeneca), FDA approved in 2009; linagliptin (Tradjenta, Eli Lilly and Boehringer Ingelheim), FDA approved in 2011; and alogliptin (Nesina, Takeda Pharmaceuticals), FDA approved in 2013.[3-6] Vildagliptin (Glavus) was approved by the European Medicine Agency in 2008 and is available in Europe. Gemigliptin, anagliptin, teneligliptin, trelagliptin, omarigliptin, evogliptin, and gosogliptin are also available in other countries. This section will review the pharmacology of DPP-4 inhibitors, as well as the properties, considerations, and role of these agents in the treatment of T2D.

PHARMACOLOGY

MECHANISM OF ACTION

The incretin effect is mediated via gut hormones that induce insulin secretion from the β-cells of the pancreas in response to oral glucose administration.[1] DPP-4 inhibitors were developed to augment the incretin effect for the treatment of T2D. Dipeptidyl peptidase-4 is an enzyme responsible for breaking down the endogenous incretin hormones GLP-1 and GIP, resulting in decreased endogenous levels of these two peptides.[7] GLP-1 and GIP are important physiological mediators of prandial insulin release and maintenance of glucose homeostasis, responsible for up to 60% of the prandial insulin response.[8] GLP-1 has been shown to lower blood glucose by several mechanisms, including induction of glucose-dependent insulin secretion, decreasing plasma glucagon concentrations, and delaying gastric emptying.[9,10] DPP-4 inhibitors ultimately contribute to improved glycemia via prolonging the half-life of endogenously produced GLP-1 and GIP by slowing enzymatic degradation of these hormones.[7] After a meal, DPP-4 inhibition has been shown to result in a two- to threefold increase in circulating levels of active GLP-1 and GIP, decreased glucagon levels, and increased glucose-dependent insulin secretion.[11]

Currently available GLP-1 RAs, such as exenatide, are susceptible to degradation within the digestive tract, thus necessitating the administration of these agents via injection. Unlike GLP-1 RAs, DPP-4 inhibitors can be administered orally, which may result in increased ease of use and patient acceptability in some circumstances.

PHARMACOKINETICS

Alogliptin

After administration of a single dose of alogliptin, peak plasma concentrations were achieved within 1–2 h.[12] Peak inhibition of DPP-4 occurred within 2–3 h after dosing, with peak inhibition ranging from 93–98%. Enzyme inhibition ranged from 74–97% 24 h after administration and from 47–83% after 72 h. At the maximum recommended clinical dose of 25 mg, alogliptin was eliminated with a mean terminal half-life of approximately 21 h.[12] Alogliptin has an absolute bioavailability of approximately 100%, even when taken with a high-fat meal, so it can be administered with or without food.[3] The volume of distribution following a 12.5 mg intravenous infusion of alogliptin was 417 L, indicating the agent is well distributed into tissues.[3] The majority of the drug, 60–71%, is excreted unchanged in the urine within 24–72 h. Alogliptin is mainly metabolized by CYP2D6 and 3A4 and is primarily excreted in urine (76%).[12]

Linagliptin

Linagliptin is rapidly absorbed and has a modest oral bioavailability of approximately 30%.[13] Peak plasma concentrations are achieved approximately 1.5 h after oral administration, and are seemingly not impacted by ingestion of a high-fat meal. Linagliptin has a long elimination half-life of 131 h, although the effective half-life is approximately 12 h. While most DPP-4 inhibitors exhibit low binding to plasma proteins, linagliptin is extensively protein-bound in a dose-dependent manner.[14] Linagliptin is primarily eliminated via the hepatic system (80%). A study of linagliptin use in patients with renal compromise concluded that dose adjustment is not required in various degrees of renal impairment.[13]

Saxagliptin

Saxagliptin reaches peak plasma concentration approximately 2 h (4 h for the active metabolite) after a 5-mg oral dose.[5] When administered with a high-fat meal, a 20-min delay to peak concentration was observed. Saxagliptin is metabolized primarily by CYP450 3A4/5, so strong CYP3A4/5 inhibitors and inducers will alter the pharmacokinetics. Both renal and hepatic elimination are involved, and the terminal half-life for saxagliptin and its active metabolite are 2.5 h and 3.1 h, respectively.[5,11] Dose adjustment is not necessary for patients with mild renal impairment, but the dosage should be reduced to 2.5 mg orally once a day for patients with an eGFR of less than 45 mL/min/1.73 m^2.[5,11] Accordingly, the manufacturer recommends the assessment of renal function prior to the initiation of saxagliptin and periodically thereafter.

Sitagliptin

Sitagliptin given orally has a bioavailability of over 85%, achieving peak concentration within 1–4 h.[15] Following administration of a single oral 100-mg dose of sitagliptin in healthy volunteers, peak serum levels were achieved in approximately 1–4 h. The mean volume of distribution at steady state is 198 L after a single dose of sitagliptin, with approximately 38% of sitagliptin reversibly bound to plasma proteins.[6] Sitagliptin is approximately 79% excreted unchanged in the urine via active tubular secretion. In vitro studies indicate that sitagliptin is modestly metabolized via CYP450 enzyme 3A4 with some contribution from the 2C8 isoenzyme.[15] Because sitagliptin is largely eliminated renally, dosage adjustment to 50 mg orally is recommended in those with moderate renal impairment (eGFR 30–49 mL/min/1.73 m^2) and to 25 mg in patients with severe renal impairment (eGFR <30 mL/min/1.73 m^2).[6] The terminal half-life of a single dose of 100 mg sitagliptin was found to be 12.4 h, on average, in healthy volunteers. When examined, the presence of moderate hepatic impairment did not show significant alterations in the pharmacokinetic profile of sitagliptin.[15]

TREATMENT ADVANTAGES/DISADVANTAGES

All four DPP-4 inhibitors currently marketed in the U.S. are generally well tolerated, with a low risk of contributing to hypoglycemia due to their glucose-dependent mechanism of action.[16] Considering their low risk of hypoglycemia, excellent tolerability profile, oral administration, and once-daily dosing, DPP-4 inhibitors can be useful antihyperglycemic agents in certain clinical circumstances where hypoglycemic risk and convenience are key considerations. That said, it should be noted that DPP-4 inhibitors result in modest A1C reduction when compared to many other antihyperglycemic medication classes. Although the risk of treatment-emergent hypoglycemia is low with the use of DPP-4 inhibitors, reducing the dose of background insulin secretagogues when beginning initial therapy with a DPP-4 inhibitor may be warranted to prevent hypoglycemia. DPP-4 inhibitors are not approved for treatment of T1D or for the treatment of DKA.[3-6]

The DPP-4 inhibitors currently available for use in the U.S. have unique differentiating factors that should be considered when selecting an agent for use in a given individual. Saxagliptin is a substrate of CYP3A4/5, and a dose reduction is recommended when given in combination with a strong CYP3A4/5 inhibitor, such as ketoconazole.[11] Linagliptin has a longer half-life (131 h) than the other

DPP-4 inhibitors due to extensive binding to plasma proteins and is primarily eliminated hepatically (~85%), with an estimated 5% of a given dose undergoing renal elimination.[13] Dose adjustment is therefore not required with linagliptin in the setting of renal impairment, which is unique when compared to other currently available DPP-4 inhibitors.[13]

The effect of DPP-4 inhibitor use on cardiovascular outcomes has also been evaluated. Dedicated CVOTs have been reported for alogliptin, sitagliptin, and saxagliptin (EXAMINE, TECOS, and SAVOR-TIMI 53, respectively), none of which showed a benefit of preventing major cardiovascular outcomes when compared to placebo.[17–19] Findings from these CVOTs have raised questions about the relationship between DPP-4 inhibitor use and HF. The SAVOR-TIMI 53 trial reported that patients treated with saxagliptin were more likely to be hospitalized for HF when compared to participants given placebo (3.5% vs. 2.85%, respectively).[19] The EXAMINE and TECOS studies, in contrast, did not show associations between DPP-4 inhibitor use and HF.[17,18] While the FDA reported that the hospital admission rates for HF in the EXAMINE trial were 3.9% for patients assigned to alogliptin, versus 3.3% for those on placebo,[20] a post hoc analysis of the trial reported that alogliptin had no effect on the composite endpoint of cardiovascular death and hospitalization for HF.[21] In support of these CVOT findings, one meta-analysis concluded that there is no statistically significant evidence that DPP-4 inhibitors reduce negative cardiovascular outcomes, including acute coronary syndrome, stroke, or overall cardiovascular mortality, and showed an increased risk of HF with DPP-4 inhibitors compared to placebo.[22] Given questions surrounding DPP-4 inhibitor use and HF risk, DPP-4 inhibitors currently carry warnings and/or precautions in their labeling related to HF and associated symptoms.

A 2015 review reported the cost-effectiveness of DPP-4 inhibitors from both a payer and societal standpoint.[23] The study concluded that DPP-4 inhibitors, when compared to sulfonylureas and insulin, are a cost-effective option for patients who are not achieving glycemic targets with monotherapy.[23] This study accounted for the costs related to side effects of insulin and sulfonylureas, such as weight gain and hypoglycemia, which are not as problematic with DPP-4 inhibitors. Of note, this study did not compare the cost-effectiveness of DPP-4 inhibitors to other agents with hypoglycemia and weight benefits, such as GLP-1 RAs or SGLT2 inhibitors. While the DPP-4 inhibitor class has clear benefits in terms of weight neutrality, low hypoglycemia risk, and general tolerability, these benefits must be weighed against cost and a generally modest A1C-lowering potential.

THERAPEUTIC CONSIDERATIONS

SIGNIFICANT WARNINGS/PRECAUTIONS

All four FDA-approved DPP-4 inhibitors carry warnings for acute pancreatitis within their respective prescribing information.[3–6] Postmarketing reports of fatal and nonfatal hemorrhagic or necrotizing pancreatitis have been reported with sitagliptin.[6] However, a large retrospective study determined the relative risk of pancreatitis in people receiving sitagliptin to be 1.0 (95% CI 0.5–2.0) compared with matched controls receiving metformin or glyburide.[24] CVOT trials with saxagliptin, alogliptin, and sitagliptin reported clear numerical imbalances in cases of acute pancreatitis, yet the numerical increase in cases of acute pancreatitis observed in patients taking a DPP-4 inhibitor did not reach statistical significance in these trials.[17–19] Although causation has not been established, manufacturers of all four products recommend monitoring for signs and symptoms of pancreatitis after initiation, and recommend immediate discontinuation of the medication if pancreatitis is suspected.[3–6] Postmarketing surveillance efforts are underway by the FDA to evaluate the risk of pancreatitis with DPP-4 inhibitor use.

Prescribing information for sitagliptin, saxagliptin, linagliptin, and alogliptin all include warnings/precautions to use with caution in patients with HF and/or to monitor patients for signs and symptoms due to CVOT findings from some agents in the DPP-4 inhibitor class.[3–6] As noted previously, a CVOT with over 16,000 participants with T2D compared the use of saxagliptin and placebo on rates of a cardiovascular-related death, MI, or ischemic stroke. Although saxagliptin did not demonstrate an increased risk of cardiovascular-related death, more participants in the saxagliptin group were hospitalized for HF, raising concerns about DPP-4 inhibitor use and HF occurrence.[19] A 2014 meta-analysis of randomized clinical trials of DPP-4 inhibitors was conducted showing the overall risk of acute HF to be higher in patients treated with DPP-4 inhibitors versus those treated with placebo or an active comparator.[25] Similar to the recommendations for pancreatitis, manufacturers of sitagliptin, alogliptin, linagliptin, and saxagliptin suggest monitoring patients who have recently begun treatment with DPP-4 inhibitors for signs and symptoms of HF.[3–6]

Renal and hepatic considerations also exist for the DPP-4 inhibitor class of medications. Sitagliptin is eliminated largely via the kidneys, and thus dose reduction is warranted in patients with renal disease. Furthermore, renal function should be assessed in patients under consideration for sitagliptin therapy prior to drug initiation.[6] Reports of fatal and nonfatal hepatic failure in patients taking alogliptin have raised concerns.[3] Patients with liver failure or elevated liver enzymes should consider one of the other DPP-4 inhibitors. Liver function tests should be conducted for any patient taking alogliptin who reports symptoms indicative of liver injury.[3]

Postmarketing reports of serious allergic and hypersensitivity reactions have been reported in patients taking all four DPP-4 inhibitors.[3–6] These reactions included cases of anaphylaxis, angioedema, and exfoliative skin conditions including Stevens-Johnson syndrome. Although the occurrences of these drug reactions are rare, patients should be aware of any abnormal skin lesions or changes upon initiation of sitagliptin, and should report any unusual reactions to their healthcare provider. DPP-4 inhibitors are contraindicated in patients with a documented hypersensitivity reaction to the medication or any of its components. Additionally, DPP-4 inhibitors are not indicated for T1D and are not intended for use in the treatment of DKA.

SPECIAL POPULATIONS

Alogliptin

The pharmacokinetic properties of alogliptin appear unaffected by age, sex, race, and BMI, although pediatric dosing has not been established.[3] Dose reduction to 12.5 mg once daily is recommended in patients with mild renal impairment (CrCl ≥30 to <60 mL/min) and 6.25 mg once daily for patients with severe renal impairment or ESRD (CrCl <30 mL/min). Alogliptin is classified as FDA pregnancy category B. In animal studies, doses of greater than 180 times the respective human dose were administered to rabbits and rats and did not demonstrate any adverse developmental effects. Alogliptin is present in rat milk during animal studies, but information about presence in human milk and impact on breast-feeding is not available.[3]

Linagliptin

Linagliptin is the only DPP-4 that does not require dose adjustment in patients with renal impairment. Adjustments for patients with hepatic impairment are also not required.[4] Pediatric use has not been established, but there are no adjustment requirements for elderly patients. Linagliptin is pregnancy category B, with no adverse developmental outcomes in animal studies. Studies in rats demonstrate the presence of linagliptin in milk, although the effects have not been tested in humans. Risks and benefits of breast-feeding should be considered.[4]

Saxagliptin

Dosage adjustments are not needed for saxagliptin based on sex, race, BMI, or age, although safe and effective use in pediatric patients has not been established. A dose of 2.5 mg once daily is recommended for patients with moderate or severe renal impairment. The 2.5-mg dose is also recommended when coadministered with strong CYP450 3A4/5 inhibitors (ketoconazole, clarithromycin, ritonavir, etc.) due to saxagliptin's metabolic pathway.[5] Lowering the dose of sulfonylureas may also be required when adding saxagliptin to reduce the risk of hypoglycemia.[5] Saxagliptin is classified as pregnancy category B. Saxagliptin crosses the placenta into the fetus in animal studies.[26] There is no information available about the presence of saxagliptin in human milk, the effect on the breast-fed infant, or the effect on milk production, although studies with rats do show presence of the drug in milk.[5]

Sitagliptin

Little clinical information is available in regard to sitagliptin use in older adults with T2D; however, dose adjustment is recommended for patients with renal compromise. Dosage adjustments are not recommended for patients with mild to moderate hepatic impairment, although sitagliptin has not been formally evaluated in patients with advanced hepatic disease.[6] Sitagliptin is a pregnancy risk category B agent, and should only be used during pregnancy if deemed necessary. Caution is advised in women who are nursing, as it is currently unknown if sitagliptin is secreted into human breast milk. Safety and efficacy in patients under 18 years of age has not been studied.[6]

ADVERSE EFFECTS AND MONITORING

Clinical trial adverse event data identified three common side effects occurring with more frequency with DPP-4 inhibitors than events seen in control subjects: nasopharyngitis, upper respiratory tract infection, and headache. In a review of 8,500 patients treated with alogliptin, the most reported side effects were nasopharyngitis (4.4%), headache (4.2%), and upper respiratory tract infection (4.2%).[16] The overall incidence of adverse event was 66%, compared to 62% with placebo and 70% with an active comparator.[16] However, the overall discontinuation was quite low, 4.7%, compared to 4.5% with placebo. Similar side-effect profiles were seen with alogliptin, saxagliptin, and sitagliptin.[3,5,6]

Additionally, the overall incidence of hypoglycemia in subjects receiving DPP-4 inhibitors as monotherapy was similar to that of placebo controls. Alogliptin monotherapy had a hypoglycemia incidence of 1.5%, and alogliptin added to insulin or glyburide did not have a statistically significant increase in incidence of hypoglycemia when compared to placebo.[16] Some of the less common but more serious side effects reported with DPP-4 inhibitors are acute pancreatitis and serious hypersensitivity, including anaphylaxis, angioedema, and severe cutaneous rash.

Therapeutic monitoring recommendations for patients receiving DPP-4 inhibitors include periodic monitoring of A1C and self-monitoring of blood glucose. Patients under consideration for DPP-4 inhibitor therapy should receive the appropriate renal and/or hepatic function testing prior to therapy and periodically during treatment.

DRUG INTERACTIONS

Alogliptin

Alogliptin is not an inducer or inhibitor of CYP450 enzymes and has not been observed to interact with any renally excreted drugs.[3] Interactions were also not observed during coadministration of alogliptin and warfarin.[27]

Linagliptin

Linagliptin efficacy may be reduced when administered with a strong CYP450 3A4 inducer, such as rifampin. Choosing an alternative treatment when the prospective patient is already taking a 3A4 inducer is strongly suggested in the prescribing information.[4] Linagliptin did not interact with ethinyl estradiol, levonorgestrel, digoxin, warfarin, glyburide, pioglitazone, simvastatin, or metformin in respective studies.[13,28-33]

Saxagliptin

Saxagliptin is significantly impacted by strong CYP3A4/5 inhibitors.[5] Ketoconazole increased saxagliptin exposure when coadministered. The dose of saxagliptin should be limited to 2.5 mg when given in combination with a strong CYP3A4/5 inhibitor.[5] Choosing an alternative DPP-4 inhibitor may also be appropriate.

Sitagliptin

Despite the limited metabolism of sitagliptin by CYP450 3A4 and 2C8, it is considered unlikely that any clinically relevant interactions exist with other drugs that utilize the CYP450 system. Sitagliptin did not alter the pharmacokinetics of metformin, glyburide, simvastatin, digoxin, rosiglitazone, warfarin, or oral contraceptives.[16] Sitagliptin given in combination with digoxin for 10 days resulted in an 11% increase in the AUC and an 18% increase in peak plasma levels of digoxin.[6] While dosage adjustments of digoxin are not recommended when given in combination with sitagliptin, patients receiving these agents in combination should receive periodic monitoring of serum digoxin levels to prevent toxicity.

DOSAGE AND ADMINISTRATION

Alogliptin

Alogliptin is available commercially in 6.25-mg (light pink), 12.5-mg (yellow), and 25-mg (light red) tablets.[3] Alogliptin is FDA approved for the treatment of T2D as an adjunct to diet and exercise to improve glycemic control in adults. The recommended dose of alogliptin is 25 mg once daily. A dose of 12.5 mg daily is recommended for patients with moderate renal impairment and 6.25 mg daily for patients with severe renal impairment. Alogliptin may be taken with or without food.[3]

Linagliptin

Linagliptin is also indicated as an adjunct to diet and exercise to improve glycemic control in adults with T2D. Linagliptin is available as a light 5-mg (red) tablet.[4] The recommended dose is 5 mg once daily with or without food. When linagliptin is coadministered with a sulfonylurea or insulin, adjusting the dose of the secretagogue or insulin may be needed.

Saxagliptin

Saxagliptin is available as a 2.5-mg pale (yellow) or 5-mg (pink) tablet.[5] Saxagliptin is indicated as monotherapy or combination therapy for treating T2D in conjunction with diet and exercise. The recommended dosage is 2.5 mg or 5 mg taken once daily regardless of meals. The 2.5-mg strength is recommended for patients taking strong CYP3A4/5 inhibitors or with moderate to severe renal impairment.[5]

Sitagliptin

Sitagliptin is available commercially in 25-mg (pink), 50-mg (light beige), and 100-mg (beige) tablets.[6] For T2D patients with normal renal function, sitagliptin is dosed at 100 mg once daily as monotherapy or in combination with metformin, a TZD, a sulfonylurea, or metformin plus a sulfonylurea. Sitagliptin can be taken with or without food, and because sitagliptin is eliminated via renal excretion, dosage adjustments are required for patients with moderate to severe renal impairment. For patients with an eGFR $\geq$30 to <45 mL/min/1.73 m^2, the recommended dose of sitagliptin is 50 mg once daily. For patients with an eGFR <30 mL/min/1.73 m^2

or with end-stage renal disease requiring dialysis, the recommended dose of sitagliptin is 25 mg once daily.[6]

Table 12.1—DPP-4 Inhibitor Dosing Recommendations

Generic (brand)	How supplied	Initial dosing	Maintenance dosing	Maximum dosing	Dosing adjustments
Alogliptin (Nesina)	6.25-mg (light pink), 12.5-mg (yellow), and 25-mg (light red) tablets	25 mg daily	25 mg daily	25 mg daily	12.5 mg if CrCl ≥30 to <60 mL/min, 6.25 mg if CrCl <30 mL/min
Linagliptin (Tradjenta)	5-mg (light red) tablet	5 mg daily	5 mg daily	5 mg daily	None
Saxagliptin (Onglyza)	2.5-mg (pale yellow) or 5-mg (pink) tablet	5 mg daily	5 mg daily	5 mg daily	2.5 mg daily if taking strong CYP3A4/5 inhibitors or eGFR <45 mL/min/1.73 m²
Sitagliptin (Januvia)	25-mg (pink), 50-mg (light beige), and 100-mg (beige) tablets	25–100 mg daily	25–100 mg daily	100 mg daily	50 mg daily if eGFR ≥30 to <45 mL/min/1.73 m², 25 mg daily if eGFR <30 mL/min/1.73 m²

Source: refs. 3–6.

COMBINATION THERAPY

Several combination products containing a DPP-4 inhibitor are available.[34–39] All four DPP-4 inhibitors are available in combination with metformin. A meta-analysis showed DPP-4 inhibitors plus metformin as initial combination therapy was associated with greater reduction in A1C, greater reduction in fasting plasma glucose level, and lower weight loss compared to metformin monotherapy.[40] The combination was also not statistically significant for any increase in gastrointestinal adverse effects or hypoglycemia.[40]

Table 12.2—DPP-4-Containing Combination Products

Brand name	Generic names	How supplied
Kazano	Alogliptin/ metformin	12.5 mg alogliptin and 500 mg metformin HCl 12.5 mg alogliptin and 1,000 mg metformin HCl
Oseni	Alogliptin/ pioglitazone	12.5 mg alogliptin and 15 mg pioglitazone 12.5 mg alogliptin and 30 mg pioglitazone 12.5 mg alogliptin and 45 mg pioglitazone 25 mg alogliptin and 15 mg pioglitazone 25 mg alogliptin and 30 mg pioglitazone 25 mg alogliptin and 45 mg pioglitazone
Glyxambi	Linagliptin/ empagliflozin	5 mg linagliptin and 10 mg empagliflozin 5 mg linagliptin and 25 mg empagliflozin
Jentadueto	Linagliptin/ metformin	2.5 mg linagliptin and 500 mg metformin HCl 2.5 mg linagliptin and 850 mg metformin HCl 2.5 mg linagliptin and 1,000 mg metformin HCl
Kombiglyze XR	Saxagliptin/ metformin	2.5 mg saxagliptin and 1,000 mg metformin HCl extended release 5 mg saxagliptin and 500 mg metformin HCl extended release 5 mg saxagliptin and 1,000 mg metformin HCl extended release
Janumet	Sitagliptin/ metformin	50 mg sitagliptin and 500 mg metformin HCl 50 mg sitagliptin and 1,000 mg metformin HCl

Source: refs. 34–39.

MONOGRAPHS

Alogliptin: https://dailymed.nlm.nih.gov/dailymed/drugInfo.cfm?setid=b25f155a-1259-47c2-aa3b-7c1356e4c7f6

Linagliptin: https://dailymed.nlm.nih.gov/dailymed/drugInfo.cfm?setid=c797ea5c-cab7-494b-9044-27eba0cfe40f

Saxagliptin: https://dailymed.nlm.nih.gov/dailymed/drugInfo.cfm?setid=c5116390-e0fe-4969-94cb-e9de5165fbab

Sitagliptin: https://dailymed.nlm.nih.gov/dailymed/drugInfo.cfm?setid=f85a48d0-0407-4c50-b0fa-7673a160bf01

REFERENCES

1. Neumiller JJ. Incretin pharmacology: a review of the incretin effect and current incretin-based therapies. *Cardiovasc Hematol Agents Med Chem* 2012;10(4):276–288

2. American Diabetes Association. 8. Pharmacologic approaches to glycemic treatment: *Standards of Medical Care in Diabetes—2018*. *Diabetes Care* 2018;41(Suppl. 1):S73–S85

3. Nesina (alogliptin) [prescribing information]. Deerfiled, IL, Takeda Pharmaceuticals America, Inc., 2016. Available from https://www.accessdata.fda.gov/drugsatfda_docs/label/2013/022271s000lbl.pdf

4. Tradjenta (linagliptin) [prescribing information]. Ridgefield, CT, Boehringer Ingelheim Pharmaceuticals, Inc., 2017. Available from https://www.accessdata.fda.gov/drugsatfda_docs/label/2012/201280s005lbl.pdf

5. Onglyza (saxagliptin) [prescribing information]. Wilmington, DE, AstraZeneca Pharmaceuticals LP, 2018. Available from https://www.accessdata.fda.gov/drugsatfda_docs/label/2009/022350lbl.pdf

6. Januvia (sitagliptin) [prescribing information]. Whitehouse Station, NJ, Merck & Co., Inc., 2018. Available from https://www.accessdata.fda.gov/drugsatfda_docs/label/2012/021995s019lbl.pdf

7. Ahrén B. Clinical results of treating type 2 diabetic patients with sitagliptin, vildagliptin or saxagliptin—diabetes control and potential adverse events. *Best Pract Res Clin Endocrinol Metab* 2009;23(4):487–498

8. Nauck MA, Homberger E, Siegel EG, Allen RC, et al. Incretin effects of increasing glucose loads in man calculated from venous insulin and C-peptide responses. *J Clin Endocrinol Metab* 1986;63(2):492–498

9. Holst JJ, Orskov C, Nielsen OV, Schwartz TW. Truncated glucagon-like peptide 1, an insulin-releasing hormone from the distal gut. *FEBS Lett* 1987;211(2):169–174

10. Kreymann B, Williams G, Ghatei MA, Bloom SR. Glucagon-like peptide-1 7–36: a physiological incretin in man. *Lancet* 1987;2(8571):1300–1304

11. Nowicki M, Rychlik I, Haller H, et al. Long-term treatment with the dipeptidyl peptidase-4 inhibitor saxagliptin in patients with type 2 diabetes mellitus and renal impairment: a randomised controlled 52-week efficacy and safety study. *Int J Clin Pract* 2011;65:1230–1239

12. Covington P, Christopher R, Davenport M, et al. Pharmacokinetic, pharmacodynamic, and tolerability profiles of the dipeptidyl peptidase–4 inhibitor alogliptin: a randomized, double-blind, placebo-controlled, multiple-dose study in adult patients with type 2 diabetes. *Clin Ther* 2008;30:499–512

13. Graefe-Mody U, Huettner S, Stähle H, Ring A, Dugi KA. Effect of linagliptin (BI 1356) on the steady-state pharmacokinetics of simvastatin. *Int J Clin Pharmacol Ther* 2010;48:367–374

14. Fuchs H, Tillement JP, Urien S, Greischel A, Roth W. Concentration-dependent plasma protein binding of the novel dipeptidyl peptidase 4 inhib-

itor BI 1356 due to saturable binding to its target in plasma of mice, rats and humans. *J Pharm Pharmacol* 2009;61:55–62

15. Subbarayan S, Kipnes M. Sitagliptin: a review. *Expert Opin Pharmacother* 2011;12:1613–1622

16. Chen XW, He ZX, Zhou ZW, Yang T, et al. Clinical pharmacology of dipeptidyl peptidase 4 inhibitors indicated for the treatment of type 2 diabetes mellitus. *Clin Exp Pharmacol Physiol* 2015;42:999–1024

17. White WB, Cannon CP, Heller SR, et al.; EXAMINE Investigators. Alogliptin after acute coronary syndrome in patients with type 2 diabetes. *N Engl J Med* 2013;369:1327–1335

18. Green JB, Bethel MA, Armstrong PW, et al.; TECOS Study Group. Effect of sitagliptin on cardiovascular outcomes in type 2 diabetes. *N Engl J Med* 2015;373:232–242

19. Scirica BM, Bhatt DL, Braunwald E, et al.; SAVOR-TIMI 53 Steering Committee and Investigators. Saxagliptin and cardiovascular outcomes in patients with type 2 diabetes mellitus. *N Engl J Med* 2013;369:1317–1326

20. U.S. Food and Drug Administration. Diabetes medications containing saxagliptin and alogliptin: drug safety communication—risk of heart failure [Internet]. Available from https://www.fda.gov/drugs/drugsafety/ucm 486096.htm. Accessed 21 November 2018

21. Zannad F, Cannon CP, Cushman WC, et al.; EXAMINE Investigators. Heart failure and mortality outcomes in patients with type 2 diabetes taking alogliptin versus placebo in EXAMINE: a multicentre , randomized, double-blind trial. *Lancet* 2015;385:2067–2076

22. Wu S, Hopper I, Skiba M, Krum H. Dipeptidyl peptidase-4 inhibitors and cardiovascular outcomes: meta-analysis of randomized clinical trials with 55,141 participants. *Cardiovascular Ther* 2014;32:147–158

23. Geng J, Yu H, Yiwei M, Zhandg P, Yingyao C. Cost effectiveness of dipeptidyl-peptidase-4 inhibitors for type 2 diabetes. *Pharmacoeconomics* 2015;33:581–597

24. Dore DD, Seeger JD, Arnold Chan K. Use of a claims-based active drug safety surveillance system to assess the risk of acute pancreatitis with exenatide or sitagliptin compared to metformin or glyburide. *Curr Med Res Opin* 2009;25(4):1019–1027

25. Monami M, Dicembrini I, Mannucci E. Dipeptidyl peptidase-4 inhibitors and heart failure: a meta-analysis of randomized clinical trials. *Nutr Metab Cardiovasc Dis* 2014;24(7):689–697

26. Lam S, Saad M. Saxagliptin: a new dipeptidyl peptidase-4 inhibitor for type 2 diabetes. *Cardiol Rev* 2010;18(4):213–217

27. Scheen AJ. Dipeptidylpeptidase-4 inhibitors (gliptins): focus on drug-drug interactions. *Clin Pharmacokinet* 2010;49:573–588

28. Friedrich C, Port A, Ring A, et al. Effect of multiple oral doses of linagliptin on the steady-state pharmacokinetics of a combination oral contraceptive in healthy female adults: an open-label, two-period, fixed-sequence, multiple-dose study. *Clin Drug Investig* 2011;31:643–653

29. Friedrich C, Ring A, Brand T, Sennewald R, et al. Evaluation of the pharmacokinetic interaction after multiple oral doses of linagliptin and digoxin in healthy volunteers. *Eur J Drug Metab Pharmacokinet* 2011;36:17–24

30. Graefe-Mody EU, Brand T, Ring A, et al. Effect of linagliptin on the pharmacokinetics and pharmacodynamics of warfarin in healthy volunteers. *Int J Clin Pharmacol Ther* 2011;49:300–310

31. Graefe-Mody U, Rose P, Ring A, Zander K, et al. Assessment of the pharmacokinetic interaction between the novel DPP-4 inhibitor linagliptin and a sulfonylurea, glyburide, in healthy subjects. *Drug Metab Pharmacokinet* 2011;26:123–129

32. Graefe-Mody EU, Jungnik A, Ring A, Woerle HJ, Dugi KA. Evaluation of the pharmacokinetic interaction between the dipeptidyl peptidase-4 inhibitor linagliptin and pioglitazone in healthy volunteers. *Int J Clin Pharmacol Ther* 2010;48:652–661

33. Scheen AJ. Linagliptin plus metformin: a pharmacokinetic and pharmacodynamic evaluation. *Expert Opin Drug Metab Toxicol* 2013;9:363–377

34. Kazano (alogliptin and metformin HCl) [prescribing information]. Deerfield, IL, Takeda Pharmaceuticals America, Inc., 2017. Available from https://general.takedapharm.com/KAZANOPI

35. Janumet (sitagliptin and metformin HCl) [prescribing information]. Whitehouse Station, NJ, Merck & Co., Inc. Available from https://www.accessdata.fda.gov/drugsatfda_docs/label/2012/022044s022lbl.pdf

36. Kombiglyze XR (saxagliptin and metformin HCl extended-release) [prescribing information]. Princeton, NJ, Bristol-Myers Squibb Company, and Wilmington, DE, AstraZeneca Pharmaceuticals LP, 2012. Available from https://www.accessdata.fda.gov/drugsatfda_docs/label/2012/200678 s003s004lbl.pdf

37. Jentadueto (linagliptin and metformin hydrochloride) [prescribing information]. Ridgefield, CT, Boehringer Ingelheim Pharmaceuticals, Inc., 2017. Available from http://docs.boehringer-ingelheim.com/Prescribing%20 Information/PIs/Jentadueto/Jentadueto.pdf

38. Oseni (alogliptin and pioglitazone) [prescribing information]. Deerfield, IL, Takeda Pharmaceuticals America, Inc., 2017. Available from https://general. takedapharm.com/OSENIPI

39. Glyxambi (empagliflozin and linagliptin) [prescribing information]. Ridgefield, CT, Boehringer Ingelheim Pharmaceuticals, Inc., and Indianapolis, IN, Eli Lilly and Company, 2015. Available from https://www.accessdata.fda.gov/drugsatfda_docs/label/2015/206073s000lbl.pdf

40. Wu D, Li L, Liu C. Efficacy and safety of dipeptidyl peptidase-4 inhibitors and metformin as initial combination therapy and as monotherapy in patients with type 2 diabetes mellitus: a meta-analysis. *Diabetes Obes Metab* 2014;16:30–37

Chapter 13
Glucagon-Like Peptide-1 Receptor Agonists

Jennifer M. Trujillo, PharmD, BCPS, FCCP, CDE, BC-ADM

INTRODUCTION

Incretin hormones are glucoregulatory neurohormones, and GLP-1 and GIP account for about 90% of the incretin effect.[1] GLP-1 and GIP are secreted in response to food ingestion and act on the pancreas to stimulate glucose-dependent insulin secretion and blunt inappropriate glucagon secretion.[2] GLP-1 is predominantly secreted from the L cells of the distal ileum and colon, but plasma levels of GLP-1 increase within minutes of eating, which suggests that GLP-1 is also released from L cells, present in small number, in the upper gut.[2,3] GLP-1 receptors are expressed on the pancreas as well as in the gastrointestinal tract, brain, and cardiac tissue.[4]

Abnormalities in the incretin system contribute to the pathophysiology of T2D. In T2D, there is a deficiency of GLP-1 and resistance to the action of GIP.[1] The deficiency of GLP-1 occurs early in the natural history of the disease and worsens as the disease progresses.[1]

At pharmacologic doses, exogenous GLP-1, administered intravenously, can restore insulin secretion in response to glucose rises and normalize glucose concentrations in patients with T2D.[3,5] However, GLP-1 is degraded within minutes by the ubiquitous DPP-4, which limits its therapeutic value. This has led to the development of GLP-1 RAs that are resistant to degradation by DPP-4.[4]

Exendin-4, a 39-amino acid GLP-1 RA, was derived from the salivary gland venom of the gila monster and is resistant to the degradation by DPP-4. It shares roughly 50% of its amino acid sequence with mammalian GLP-1. Exenatide is a synthetically derived peptide of exendin-4 and was the first GLP-1 RA approved in the U.S. by the FDA in 2005.[3] Since then, several additional GLP-1 RAs have been developed to provide similar effects of GLP-1 while being resistant to the degradation by DPP-4, thereby extending the duration of action.[5] Currently available GLP-1 RAs, in order of approval by the FDA, include exenatide (Byetta), liraglutide (Victoza, approved 2010), exenatide XR (Bydureon, approved 2012; BCise pen approved 2017), dulaglutide (Trulicity, approved 2014), lixisenatide (Adlyxin, approved 2016), and semaglutide (Ozempic, approved 2017). Of note, due to steady decline in sales, the manufacturing of albiglutide (Tanzeum, approved 2014) was discontinued in 2017. For this reason, albiglutide will not be discussed in detail within this chapter.

GLP-1 RAs are treatment options at multiple points in the T2D disease process and can be used in combination with many other agents including metformin,

TZDs, sulfonylureas, SGLT2 inhibitors, and basal insulin. They are not currently recommended as first-line agents, but can be used as monotherapy in patients who cannot tolerate or take first-line therapy.[6-8] GLP-1 RAs are administered via subcutaneous injections with varying dosing schedules ranging from twice daily to once weekly. They are attractive treatment options as they target multiple pathophysiologic defects and reduce glucose and weight with minimal risk of hypoglycemia. Some agents have also demonstrated CV benefit.[9] Disadvantages such as gastrointestinal adverse effects, subcutaneous administration requirements, and cost can impact adherence and persistence, and may limit their use.

PHARMACOLOGY

MECHANISM OF ACTION

The GLP-1 RA class mimics the action of endogenous GLP-1. GLP-1 RAs stimulate insulin secretion from pancreatic β-cells in a glucose-dependent manner. In addition, during hyperglycemia, GLP-1 RAs reduce inappropriately elevated levels of glucagon, which results in decreased hepatic glucose output. These agents also have a direct effect on the stomach through the autonomic nervous system to slow gastric emptying, thereby reducing meal-related glucose excursions. Additionally, agents that penetrate the blood-brain barrier increase satiety via the central nervous system (CNS). These actions result in both a reduction in glucose and weight.[1,3,6-8,10] GLP-1 RAs also potentially preserve pancreatic β-cell function and protect against cytokine-induced apoptosis.[1-3,11]

PHARMACOKINETICS

Multiple differences exist in the characteristics of the individual agents within the GLP-1 RA class, including molecular structure and size, half-life, duration of action, ability to penetrate different tissue compartments, and homology to native GLP-1, which, in turn, lead to important clinical differences such as efficacy, rates of adverse events, dosing schedule, and impact on glucose profile (see Table 13.1).[12-17]

GLP-1 RAs can be categorized as either exendin-4 based or human GLP-1 based. They can also be categorized as short-acting or long-acting. Short-acting GLP-1 RAs predominantly lower PPG levels, likely due to their effect on gastric emptying. Long-acting GLP-1 RAs demonstrate larger effects on FPG levels and appear to lower both FPG and PPG.[4]

SHORT-ACTING GLP-1 RAs

Exenatide

Exenatide is a synthetic form of exendin-4 that shares 53% amino acid homology with mammalian GLP. It is a short-acting, twice-daily GLP-1 RA that has a

Table 13.1 — Pharmacology/Pharmacokinetics/Pharmacodynamics of GLP-1 RAs

	Name	Base	Homology to native GLP-1	Dose/range	T_{max}	Half-life	Antidrug antibodies (%)
Short-acting	Exenatide	Exendin-4	53%	5–10 µg twice daily	2.1 h	2.4 h	44
	Lixisenatide	Exendin-4	50%	10–20 µg once daily	1–3.5 h	3 h	70
Long-acting	Liraglutide	Human GLP-1	97%	0.6–1.8 mg once daily	8–12 h	13 h	8.6
	Exenatide XR	Exendin-4	53%	2 mg once weekly	2.1–5.1 h	NR	42.2
	Dulaglutide	Human GLP-1	90%	0.75–1.5 mg once weekly	24–72 h	5 days	1.6
	Semaglutide	Human GLP-1	94%	0.25–1 mg once weekly	1–3 days	1 week	1.0

Source: refs. 11–17.

more pronounced effect on PPG levels than FPG levels.[3,4,12,18] At therapeutic concentrations, exenatide restores both first- and second-phase insulin secretion in response to food in patients with T2D.[4] Exenatide has a terminal half-life of 2.4 h, and, in most individuals, concentrations are measurable for approximately 10 h post dose. Rate of absorption is similar when injected into the upper arm, abdomen, or thigh. Exenatide is predominantly eliminated by glomerular filtration with subsequent proteolytic degradation. Mean exenatide exposure increased by 3.37 times in patients with ESRD on dialysis; therefore, exenatide is not recommended in this patient population.[12,18]

Lixisenatide

Lixisenatide is a once-daily, exendin-4-based GLP-1 RA composed of a 44-amino-acid peptide that differs from exendin-4 by the addition of 6 lysine residues at the C-terminal. It presents an approximately fourfold higher affinity for the GLP-1 receptor than native human GLP-1. Lixisenatide reaches peak concentrations after 1–3.5 h and has an elimination half-life of 3 h. Rate of absorption is similar when injected into the upper arm, abdomen, or thigh.[13,19] Lixisenatide has been shown to cross the blood-brain barrier to bind to GLP-1 receptors. Because of its shorter duration of action, it primarily improves glucose by a pronounced effect on PPG levels following administration. The PPG reductions are most notable after the first meal of the day, and effects attenuate with later meals in the day.[13,19,20] Lixisenatide is presumed to be eliminated through glomerular filtration and proteolytic degradation. Plasma AUC was increased by 34%, 69%, and 124% in patients with mild, moderate, and severe renal impairment, respectively. Close monitoring is recommended in patients with mild to moderate renal insufficiency, and lixisenatide use is not recommended in patients with ESRD.[13,19]

LONG-ACTING GLP-1 RAs

Liraglutide

Liraglutide is a once-daily, acylated human GLP-1 RA with 97% homology to native GLP-1. Liraglutide is made by substituting arginine for lysine at position 34 and attaching a C-16 fatty acid with a glutamic acid spacer to lysine at position 26. Following subcutaneous administration, maximum concentrations are achieved at 8–12 h post dosing. The elimination half-life is approximately 13 h. Absorption was similar between upper arm and abdomen and between upper arm and thigh, but was 22% lower from the thigh than from the abdomen.[14,21] Liraglutide restores both first- and second-phase insulin response. It also crosses the blood-brain barrier and binds to GLP-1 receptors in the hypothalamus.[4] Because of its half-life of 13 h, liraglutide reduces both PPG and FPG and is thus considered a long-acting GLP-1 RA. Liraglutide is endogenously metabolized in a similar manner to large proteins without a specific organ as a major route of elimination.[14,21]

Exenatide Extended Release (XR)

Exenatide XR is a once-weekly, extended-release formulation of the exendin-4-based GLP-1 RA exenatide. The product contains microspheres of exenatide encapsulated in a biodegradable polymer for gradual drug delivery. Following a single subcutaneous dose of exenatide XR, there is an initial period of release of surface-bound exenatide followed by gradual release from the microspheres. This results in a peak concentration at week 6–7 following once-weekly administration and a steady-state concentration reached at week 10. Concentrations of exenatide XR are below minimal quantifiable concentrations approximately 10 weeks after discontinuation. Exenatide is predominantly eliminated by glomerular filtration with subsequent proteolytic degradation. Exenatide XR is not recommended for use in patients with severe renal impairment or ESRD.[15,22]

Dulaglutide

Dulaglutide is a long-acting, once-weekly GLP-1 RA consisting of two GLP-1 analogs that have been linked to a human immunoglobulin class 4 constant fragment. This reduced the renal clearance of the drug because of the increased size of the protein. The amino acid sequence has been modified in both analogs at positions 8, 22, and 26 to protect from DPP-4 degradation. Dulaglutide decreases both FPG and PPG. Maximum concentrations of dulaglutide are seen 24–72 h after dosing. Steady-state concentrations are achieved after 2–4 weeks with once-weekly administration. The site of subcutaneous injection (abdomen, upper arm, or thigh) does not change the exposure to dulaglutide. The elimination half-life is approximately 5 days. Dulaglutide is presumed to be degraded by general protein catabolism pathways, and no dose adjustments are needed for renal or hepatic impairment.[16,23]

Semaglutide

Semaglutide is a long-acting, once-weekly GLP-1 RA with 94% structural homology to native human GLP-1. It is structurally similar to liraglutide; however, it has structural modifications, which give it a longer half-life and make it suitable for once-weekly dosing. Amino acid substitutions occur at positions 8 and 34, with the substitution at position 8 rendering semaglutide less susceptible to degradation by DPP-4. Acylation of the lysine at position 26, a spacer, and a C-18 fatty diacid chain improve binding to albumin. Like other long-acting GLP-1 RAs, semaglutide lowers both FPG and PPG. Maximum concentrations are reached 1–3 days post dose. Steady state is achieved following 4–5 weeks of once-weekly administration. The elimination half-life is approximately 1 week, so semaglutide will be present in the circulation for about 5 weeks after the last dose. The primary route of elimination is metabolism following proteolytic cleavage of the peptide and sequential β-oxidation of the fatty acid sidechain. Renal impairment does not have significant effects on the pharmacokinetics of semaglutide.[17,24]

An oral formulation of semaglutide is currently being studied to treat T2D. This would be the first-in-class GLP-1 RA delivered as an oral agent. The long half-life and molecular stability of semaglutide along with the use of a carrier, which facilitates absorption, provide the potential for effective oral delivery of a GLP-1 RA protein. Oral semaglutide was evaluated in 10 phase 3 clinical studies, which included 9,543 adults with T2D. The new drug application was submitted to the FDA in early 2019.

TREATMENT ADVANTAGES/DISADVANTAGES

The GLP-1 RAs are suggested by the American Diabetes Association and the EASD Consensus Report and by the American Diabetes Association *Standards of Medical Care in Diabetes* as a treatment option that may be combined with metformin when additional therapy is needed to achieve glucose control.[6,7] GLP-1 RAs with evidence supporting a reduction in major adverse cardiovascular outcomes are considered preferred agents (along with SGLT2 inhibitors) in patients with established ASCVD. The American Association of Clinical Endocrinologists (AACE) guidelines recommend the use of GLP-1 RAs as the first therapeutic choice after metformin.[8]

The GLP-1 RAs have many favorable attributes compared to other second-line therapies. First, the GLP-1 RAs potentially preserve β-cell function and target multiple pathophysiologic defects caused by T2D including insulin secretion, glucagon secretion, gastric motility, and satiety. The GLP-1 RAs have demonstrated robust A1C-lowering efficacy in a wide array of patients with T2D. The class has been studied extensively with varying background therapies and in comparison with a variety of active comparators, and reductions in A1C range generally from 0.4–2.2%. Studies have consistently shown better A1C lowering with GLP-1 RAs than with DPP-4 inhibitors[25] and similar or better A1C lowering with GLP-1 RAs than with sulfonylureas, TZDs, and basal insulin.[4,18–24,26,27] The GLP-1 RAs also have a body-weight advantage and are associated with changes in weight ranging from +0.3 to –6.5 kg. The GLP-1 RAs also confer a low risk of hypoglycemia because their effect on insulin secretion is glucose-dependent.[4] Efficacy and safety results of phase 3 clinical trials are summarized in Table 13.2.

Several phase 3 trials have compared GLP-1 RAs in a head-to-head fashion and have demonstrated that differences exist in terms of magnitude of effect on A1C and weight, as well as frequency and severity of adverse effects. Semaglutide appears to offer the best A1C and weight reduction, followed by liraglutide, dulaglutide, and exenatide XR. Lixisenatide results in the smallest reductions in A1C and weight.[5,28,29]

Through large-scale outcome trials, two of the GLP-1 RAs (liraglutide and semaglutide) have also demonstrated CV benefits in addition to their benefits in glycemic control and weight. In the Liraglutide Effect and Action in Diabetes: Evaluation of Cardiovascular Outcome Results (LEADER) trial, liraglutide reduced the risk of a composite endpoint of CV death, nonfatal MI, and nonfatal stroke by 17% compared to placebo (HR 0.87 [95% CI 0.78–0.97]) in patients with T2D at high CV risk. This result was driven by a significant reduction in CV death (HR 0.78 [95% CI 0.66–0.93]). Liraglutide also resulted in a reduction in

Table 13.2—Efficacy and Safety of GLP-1 RAs in Phase 3 Clinical Studies

Drug	Phase 3 clinical program	Change in A1C (%)	Change in weight (kg)	Gastrointestinal adverse effects (%)^	Injection site reactions (%)
Exenatide	AMIGO	−0.4 to −1.1	−0.3 to −2.8	Nausea 8–44* Vomiting 4–18* Diarrhea 6–18*	5.1
Lixisenatide	GETGOAL	−0.46 to −0.99	+0.3 to −2.96	Nausea 25 Vomiting 10 Diarrhea 8	3.9
Liraglutide	LEAD	−0.84 to −1.5	+0.3 to −3.24	Nausea 18–20 Vomiting 6–9 Diarrhea 10–12	2.0
Exenatide XR	DURATION	−1.48 to −1.9	−2.0 to −4.0	Nausea 8.2 Vomiting 3.4 Diarrhea 4	23.9
Dulaglutide	AWARD	−0.71 to −1.64	+0.2 to −3.03	Nausea 12.4–21.1 Vomiting 6–12.7 Diarrhea 8.9–12.6	0.5
Semaglutide	SUSTAIN	−1.1 to −2.2	−1.4 to −6.5	Nausea 15.8–20.3 Vomiting 5–9.2 Diarrhea 8.8–8.9	0.2

^ Averages from phase 3 trials taken from prescribing information. Ranges based on different doses, except for exenatide. * Ranges based on reported data from separate studies based on background therapy. *Source*: refs. 4,11–24,26.

all-cause mortality and a reduction in the progression of renal disease. Because of these results, the FDA approved an additional indication for liraglutide to reduce the risk of major adverse CV events in adults with T2D and established CV disease.[9,30]

In the Trial to Evaluate Cardiovascular and Other Long-Term Outcomes with Semaglutide in Subjects with Type 2 Diabetes (SUSTAIN-6) trial, semaglutide reduced the risk of a composite endpoint of CV death, nonfatal MI, and nonfatal stroke by 26% compared to placebo (HR 0.74 [95% CI 0.58–0.95]) in patients with T2D at high CV risk. There was also a reduction in the individual endpoint of nonfatal stroke with semaglutide compared to placebo and a reduction in the progression of renal disease. No significant differences were seen between groups in CV death or all-cause mortality.[9,31]

Two additional CV outcome trials have been published and have demonstrated safety, but not benefit, with exenatide XR and lixisenatide. The study evaluating CV outcomes with dulaglutide has not yet been published.[9]

GLP-1 RAs can be used in combination with many other antidiabetic agents to provide glycemic control and target multiple pathophysiologic defects. Current guidelines, however, do not recommend using GLP-1 RAs in combination with DPP-4 inhibitors due to duplication of mechanism of action and lack of clinical outcomes and experience with this combination.[6-8,27] A significant amount of evidence shows the beneficial effect of the combination of a GLP-1 RA and a basal insulin. This combination offers complementary effects on the glucose profile and improved glycemic control with potentially lower risks of hypoglycemia and weight gain, providing a safe and effective alternative to basal-bolus insulin with lower treatment burden.[32] Current guidelines recommend the addition of a GLP-1 RA as an alternative to bolus insulin in patients not adequately controlled on basal insulin.[6-8] Two fixed-ratio combination products have been approved by the FDA and contain both a basal insulin and a GLP-1 RA in one delivery device. iDegLira combines insulin degludec and liraglutide (Xultophy, approved 2016) and iGlarLixi combines insulin glargine and lixisenatide (Soliqua, approved 2017).[33,34] These agents are approved for use in patients with T2D who have not achieved adequate glycemic control on basal insulin or a GLP-1 RA. They offer better glycemic control than the individual components, less required injections, and lower rates of gastrointestinal adverse effects, likely due to the slow dose titration.[35-38]

Disadvantages of GLP-1 RAs are the gastrointestinal adverse effects, including nausea, vomiting, and diarrhea, which usually occur early in the treatment course, are mild in nature, and are transient. But, in a small number of patients, the adverse effects are significant enough to require discontinuation. The shorter-acting agents, exenatide and lixisenatide, have more effect on gastric emptying and therefore cause more gastrointestinal adverse effects than the once-weekly options. Other disadvantages include safety concerns such as the immunogenicity risk, the potential risk of pancreatitis, and the black box warning regarding thyroid C-cell tumors. These risks are discussed in more detail in the following section. The GLP-1 RAs require subcutaneous administration, which is a disadvantage for patients who are resistant to injections. Each agent uses a unique injection pen device with unique administration requirements. In addition, the short-acting agents require specific dosing schedules before meals. Another potential disadvantage is cost. The GLP-1 RAs are expensive treatment options with out-of-pocket cost for a 1-month supply ranging from $500 to $775.[6] Finally, although this medication class is appealing for many reasons, the uptake of prescribing has been slow. For reasons not entirely clear, the GLP-1 RAs are still not commonly used, especially in the primary care setting, and long-term persistence is low.

THERAPEUTIC CONSIDERATIONS

SIGNIFICANT WARNINGS/PRECAUTIONS

Thyroid C-Cell Carcinoma

Most of the GLP-1 RAs, excluding exenatide twice daily and lixisenatide, carry a black box warning for potential risk of thyroid C-cell tumors. GLP-1 RAs cause an increase in the incidence of thyroid C-cell tumors in rodents in a dose-related, duration-dependent fashion. Medullary thyroid carcinoma (MTC) in humans is very rare, and no cases of thyroid C-cell tumors or MTC have been reported in humans to date. Nonetheless, dulaglutide, exenatide XR, liraglutide, and semaglutide are all contraindicated in patients with a personal or family history of MTC or multiple endocrine neoplasia type 2 (MEN2).[12–17]

Acute Pancreatitis

Cases of acute pancreatitis have been reported in animals and humans taking GLP-1 RAs as well as DPP-4 inhibitors. Retrospective and observational studies have been inconsistent, with some showing positive associations and some showing no association between incretin agents and pancreatitis. Some studies suggested that the risk may be related to T2D itself and not the specific drug treatment. However, early postmarketing reports led the FDA to release warnings that there may be a link between the use of these medication classes and acute pancreatitis. Ultimately, the FDA concluded that a causal relationship could not be established and there was insufficient evidence to modify treatment. The large-scale, prospective CV outcome trials have provided more insight into this potential association. Recent systematic reviews and meta-analyses of randomized controlled trials have concluded that treatment with GLP-1 RAs was not associated with an increased risk of acute pancreatitis or pancreatic cancer.[39,40] Nonetheless, current prescribing information, FDA guidance, and treatment guidelines recommend to use GLP-1 RAs cautiously in patients with a history of pancreatitis. Patients treated with GLP-1 RAs should be monitored for signs and symptoms of pancreatitis and, if pancreatitis develops while taking a GLP-1 RA, therapy should be discontinued and not re-initiated.[6,12–17,41]

Diabetic Retinopathy Complications

A significant increase in retinopathy complications including vitreous hemorrhage, blindness, or need for treatment with photocoagulation or an intravitreal agent was seen in patients receiving semaglutide during the SUSTAIN-6 trial (3% vs. 1.8%; $P = 0.02$).[31] Of the patients with retinopathy complications, 83.5% had a history of retinopathy at baseline. Rapid glucose lowering has previously been associated with worsening of diabetic retinopathy. It is unclear if this is due to the drug itself or an effect of the change in blood glucose levels. Caution should be taken when using semaglutide in patients with a history of diabetic retinopathy, and the patient should be monitored closely for progression of retinopathy.[17]

Hypoglycemia

Although GLP-1 RAs independently carry a low risk of hypoglycemia, the risk of hypoglycemia is increased when they are used in combination with insulin or insulin secretagogues. Patients may require a lower dose of insulin or the secretagogue to reduce the risk of hypoglycemia in this situation.[12–17]

Acute Kidney Injury

There have been postmarketing reports of acute kidney injury and worsening of chronic renal failure in patients taking GLP-1 RAs. Some reports were in patients who did not have existing kidney disease. A majority of the cases occurred in patients who experienced nausea, vomiting, diarrhea, or dehydration. It remains unclear whether a true causal relationship exists in these case reports, but it is recommended to use caution when starting or increasing the dose of GLP-1 RAs in patients with renal insufficiency.[12–17]

Hypersensitivity

Hypersensitivity reactions have been reported with GLP-1 RAs. If a hypersensitivity reaction occurs, the drug should be stopped immediately, and the patient should be promptly treated until symptoms resolve.

SPECIAL POPULATIONS

T1D

GLP-1 RAs are not indicated for the treatment of T1D or DKA, and cannot replace insulin therapy in this population. The physiologic actions and secretion of GLP-1 in T1D are not well understood, but it is appreciated that T1D is associated with defective counterregulation, including unregulated secretion of glucagon postprandially. Thus, GLP-1 RA therapy has the potential for benefit in T1D by inhibiting inappropriate glucagon secretion after a meal.[20] To date, studies of GLP-1 RAs in combination with insulin in T1D have shown modest improvements in A1C and weight, but currently, no agent has an FDA indication for use in T1D.[42]

Pregnancy and Lactation

Limited data are available to guide the use of GLP-1 RAs in pregnant women. Based on animal studies, there may be risks to the fetus from exposure to GLP-1 RAs during pregnancy. Animal studies demonstrated embryo-fetal mortality as well as structural abnormalities, birth defects, growth alterations, and marked maternal weight loss. Women using GLP-1 RAs should discontinue use prior to a planned pregnancy to allow for washout of the medication. This time frame varies between products, with requirements of 1–2 months for once-weekly agents. No data exists with use of GLP-1 RAs in lactation, and it is not known whether GLP-1 RAs are excreted in human milk.[12-17]

Pediatrics

Safety and efficacy of GLP-1 RAs have not been established in the pediatric population. They are not recommended for use in patients under the age of 18 years. There are, however, several ongoing phase 3 clinical studies evaluating the use of GLP-1 RAs in youth.[43]

Geriatrics

The phase 3 clinical trials of all GLP-1 RAs did include patients over the age of 65 and a small percentage of patients over the age of 75. No meaningful differences were observed in safety and efficacy between younger and older adults. Small sample sizes could limit these conclusions. Since older patients may have declined renal function, care should be taken with product and dose selection based on renal function status.[12-17]

Renal or Hepatic Impairment

Dose adjustments are not recommended for most of the GLP-1 RAs with the exception of exenatide and exenatide XR, which are not recommended for use in patients with severe renal impairment (CrCl <30 mL/min). There is limited experience with the use of GLP-1 RAs in patients with ESRD. Clinicians should use caution in this patient population and in those at risk for worsening renal function, such as patients experiencing dehydration. Recommendations on the use and dose of specific GLP-1 RAs in renal impairment are in Table 13.3. There is limited experience in patients with hepatic impairment, and dose adjustments are not recommended in this patient population. Exenatide and exenatide XR undergo renal elimination, so hepatic impairment would not be expected to affect blood concentrations.[27]

Gastroparesis

GLP-1 RAs have not been studied in patients with severe gastrointestinal disease, including gastroparesis. Since these agents delay gastric emptying, they are not recommended in patients with gastroparesis.

Table 13.3—Availability, Dosing, and Administration Requirements of GLP-1 RAs

Drug	Availability, storage, preparation	Dosing	Missed dose recommendations	Use in renal impairment
Exenatide	■ Multidose pen (5 µg/dose, 10 µg/dose, 60 doses per pen) ■ Pen needles not supplied with pen ■ Keep refrigerated ■ After first use, store at room temperature; discard 30 days after first use ■ No reconstitution required	■ Start with 5 µg twice daily ■ Increase to 10 µg twice daily after one month if needed for additional A1C lowering ■ Inject within 60 min prior to morning and evening meals (or before the two main meals of the day; ≥6 h apart)	■ Skip the dose and resume next dose at the pre-scribed time	■ Not recommended with severe renal impairment (eGFR or CrCl <30 mL/min)
Lixisenatide	■ Multidose pen (10 µg/dose, 20-µg/dose, 14 doses per pen) ■ Pen needles not supplied with pen ■ Keep refrigerated ■ After first use, store at room temperature; discard 14 days after first use ■ No reconstitution required	■ Start with 10 µg once daily for 14 days ■ Increase to 20 µg once daily ■ Inject within 1 h prior to first meal of the day	■ Skip the dose and resume next dose at the pre-scribed time	■ No dose adjustment recommended; limited experience in severe renal impairment; avoid if eGFR <15 mL/min/1.73 m²
Liraglutide	■ Multidose pen (6 mg/mL, 3 mL; each pen delivers doses of 0.6 mg, 1.2 mg, or 1.8 mg) ■ Pen needles not supplied with pen ■ Keep refrigerated ■ After first use, store at room temperature; discard 30 days after first use ■ No reconstitution required	■ Start with 0.6 mg once daily for 1 week; then increase to 1.2 mg once daily ■ Increase to 1.8 mg once daily if needed for additional A1C lowering ■ Inject at any time of day, with or without meals	■ Skip the dose and resume next dose at the pre-scribed time	■ No dose adjustment recommended; limited experience in severe renal impairment

(continued)

Table 13.3 (continued)

Drug	Availability, storage, preparation	Dosing	Missed dose recommendations	Use in renal impairment
Exenatide XR	■ Single-dose pen (2 mg) ■ Pen needle supplied with pen ■ Keep refrigerated ■ Store flat in original packaging, protected from light ■ May store at room temperature for 4 weeks ■ Remove from refrigerator 15 min prior to mixing ■ Requires reconstitution ■ Dose should be administered immediately once reconstituted	■ 2 mg once weekly ■ Inject at any time of day, with or without meals	■ If within 3 days of missed dose, give right away; resume dosing on usual day of administration ■ If 3 days have passed, skip dose and resume on usual day of administration	■ Not recommended with severe renal impairment (eGFR or CrCl <30 mL/min)
Dulaglutide	■ Single-dose pen (0.75 mg, 1.5 mg) ■ Pen needle attached ■ Keep refrigerated ■ May store at room temperature for 14 days ■ No reconstitution required	■ Start with 0.75 mg once weekly ■ Increase to 1.5 mg once weekly if needed for additional A1C lowering ■ Inject at any time of day, with or without meals	■ If within 3 days of missed dose, give right away. Resume dosing on usual day of administration ■ If 3 days have passed, skip dose and resume on usual day of administration	■ No dose adjustment recommended; limited experience in severe renal impairment
Semaglutide	■ Multidose pen (1.34 mg/mL; 1.5 mL; lower-dose pen delivers 0.25 mg or 0.5 mg doses; higher-dose pen delivers 1 mg dose) ■ Pen needles supplied with pen ■ Keep refrigerated ■ After first use, store at room temperature; discard 56 days after first use ■ No reconstitution required	■ Start with 0.25 mg once weekly ■ Increase to 0.5 mg once weekly after 4 weeks ■ May increase to 1 mg once weekly after 4 weeks, if needed for additional A1C lowering ■ Inject at any time of day, with or without meals	■ If within 5 days of missed dose, give right away; resume dosing on usual day of administration ■ If 5 days have passed, skip dose and resume on usual day of administration	■ No dose adjustment recommended

Source: refs. 11–17.

ADVERSE EFFECTS AND MONITORING

Gastrointestinal Adverse Effects

The most commonly reported adverse effects of the GLP-1 RAs are gastrointestinal in nature, including nausea, vomiting, and diarrhea, which usually occur early in the treatment course, are transient, are mild in nature, and rarely require discontinuation.[4] Rates of nausea, vomiting, and diarrhea range from 8–44% for nausea, from 3.4–18% for vomiting, and from 4–18% for diarrhea with the GLP-1 RAs (Table 13.2).[12–17] These varying rates are dependent not only on the specific drug, but also on the dose, background therapy, and adverse event reporting process in each clinical trial. In head-to-head clinical studies, exenatide XR was associated with lower rates of nausea and vomiting than liraglutide and exenatide twice daily. Lixisenatide had lower rates compared to exenatide twice daily; dulaglutide and liraglutide had similar rates.[4,5,28] The shorter-acting agents, exenatide and lixisenatide, have more effect on gastric emptying and therefore may cause more gastrointestinal adverse effects than the once-weekly options.[28] Slow dose titration can minimize the gastrointestinal adverse effects. Patients should also be encouraged to eat slowly and reduce portion sizes to help minimize the gastrointestinal adverse effects.

Hypoglycemia

Because GLP-1 RAs increase insulin secretion from pancreatic β-cells in a glucose-dependent manner in response to food intake, the risk of hypoglycemia is low. Clinical studies done with GLP-1 RAs alone or in combination with other low hypoglycemia risk agents such as metformin have reported low rates of hypoglycemia, typically under 5%.[18–24] Episodes of severe hypoglycemia are rare. Rates of hypoglycemia are consistently lower with GLP-1 RAs than with insulin or sulfonylureas in clinical studies. In head-to-head trials, there have been no significant differences in the rates of hypoglycemia among GLP-1 RAs.[5,28,29]

The risk of hypoglycemia is increased when GLP-1 RAs are used in combination with insulin or insulin secretagogues such as sulfonylureas or meglitinides. However, a meta-analysis evaluating the combination of a GLP-1 RA and basal insulin showed no significant increase in hypoglycemia in patients taking the combination versus other treatments.[44] Studies have also demonstrated that the fixed-ratio combinations of basal insulin and GLP-1 RAs can achieve better A1C lowering with similar or lower rates of hypoglycemia compared to basal insulin alone.[35–37] Nonetheless, care should be taken when initiating a GLP-1 RA in a patient already taking basal insulin. The basal insulin dose may need to be decreased as the GLP-1 RA starts to take effect.[32] Across clinical studies, there were varying approaches to adjusting basal insulin doses, with some empirically decreasing the dose by 10–20% when the GLP-1 RA was initiated. This dose adjustment should depend on baseline glucose and A1C levels, as well as the onset of action, dose titration schedule, and expected impact on glucose profile of the specific GLP-1 RA.[32]

Injection Site Reactions

Injection site reactions range from 0.2–23.9% in patients taking GLP-1 RAs (Table 13.2).[12–17] Some evidence suggests that injection site reactions are more common in patients with high drug antibody titers.[4] Rates were also more pronounced with exenatide than other GLP-1 RAs. Exenatide XR can also cause injection site nodules, likely due to its formulation. Exenatide XR is encapsulated in microspheres made of a biodegradable polymer that release the drug over a sustained time interval. The microspheres can lead to injection site nodules described as pea-sized, hard, subcutaneous, lumps, masses, or indurations.[45]

Immunogenicity

Immunogenicity is a potential concern with all therapeutic proteins. The detection of antibody formation in assays is influenced by several factors including assay methodology, sample handling, concomitant medications, and underlying disease; therefore, caution must be taken when comparing rates of antibody formation between studies. Antidrug antibodies occurred in 1–70% of patients taking GLP-1 RAs during phase 3 clinical trials and occurred more frequently with the exendin-4-based agents (exenatide and lixisenatide) than with other agents (Table 13.1).[4,12–17] Patients with antibody formation may have an attenuated A1C response. In the phase 3 clinical program, 70% of patients taking lixisenatide had antibody formation, and an attenuated glycemic response was seen in the subset of patients with the highest antibody titers.[13] Similarly, 20–38% of patients taking exenatide twice daily had low titer antibodies in the phase 3 studies and 2–9% had high titer antibodies, with about half of the patients with high titer antibodies having an attenuated glycemic response.[12]

Increased Heart Rate

Although GLP-1 RAs have been associated with a mild decrease in blood pressure, they also are associated with an increased heart rate of 2–4 beats per minute. The clinical significance of this effect has not been established.[46]

Cholelithiasis

In an evaluation of over 90 clinical trials involving 17,232 patients taking a GLP-1 RA versus 14,872 patients taking a comparator, there was a small but significantly increased risk of cholelithiasis in patients taking a GLP-1 RA versus a comparator (141 vs. 99 cases; HR 1.3 [95% CI 1.01–1.68, $P = 0.041$]).[40] The mechanism of this adverse effect is not understood and warrants further investigation.

Monitoring

Monitoring for efficacy should include A1C every 3–6 months and weight. Self-monitoring of blood glucose (SMBG) can be useful to determine whether FPG or PPG levels are more problematic. Since some of the GLP-1 RAs are affected by renal impairment, routine monitoring of serum creatinine is warranted. Although hypoglycemia is rare with GLP-1 RAs, the risk is increased when used with insulin or secretagogues. Therefore, hypoglycemia occurrence, frequency, and severity should be evaluated. Other monitoring should include close follow-up to assess injection site reactions and gastrointestinal adverse effects such as nausea, vomiting, and diarrhea. Although pancreatitis and cholelithiasis are rare, patients should be educated about the symptoms, including extreme abdominal pain.[27]

DRUG INTERACTIONS

The risk of hypoglycemia is increased when GLP-1 RAs are used concomitantly with insulin or insulin secretagogues (e.g., sulfonylureas or meglitinides). The risk can be decreased by reducing the dose of the concomitant medication.[12–17]

GLP-1 RAs cause delayed gastric emptying and thereby have the potential to impact the absorption of other medications administered concomitantly. In clinical trials, most of the GLP-1 RAs did not affect the absorption of orally administered drugs to any clinically meaningful degree. However, since GLP-1 RAs delay gastric emptying, caution should be taken when oral medications are given concomitantly with GLP-1 RAs, particularly when a slower rate of absorption could be clinically meaningful.[12–17] Drugs that have a narrow therapeutic index should be adequately monitored when being given with a GLP-1 RA. A drug interaction study of exenatide and warfarin did not show any significant interaction; however, there have been postmarketing reports of increased international normalized ratio (INR) with concomitant use of exenatide and warfarin. Therefore, INR should be monitored more frequently after initiating exenatide and can return to normal intervals once stable.[15]

For patients taking a short-acting GLP-1 RA (exenatide and lixisenatide), oral medications that are dependent on threshold concentrations (e.g., antibiotics and contraceptives) should be taken at least 1 h prior to the GLP-1 RA injection (or at least 11 h after the dose for lixisenatide). Drugs that should be taken with food should be taken with a meal or snack when the GLP-1 RA is not administered.[12,13]

DOSING AND ADMINISTRATION

The availability, storage, dosing, and administration requirements for the GLP-1 RAs are compared in Table 13.3. Availability and dosing of fixed-ratio combination products are summarized in Table 13.4. The GLP-1 RAs are all available in injectable pen devices and administered subcutaneously into the abdomen, thigh, or upper arm. Dosing schedules vary between agents and range from twice daily to once weekly. The short-acting agents, exenatide and lixisenatide, have specific timing requirements in relation to meals since their mechanisms are more targeted toward slowing gastric emptying postprandially. If the dose of exenatide or lixisenatide is missed, it should not be taken after the meal. The long-acting agents have more flexibility with timing of doses and can be taken at any time of day, with or without food. Most of the GLP-1 RAs have recommended lower doses when initiating the drug, followed by titration to higher doses if needed for glycemic control. This is to minimize gastrointestinal adverse effects, since studies have found that the gastrointestinal adverse effects are dose related and transient.

Each GLP-1 RA requires medication counseling and self-administration education specific to the product. Preparation steps, administration, and storage requirements are all unique to each product. Some pen devices are single use, while others are multi-use. Exenatide XR requires reconstitution prior to administering the dose, which involves several steps including shaking the pen vigorously for at least 15 seconds. Some require pen needle attachment, while others come with the pen already attached. Therefore, each patient requires education

Table 13.4—Combination GLP-1 RA and Basal Insulin Products

Drug	Availability, storage, preparation	Dosing
iDegLira 100/3.6 (Insulin degludec and liraglutide)	■ Multi-dose pens (insulin degludec 100 units/mL and liraglutide 3.6 mg/mL; 3 mL) ■ Each pen delivers doses based on insulin units; doses range from 10–50 units ■ Pen needles not supplied with pen ■ Keep refrigerated ■ After first use, store at room temperature; discard 21 days after first use	■ Start with 16 units insulin degludec/0.58 mg liraglutide once daily ■ Increase dose by 2 units every 3–4 days until FPG goal is reached; maximum dose is 50 units insulin degludec/1.8 mg liraglutide ■ Inject at any time of day, with or without meals
iGlarLixi 100/33 (Insulin glargine and lixisenatide)	■ Multi-dose pens (insulin glargine 100 units/mL and lixisenatide 33 µg/mL; 3 mL) ■ Each pen delivers doses based on insulin units; doses range from 15–60 units ■ Pen needles not supplied with pen ■ Keep refrigerated ■ After first use, store at room temperature; discard 14 days after first use	■ If on <30 units of basal insulin or lixisenatide: start with 15 units insulin glargine/5 µg lixisenatide once daily ■ If on ≥30 units of basal insulin: start with 30 units insulin glargine/10 µg lixisenatide once daily ■ Increase dose by 2–4 units every week until FPG goal is reached; maximum dose is 60 units insulin glargine/20 µg lixisenatide ■ Inject within 1 h before first meal of the day

Source: Xultophy [product information][33] and Soliqua [product information].[34]

on the agent prescribed and occasional review of administration technique and medication-taking behaviors. Regardless of product, all patients should be instructed that pen devices should never be shared between patients, even if the needle is changed, as it poses a risk for the transmission of blood-borne pathogens.

Adherence and persistence are particularly challenging with the GLP-1 RAs. Several barriers have been identified to consistent use of these agents, including clinical inertia, cost, gastrointestinal adverse effects, and injection concerns. These issues underscore the need for better provider-patient communication to set expectations appropriately, discuss the patient's willingness and ability to take the medication, and address additional barriers that may arise.[47] Several real-world studies have demonstrated variability in patient preference, adherence, and persistence among GLP-1 RA agents. Higher adherence and persistence rates have been demonstrated with dulaglutide than with exenatide XR and liraglutide.[48] Higher adherence has been demonstrated with exenatide XR than with exenatide and liraglutide.[49,50]

The GLP-1 RAs offer an attractive treatment option for T2D with high glycemic-lowering efficacy, weight loss, and low risk of hypoglycemia. Some agents also lower major adverse cardiovascular outcomes. Clinicians should use a patient-centered approach when considering the utility, advantages, and disadvantages of a GLP-1 RA compared to other medication classes for the treatment of T2D. When selecting a specific GLP-1 RA within the class, the decision-making process should incorporate evidence on comparative efficacy (A1C, weight, CV outcomes), safety (gastrointestinal adverse effects, injection site reactions), as well as other practical considerations such as self-administration requirements, ease of use, and cost.

MONOGRAPHS

Adlyxin: https://dailymed.nlm.nih.gov/dailymed/drugInfo.cfm?setid=1727cc16-4f86-4f13-b8b5-804d4984fa8c

Bydureon BCise: https://dailymed.nlm.nih.gov/dailymed/drugInfo.cfm?setid=2d18cfc4-e0de-4814-a712-c1b7c504bff5

Byetta: https://dailymed.nlm.nih.gov/dailymed/drugInfo.cfm?setid=53d03c03-ebf7-418d-88a8-533eabd2ee4f

Ozempic: https://dailymed.nlm.nih.gov/dailymed/drugInfo.cfm?setid=adec4fd2-6858-4c99-91d4-531f5f2a2d79

Soliqua: https://dailymed.nlm.nih.gov/dailymed/drugInfo.cfm?setid=4bba538b-cf7c-4310-ae8f-cb711ed21bcc

Trulicity: https://dailymed.nlm.nih.gov/dailymed/drugInfo.cfm?setid=463050bd-2b1c-40f5-b3c3-0a04bb433309

Victoza: https://dailymed.nlm.nih.gov/dailymed/drugInfo.cfm?setid=5a9ef4ea-c76a-4d34-a604-27c5b505f5a4

Xultophy: https://dailymed.nlm.nih.gov/dailymed/drugInfo.cfm?setid=21335fe4-d395-4501-ac2a-2f20d7520da9

REFERENCES

1. DeFronzo RA. From the triumvirate to the ominous octet: a new paradigm for the treatment of type 2 diabetes mellitus. *Diabetes* 2009;58:773–795

2. Mudaliar S, Henry RR. The incretin hormones: from scientific discovery to practical therapeutics. *Diabetologia* 2012;55:1865–1868

3. Drucker DJ, Nauck MA. The incretin system: glucagon-like peptide-1 receptor agonists and dipeptidyl peptidase-4 inhibitors in type 2 diabetes. *Lancet* 2006;368:1696–1705

4. Leiter LA, Nauck MA. Efficacy and safety of GLP-1 receptor agonists across the spectrum of type 2 diabetes mellitus. *Exp Clin Endocrinol Diabetes* 2017;125:419–435

5. Madsbad S. Review of head-to-head comparisons of glucagon-like peptide-1 receptor agonists. *Diabetes Obes Metab* 2016;18:317–332

6. American Diabetes Association. 8. Pharmacologic approaches to glycemic treatment: *Standards of Medical Care in Diabetes—2018. Diabetes Care* 2018;41(Suppl. 1):S73–S85

7. Davies MJ, D'Alessio DA, Fradkin J, et al. Management of hyperglycemia in type 2 diabetes, 2018. A consensus report by the American Diabetes Association (ADA) and the European Association for the Study of Diabetes (EASD). *Diabetes Care* 2018;41(12):2669–2701

8. Garber AJ, Abrahamson MJ, Barzilay JI, et al. Consensus statement by the American Association of Clinical Endocrinologists and American College of Endocrinology on the comprehensive type 2 diabetes management algorithm. *Endocr Pract* 2018;24(1):91–120

9. Cefalu WT, Kaul S, Gerstein HC, et al. Cardiovascular outcomes trials in type 2 diabetes: where do we go from here? Reflections from a *Diabetes Care* editors' expert forum. *Diabetes Care* 2018;41:14–31

10. Nauck M. Incretin therapies: highlighting common features and differences in the modes of action of glucagon-like peptide-1 receptor agonists and dipeptidyl peptidase-4 inhibitors. *Diabetes Obes Metab* 2016;18:203–216

11. DeFronzo RA, Eldor R, Abdul-Ghani M. Pathophysiologic approach to therapy in patients with newly diagnosed type 2 diabetes. *Diabetes Care* 2013;36(Suppl. 2):S127–S138

12. Byetta (exenatide) injection [product information]. Wilmington, DE, AstraZeneca Pharmaceuticals LP, February 2015

13. Adlyxin (lixisenatide) injection [product information]. Bridgewater, NJ, Sanofi-aventis U.S. LLC, July 2017

14. Victoza (liraglutide) injection [product information]. Plainsboro, NJ, Novo Nordisk Inc., January 2018

15. Bydureon BCise (exenatide extended release) injectable suspension [product information]. Wilmington, DE, AstraZeneca Pharmaceuticals LP, December 2017

16. Trulicity (dulaglutide) injection [product information]. Indianapolis, IN, Eli Lilly and Company, August 2017

17. Ozempic (semaglutide) injection [product information]. Plainsboro, NJ, Novo Nordisk Inc., December 2017

18. Yoo BK, Triller DM, Yoo DJ. Exenatide: a new option for the treatment of type 2 diabetes. *Ann Pharmacother* 2006;40:1777–1784

19. Trujillo JM, Goldman J. Lixisenatide, a once-daily prandial glucagon-like peptide-1 receptor agonist for the treatment of adults with type 2 diabetes. *Pharmacotherapy* 2017;37(8):927–943

20. Trujillo JM, Nuffer W. GLP-1 receptor agonists for type 2 diabetes mellitus: recent developments and emerging agents. *Pharmacotherapy* 2014;34(11):1174–1186

21. Montanya E, Sesti G. A review of efficacy and safety data regarding the use of liraglutide, a once-daily human glucagon-like peptide 1 analogue, in the treatment of type 2 diabetes. *Clin Ther* 2009;31(11):2472–2488

22. Genovese S, Mannucci E, Ceriello A. A review of the long-term efficacy, tolerability, and safety of exenatide once weekly for type 2 diabetes. *Adv Ther* 2017;34:1791–1814

23. Thompson AM, Trujillo JM. Advances in the treatment of type 2 diabetes: impact of dulaglutide. *Diabetes Metab Syndr Obes* 2016;9:125–136

24. Tuchscherer RM, Thompson AM, Trujillo JM. Semaglutide: the newest once-weekly GLP-1 RA for type 2 diabetes. *Ann Pharmacother* 2018;52(12):1224–1232

25. Tran S, Retnakaran R, Zinman B, Kramer CK. Efficacy of glucagon-like peptide-1 receptor agonists compared to dipeptidyl peptidase-4 inhibitors for the management of type 2 diabetes: a meta-analysis of randomized clinical trials. *Diabetes Obes Metab* 2018;20(Suppl. 1):68–76

26. Tran KL, Park YI, Pandya S, et al. Overview of glucagon-like peptide-1 receptor agonists for the treatment of patients with type 2 diabetes. *Am Health Drug Benefits* 2017;10(4):178–188

27. Prasad-Reddy L, Isaacs D. A clinical review of GLP-1 receptor agonists: efficacy and safety in diabetes and beyond. *Drugs Context* 2015;4:212283. DOI:10.7573/dic.212283

28. Trujillo JM, Nuffer W, Ellis SL. GLP-1 receptor agonists: a review of head-to-head clinical studies. *Ther Adv Endocrinol Metab* 2015;6:19–28

29. Pratley RE, Aroda VR, Lingvay I, et al. Semaglutide versus dulaglutide once weekly in patients with type 2 diabetes (SUSTAIN 7): a randomized, open-label phase 3b trial. *Lancet Diabetes Endocrinol.* 31 January 2018 [Epub ahead of print]. Available from http://dx.doi.org/10.1016/S2213-8587(18)30024-X

30. Marso SP, Daniels GH, Brown-Frandsen K, et al. Liraglutide and cardiovascular outcomes in type 2 diabetes. *N Engl J Med* 2016;375:311–322

31. Marso SP, Bain SC, Consoli A, et al. Semaglutide and cardiovascular outcomes in patients with type 2 diabetes. *N Engl J Med* 2016;375:1834–1844

32. Anderson SL, Trujillo JM. Basal insulin use with GLP-1 receptor agonists. *Diabetes Spectr* 2016;29(3):152–160

33. Xultophy 100/3.6 (insulin degludec and liraglutide) injection [product information]. Plainsboro, NJ, Novo Nordisk Inc., November 2016

34. Soliqua 100/33 (insulin glargine and lixisenatide) injection [product information]. Bridgewater, NJ, Sanofi-aventis U.S. LLC, October 2017

35. Goldman J, Trujillo JM. iGlarLixi: a fixed-ratio combination of insulin glargine 100 U/mL and lixisenatide for the treatment of type 2 diabetes. *Ann Pharmacother* 2017;51(11):990–999

36. Gough SCL, Jain R, Woo VC. Insulin degludec/liraglutide (iDegLira) for the treatment of type 2 diabetes. *Expert Rev Endocrinol Metab* 2016; 11(1):7–18

37. Nuffer W, Guesnier A, Trujillo JM. A review of the new GLP-1 receptor agonist/basal insulin fixed-ratio combination products. *Ther Adv Endocrinol Metab* 2018;9(3):69–79

38. Trujillo JM, Roberts M, Dex T, et al. Low incidence of gastrointestinal adverse events over time with a fixed-ratio combination of insulin glargine and lixisenatide versus lixisenatide alone. *Diabetes Obes Metab* 2018;20(11):2690–2694

39. Storgaard H, Cold F, Gluud LL, et al. Glucagon-like peptide-1 receptor agonists and risk of acute pancreatitis in patients with type 2 diabetes. *Diabetes Obes Metab* 2017;19:906–908

40. Monami M, Nreu B, Scatena A, et al. Safety issues with glucagon-like peptide-1 receptor agonists (pancreatitis, pancreatic cancer and cholelithiasis): data from randomized controlled trials. *Diabetes Obes Metab* 2017; 19:1233–1241

41. FDA Drug Safety Communication: FDA investigating reports of possible increased risk of pancreatitis and pre-cancerous findings of the pancreas from incretin mimetic drugs for type 2 diabetes. Available from https://www.fda.gov/Drugs/DrugSafety/ucm343187.htm. Accessed 20 April 2018

42. Wang W, Liu H, Xiao S, et al. Effects of insulin plus glucagon-like peptide-1 receptor agonists (GLP-1RAs) in treating type 1 diabetes mellitus: a systematic review and meta-analysis. *Diabetes Ther* 2017;8(4):727–738

43. Tamborlane WV, Haymond MW, Dunger D, et al. Expanding treatment options for youth with type 2 diabetes: current problems and proposed solutions: a white paper from the NICHD Diabetes Working Group. *Diabetes Care* 2016;39(3):323–329

44. Eng C, Kramer CK, Zinman B, Retnakaran R. Glucagon-like peptide-1 receptor agonist and basal insulin combination treatment for the management of type 2 diabetes: a systematic review and meta-analysis. *Lancet* 2014;384(9961):2228–2234

45. Jones SC, Ryan DL, Pratt VSW, et al. Injection site nodules associated with the use of exenatide extended-release reports to the U.S. Food and Drug Administration adverse event reporting system. *Diabetes Spectr* 2015;28(4):283–288

46. Sun F, Wu S, Guo S, et al. Impact of GLP-1 receptor agonists on blood pressure, heart rate, and hypertension among patients with type 2 diabetes: a systematic review and network meta-analysis. *Diabetes Res Clin Pract* 2015;110:26–37

47. Spain CV, Wright JJ, Hahn RM, et al. Self-reported barriers to adherence and persistence to treatment with injectable medications for type 2 diabetes. *Clin Ther* 2016;38(7):1653–1664

48. Alatorre C, Fernández Landó L, Yu M, et al. Treatment patterns in patients with type 2 diabetes mellitus treated with glucagon-like peptide-1 receptor agonists: higher adherence and persistence with dulaglutide compared with once-weekly exenatide and liraglutide. *Diabetes Obes Metab* 2017; 19:953–961

49. Nguyen H, Dufour R, Caldwell-Tarr A. Glucagon-like peptide-1 receptor agonist (GLP-1RA) therapy adherence for patients with type 2 diabetes in a Medicare population. *Adv Ther* 2017;34(3):658–673

50. Qiao Q, Ouwens MJ, Grandy S, et al. Adherence to GLP-1 receptor agonist therapy administered by once-daily or once-weekly injection in patients with type 2 diabetes in Germany. *Diabetes Metab Syndr Obes* 2016;9:201–205

Chapter 14
Pramlintide

JENNIFER M. TRUJILLO, PHARMD, BCPS, FCCP, CDE, BC-ADM

INTRODUCTION

Pramlintide is an amylin analog and is the only approved medication in this class. Amylin is a 37-amino acid peptide neurohormone that is co-secreted with insulin from pancreatic β-cells. Amylin plasma levels, similar to insulin, are lower during the fasting state and rise in response to caloric intake. Amylin works in concert with insulin and glucagon to maintain glucose homeostasis by blunting inappropriate glucagon secretion after meals, slowing gastric emptying, and increasing satiety via a centrally mediated mechanism.[1,2]

Amylin secretion is significantly altered in both T1D and T2D. In normal healthy adults, amylin levels rise after calorie intake and return to baseline by 2 h. In patients with T1D, the amylin rise after calorie intake is absent, similar to insulin, due to the destruction of the pancreatic β-cells.[3] Similar to the insulin response in T2D, amylin levels could be increased, normal, or reduced in patients with T2D, depending on the level of β-cell function. In patients with impaired glucose tolerance, amylin increases after calorie intake and remains above baseline 2 h later. Patients with T2D who require insulin therapy have a diminished amylin response to calorie intake.[2]

Amylin can play an additional role in the pathophysiology of T2D when the native type aggregates to form amyloid fibrils in the pancreas. These amylin deposits are thought to be cytotoxic and may contribute to pancreatic β-cell death in T2D.[2]

Amylin is insoluble and viscous and tends to aggregate; thus, it is not viable as an injectable medication. Pramlintide is a synthetic analog of amylin, differing from amylin by three amino acids. It was approved by the FDA in 2005 and is indicated for patients with T1D or T2D who use mealtime insulin and have failed to achieve desired glycemic control despite optimal insulin therapy.[4] Pramlintide was the first noninsulin agent approved for patients with T1D. Pramlintide is effective at lowering PPG levels and A1C and can be an attractive option for some patients, as it can also decrease weight and may allow for lower mealtime insulin doses. It is administered by subcutaneous injection immediately before meals.

MECHANISM OF ACTION

Pramlintide mimics the action of amylin and regulates glucose by three key mechanisms: reducing glucagon secretion, slowing gastric emptying, and increasing satiety.

In normal glucose homeostasis, glucagon is secreted from pancreatic α-cells to signal the liver to stimulate glycogenolysis and gluconeogenesis to ultimately increase glucose output from the liver. This counter-regulatory hormone response is to maintain normal glucose levels during fasting conditions or times of high energy consumption. In patients with diabetes, glucagon secretion occurs inappropriately after meals, ultimately leading to excessive hepatic glucose output postprandially. Pramlintide reduces the release of glucagon from the pancreas, and thus decreases this postprandial hepatic glucose output. Importantly, pramlintide does not appear to blunt the counter-regulatory glucagon response to hypoglycemia.[1,2]

Pramlintide signals the stomach to slow gastric emptying, which allows for more gradual absorption of glucose from the small intestine into the circulation and thereby reduces postprandial spikes in blood glucose levels. Slowing gastric emptying may also lead to a quicker feeling of fullness, which could decrease calorie intake and ultimately promote weight loss.[1,2]

Pramlintide also increases satiety by stimulating the satiety center of the brain. This effect may decrease PPG levels by decreasing the amount of carbohydrates and calories consumed in the meal. This reduction may ultimately promote weight loss, which may further improve glucose control.[1,2]

PHARMACOKINETICS

The bioavailability of pramlintide after a single subcutaneous injection is 30–40%. There is a linear dose-dependent increase in the maximum plasma concentration and overall exposure (AUC) of pramlintide after subcutaneous administration into the abdomen or thigh (Table 14.1).[4] In healthy individuals, the plasma half-life of pramlintide is approximately 48 min and maximum concentration occurs about 20 min after injection. Overall exposure to pramlintide is relatively constant with repeat dosing, indicating no accumulation.[4]

Injection into the arm in obese patients with T1D or T2D showed higher exposure and greater variability compared to injection into the abdomen or thigh. Bioavailability was not significantly different between obese and nonobese patients and was not impacted by skin thickness or injection needle size.[4]

The advantages of pramlintide in the treatment of diabetes include modest reductions in A1C and PPG levels in patients not able to achieve glucose control with insulin alone. In addition, pramlintide may allow for lower doses of insulin and has

Table 14.1—Pharmacokinetics of Pramlintide Following a Single Subcutaneous Dose (Product Information)

Dose (µg)	AUC (pmol*min/L)	C_{max} (pmol/L)	T_{max} (min)	Half-life (min)
30	3,750	39	21	55
60	6,778	79	20	49
90	8,507	102	19	51
120	11,970	147	21	48

more favorable effects on weight compared to continued insulin titration. Pramlintide may also result in less glucose variability.

The efficacy and safety of pramlintide in patients with T1D was evaluated in three large, randomized controlled trials (Table 14.2).[5-7] Reductions in A1C were significantly better in patients taking pramlintide compared to placebo, and mean body weight was decreased in patients taking pramlintide compared to placebo. These improvements were not accompanied by increased rates of severe hypoglycemia. However, in the study conducted by Whitehouse et al., the A1C lowering was more significant earlier in the study and waned over the 52 weeks. Changes in A1C from baseline with pramlintide versus placebo were –0.67% versus –0.16% at week 13, –0.58% versus –0.18% at week 26, and –0.39% versus –0.12% at week 52. The open-label extension of that study showed that patients who continued pramlintide maintained reductions in A1C from week 52 to week 104.[5] Similarly, in the study conducted by Ratner et al., the A1C lowering was most pronounced in the earlier weeks of the study and waned at the end of the study.[6] The study conducted by Edelman et al. specifically investigated whether increasing the pramlintide dose progressively with concomitant reduction in mealtime insulin would increase tolerability and reduce the risk of severe hypoglycemia. Both the pramlintide and placebo groups achieved similar A1C reductions and low rates of severe hypoglycemia, but pramlintide led to reductions in PPG and weight beyond that seen with insulin alone. The authors concluded that pramlintide dose escalation with simultaneous reduced mealtime insulin was effective during therapy initiation in T1D compared to placebo.[7]

Smaller studies have also demonstrated reductions in PPG in patients taking pramlintide.[8,9] Weyer et al. showed reductions in postprandial excursions by more than 100% versus placebo in patients taking regular insulin and by 75% versus placebo in patients taking insulin lispro. The optimal time of administration was immediately with the meal.[8] Hinshaw et al. also demonstrated significant reductions in PPG levels in patients with T1D and determined this effect was due to inhibition of glucagon and gastric emptying.[9]

In a post hoc analysis of the clinical studies in T1D, pramlintide was found to be safe and effective in patients specifically on insulin pump therapy. Pramlintide improved glycemic control while significantly reducing the patient's daily insulin dose and body weight. Thus, pramlintide can be a treatment option in patients on insulin pump therapy who are not achieving optimal glycemic control with insulin alone. Similar to patients on multiple daily injections, pramlintide would be an

Table 14.2—Efficacy and Safety of Pramlintide in Patients with T1D and T2D

Study	Patients and study duration	Treatment arms	A1C, change from baseline (%)	Weight, change from baseline (kg)	Insulin TDD, change from baseline (%)	Severe hypoglycemia (%)	Nausea (%)
T1D (added to premeal insulin)							
Whitehouse F, et al.	n = 480 52 weeks	30–60 µg t.i.d. Placebo	-0.39 -0.12	+0.5 +1.0	+2.3 +10.3	2.12, 0.74, 0.43* 2, 1.37, 1.24*	46.5 21.9
Ratner RE, et al.	n = 479 52 weeks	60 µg t.i.d. 60 µg q.i.d. Placebo	-0.29 -0.34 -0.04	-0.4 -0.4 +0.7	-3.0 -6.0 ±0.0	3.78, 1.13, 0.74* 3.41, 0.98, 0.79* 0.87, 0.80, 0.45*	47 47 12
Edelman S, et al.	n = 296 29 weeks	60 µg t.i.d. Placebo	-0.5 -0.5	-1.3 +1.2	-28.0 +4.0	0.57 0.30	63 36
T2D (added to premeal insulin)							
Ratner RE, et al.	n = 538 52 weeks	30 µg t.i.d. 75 µg t.i.d. 150 µg t.i.d. Placebo	-0.3 -0.5 -0.6 -0.2	-0.3 -0.4 -1.2 +1.0	+10.9 +7.9 NR +15.4	1.5 4.1 2.2 2.8	16.9 14.8 26.5 22.9
Hollander PA, et al.	n = 498 52 weeks	90 µg b.i.d. 120 µg b.i.d. Placebo	-0.35 -0.62 -0.22	-0.5 -1.4 +0.7	2.9 1.4 2.7	0.1 0.3 0.3	31 30 14
T2D (added to basal insulin)							
Riddle M, et al. 2007	n = 212 16 weeks	60–120 µg b.i.d./t.i.d. Placebo	-0.7 -0.36	-1.6 +0.7	+11.7 units +13.1 units	1 event 0	31 10
Riddle M, et al. 2009	n = 113 24 weeks	120 µg t.i.d. RAIA	-1.1 -1.3	+0.0 +4.7	+28 units +67 units	0 0	21 0

RAIA, rapid-acting insulin analog; TDD, total daily dose. * Reported for weeks 0–4, weeks 4–26, weeks 26–52, respectively.

appealing option for patients on insulin pump therapy with continued difficulty controlling PPG levels or body weight.[10]

Another post hoc analysis of clinical studies in T1D demonstrated that pramlintide was effective at lowering A1C regardless of diabetes duration at baseline. Longer disease duration appeared to augment the insulin sparing and weight loss seen with pramlintide. Therefore, pramlintide could be a therapeutic option at any point in the disease.[11]

The efficacy and safety of pramlintide in patients with T2D was evaluated in four large randomized controlled trials (Table 14.2).[12–15] Two of these studies evaluated pramlintide versus placebo in addition to background insulin therapy, which usually included mealtime insulin.[12,13] Both studies found that pramlintide in conjunction with insulin resulted in significant reductions in A1C that were sustained throughout the study. The improvements were achieved without increases in insulin dose or additional hypoglycemia risk. Modest weight loss was also achieved.[12,13] The other two studies evaluated pramlintide versus rapid-acting insulin added to basal insulin.[14,15] In this setting, pramlintide resulted in less hypoglycemia and lower total daily doses of insulin compared to the rapid-acting insulin group.[14,15] Despite these results, pramlintide does not have a specific FDA indication for use with basal insulin alone.

Disadvantages of pramlintide include the potential risk of hypoglycemia when added to insulin therapy and the need for insulin dose adjustments, close glucose monitoring, subsequent dose titrations, and routine follow-up to ensure the safety and efficacy of this combination. Other disadvantages include the subcutaneous injection requirement, increased total number of daily injections, inconvenience, nausea, and cost. Although pramlintide use requires up to three additional daily injections, in one study, pramlintide-treated patients reported greater treatment satisfaction than did patients in the placebo group despite similar reductions in A1C. This suggests that reductions in insulin dose and weight may be more meaningful to many patients than number of injections per day or overall A1C reductions.[16]

Another disadvantage is that the overall efficacy of pramlintide is small with mild reductions in PPG, A1C, and weight, which may not persist. Current treatment guidelines also do not classify pramlintide as a preferred agent for T2D because of its lower effectiveness compared to other agents, the limited clinical evidence, the benefit/risk ratio, and the cost.[17,18]

THERAPEUTIC CONSIDERATIONS

SIGNIFICANT WARNINGS/PRECAUTIONS

The prescribing information for pramlintide includes a black box warning for severe hypoglycemia. Pramlintide itself has a low risk of hypoglycemia. However, pramlintide is only indicated for use in conjunction with insulin, and this combination has been associated with an increased risk of hypoglycemia, particularly in patients with T1D. Hypoglycemia usually occurs within the first 2–3 h following injection. The manufacturer suggests that the hypoglycemia risk can be reduced by appropriate patient selection, patient education, frequent blood glucose monitoring, and an initial insulin dose reduction. The prescribing information recommends an initial insulin dose reduction of 50% when pramlintide is initiated.[4]

Pramlintide slows gastric emptying; therefore, it is contraindicated in patients who have confirmed gastroparesis. Pramlintide is also contraindicated in patients who have had a prior serious hypersensitivity reaction to pramlintide. The prescribing information also warns against mixing pramlintide with insulin due to the potential for altered pharmacokinetics and warns against the potential for drug interactions due to slowed gastric motility. Both of these are discussed in more detail in the "Drug Interactions" section.[4]

Appropriate patient selection is important to ensure the efficacy and safety of pramlintide. Before initiating pramlintide, the patient's A1C, glucose monitoring data, hypoglycemia history, current insulin regimen, and body weight should be reviewed. Pramlintide should be considered only in patients with T1D or T2D who are using mealtime insulin and have failed to achieve glycemic control despite individualized insulin management and are receiving consistent, ongoing diabetes care by a healthcare provider skilled in insulin management and supported by a diabetes educator. Pramlintide should not be used in the following patients:[2,4]

- Poor compliance with insulin regimen.
- Poor compliance with SMBG.
- A1C >9%.
- Recurrent severe hypoglycemia requiring assistance within the past 6 months.
- Hypoglycemia unawareness.
- Confirmed diagnosis of gastroparesis.
- Requiring the use of drugs that stimulate gastric motility.
- Pediatric patients.

SPECIAL POPULATIONS

Pregnancy and Lactation

Pramlintide is a pregnancy category C medication. Studies in pregnancy have not been conducted. Pramlintide has a low potential to cross the maternal/fetal placental barrier. Embryofetal studies in rats and rabbits show increases in congenital abnormalities (neural tube defect, cleft palate, exencephaly) with 10 and 47 times the exposure resulting from the human dose of 360 μg/day. Doses up to nine times the human dose of 360 μg/day given to pregnant rabbits had no effect on embryofetal development.[4]

It is unknown whether pramlintide is excreted in human milk, but there is a high likelihood that it is, based on its structure. Pramlintide should only be used in women who are breast-feeding if it is determined that the benefit outweighs the potential risk to the infant.[4]

Pediatrics

Pramlintide has shown promise in a few small studies in children and adolescents with T1D. PPG levels improved, and pramlintide demonstrated reasonable tolerability in these studies.[19,20] However, the safety and efficacy of pramlintide have not been established in large-scale, long-term studies in this patient population. Thus, pramlintide is not currently recommended in pediatric patients.

Geriatrics

Pramlintide has been studied in patients up to age 85 years. No consistent differences in efficacy and safety were observed in older patients. However, older patients may be more susceptible to hypoglycemia; therefore, caution should still be taken when using pramlintide in this population.[4] It may be appropriate to start with a lower dose and titrate the dose more slowly than for a younger adult. Because pramlintide is administered subcutaneously using an injection pen device, the clinician should ensure that the patient has adequate vision and dexterity to allow for correct self-administration.

Renal Insufficiency

Dose adjustments are not needed in patients with mild (CrCl 60–89 mL/min), moderate (CrCl 30–59 mL/min), or severe (CrCl 15–29 mL/min) renal insufficiency. Pramlintide has not been studied in patients with ESRD.[4]

Hepatic Insufficiency

Studies have not been conducted in patients with hepatic impairment. No changes would be expected, however, since pramlintide is almost exclusively eliminated through the kidneys.[4]

Sex, Race, Ethnicity

No consistent differences in efficacy and safety were observed between men and women in initial pramlintide clinical studies. Similarly, no consistent differences were observed among differing races or ethnicities included in the studies (Caucasian, black, Hispanic, and Asian populations), though smaller sample sizes for non-Caucasian subjects may limit this conclusion.[4]

ADVERSE EFFECTS AND MONITORING

Hypoglycemia

Although hypoglycemia is a concern with pramlintide used in conjunction with insulin, the rates of severe hypoglycemia in clinical studies are low (Table 14.2).

As discussed in the "Significant Warnings/Precautions" section, to minimize the risk of hypoglycemia, patients should be screened carefully to determine if pramlintide is appropriate. Patients must be willing and able to self-monitor their blood glucose, recognize signs and symptoms of hypoglycemia and adhere to patient instructions. The mealtime insulin dose should be reduced by 50% when initiating pramlintide. The dose can be titrated up if needed after a stable dose of pramlintide is reached. Patients should SMBG frequently and should be educated on the prevention, detection, and treatment of hypoglycemia.

Gastrointestinal Effects

The most common adverse effects of pramlintide in clinical trials were gastrointestinal in nature and included nausea, anorexia, vomiting, and abdominal pain. Nausea occurred in 14.8–63% of patients taking pramlintide compared to 10–36% of patients taking placebo (Table 14.2).[5–7,12–15] Nausea can be minimized by initiating pramlintide at a low dose and titrating the dose gradually. If nausea is a significant concern, pramlintide can be initiated with just one meal of the day and increased from there. Administering the first dose before the evening meal may allow patients to evaluate how well they tolerate pramlintide and better manage symptoms of nausea while they are at home.[21]

Injection Site Reactions

Injection site reactions have been reported by patients taking pramlintide. Patients should use proper technique when administering pramlintide and should rotate injection sites.[4]

Cardiovascular Safety

The cardiovascular safety of pramlintide was evaluated in a post hoc analysis of five randomized, controlled phase 3 and 4 trials. The incidence of major adverse cardiovascular outcomes was similar between pramlintide and comparator arms (4.7% vs. 4.5%; RR 1.034 [95% CI 0.694–1.540]). The authors concluded that pramlintide conferred no increased risk of cardiovascular adverse events in patients with diabetes using insulin.[22]

DRUG INTERACTIONS

Because the pH of pramlintide is 4.0 and the pH of most insulin products is 7.8, it is assumed that pramlintide is not compatible with insulin. However, studies evaluating the pharmacokinetic effects of mixing pramlintide with different insulins (regular, NPH, 70/30 premixed, and recombinant human) have produced variable results, with decreases up to 40% in maximum concentrations of pramlintide, increases up to 36% in pramlintide AUC, increases up to 15% in maximum concentrations of insulin, and increases up to 20% in insulin AUC. One randomized, controlled study in 51 patients with T1D did show that mixing pramlintide in the same syringe with regular insulin did not affect the pharmacokinetics or efficacy of either the insulin or pramlintide. Ultimately, mixing pramlintide and insulin in the same syringe is not recommended.[4,23]

Since pramlintide slows gastric emptying, it has the potential to impact the absorption of other medications administered concomitantly. Caution should be taken when oral medications are given concomitantly with pramlintide, particularly when a slower rate of absorption could be clinically meaningful. Other oral medications should be administered at least 1 h before or 2 h after administration of pramlintide, particularly if the onset of effect or threshold concentration is critical. Pramlintide may also impair the efficacy of agents that stimulate gastric motility.[4]

Table 14.3—Availability, Dosing, and Administration Requirements of Pramlintide

Availability, storage, preparation	Dosing	Missed-dose recommendations	Use in renal impairment
■ Multi-dose pen (1,000 μg/mL, 1.5 mL for 15-μg, 30-μg, 45-μg, and 60-μg doses or 1,000 μg/mL, 2.7 mL for 60-μg and 120-μg doses) ■ Pen needles not supplied ■ Keep refrigerated ■ After first use, store in refrigerator or at room temperature; bring to room temperature before injecting; discard 30 days after first use ■ No reconstitution needed	■ T1D: Start with 15 μg before major meals; increase in 15-μg increments to a maximum of 30–60 μg before major meals ■ T2D: Start with 60 μg before major meals; increase to 120 μg before meals, as tolerated ■ Upon initiation, reduce mealtime insulin by 50%; monitor glucose frequently and adjust insulin do,ses as needed ■ Wait at least 3 days between dose titrations to minimize nausea ■ Do not inject if you have hypoglycemia, do not plan to eat, plan to eat less than 250 calories or 30 g carbohydrates, or are sick and cannot eat usual meal	■ Skip the dose and resume next dose at the prescribed time	■ No dose adjustment recommended; has not been studied in patients with ESRD (CrCl <15 mL/min)

DOSAGE AND ADMINISTRATION

A summary of the dosage and administration recommendations for pramlintide are in Table 14.3. Different doses are recommended for T1D and T2D. However, in both groups, the dose of mealtime insulin should be initially reduced by 50% when pramlintide is initiated to avoid hypoglycemia. The dose of basal insulin does not usually need to be adjusted. The pramlintide dose is then titrated over time based on efficacy and tolerability. Once the maintenance dose of pramlintide is reached, mealtime insulin dose adjustments can be made according to standard clinical practice based on glucose profile data.[2,4]

The recommended starting dose for patients with T1D is 15 μg given with each major meal (at least 250 calories or 30 g carbohydrates). If the patient is tolerating the medication without significant nausea after 3–7 days, the dose can be increased by 15-μg increments to a maximum dose of 30–60 μg before major meals. For patients with T2D, the recommended starting dose is 60 μg before major meals. This can be increased to 120 μg as tolerated after 3–7 days. If a meal has fewer than 250 calories or 30 g carbohydrates, or if the patient does not plan to eat or has hypoglycemia, then the pramlintide dose should be skipped. The dose of pramlintide should be taken immediately prior to major meals.[4]

Pramlintide is available in two different pen devices: one with a maximum dose of 60 μg, primarily indicated for T1D, and one with a maximum dose of 120 μg, primarily indicated for T2D. Pramlintide should be injected into either the abdomen or the thigh. It is not recommended for injection into the arm due to inconsistent absorption from that site. Pramlintide and insulin should not be injected into the same site. Patients should be instructed to inject pramlintide into a site at least 2 inches away from the site of insulin injection. The pen device that is actively being used can be stored at room temperature or in the refrigerator for up to 30 days. If stored in the refrigerator, it should be brought up to room temperature before injecting. Additional pens should be stored in the refrigerator.[4]

MONOGRAPHS

Pramlintide: https://dailymed.nlm.nih.gov/dailymed/drugInfo.cfm?setid=4aea30ff-eb0d-45c1-b114-3127966328ff

REFERENCES

1. Ryan GJ, Jobe LJ, Martin R. Pramlintide in the treatment of type 1 and type 2 diabetes mellitus. *Clin Ther* 2005;27(10):1500–1512

2. Hieronymus L, Griffin S. Role of amylin in type 1 and type 2 diabetes. *Diabetes Educ* 2015;41(Suppl. 1):47S–56S

3. Koda JE, Fineman M, Rink TJ, et al. Amylin concentrations and glucose control. *Lancet* 1992;339:1179–1180

4. Symlin (pramlintide acetate injection) [product information]. Wilmington, DE, AstraZeneca Pharmaceuticals LP, June 2014

5. Whitehouse F, Kruger DF, Fineman M, et al. A randomized study and open-label extension evaluating the long-term efficacy of pramlintide as an adjunct to insulin therapy in type 1 diabetes. *Diabetes Care* 2002;25:724–730

6. Ratner RE, Dickey R, Fineman M, et al. Amylin replacement with pramlintide as an adjunct to insulin therapy improves long-term glycemic and weight control in type 1 diabetes mellitus: a 1-year, randomized controlled trial. *Diabet Med* 2004;21:1204–1212

7. Edelman S, Garg S, Frias J, et al. A double-blind, placebo-controlled trial assessing pramlintide treatment in the setting of intensive insulin therapy in type 1 diabetes. *Diabetes Care* 2006;29:2189–2195

8. Weyer C, Gottlieb A, Kim DD, et al. Pramlintide reduces postprandial glucose excursions when added to regular insulin or insulin lispro in subjects with type 1 diabetes: a dose-timing study. *Diabetes Care* 2003;26:3074–3079

9. Hinshaw L, Schiavon M, Dadlani V, et al. Effect of pramlintide on postprandial glucose fluxes in type 1 diabetes. *J Clin Endocrinol Metab* 2016;101(5):1954–1962

10. Herrmann K, Frias JP, Edelman SV, et al. Pramlintide improved measures of glycemic control and body weight in patients with type 1 diabetes mellitus undergoing continuous subcutaneous insulin infusion therapy. *Postgrad Med* 2013;125(3):136–144

11. Herrmann K, Brunell SC, Li Y, et al. Impact of disease duration on the effects of pramlintide in type 1 diabetes: a post hoc analysis of three clinical trials. *Adv Ther* 2016;33:848–861

12. Ratner RE, Want LL, Fineman MS, et al. Adjunctive therapy with the amylin analogue pramlintide leads to a combined improvement in glycemic and weight control in insulin-treated subjects with type 2 diabetes. *Diabetes Technol Ther* 2002;4:51–61

13. Hollander PA, Levy P, Fineman MS, et al. Pramlintide as an adjunct to insulin therapy improves long-term glycemic and weight control in patients with type 2 diabetes: a 1-year randomized controlled trial. *Diabetes Care* 2003;26:784–790

14. Riddle M, Frias J, Zhang B, et al. Pramlintide improved glycemic control and reduced weight in patients with type 2 diabetes using basal insulin. *Diabetes Care* 2007;30:2794–2799

15. Riddle M, Pencek R, Charenkavanich S, et al. Randomized comparison of pramlintide or mealtime insulin added to basal insulin treatment for patients with type 2 diabetes. *Diabetes Care* 2009;32:1577–1582

16. Marrero DG, Crean J, Zhang B, et al. Effect of adjunctive pramlintide treatment on treatment satisfaction in patients with type 1 diabetes. *Diabetes Care* 2007;30(2):210–216

17. American Diabetes Association. 8. Pharmacologic approaches to glycemic treatment: *Standards of Medical Care in Diabetes—2018. Diabetes Care* 2018;41(Suppl. 1):S73–S85

18. Garber AJ, Abrahamson MJ, Barzilay JI, et al. Consensus statement by the American Association of Clinical Endocrinologists and American College of Endocrinology on the comprehensive type 2 diabetes management algorithm. *Endocr Pract* 2018;24(1):91–120

19. Chase HP, Lutz K, Pencek R, et al. Pramlintide lowered glucose excursions and was well-tolerated in adolescents with type 1 diabetes: results from a randomized, single-blind, placebo-controlled, crossover study. *J Pediatr* 2009;155:369–373

20. Hassan K, Heptulla RA. Reducing postprandial hyperglycemia with adjuvant premeal pramlintide and postmeal insulin in children with type 1 diabetes mellitus. *Pediatr Diabetes* 2009;10:264–268

21. Alrefai HA, Latif KA, Hieronymus LB, et al. Pramlintide: clinical strategies for success. *Diabetes Spectr* 2010;23:124–130

22. Herrmann K, Zhou M, Wang A, de Bruin TWA. Cardiovascular safety assessment of pramlintide in type 2 diabetes: results from a pooled analysis of five clinical trials. *Clin Diabetes Endocrinol* 2016;2(12):1–8

23. Weyer C, Fineman M, Strobel S, et al. Properties of pramlintide and insulin upon mixing. *Am J Health Syst Pharm* 2005;62:816–822

Chapter 15
Bile Acid Sequestrants

CHRISTINA R. BUCHMAN, PHARMD, BCACP

INTRODUCTION

Bile acid sequestrants (BAS), also known as bile acid resins, were initially approved in 1973 to treat hyperlipidemia—more specifically, to reduce LDL-C levels.[1] BAS are most frequently used in combination with statins for hyperlipidemia (although their use is declining) and have been associated with modest decreases in A1C in patients with T2D as monotherapy or in combination with other antidiabetic agents.[2-4] There are three FDA-approved BAS in use in the U.S.[1] Of these, the first-generation agents include cholestyramine and colestipol, while the only second-generation agent is colesevelam.[1] There is another second-generation BAS, colestimide, that is available only in Japan and has a similar safety and efficacy profile to colesevelam.[4] Colesevelam is the only BAS that has received FDA approval to treat T2D, but is not indicated for T1D.[1] Although colesevelam is the only FDA-approved agent for patients with T2D, all agents in the class have been shown in studies to decrease FPG and A1C.[5] BAS decreased A1C by 0.5–1% in clinical studies and can be used safely in conjunction with other antidiabetic agents.[4,6] In patients with elevated LDL-C who have not been able to reach target A1C levels, adding a BAS may be a valuable option in helping patients reach their goals and possibly in reducing micro- and macrovascular complications of T2D and hypercholesterolemia.

PHARMACOLOGY

The studies that showed treatment with BAS reduced LDL and cardiovascular risk also showed a reduction in FPG and A1C in patients with T2D.[4,5] This improvement led to further studies in patients with T2D and the eventual FDA approval of colesevelam to treat T2D. Studies have demonstrated an average decrease in A1C of 0.5% with a range of 0.4–1%, depending on the agent taken.[4,5] Among the BAS that are approved in the U.S., colesevelam produces the most marked decrease in FPG and A1C due to its higher affinity for binding bile acids.[5]

MECHANISM OF ACTION

BAS are highly polarized large molecules that tightly bind bile acids to form a nonabsorbable complex that is then excreted in the feces.[7-10] As a response to the increased excretion of bile acids, the body compensates by increasing the synthesis of new bile acids and consumption of LDL-C. The exact mechanism of lowering blood glucose is not completely understood, but it is thought to be multifactorial and surprisingly complex.[7-10]

Historically, it has been hypothesized that BAS administration decreases glucose and carbohydrate absorption, but this proposed mechanism has since been disproven in several studies.[9] Instead of this classical model of blocked absorption, current evidence suggests a much more complex, hormone-related mechanism that involves multiple receptors and organs.[9]

Bile acids are known to be independent signaling molecules that activate farnesoid X receptors (FXR) and a transmembrane G-protein coupled receptor (TGR5).[7-10] FXR is located in the gastrointestinal tract and liver and is involved in the feedback loop of bile acid synthesis. When bile acids interact with FXR, they act as the "brakes" by inhibiting further synthesis of bile acids. Essentially, the body uses FXR to sense existing bile acid levels, and when levels are high, there is no need for further production. When bile acids are bound to BAS, they can no longer interact with FXR, and this leads to the body continuing to synthesize bile acids, leading to changes in the bile acid pool and alterations in bile acid composition. TGR5 is widely expressed in the gastrointestinal tract, liver, pancreas, and gallbladder, and activation of TGR5 leads to increases in cyclic adenosine monophosphate (cAMP), activation of protein kinase A, and many subsequent downstream effects. TGR5 activation is involved in incretin hormone secretion via GLP-1 secretion, leading to decreases in plasma glucose and A1C. Interestingly, unlike with FXR, bile acids continue to interact and activate TGR5 even while bound to BAS, leading to increases in GLP-1 and subsequent decreases in plasma glucose. In conclusion, the lack of FXR activation and the preserved activation of TGR5 (and the related increase of GLP-1 activity) are key to the lowering of plasma glucose and A1C that is observed in studies of patients treated with BAS.[7-10]

PHARMACOKINETICS/PHARMACODYNAMICS

BAS are hydrophilic polymers that are not hydrolyzed by digestive enzymes and are largely not absorbed from the gastrointestinal tract.[11,12] Since BAS are primarily unabsorbed, the distribution is limited to the gastrointestinal tract. BAS are not metabolized systemically and do not interfere with any metabolizing enzymes or CYPs. Excretion is primarily in the feces. Cholestyramine is 100% excreted in the feces. Approximately 0.05% of the doses of colesevelam and colestipol are excreted renally, while the remainder is excreted in the feces. Onset of action in the gastrointestinal tract is immediate for bile acid sequestration, but it takes 4–6 weeks to see initial changes in A1C and 12–18 weeks for maximal effect.[11,12]

TREATMENT ADVANTAGES/DISADVANTAGES

Per the American Diabetes Association *Standards of Medical Care in Diabetes*, BAS are not recommended as a standard part of therapy but may be tried in patients resistant to other treatments or in whom there are other indications for BAS therapy.[2] Per the AACE/American College of Endocrinology (ACE) guidelines, BAS are an acceptable add-on therapy, but BAS are the sixth class of agents in order of preference, falling just ahead of bromocriptine, α-glucosidase inhibitors, and sulfonylureas.[13]

BAS only have modest efficacy on FPG and A1C. In recent meta-analyses, the average decrease in FPG was found to be between 19.3 and 37.8 mg/dL.[4,2] The average decrease in A1C was found to be between 0.55 and 0.83% with a range of 0.3–1.4%. BAS are associated with an LDL decrease of 15–25% and moderate increases in triglycerides.[14] The combination of effects on LDL and A1C make the use of BAS appealing in patients with comorbid T2D and hyperlipidemia not achieving their goals on standard therapies.

BAS have been used safely with many different oral antidiabetic agents and insulin, as well as monotherapy in diabetes. In the initial study that discovered the A1C-lowering effects of cholestyramine, the patients were stable on either glyburide or insulin therapy with no instances of drug interactions or hypoglycemia noted.[14] In studies, colesevelam was used as an add-on therapy with sulfonylureas, TZDs, metformin, and insulin, with only rare, mild cases of hypoglycemia noted.[15-19] BAS are not recommended in the treatment of prediabetes or as monotherapy for the treatment of T2D due to the modest effects and the presence of better alternative therapies.[2]

BAS should not be used in the treatment of T1D or DKA.[20] They were not studied in this population. If a patient with T1D has comorbid hyperlipidemia that is not responding to statin therapy, the use of BAS is not contraindicated and can be recommended.[20-22] BAS may theoretically affect FPG and A1C in patients with T1D due to the potential effects of GLP-1 action, but further research is needed to determine if this conceptual benefit holds true.

Both T2D and hyperlipidemia are independent risk factors for cardiovascular events, but the use of BAS has not consistently been shown to decrease this risk.[23-25] However, there are several studies and models that propose there are cardiovascular benefits when BAS are used in patients with comorbid diabetes and hyperlipidemia.[23-25] Although it is assumed that BAS may contribute to decreased cardiovascular risk, further studies are needed to verify this assumption.

The major barriers to the consistent use of BAS in standard practice are the undesirably large tablets or taste of the suspensions, dosing frequency, and the side effects and possible drug interactions.[20-22] The tablets of colesevelam are rather large and have been associated with dysphagia; when combined with the number of tablets needed to reach a therapeutic dose, this is a significant barrier to patient adherence.[20] The other BAS are all powder formulations for suspension; for cholestyramine and colestipol, several packets/scoops are needed for a therapeutic dose, leading to patient nonadherence.[21,22] The primary side effects of gastrointestinal disturbances, although generally mild, may inhibit some patients from wanting to take BAS.[20-22] The last barrier is the large list of drug interactions seen with BAS, which may limit the patient population able to take them.[20-22]

In general, BAS are a useful drug class to have in the tool chest of T2D oral antidiabetic agents, and they are especially important for patients with comorbid hyperlipidemia.

THERAPEUTIC CONSIDERATIONS

SIGNIFICANT WARNINGS/PRECAUTIONS

Decreased Absorption of Fat-Soluble Vitamins

BAS have been shown to cause decreased absorption of fat-soluble vitamins A, D, E, and K.[20-22] To avoid this interaction, patients should take any supplements at least 4 h prior to or after BAS administration and, when reasonable, the longest dosing gap possible is recommended. Caution should be used when treating any patient susceptible to deficiencies or changes in vitamin K absorption (e.g., patient taking warfarin or with malabsorption syndromes). Chronic use of BAS may be associated with an increased risk of bleeding due to hyper-prothrombinemia from vitamin K deficiency, which is typically corrected by intravenous administration of vitamin K and further oral supplementation with vitamin K.[20-22]

Serum Triglycerides

BAS are contraindicated in patients with serum triglyceride concentrations greater than 500 mg/dL, and caution should be used for any patient with triglyceride concentrations greater than 300 mg/dL.[20-22] BAS are associated with elevations in serum triglycerides, with the average elevation observed to be 5%, but larger elevations have been observed when added to other antidiabetic agents (up to 20%).[20-22] This elevation is of greater concern in patients with preexisting high triglycerides and patients with a history of familial hypertriglyceridemia. Serum triglycerides above 500 mg/dL are associated with increased risk of pancreatitis, and levels over 1,000 mg/dL have a 5% risk of pancreatitis.[26] Lipid levels, including triglycerides, LDL, and non-HDL, should be obtained prior to initiating therapy with a BAS, at 3 months after initiation, and then at 6-month intervals thereafter to monitor triglyceride levels. If a patient experiences pancreatitis or serum triglyceride levels exceeding 400 mg/dL, the BAS should be promptly discontinued.[3,20-22]

Gastrointestinal Disorders

BAS can cause gastrointestinal problems, including constipation, so patients with preexisting gastroparesis or motility disorders or a history of gastrointestinal tract surgery may be at risk of bowel obstruction.[20-22] All patients should be instructed to take their BAS with food and plenty of fluid to alleviate the risk of constipation. If a patient reports constipation, treatment with a stool softener may be indicated. In patients with preexisting constipation, the starting dose should be reduced and, if tolerated, the dose may be titrated to the maximum tolerated dose or until constipation is exacerbated. BAS-associated constipation may aggravate preexisting hemorrhoids. Constipation should be avoided in patients with symptomatic coronary artery disease due to the risk of straining with hard stool. These patients will need to be monitored closely and treatment modified if constipation occurs during BAS treatment.[20-22]

Dysphagia

Colesevelam tablets are rather large and should be used with caution in patients with preexisting dysphagia or patients with swallowing disorders, due to risk of new or worsening dysphagia and esophageal obstruction.[20–22]

Phenylketonurics

All marketed BAS contain phenylalanine and so are contraindicated in patients with phenylketonuria.[20–22]

Hypothyroidism

There is a theoretical risk of developing hypothyroidism when taking BAS for patients with a limited thyroid reserve.[12] BAS, specifically cholestyramine and colestipol, have been used off-label for adjunctive treatment of Graves' disease and hyperthyroidism.[12]

SPECIAL POPULATIONS

Pregnancy

BAS as a class are pregnancy category B or C drugs and should be relatively safe since they are not absorbed from the gastrointestinal tract.[20–22] However, because BAS interfere with absorption of fat-soluble vitamins, they should be used with caution in pregnant women.[27] Briggs's *Drugs in Pregnancy and Lactation* rates BAS as *potentially toxic*.[27] This is due to a case report of a vitamin K deficiency-induced hemorrhage in a mother and fetus attributed to use of cholestyramine in pregnancy.[27] If BAS treatment is continued during pregnancy, it is recommended to take all fat-soluble vitamins, including vitamin-K containing supplements, at least 4 h before BAS administration.[27]

Lactation

There are not reports describing the use of BAS in lactation, but as they are not absorbed from the gastrointestinal tract, BAS are classified as *probably compatible*.[20–22,26] Since BAS interfere with the absorption of fat-soluble vitamins, milk produced by women taking BAS may be deficient in these vitamins and supplementation of the woman and infant may be necessary.[20–22,27]

Pediatrics

BAS are not approved to treat diabetes in children and have not been studied in this population.[20–22] However, BAS are used to treat heterozygous familial hypercholesterolemia in children ≥10 years at typical adult dosing and show equivalent safety and efficacy to adult use. Of note, due to the large tablet sizes of colesevelam, it is recommended that children receive the oral suspension or powder formulations of BAS.[20–22]

Geriatrics

In studies, only a small percentage of patients enrolled were over 65 years and very few were over 75 years; among patients that were enrolled, no differences in safety of efficacy were observed between geriatric and younger patients.[20-22] Due to the small sample sizes, greater sensitivity to adverse effects in some individuals cannot be ruled out.[20-22]

Hepatic Impairment

No dosage adjustments are needed as BAS are not absorbed from the gastrointestinal tract.[20-22]

Renal Impairment

No dosage adjustments are needed as BAS are not absorbed from the gastrointestinal tract.[20-22]

PHARMACOGENOMICS

There are no clinically significant pharmacogenomic polymorphisms that lead to altered dosing.[12]

ADVERSE EFFECTS AND MONITORING

BAS are generally well tolerated, and most side effects are mild and subside with continued use or a decrease in dose.[20-22] The most common adverse effect associated with BAS use is constipation, reported by 6–11% of patients. Constipation associated with BAS is typically mild, transient, and easily controlled with a standard regimen of increased fluid and fiber intake and, if necessary, by adding a stool softener. In some patients, the constipation can be severe and lead to fecal impaction or bowel obstruction. Therefore, patients with a history of bowel obstruction or gastrointestinal tract surgery should be treated very cautiously with BAS, and the benefits may not outweigh the risks. For patients with preexisting constipation due to other medical conditions, the use of BAS should be weighed to determine whether the benefits of treatment outweigh the risks. If treatment is initiated, the dose should be decreased and then titrated slowly with frequent monitoring for increased constipation. If constipation presents and does not resolve with increased fluid and fiber, the patient may need to have the dose decreased or to discontinue therapy.

Most of the other frequently reported adverse effects are related to the gastrointestinal tract and include dyspepsia, abdominal discomfort, bloating, flatulence, nausea, and vomiting. These are also generally mild and resolve with continued use or with a decrease in dose.

Rare but serious adverse effects include hypersensitivity reactions (primarily rash and urticaria), cholecystitis, cholelithiasis, and pancreatitis. These effects were noted in less than 2% of patients taking BAS and resolved after discontinuing the BAS.

Patients using BAS should receive the typical monitoring of their diabetes and should be instructed to self-monitor their blood glucose. Other suggested monitoring includes regular (every 3–6 months) monitoring of serum triglycerides and other lipid markers. Patients should also self-monitor for signs and symptoms of pancreatitis (severe abdominal pain with or without nausea and vomiting). Patients with a history of hyper- or hypothyroidism should have their thyroid function monitored before starting BAS treatment and then every 6 months afterward.

BAS have also been associated with transient changes to liver function enzymes (aspartate transaminase [AST], ALT, and alkaline phosphatase), but routine monitoring is not recommended.[20-22]

DRUG INTERACTIONS

BAS are positively charged anion resins that have the potential to bind to any negatively charged oral drug molecules that are coadministered.[20-22] Since there is a potential for many drugs to interact with BAS, the manufacturers recommend administering any drug with a narrow therapeutic window at least 4 h prior to or after BAS administration, and if the coadministered medication has a high risk profile, monitoring therapeutic drug levels is recommended.

Table 15.1 — Drug Interactions

Drug/class	Degree of interaction	Interaction type
Cyclosporine	Major	Decreased cyclosporine levels
Deferasirox	Major	Decreased deferasirox levels and corresponding increase in iron levels
Digoxin	Major	Decreased digoxin levels
Mycophenolate	Major	Decreased mycophenolate levels
Pravastatin	Major	Decreased pravastatin levels
Amiodarone	Moderate	Decreased amiodarone levels
Antibiotics (metronidazole, penicillin, cephalexin, tetracycline, etc.)	Moderate	Decreased absorption and decreased efficacy
Oral Contraceptives	Moderate	Decreased contraception efficacy
Diltiazem	Moderate	Decreased diltiazem levels
Levothyroxine	Moderate	Decreased levothyroxine levels and decreased efficacy; may also elevate thyroid-stimulating hormone (TSH) levels
NSAIDs (meloxicam and diclofenac)	Moderate	Decreased efficacy
Phenytoin	Moderate	Decreased phenytoin levels
Propranolol	Moderate	Decreased propranolol levels and decreased efficacy
Sulfonylureas	Moderate	Decreased sulfonylurea levels
Valproic Acid	Moderate	Decreased serum valproic acid levels
Warfarin	Moderate	Variable/reduced INR levels due to changes in vitamin K absorption

INR, international normalized ratios. *Source*: Micromedex.[10]

DOSAGE AND ADMINISTRATION

The recommended dose of BAS varies by agent, but the dosing required to show benefit in diabetes appears to be the same as the dosing recommended to treat hyperlipidemia.[4,6] Since the primary adverse effect that limits treatment for all agents in the class is constipation, titration of dosing is generally slow, and many patients never reach the maximum dosing for any of the agents.[20-22] All agents need to be taken with food to minimize gastrointestinal upset and should be taken with plenty of fluids to prevent constipation. The powder formulations of BAS need to be mixed with 2–6 ounces of noncarbonated fluid or applesauce and consumed completely.[20-22]

Table 15.2—Doses and Dose Adjustments

Generic (brand)	Form/strength	Dosage
Colesevelam (Welchol)	Oral: 625-mg tablet and 3.75-g powder packet for suspension	▪ Once-daily dosing: 3.75 g (6 tablets or 1 packet for suspension); twice-daily dosing: 1.875 g (3 tablets).
Cholestyramine (Questran)	Oral: 4 g powder for suspension (packets and loose powder)	▪ Initial: 4 g once or twice daily. Titrate: may increase dose every month to effective or max tolerated dose; maximum dose of 24 g/day.
Colestipol (Colestid)	Oral: 1-g tablets and 5 g powder for suspension (packets and loose granules)	▪ Initial (tablets): 2 g (2 tablets) once or twice daily. Titrate: may increase dose every month to effective or max tolerated dose; maximum dose of 16 g/day. ▪ Initial (granules): 5 g once or twice daily. Titrate: may increase dose every month to effective or max tolerated dose; maximum dose of 30 g/day.

MONOGRAPHS

Cholestyramine (Questran): https://dailymed.nlm.nih.gov/dailymed/drugInfo.cfm?setid=362ddd91-a63f-4ec6-841a-75785dd208c8

Colestipol (Colestid): https://dailymed.nlm.nih.gov/dailymed/drugInfo.cfm?setid=21b37725-fc0c-4365-a7dc-1a473d42502d

Colesevelam (Welchol): https://dailymed.nlm.nih.gov/dailymed/drugInfo.cfm?setid=fc274f83-4cd6-47bd-b43e-53a0bf345f11

REFERENCES

1. Drugs@FDA. U.S. Food & Drug Administration website. Available from https://www.accessdata.fda.gov/scripts/cder/daf/index.cfm. Accessed 31 May 2018

2. American Diabetes Association. 8. Pharmacologic approaches to glycemic treatment: *Standards of Medical Care in Diabetes—2018. Diabetes Care* 2018;41(Suppl. 1):S73–S85

3. Stone NJ, Robinson JG, Lichtenstein AH, et al. 2013 ACC/AHA Guideline on the treatment of blood cholesterol to reduce atherosclerotic cardiovascular risk in adults. *J Am Coll Cardiol* 2013;63(25PartB):2889–2934

4. Hansen M, Sonne DP, Mikkelsen KH, et al. Bile acid sequestrants for glycemic control in patients with type 2 diabetes: a systematic review with meta-analysis of randomized controlled trials. *J Diabetes Complications* 2017;31(5):918–927

5. Mazidi M, Rezaie P, Karimi E, Kengne AP. The effects of bile acid sequestrants on lipid profile and blood glucose concentrations: a systematic review and meta-analysis of randomized controlled trials. *Int J Cardiol* 2017;15(227):850–857

6. Bays HE, Goldberg RB, Truitt KE, Jones MR. Colesevelam hydrochloride therapy in patients with type 2 diabetes mellitus treated with metformin: glucose and lipid effects. *Arch Intern Med.* 2008;168(18):1975–1983

7. Hansen M, Sonne DP, Knop FK. Bile acid sequestrants: glucose-lowering mechanisms and efficacy in type 2 diabetes. *Curr Diab Rep* 2014;14(5):482

8. Chávez-Talavera O, Tailleux A, Lefebvre P, Staels B. Bile acid control of metabolism and inflammation in obesity, type 2 diabetes, dyslipidemia, and nonalcoholic fatty liver disease. *Gastroenterology* 2017;152(7):1679–1694

9. Sonne DP, Hansen M, Knop FK. Bile acid sequestrants in type 2 diabetes: potential effects on GLP1 secretion. *Eur J Endocrinol* 2014;171(2):R47–65

10. Kårhus ML, Brønden A, Sonne DP, et al. Evidence connecting old, new and neglected glucose-lowering drugs to bile acid-induced GLP-1 secretion: a review. *Diabetes Obes Metab* 2017;19(9):1214–1222

11. Micromedex Healthcare Series. Colesevelam. Greenwood Village, CO, Truven Health Analytics, 2018. Available from www.micromedexsolutions.com. Accessed 16 May 2018

12. Lexicomp Online, Lexi-Drugs Online. Hudson, OH, Lexi-Comp, Inc., 2018. Accessed 16 May 2018.

13. Garber AJ, Abrahamson MJ, Barzilay JI, et al. Consensus statement by the American Association of Clinical Endocrinologists and American College of Endocrinology on the comprehensive type 2 diabetes management algorithm—2018 executive summary. *Endocr Pract* 2018;24(1):91–120

14. Jellinger PS, Handelsman Y, Rosenblit PD, et al. American Association of Clinical Endocrinologists and American College of Endocrinology guidelines for management of dyslipidemia and prevention of cardiovascular disease. *Endocr Pract* 2017;23(Suppl. 2):1–87

15. Garg A, Grundy SM. Cholestyramine therapy for dyslipidemia in non-insulin-dependent diabetes mellitus: a short-term, double-blind, crossover trial. *Ann Intern Med* 1994;121:416–422

16. Zema MJ. Colesevelam hydrochloride: evidence for its use in the treatment of hypercholesterolemia and type 2 diabetes mellitus with insights into mechanism of action. *Core Evid* 2012;7:61–75

17. Ooi CP, Loke SC. Colesevelam for type 2 diabetes mellitus: an abridged Cochrane review. *Diabet Med* 2014;31(1):2–14

18. Brunetti L, Hermes-Desantis ER. The role of colesevelam hydrochloride in hypercholesterolemia and type 2 diabetes mellitus. *Ann Pharmacother* 2010;44(7–8):1196–1206

19. Fonseca VA, Rosenstock J, Wang AC, et al. Colesevelam HCl improves glycemic control and reduces LDL cholesterol in patients with inadequately controlled type 2 diabetes on sulfonylurea-based therapy. *Diabetes Care* 2008;31(8):1479–1484

20. Welchol [package insert]. Basking Ridge, NJ, Daiichi Sankyo, Inc., July 2017

21. Colestid [package insert]. New York, Pfizer, May 2018

22. Questran [package insert]. Spring Valley, NY, Par Pharmaceutical Co., October 2017

23. Ganda OP. The role of bile acid sequestrants in the management of type 2 diabetes mellitus. *Metab Syndr Relat Disord* 2010;8(Suppl. 1):S15–S21

24. Ross S, D'Mello M, Anand SS, et al. Effect of bile acid sequestrants on the risk of cardiovascular events: a mendelian randomization analysis. *Circ Cardiovasc Genet* 2015;8(4):618–627

25. Spinelli V, Chávez-Talavera O, Tailleux A, Staels B. Metabolic effects of bile acid sequestration: impact on cardiovascular risk factors. *Curr Opin Endocrinol Diabetes Obes* 2016;23(2):138–144

26. Scherer J, Singh VP, Pitchumoni CS, Yadav D. Issues in hypertriglyceridemic pancreatitis: an update. *J Clin Gastroenterol* 2014;48(3):195–203

27. Briggs GG, Freeman RK, Yaffe SJ. *Drugs in Pregnancy and Lactation: A Reference Guide to Fetal and Neonatal Risk*, 11th ed. Philadelphia, Lippincott Williams & Wilkins, 2017

Chapter 16
Dopamine-2 Receptor Agonists

CHRISTINA R. BUCHMAN, PHARMD, BCACP

B romocriptine is the only dopamine agonist that is approved for treatment of diabetes.[1] Other dopamine agonists include cabergoline, ropinirole, and pramipexole, but their usefulness in diabetes has not been demonstrated. Bromocriptine quick release (QR) was first approved for T2D on 5 May 2009 under the brand name Cycloset.[1] Bromocriptine is not a new drug, and has in fact been used since the late 1970s in the treatment of Parkinson's disease, hyperprolactinemia, and acromegaly. Patients with Parkinson's disease and comorbid diabetes treated with bromocriptine showed decreases in plasma glucose and A1C.[2] This prompted research looking into bromocriptine for diabetes. The new formulation of bromocriptine that was developed and approved for the treatment of diabetes is designed to rapidly release and be absorbed to quickly achieve elevated plasma levels.[3] The absorption timing of this quick-release formulation turns out to be vital for the treatment of diabetes as it is thought that low endogenous levels of dopamine upon waking contribute to insulin resistance.[4,5] Bromocriptine is not indicated for T1D or DKA.[3]

MECHANISM OF ACTION

Bromocriptine is a semisynthetic ergot alkaloid derivative and is classified as a sympatholytic, semiselective dopamine-2 (D2) receptor agonist, but its mechanism in diabetes is not thoroughly understood.

Dopamine is an endogenous neurotransmitter that performs many actions in the body and targets many different receptors that potentially play a role in diabetes.[4-7] Dopamine interacts primarily with dopamine receptors, but also with serotonin receptors related to the control of appetite and glucose tolerance. Dopamine's primary actions include control of many physiologic processes, such as motivation, appetite, weight gain, circadian rhythms, and insulin sensitization. These actions are primarily mediated by the D2 receptor pathway, which is the main target of bromocriptine. The majority of D2 receptors involved in processes important for diabetes are in the hypothalamus; these receptors control circadian rhythms and contribute to insulin resistance and dyslipidemia. Persons diagnosed with T2D have been shown to have lower-than-normal hypothalamic dopamine levels upon waking. Low dopamine levels are associated with glucose intolerance, dyslipidemia, increased hepatic gluconeogenesis, and increased risk of CVD.[4-7]

Administration of bromocriptine within 2 h of waking is thought to reset the sympathetic system in the CNS by increasing morning dopamine levels to a point that is similar to the levels in nondiabetic persons.[3,5,6] In studies, the administration of bromocriptine has been associated with decreased fasting and postprandial blood glucose levels without increasing plasma insulin levels. This resulted in modest decreases in A1C (0.6–0.7%). Bromocriptine also decreases plasma free fatty acids and triglycerides. Studies also show that bromocriptine is associated with a decreased risk of cardiovascular events, though the mechanism is unknown.[3,5,6]

PHARMACOKINETICS

Approximately 65–95% of bromocriptine-QR is absorbed, but it undergoes extensive first-pass metabolism, and only 5–10% of the dose reaches the target tissues.[2,5,6] Time to peak concentration is approximately 45–60 min when fasting. Bioavailability is increased by 55–65% and the time to peak concentration is delayed with the intake of food. This pharmacokinetic profile is unique to the QR formulation, and the two formulations are not interchangeable.[2,5,6]

Bromocriptine is highly protein bound with a volume of distribution of 61 L.[2,5,6] It undergoes extensive metabolism in the gastrointestinal tract; CYP3A4 is the primary metabolism pathway through the liver. The metabolites are all inactive and primarily excreted in the bile and feces, with only 2–6% excreted in the urine. The half-life of bromocriptine is approximately 6 h.[2,5,6]

TREATMENT ADVANTAGES/DISADVANTAGES

Per the American Diabetes Association *Standards of Medical Care in Diabetes—2018*, bromocriptine is not recommended as a standard part of therapy in T2D, but may be tried in patients resistant to other treatments or in whom there are other indications for its use.[8] Per the AACE/ACE guidelines, it is an acceptable add-on therapy, but it is the seventh agent in the list in order of preference, falling just behind BAS but ahead of α-glucosidase inhibitors and sulfonylureas.[9]

Bromocriptine should not be used in the treatment of T1D or DKA.[3] It has been studied as monotherapy for the treatment of T2D, showing small decreases in A1C of 0.4–0.6% more than placebo.[10] It has also been studied as add-on therapy with sulfonylureas, with and without metformin, leading to decreases in A1C of 0.4–1.2%.[10] It has been studied in small pilot studies as add-on to insulin therapy with good preliminary results and no increased risk of hypoglycemia.[11] It has not been studied in combination with TZDs, SGLT2 inhibitors, or DPP-4 inhibitors.[3]

One significant advantage of bromocriptine is the cardiovascular risk benefits. Bromocriptine shows a 40% risk reduction of heart attack, stroke, and other major cardiovascular events in patients with preexisting CVD compared to those receiving standard therapy.[12-14] The relative risk reduction was found to be 40%. In this study, the patients were allowed to take no more than two oral antidiabetics, or insulin plus one oral agent, in addition to the bromocriptine and were allowed to change the underlying antidiabetic regimen at the discretion of the study investigators.[12-14] Further studies and observations need to be done to see if this benefit holds true outside of the studies and if the use of bromocriptine is limited by the incidence of side effects.

The barriers to bromocriptine therapy include the high cost of the QR formulation approved for diabetes as well as the relatively high number of tablets that need to be taken to achieve the therapeutic dose.[3] Other barriers include the relatively high incidence of gastrointestinal side effects, leading to discontinuation.[3]

In general, bromocriptine is a useful drug to have in the tool chest of oral antidiabetic agents for T2D and is especially important for patients who have comorbid conditions or cardiovascular risk factors.

THERAPEUTIC CONSIDERATIONS

Patients using bromocriptine need to be instructed to follow the administration timing carefully and to take bromocriptine with food to increase the absorption and half-life, as well as to decrease the incidence of gastrointestinal side effects.

SIGNIFICANT WARNINGS/PRECAUTIONS

Hypotension

In studies, hypotension (including orthostatic hypotension) was reported in patients taking bromocriptine and is particularly seen upon initiation of therapy and with dose increases.[3] Prior to initiation of bromocriptine, patients should be assessed for orthostatic changes and should be advised on the risks of orthostatic hypotension. Caution should be used in patients who are also taking antihypertensives.[3]

Psychiatric Disorders

Patients with severe psychiatric disorders should not receive bromocriptine therapy due to the possibility that bromocriptine may exacerbate the disorder and decrease the efficacy of the neuroleptic treatments they are receiving.[3]

Somnolence

Bromocriptine has been known to cause somnolence, reported as sudden sleep onset, sometimes during activities.[3] This side effect is more common in patients being treated for Parkinson's disease, but was reported in clinical trials for diabetes. Patients should be made aware of the potential for somnolence on bromocriptine therapy and counseled not to drive or operate heavy machinery until they know how the drug affects them.[3]

Syncopal Migraines

Patients who have a known history of syncopal migraines should not take bromocriptine due to an increased risk of syncope.[3] Bromocriptine increases the risk of hypotension among patients with syncopal migraines. Loss of consciousness during a migraine for patients treated with bromocriptine may represent hypersensitivity, and these patients should no longer receive bromocriptine therapy.[3]

SPECIAL POPULATIONS

Pregnancy

Bromocriptine is a pregnancy category B drug, with inadequate studies in humans.[3] Briggs's *Drugs in Pregnancy and Lactation* rates bromocriptine as *compatible*.[15] Observational data from pregnant women who used bromocriptine throughout pregnancy showed safety similar to other medications, and children exposed to intrauterine bromocriptine did not have a higher rate of birth defects than the general population. Because the possibility of harm cannot be ruled out, the use of bromocriptine during pregnancy should be avoided in diabetic patients unless there is a compelling indication without other safer treatment options.[15]

Lactation

Bromocriptine is contraindicated in lactation because it inhibits lactation and decreases levels of prolactin.[3,15]

Pediatrics

Bromocriptine has not been studied in children for the treatment of diabetes.[3] Bromocriptine has been used in children as young as 11 years to treat other conditions and has generally been found to be safe.[16,17]

Geriatrics

No differences in efficacy or safety were noted in geriatric patients taking bromocriptine to treat either diabetes or other approved indications.[3,16,17] Some sensitive populations cannot be ruled out and so use should be monitored in fragile patients.

Sex

Females have an increased plasma exposure of 18–30% compared to males.[3] It is not known if this is clinically relevant.

Hepatic Impairment

Bromocriptine has not been studied in hepatic impairment, but since it primarily undergoes hepatic metabolism, its use is cautioned in hepatic impairment.[3]

Renal Impairment

Bromocriptine has not been studied in renal impairment and has no reported adjustments for impaired renal function.[3]

PHARMACOGENOMICS

There are no known clinically significant pharmacogenomic polymorphisms that lead to altered dosing.[17]

ADVERSE EFFECTS AND MONITORING

Bromocriptine is generally well tolerated, and most side effects are mild and subside with continued use.[3,18–20] The most frequently reported adverse effects associated with bromocriptine are all gastrointestinal related. The most common adverse effect is nausea, affecting 25–30% of patients and lasting for an average of 14 days. In studies, nausea was cited as the primary reason for discontinuing the drug. Other gastrointestinal effects include vomiting (5–8%), constipation (5–11%), diarrhea (8%), dyspepsia (7.5%), and anorexia (5%). Taking bromocriptine with food reduces the incidence of gastrointestinal adverse effects. Other side effects reported in clinical trials that rarely lead to discontinuation include dizziness (14%), drowsiness (6%), fatigue (14%), headache (14%), asthenia (14%), and rhinitis (12%).[3,18–20]

Rare but serious adverse effects include syncope (1.5%) and hypotension (2.2%). Other serious side effects that have been observed with higher doses, but have not been reported with the QR formulation or the doses used to treat diabetes, include hallucinations, fibrotic complications (pulmonary and pleural), stroke, and neuroleptic-like malignant syndrome.[3,18–20] Anaphylaxis has been reported; if a patient has a known reaction to other ergot derivatives, he or she should be cautioned that anaphylaxis is more likely with bromocriptine.[3]

Patients taking bromocriptine should receive the typical monitoring of their diabetes and should be instructed to self-monitor their blood glucose.[3,18–20] Patients should have their blood pressure monitored periodically, with special attention paid during the initiation phase and whenever doses are titrated. Patients should also be evaluated for orthostatic changes prior to initiation and periodically during use. It may also be recommended to monitor serum prolactin levels, although no cases of hypoprolactinemia have been reported with use.[3,18–20]

DRUG INTERACTIONS

Bromocriptine has several clinically relevant drug interactions due to its pharmacology and metabolism by CYP enzymes.[3,16] Bromocriptine is contraindicated with concomitant use of other ergot derivatives, sympathomimetic drugs (e.g., phenylpropanolamine and isometheptene), and selective 5-hydroxytryptamine$_{1B}$ (5-HT$_{1B}$) agonists (e.g., "-triptans"). Bromocriptine is also highly protein-bound, and may increase the unbound fraction of other highly protein-bound drugs (e.g., salicylates, sulfonamides, and probenecid) and alter the efficacy and risk for side effects, so concomitant use is not recommended. Concomitant use of other dopamine agonists is not recommended due to an increased risk for side effects. Bromocriptine is primarily metabolized by CYP3A4, and so it is not recommended for patients to take either strong CYP3A4 inducers or inhibitors while taking bromocriptine due to the potential for changes in efficacy and risk of side effects. Doses should not exceed 1.6 mg daily if used with a moderate inhibitor of CYP3A4 (e.g., erythromycin).[3,16]

DOSAGE AND ADMINISTRATION

The recommended dose of bromocriptine for the treatment of T2D is 1.6–4.8 mg once a day within 2 h of waking.[3] Bromocriptine should be initiated at 0.8 mg (1 tablet) and then titrated slowly by increasing the dose by 0.8 mg (1 tablet) per week until the maximum dose of 4.8 mg (6 tablets) or the maximally tolerated dose is reached. The average dose achieved in clinical trials was 4.0 mg daily, but in postmarketing surveillance, the most common dose used is 3.2 mg daily.[3]

Table 16.1 — Dosage

Generic (brand)	Form/strength	Dosage
Bromocriptine mesylate (Cycloset)	Oral: 0.8-mg tablet	■ Initial: 0.8 mg p.o. daily within 2 h of waking. ■ Titrate: May increase by 0.8 mg every week to a max of 4.8 mg daily, or the maximum tolerated dose.

MONOGRAPHS

Bromocriptine mesylate (Cylcoset): https://dailymed.nlm.nih.gov/dailymed/drugInfo.cfm?setid=3e719d6a-342e-428b-93d3-377d31cb15c7

REFERENCES

1. Drugs@FDA. U.S. Food & Drug Administration website. Available from https://www.accessdata.fda.gov/scripts/cder/daf/index.cfm. Accessed 31 May 2018

2. Valiquette G. Bromocriptine for diabetes mellitus type II. *Cardiol Rev* 2011;19(6):272–275

3. Cycloset (bromocriptine mesylate) [package insert]. Tiverton, RI, Santarus, Inc., February 2017

4. Lopez Vicchi F, Luque GM, Brie B, et al. Dopaminergic drugs in type 2 diabetes and glucose homeostasis. *Pharmacol Res* 2016;109:74–80

5. Holt RI, Barnett AH, Bailey CJ. Bromocriptine: old drug, new formulation and new indication. *Diabetes Obes Metab* 2010;12(12):1048–1057

6. Grunberger, G. Bromocriptine mesylate QR in treatment of type 2 diabetes. *Diabetes Manag* 2014;4(2);203–211

7. Grunberger G. Novel therapies for the management of type 2 diabetes mellitus: part 1. pramlintide and bromocriptine-QR. *J Diabetes* 2013;5(2): 110–117

8. American Diabetes Association. 8. Pharmacologic approaches to glycemic treatment: *Standards of Medical Care in Diabetes—2018*. *Diabetes Care* 2018;41(Suppl. 1):S73–S85

9. Garber AJ, Abrahamson MJ, Barzilay JI, et al. Consensus statement by the American Association of Clinical Endocrinologists and American College of Endocrinology on the comprehensive type 2 diabetes management algorithm—2018 executive summary. *Endocr Pract* 2018;24(1):91–120

10. DeFronzo RA. Bromocriptine: a sympatholytic, d2-dopamine agonist for the treatment of type 2 diabetes [erratum, *Diabetes Care* 2011;34(6):1442]. *Diabetes Care* 2011;34(4):789–794

11. Roe ED, Chamarthi B, Raskin P. Impact of bromocriptine-QR therapy on glycemic control and daily insulin requirement in type 2 diabetes mellitus subjects whose dysglycemia is poorly controlled on high-dose insulin: a pilot study. *J Diabetes Res* 2015:834903

12. Lamos EM, Levitt DL, Munir KM. A review of dopamine agonist therapy in type 2 diabetes and effects on cardio-metabolic parameters. *Prim Care Diabetes* 2016;10(1):60–65

13. Gaziano JM, Cincotta AH, O'Connor CM, et al. Randomized clinical trial of quick-release bromocriptine among patients with type 2 diabetes on overall safety and cardiovascular outcomes [erratum, *Diabetes Care* 2016;39(10):1846]. *Diabetes Care* 2010;33(7):1503–1508

14. Gaziano JM, Cincotta AH, Vinik A, et al. Effect of bromocriptine-QR (a quick-release formulation of bromocriptine mesylate) on major adverse cardiovascular events in type 2 diabetes subjects [erratum, *J Am Heart Assoc* 2015;4(10)]. *J Am Heart Assoc* 2012;1(5):e002279

15. Briggs GG, Freeman RK, Yaffe SJ. *Drugs in Pregnancy and Lactation: A Reference Guide to Fetal and Neonatal Risk*, 11th ed. Philadelphia, Lippincott Williams & Wilkins, 2017

16. Micromedex Healthcare Series. Bromocriptine. Greenwood Village, CO, Truven Health Analytics, 2018. Available from www.micromedexsolutions.com. Accessed 16 May 2018

17. Lexicomp Online, Lexi-Drugs Online. Hudson, OH, Lexi-Comp, Inc., 2018. Accessed 16 May 2018

18. Kerr JL, Timpe EM, Petkewicz KA. Bromocriptine mesylate for glycemic management in type 2 diabetes mellitus. *Ann Pharmacother* 2010;44(11): 1777–1785

19. Sando KR, Taylor J. Bromocriptine: its place in type 2 diabetes Tx. *J Fam Pract* 2011;60(11):E1–E5

20. Schwartz SS, Zangeneh F. Evidence-based practice use of quick-release bromocriptine across the natural history of type 2 diabetes mellitus. *Postgrad Med* 2016;128(8):828–838

Chapter 17
Cardiovascular Disease and Risk Management

The American Diabetes Association *Standards of Medical Care in Diabetes* includes ADA's current clinical practice recommendations and is intended to provide the components of diabetes care, general treatment goals and guidelines, and tools to evaluate quality of care. Members of the ADA Professional Practice Committee, a multidisciplinary expert committee, are responsible for updating the *Standards of Care* annually, or more frequently as warranted. For a detailed description of ADA standards, statements, and reports, as well as the evidence-grading system for ADA's clinical practice recommendations, please refer to the Introduction to *Standards of Medical Care in Diabetes*. Readers who wish to comment on the *Standards of Care* are invited to do so at professional.diabetes.org/SOC.

For prevention and management of diabetes complications in children and adolescents, please refer to Section 13 "Children and Adolescents" in *Standards of Medical Care in Diabetes*.

Atherosclerotic cardiovascular disease (ASCVD)—defined as coronary heart disease, cerebrovascular disease, or PAD presumed to be of atherosclerotic origin—is the leading cause of morbidity and mortality for individuals with diabetes and results in an estimated $37.3 billion in cardiovascular-related spending per year associated with diabetes.[1] Common conditions coexisting with type 2 diabetes (e.g., hypertension and dyslipidemia) are clear risk factors for ASCVD, and diabetes itself confers independent risk. Numerous studies have shown the efficacy of controlling individual cardiovascular risk factors in preventing or slowing ASCVD in people with diabetes. Furthermore, large benefits are seen when multiple cardiovascular risk factors are addressed simultaneously. Under the current paradigm of aggressive risk factor modification in patients with diabetes, there is evidence that measures of 10-year coronary heart disease (CHD) risk among U.S. adults with diabetes have improved significantly over the past decade[2] and that ASCVD morbidity and mortality have decreased.[3,4]

HF is another major cause of morbidity and mortality from cardiovascular disease. Recent studies have found that rates of incident HF hospitalization (adjusted for age and sex) were twofold higher in patients with diabetes compared

Chapter 17 is an excerpt from American Diabetes Association, 10. Cardiovascular Disease and Risk Management: *Standards of Medical Care in Diabetes—2019. Diabetes Care* 2019; 42(Suppl. 1):S103–S123. DOI:10.2337/dc19S010. This section has received endorsement from the American College of Cardiology.

with those without.[5,6] People with diabetes may have heart failure with preserved ejection fraction (HFpEF) or with reduced ejection fraction (HFrEF). Hypertension is often a precursor of heart failure of either type, and ASCVD can coexist with either type,[7] whereas prior myocardial infarction (MI) is often a major factor in HFrEF. Rates of heart failure hospitalization have been improved in recent trials including patients with type 2 diabetes, most of whom also had ASCVD, with sodium–glucose cotransporter 2 (SGLT2) inhibitors.[8–10]

For prevention and management of both ASCVD and heart failure, cardiovascular risk factors should be systematically assessed at least annually in all patients with diabetes. These risk factors include obesity/overweight, hypertension, dyslipidemia, smoking, a family history of premature coronary disease, chronic kidney disease, and the presence of albuminuria. Modifiable abnormal risk factors should be treated as described in these guidelines.

THE RISK CALCULATOR

The American College of Cardiology/American Heart Association ASCVD risk calculator (Risk Estimator Plus) is generally a useful tool to estimate 10-year ASCVD risk (http://tools.acc.org/ASCVD-Risk-Estimator-Plus). These calculators have diabetes as a risk factor, since diabetes itself confers increased risk for ASCVD, although it should be acknowledged that these risk calculators do not account for the duration of diabetes or the presence of diabetes complications, such as albuminuria. Although some variability in calibration exists in various subgroups, including by sex, race, and diabetes, the overall risk prediction does not differ in those with or without diabetes,[11–14] validating the use of risk calculators in people with diabetes. The 10-year risk of a first ASCVD event should be assessed to better stratify ASCVD risk and help guide therapy, as described below.

Recently, risk scores and other cardiovascular biomarkers have been developed for risk stratification of secondary prevention patients (i.e., those who are already high risk because they have ASCVD) but are not yet in widespread use.[15,16] With newer, more expensive lipid-lowering therapies now available, use of these risk assessments may help target these new therapies to "higher risk" ASCVD patients in the future.

HYPERTENSION/BLOOD PRESSURE CONTROL

Hypertension, defined as a sustained blood pressure ≥140/90 mmHg, is common among patients with either type 1 or type 2 diabetes. Hypertension is a major risk factor for both ASCVD and microvascular complications. Moreover, numerous studies have shown that antihypertensive therapy reduces ASCVD events, heart failure, and microvascular complications. Please refer to the American Diabetes Association position statement "Diabetes and Hypertension" for a detailed review of the epidemiology, diagnosis, and treatment of hypertension.[17] The recommendations presented here reflect ADA's updated stance on blood pressure.

SCREENING AND DIAGNOSIS

Recommendations

10.1 Blood pressure should be measured at every routine clinical visit. Patients found to have elevated blood pressure (≥140/90 mmHg) should have blood pressure confirmed using multiple readings, including measurements on a separate day, to diagnose hypertension. **B***

10.2 All hypertensive patients with diabetes should monitor their blood pressure at home. **B**

Blood pressure should be measured by a trained individual and should follow the guidelines established for the general population: measurement in the seated position, with feet on the floor and arm supported at heart level, after 5 min of rest. Cuff size should be appropriate for the upper-arm circumference. Elevated values should be confirmed on a separate day. Postural changes in blood pressure and pulse may be evidence of autonomic neuropathy and therefore require adjustment of blood pressure targets. Orthostatic blood pressure measurements should be checked on initial visit and as indicated.

Home blood pressure self-monitoring and 24-h ambulatory blood pressure monitoring may provide evidence of white coat hypertension, masked hypertension, or other discrepancies between office and "true" blood pressure.[17] In addition to confirming or refuting a diagnosis of hypertension, home blood pressure assessment may be useful to monitor antihypertensive treatment. Studies of individuals without diabetes found that home measurements may better correlate with ASCVD risk than office measurements.[18,19] Moreover, home blood pressure monitoring may improve patient medication adherence and thus help reduce cardiovascular risk.[20]

TREATMENT GOALS

Recommendations

10.3 For patients with diabetes and hypertension, blood pressure targets should be individualized through a shared decision-making process that addresses cardiovascular risk, potential adverse effects of antihypertensive medications, and patient preferences. **C**

10.4 For individuals with diabetes and hypertension at higher cardiovascular risk (existing atherosclerotic cardiovascular disease or 10-year atherosclerotic cardiovascular disease risk >15%), a blood pressure target of <130/80 mmHg may be appropriate, if it can be safely attained. **C**

10.5 For individuals with diabetes and hypertension at lower risk for cardiovascular disease (10-year atherosclerotic cardiovascular disease risk >15%), treat to a blood pressure target of <140/90 mmHg. **A**

10.6 In pregnant patients with diabetes and preexisting hypertension who are treated with antihypertensive therapy, blood pressure targets of 120–160/80–105 mmHg are suggested in the interest of optimizing long-term maternal health and minimizing impaired fetal growth. **E**

---

* See Table 1.1 (p. 4) for an explanation of the American Diabetes Association evidence-grading system for *Standards of Medical Care in Diabetes*.

Randomized clinical trials have demonstrated unequivocally that treatment of hypertension to blood pressure <140/90 mmHg reduces cardiovascular events as well as microvascular complications.[21-27] Therefore, patients with type 1 or type 2 diabetes who have hypertension should, at a minimum, be treated to blood pressure targets of <140/90 mmHg. The benefits and risks of intensifying antihypertensive therapy to target blood pressures <140/90 mmHg (e.g., <130/80 or <120/80 mmHg) have been evaluated in large randomized clinical trials and meta-analyses of clinical trials. Notably, there is an absence of high-quality data available to guide blood pressure targets in type 1 diabetes.

Randomized Controlled Trials of Intensive Versus Standard Blood Pressure Control

The Action to Control Cardiovascular Risk in Diabetes blood pressure (ACCORD BP) trial provides the strongest direct assessment of the benefits and risks of intensive blood pressure control among people with type 2 diabetes.[28] In ACCORD BP, compared with standard blood pressure control (target systolic blood pressure <140 mmHg), intensive blood pressure control (target systolic blood pressure <120 mmHg) did not reduce total major atherosclerotic cardiovascular events but did reduce the risk of stroke, at the expense of increased adverse events (Table 17.1). The ACCORD BP results suggest that blood pressure targets more intensive than <140/90 mmHg are not likely to improve cardiovascular outcomes among most people with type 2 diabetes but may be reasonable for patients who may derive the most benefit and have been educated about added treatment burden, side effects, and costs, as discussed below.

Additional studies, such as the Systolic Blood Pressure Intervention Trial (SPRINT) and the Hypertension Optimal Treatment (HOT) trial, also examined effects of intensive versus standard control (Table 17.1), though the relevance of their results to people with diabetes is less clear. The Action in Diabetes and Vascular Disease: Preterax and Diamicron MR Controlled Evaluation–Blood Pressure (ADVANCE BP) trial did not explicitly test blood pressure targets;[29] the achieved blood pressure in the intervention group was higher than that achieved in the ACCORD BP intensive arm and would be consistent with a target blood pressure of <140/90 mmHg. Notably, ACCORD BP and SPRINT measured blood pressure using automated office blood pressure measurement, which yields values that are generally lower than typical office blood pressure readings by approximately 5–10 mmHg,[30] suggesting that implementing the ACCORD BP or SPRINT protocols in an outpatient clinic might require a systolic blood pressure target higher than <120 mmHg, such as <130 mmHg.

A number of post hoc analyses have attempted to explain the apparently divergent results of ACCORD BP and SPRINT. Some investigators have argued that the divergent results are not due to differences between people with and without diabetes but rather are due to differences in study design or to characteristics other than diabetes.[31-33] Others have opined that the divergent results are most readily explained by the lack of benefit of intensive blood pressure control on cardiovascular mortality in ACCORD BP, which may be due to differential mechanisms underlying cardiovascular disease in type 2 diabetes, to chance, or both.[34.]

Table 17.1—Randomized Controlled Trials of Intensive Versus Standard Hypertension Treatment Strategies

Clinical trial	Population	Intensive	Standard	Outcomes
ACCORD BP (28)	4,733 participants with T2D aged 40–79 years with prior evidence of CVD or multiple cardiovascular risk factors	Systolic blood pressure target: <120 mmHg Achieved (mean) systolic/diastolic: 119.3/64.4 mmHg	Systolic blood pressure target: 130–140 mmHg Achieved (mean) systolic/diastolic: 133.5/70.5 mmHg	■ No benefit in primary endpoint: composite of nonfatal MI, nonfatal stroke, and CVD death ■ Stroke risk reduced 41% with intensive control, not sustained through follow-up beyond the period of active treatment ■ Adverse events more common in intensive group, particularly elevated serum creatinine and electrolyte abnormalities
ADVANCE BP (29)	11,140 participants with T2D aged 55 years and older with prior evidence of CVD or multiple cardiovascular risk factors	Intervention: a single-pill, fixed-dose combination of perindopril and indapamide Achieved (mean) systolic/diastolic: 136/73 mmHg	Control: placebo Achieved (mean) systolic/diastolic: 141.6/75.2 mmHg	■ Intervention reduced risk of primary composite endpoint of major macrovascular and microvascular events (9%), death from any cause (14%), and death from CVD (18%) ■ 6-year observational follow-up found reduction in risk of death in intervention group attenuated but still significant (174)
HOT (173)	18,790 participants, including 1,501 with diabetes	Diastolic blood pressure target: ≤80 mmHg	Diastolic blood pressure target: ≤90 mmHg	■ In the overall trial, there was no cardiovascular benefit with more intensive targets ■ In the subpopulation with diabetes, an intensive diastolic target was associated with a significantly reduced risk (51%) of CVD events
SPRINT (39)	9,361 participants without diabetes	Systolic blood pressure target: <120 mmHg Achieved (mean): 121.4 mmHg	Systolic blood pressure target: <140 mmHg Achieved (mean): 136.2 mmHg	■ Intensive systolic blood pressure target lowered risk of the primary composite outcome 25% (MI, ACS, stroke, HF, and death due to CVD) ■ Intensive target reduced risk of death 27% ■ Intensive therapy increased risks of electrolyte abnormalities and AKI

ACS, acute coronary syndrome; AKI, acute kidney injury; CVD, cardiovascular disease; HF, heart failure; MI, myocardial infarction; T2D, type 2 diabetes.

Data from this table can also be found in the ADA position statement "Diabetes and Hypertension".[17]

Meta-Analyses of Trials

To clarify optimal blood pressure targets in patients with diabetes, meta-analyses have stratified clinical trials by mean baseline blood pressure or mean blood pressure attained in the intervention (or intensive treatment) arm. Based on these analyses, antihypertensive treatment appears to be beneficial when mean baseline blood pressure is ≥140/90 mmHg or mean attained intensive blood pressure is ≥130/80 mmHg.[17,21,22,24-26] Among trials with lower baseline or attained blood pressure, antihypertensive treatment reduced the risk of stroke, retinopathy, and albuminuria, but effects on other ASCVD outcomes and heart failure were not evident. Taken together, these meta-analyses consistently show that treating patients with baseline blood pressure ≥140 mmHg to targets <140 mmHg is beneficial, while more intensive targets may offer additional (though probably less robust) benefits.

Individualization of Treatment Targets

Patients and clinicians should engage in a shared decision-making process to determine individual blood pressure targets.[17] This approach acknowledges that the benefits and risks of intensive blood pressure targets are uncertain and may vary across patients and is consistent with a patient-focused approach to care that values patient priorities and provider judgment.[35] Secondary analyses of ACCORD BP and SPRINT suggest that clinical factors can help determine individuals more likely to benefit and less likely to be harmed by intensive blood pressure control.[36]

Absolute benefit from blood pressure reduction correlated with absolute baseline cardiovascular risk in SPRINT and in earlier clinical trials conducted at higher baseline blood pressure levels.[11,37] Extrapolation of these studies suggests that patients with diabetes may also be more likely to benefit from intensive blood pressure control when they have high absolute cardiovascular risk. Therefore, it may be reasonable to target blood pressure <130/80 mmHg among patients with diabetes and either clinically diagnosed cardiovascular disease (particularly stroke, which was significantly reduced in ACCORD BP) or 10-year ASCVD risk ≥15%, if it can be attained safely. This approach is consistent with guidelines from the American College of Cardiology/American Heart Association, which advocate a blood pressure target <130/80 mmHg for all patients, with or without diabetes.[38]

Potential adverse effects of antihypertensive therapy (e.g., hypotension, syncope, falls, acute kidney injury, and electrolyte abnormalities) should also be taken into account.[28,39-41] Patients with older age, CKD, and frailty have been shown to be at higher risk of adverse effects of intensive blood pressure control.[41] In addition, patients with orthostatic hypotension, substantial comorbidity, functional limitations, or polypharmacy may be at high risk of adverse effects, and some patients may prefer higher blood pressure targets to enhance quality of life. Patients with low absolute cardiovascular risk (10-year ASCVD risk <15%) or with a history of adverse effects of intensive blood pressure control or at high risk of such adverse effects should have a higher blood pressure target. In such patients, a blood pressure target of <140/90 mmHg is recommended, if it can be safely attained.

Pregnancy and Antihypertensive Medications

Since there is a lack of randomized controlled trials of antihypertensive therapy in pregnant women with diabetes, recommendations for the management of hypertension in pregnant women with diabetes should be similar to those for all pregnant women. The American College of Obstetricians and Gynecologists (ACOG) has recommended that women with mild to moderate gestational hypertension (systolic blood pressure <160 mmHg or diastolic blood pressure <110 mmHg) do not need to be treated with antihypertensive medications as there is no benefit identified that clearly out weighs potential risks of therapy.[42] A 2014 Cochrane systematic review of antihypertensive therapy for mild to moderate chronic hypertension that included 49 trials and over 4,700 women did not find any conclusive evidence for or against blood pressure treatment to reduce the risk of preeclampsia for the mother or effects on perinatal outcomes such as preterm birth, small-for-gestational-age infants, or fetal death.[43] For pregnant women who require antihypertensive therapy, systolic blood pressure levels of 120–160 mmHg and diastolic blood pressure levels of 80–105 mmHg are suggested to optimize maternal health without risking fetal harm. Lower targets (systolic blood pressure 110–119 mmHg and diastolic blood pressure 65–79 mmHg) may contribute to improved long-term maternal health; however, they may be associated with impaired fetal growth. Pregnant women with hypertension and evidence of end-organ damage from cardiovascular and/or renal disease may be considered for lower blood pressure targets to avoid progression of these conditions during pregnancy.

During pregnancy, treatment with ACE inhibitors, angiotensin receptor blockers (ARBs), and spironolactone are contraindicated as they may cause fetal damage. Antihypertensive drugs known to be effective and safe in pregnancy include methyldopa, labetalol, and long-acting nifedipine, while hydralzine may be considered in the acute management of hypertension in pregnancy or severe preeclampsia.[42] Diuretics are not recommended for blood pressure control in pregnancy but may be used during late-stage pregnancy if needed for volume control.[42,44] ACOG also recommends that postpartum patients with gestational hypertension, preeclampsia, and superimposed preeclampsia have their blood pressures observed for 72 h in the hospital and for 7–10 days postpartum. Long-term follow-up is recommended for these women as they have increased lifetime cardiovascular risk.[45] See Section 14 "Management of Diabetes in Pregnancy" in the *Standards of Medical Care in Diabetes—2019* (DOI:10.2337/dc19-S014) for additional information.

TREATMENT STRATEGIES

Lifestyle Intervention

Recommendations

10.7 For patients with blood pressure >120/80 mmHg, lifestyle intervention consists of weight loss if overweight or obese, a Dietary Approaches to Stop Hypertension (DASH)-style dietary pattern including reducing sodium and increasing potassium intake, moderation of alcohol intake, and increased physical activity. **B**

Lifestyle management is an important component of hypertension treatment because it lowers blood pressure, enhances the effectiveness of some antihypertensive medications, promotes other aspects of metabolic and vascular health, and generally leads to few adverse effects. Lifestyle therapy consists of reducing excess body weight through caloric restriction, restricting sodium intake (<2,300 mg/day), increasing consumption of fruits and vegetables (8–10 servings per day) and low-fat dairy products (2–3 servings per day), avoiding excessive alcohol consumption (no more than 2 servings per day in men and no more than 1 serving per day in women),[46] and increasing activity levels.[47]

These lifestyle interventions are reasonable for individuals with diabetes and mildly elevated blood pressure (systolic >120 mmHg or diastolic >80 mmHg) and should be initiated along with pharmacologic therapy when hypertension is diagnosed (Figure 17.1).[47] A lifestyle therapy plan should be developed in collaboration with the patient and discussed as part of diabetes management.

Pharmacologic Interventions

Recommendations

10.8   Patients with confirmed office-based blood pressure ≥140/90 mmHg should, in addition to lifestyle therapy, have prompt initiation and timely titration of pharmacologic therapy to achieve blood pressure goals. **A**

10.9   Patients with confirmed office-based blood pressure ≥160/100 mmHg should, in addition to lifestyle therapy, have prompt initiation and timely titration of two drugs or a single-pill combination of drugs demonstrated to reduce cardiovascular events in patients with diabetes. **A**

10.10 Treatment for hypertension should include drug classes demonstrated to reduce cardiovascular events in patients with diabetes (ACE inhibitors, angiotensin receptor blockers, thiazide-like diuretics, or dihydropyridine calcium channel blockers). **A**

10.11 Multiple-drug therapy is generally required to achieve blood pressure targets. However, combinations of ACE inhibitors and ARBs and combinations of ACE inhibitors or angiotensin receptor blockers with direct renin inhibitors should not be used. **A**

10.12 An ACE inhibitor or angiotensin receptor blocker, at the maximum tolerated dose indicated for blood pressure treatment, is the recommended first-line treatment for hypertension in patients with diabetes and urinary albumin-to-creatinine ratio ≥300 mg/g creatinine **A** or 30–299 mg/g creatinine. **B** If one class is not tolerated, the other should be substituted. **B**

10.13 For patients treated with an ACE inhibitor, angiotensin receptor blocker, or diuretic, serum creatinine/estimated glomerular filtration rate and serum potassium levels should be monitored at least annually. **B**

Initial Number of Antihypertensive Medications. Initial treatment for people with diabetes depends on the severity of hypertension (Figure 17.1). Those with blood pressure between 140/90 mmHg and 159/99 mmHg may begin with a single drug. For patients with blood pressure ≥160/100 mmHg, initial pharmacologic treatment with two antihypertensive medications is recommended in order to more effectively achieve adequate blood pressure control.[48-50] Single-pill antihypertensive combinations may improve medication adherence in some patients.[51]

Classes of Antihypertensive Medications. Initial treatment for hypertension should include any of the drug classes demonstrated to reduce cardiovascular events in patients with diabetes: ACE inhibitors,[52,53] ARBs,[52,53] thiazide-like diuret-

Recommendations for the Treatment of Confirmed Hypertension in People With Diabetes

Figure 17.1—Recommendations for the treatment of confirmed hypertension in people with diabetes. *An ACE inhibitor (ACEi) or angiotensin receptor blocker (ARB) is suggested to treat hypertension for patients with urine albumin-to-creatinine ratio 30–299 mg/g creatinine and strongly recommended for patients with urine albumin-to-creatinine ratio ≥300 mg/g creatinine. **Thiazide-like diuretic; long-acting agents shown to reduce cardiovascular events, such as chlorthalidone and indapamide, are preferred. ***Dihydropyridine calcium channel blocker (CCB). BP, blood pressure. *Source*: Adapted from de Boer et al.[17]

ics,[54] or dihydropyridine calcium channel blockers.[55] For patients with albuminuria (urine albumin-to-creatinine ratio ≥30 mg/g), initial treatment should include an ACE inhibitor or ARB in order to reduce the risk of progressive kidney disease[17] (Figure 17.1). In the absence of albuminuria, risk of progressive kidney disease is low, and ACE inhibitors and ARBs have not been found to afford superior cardioprotection when compared with thiazide-like diuretics or dihydropyridine calcium channel blockers.[56] β-Blockers may be used for the treatment of prior MI, active angina, or heart failure but have not been shown to reduce mortality as blood pressure-lowering agents in the absence of these conditions.[23,57]

Multiple-Drug Therapy. Multiple-drug therapy is often required to achieve blood pressure targets (Figure 17.1), particularly in the setting of diabetic kidney disease. However, the use of both ACE inhibitors and ARBs in combination, or the combination of an ACE inhibitor or ARB and a direct renin inhibitor, is not recommended given the lack of added ASCVD benefit and increased rate of adverse events—namely, hyperkalemia, syncope, and acute kidney injury (AKI).[58-60] Titration of and/or addition of further blood pressure medications should be made in a timely fashion to overcome clinical inertia in achieving blood pressure targets.

Bedtime Dosing. Growing evidence suggests that there is an association between the absence of nocturnal blood pressure dipping and the incidence of ASCVD. A meta-analysis of randomized clinical trials found a small benefit of evening versus morning dosing of antihypertensive medications with regard to blood pressure control but had no data on clinical effects.[61] In two subgroup analyses of a single subsequent randomized controlled trial, moving at least one antihypertensive medication to bedtime significantly reduced cardiovascular events, but results were based on a small number of events.[62]

Hyperkalemia and Acute Kidney Injury. Treatment with ACE inhibitors or ARBs can cause AKI and hyperkalemia, while diuretics can cause AKI and either hypokalemia or hyperkalemia (depending on mechanism of action).[63,64] Detection and management of these abnormalities is important because AKI and hyperkalemia each increase the risks of cardiovascular events and death.[65] Therefore, serum creatinine and potassium should be monitored during treatment with an ACE inhibitor, ARB, or diuretic, particularly among patients with reduced glomerular filtration who are at increased risk of hyperkalemia and AKI.[63,64,66]

Resistant Hypertension

Recommendation

10.14 Patients with hypertension who are not meeting blood pressure targets on three classes of antihypertensive medications (including a diuretic) should be considered for mineralocorticoid receptor antagonist therapy. **B**

Resistant hypertension is defined as blood pressure ≥140/90 mmHg despite a therapeutic strategy that includes appropriate lifestyle management plus a diuretic and two other antihypertensive drugs belonging to different classes at adequate doses. Prior to diagnosing resistant hypertension, a number of other conditions should be excluded, including medication nonadherence, white coat hypertension, and secondary hypertension. In general, barriers to medication adherence (such as cost and side effects) should be identified and addressed (Figure 17.1). Mineralocorticoid receptor antagonists are effective for management of resistant hypertension in patients with type 2 diabetes when added to existing treatment with an ACE inhibitor or ARB, thiazide-like diuretic, and dihydropyridine calcium channel blocker.[67] Mineralocorticoid receptor antagonists also reduce albuminuria and have additional cardiovascular benefits.[68–71] However, adding a mineralocorticoid receptor antagonist to a regimen including an ACE inhibitor or ARB may increase the risk for hyperkalemia, emphasizing the importance of regular monitoring for serum creatinine and potassium in these patients, and long-term outcome studies are needed to better evaluate the role of mineralocorticoid receptor antagonists in blood pressure management.

LIPID MANAGEMENT

Lifestyle Intervention

Recommendations

10.15 Lifestyle modification focusing on weight loss (if indicated); application of a Mediterranean diet or Dietary Approaches to Stop Hypertension (DASH) dietary pattern; reduction of saturated fat and trans fat; increase of dietary n-3 fatty acids, viscous fiber, and plant stanols/sterols intake; and increased physical activity should be recommended to improve the lipid profile and reduce the risk of developing atherosclerotic cardiovascular disease in patients with diabetes. **A**

10.16 Intensify lifestyle therapy and optimize glycemic control for patients with elevated triglyceride levels (≥150 mg/dL [1.7 mmol/L]) and/or low HDL cholesterol (<40 mg/dL [1.0 mmol/L] for men, <50 mg/dL [1.3 mmol/L] for women). **C**

Lifestyle intervention, including weight loss,[72] increased physical activity, and medical nutrition therapy, allows some patients to reduce ASCVD risk factors. Nutrition intervention should be tailored according to each patient's age, diabetes type, pharmacologic treatment, lipid levels, and medical conditions.

Recommendations should focus on application of a Mediterranean diet[73] or Dietary Approaches to Stop Hypertension (DASH) dietary pattern, reducing saturated and trans fat intake, and increasing plant stanols/sterols, n-3 fatty acids, and viscous fiber (such as in oats, legumes, and citrus) intake.[74] Glycemic control may also beneficially modify plasma lipid levels, particularly in patients with very high triglycerides and poor glycemic control. See Section 5 "Lifestyle Management" in the *Standards of Medical Care in Diabetes—2019* (DOI:10.2337/dc19-S005) for additional nutrition information.

Ongoing Therapy and Monitoring with Lipid Panel

Recommendations

10.17 In adults not taking statins or other lipid-lowering therapy, it is reasonable to obtain a lipid profile at the time of diabetes diagnosis, at an initial medical evaluation, and every 5 years thereafter if under the age of 40 years, or more frequently if indicated. **E**

10.18 Obtain a lipid profile at initiation of statins or other lipid-lowering therapy, 4–12 weeks after initiation or a change in dose, and annually thereafter as it may help to monitor the response to therapy and inform medication adherence. **E**

In adults with diabetes, it is reasonable to obtain a lipid profile (total cholesterol, LDL cholesterol, HDL cholesterol, and triglycerides) at the time of diagnosis, at the initial medical evaluation, and at least every 5 years thereafter in patients under the age of 40 years. In younger patients with longer duration of disease (such as those with youth-onset type 1 diabetes), more frequent lipid profiles may be reasonable. A lipid panel should also be obtained immediately before initiating statin therapy. Once a patient is taking a statin, LDL cholesterol levels should be assessed 4–12 weeks after initiation of statin therapy, after any change in dose, and on an individual basis (e.g., to monitor for medication adherence and efficacy). If LDL cholesterol levels are not responding in spite of medication adherence, clinical judgment is recommended to determine the need for and timing of lipid panels. In individual patients, the highly variable LDL cholesterol–lowering response seen with statins is poorly understood.[75] Clinicians should attempt to find a dose or alternative statin that is tolerable if side effects occur. There is evidence for benefit from even extremely low, less-than-daily statin doses.[76]

Statin Treatment

Recommendations

10.19 For patients of all ages with diabetes and atherosclerotic cardiovascular disease or 10-year atherosclerotic cardiovascular disease risk >20%, high-intensity statin therapy should be added to lifestyle therapy. **A**

10.20 For patients with diabetes aged <40 years with additional atherosclerotic cardiovascular disease risk factors, the patient and provider should consider using moderate-intensity statin in addition to lifestyle therapy. **C**

10.21 For patients with diabetes aged 40–75 years **A** and >75 years **B** without atherosclerotic cardiovascular disease, use moderate-intensity statin in addition to lifestyle therapy.

10.22 In patients with diabetes who have multiple atherosclerotic cardiovascular disease risk factors, it is reasonable to consider high-intensity statin therapy. **C**

10.23 For patients who do not tolerate the intended intensity, the maximally tolerated statin dose should be used. **E**

10.24 For patients with diabetes and atherosclerotic cardiovascular disease, if LDL cholesterol is ≥70 mg/dL on maximally tolerated statin dose, consider adding additional LDL-lowering therapy (such as ezetimibe or PCSK9 inhibitor). **A** Ezetimibe may be preferred due to lower cost.

10.25 Statin therapy is contraindicated in pregnancy. **B**

Initiating Statin Therapy Based on Risk

Patients with type 2 diabetes have an increased prevalence of lipid abnormalities, contributing to their high risk of ASCVD. Multiple clinical trials have demonstrated the beneficial effects of statin therapy on ASCVD outcomes in subjects with and without CHD.[77,78] Subgroup analyses of patients with diabetes in larger trials[79–83] and trials in patients with diabetes[84,85] showed significant primary and secondary prevention of ASCVD events and CHD death in patients with diabetes. Meta-analyses, including data from over 18,000 patients with diabetes from 14 randomized trials of statin therapy (mean follow-up 4.3 years), demonstrate a 9% proportional reduction in all-cause mortality and 13% reduction in vascular mortality for each mmol/L (39 mg/dL) reduction in LDL cholesterol.[86]

Accordingly, statins are the drugs of choice for LDL cholesterol lowering and cardioprotection. Table 17.2 shows recommended lipid-lowering strategies, and Table 17.3 shows the two statin dosing intensities that are recommended for use in clinical practice: high-intensity statin therapy will achieve approximately a 50% reduction in LDL cholesterol, and moderate-intensity statin regimens achieve 30–50% reductions in LDL cholesterol. Low-dose statin therapy is generally not recommended in patients with diabetes but is sometimes the only dose of statin that a patient can tolerate. For patients who do not tolerate the intended intensity of statin, the maximally tolerated statin dose should be used.

As in those without diabetes, absolute reductions in ASCVD outcomes (CHD death and nonfatal MI) are greatest in people with high baseline ASCVD risk (known ASCVD and/or very high LDL cholesterol levels), but the overall benefits of statin therapy in people with diabetes at moderate or even low risk for ASCVD are convincing.[87,88] The *relative* benefit of lipid-lowering therapy has been uniform across most subgroups tested,[78,86] including subgroups that varied with respect to age and other risk factors.

Primary Prevention (Patients without ASCVD)

For primary prevention, moderate-dose statin therapy is recommended for those 40 years and older,[80,87,88] though high-intensity therapy may be considered on an individual basis in the context of additional ASCVD risk factors. The evidence is strong for patients with diabetes aged 40–75 years, an age-group well represented in statin trials showing benefit. Since risk is enhanced in patients with diabetes, as noted above, patients who also have multiple other coronary risk factors have increased risk, equivalent to that of those with ASCVD. As such, recent guidelines recommend that in patients with diabetes who have multiple ASCVD risk factors, it is reasonable to prescribe high-intensity statin therapy.[12,89] Furthermore, for patients with diabetes whose ASCVD risk is >20%, i.e., an ASCVD risk equivalent, the same high-intensity statin therapy is recommended as for those with documented ASCVD.[12]

The evidence is lower for patients aged >75 years; relatively few older patients with diabetes have been enrolled in primary prevention trials. However, heterogeneity by age has not been seen in the relative benefit of lipid-lowering therapy in trials that included older participants,[78,85,86] and because older age confers higher risk, the absolute benefits are actually greater.[78,90] Moderate-intensity statin therapy is recommended in patients with diabetes that are 75 years or older. However, the risk-benefit profile should be routinely evaluated in this population, with downward titration of dose performed as needed. See Section 12 "Older Adults" in the *Standards of Medical Care in Diabetes—2019* (DOI:10.2337/dc19-S012) for more details on clinical considerations for this population.

Age <40 Years and/or Type 1 Diabetes.

Very little clinical trial evidence exists for patients with type 2 diabetes under the age of 40 years or for patients with type 1 diabetes of any age. For pediatric recommendations, see Section 13 "Children and Adolescents" in the *Standards of Medical Care in Diabetes—2019* (DOI:10.2337/dc19-S013). In the Heart Protection Study (lower age limit 40 years), the subgroup of ~600 patients with type 1 diabetes had a proportionately similar, although not statistically significant, reduction in risk as patients with type 2 diabetes.[80] Even though the data are not definitive, similar statin treatment approaches should be considered for patients with type 1 or type 2 diabetes, particularly in the presence of other cardiovascular risk factors. Patients below the age of 40 have lower risk of developing a cardiovascular event over a 10-year horizon; however, their lifetime risk of developing cardiovascular disease and suffering an MI, stroke, or cardiovascular death is high. For patients under the age of 40 years and/or who have type 1 diabetes with other ASCVD risk factors, we recommend that the patient and healthcare provider discuss the relative benefits and risks and consider the use of moderate-intensity statin therapy. Please refer to "Type 1 Diabetes Mellitus and Cardiovascular Disease: A Scientific Statement From the American Heart Association and American Diabetes Association"[91] for additional discussion.

Secondary Prevention (Patients with ASCVD)

Because risk is high in patients with ASCVD, intensive therapy is indicated and has been shown to be of benefit in multiple large randomized cardiovascular outcomes trials.[86,90,92,93] High-intensity statin therapy is recommended for all patients with diabetes and ASCVD. This recommendation is based on the Cholesterol Treatment Trialists' Collaboration involving 26 statin trials, of which 5 compared high-intensity versus moderate-intensity statins. Together, they found reductions in nonfatal cardiovascular events with more intensive therapy, in patients with and without diabetes.[78,82,92]

Over the past few years, there have been multiple large randomized trials investigating the benefits of adding nonstatin agents to statin therapy, including those that evaluated further lowering of LDL cholesterol with ezetimibe[90,94] and proprotein convertase subtilisin/kexin type 9 (PCSK9) inhibitors.[93] Each trial found a significant benefit in the reduction of ASCVD events that was directly related to the degree of further LDL cholesterol lowering. These large trials included a significant number of participants with diabetes. For patients with ASCVD who are on high-intensity (and maximally tolerated) statin therapy and have an LDL cholesterol ≥70 mg/dL, the addition of nonstatin LDL-lowering therapy is recommended following a clinician-patient discussion about the net benefit, safety, and cost (Table 17.2).

Combination Therapy for LDL Cholesterol Lowering

Statins and Ezetimibe

The IMProved Reduction of Outcomes: Vytorin Efficacy International Trial (IMPROVE-IT) was a randomized controlled trial in 18,144 patients comparing the addition of ezetimibe to simvastatin therapy versus simvastatin alone. Individuals were ≥50 years of age, had experienced a recent acute coronary syndrome (ACS), and were treated for an average of 6 years. Overall, the addition of ezetimibe led to a 6.4% relative benefit and a 2% absolute reduction in major adverse cardiovascular events, with the degree of benefit being directly proportional to the change in LDL cholesterol, which was 70 mg/dL in the statin group on average and 54 mg/dL in the combination group.[90] In those with diabetes (27% of par-

Table 17.2—Recommendations for Statin and Combination Treatment in Adults with Diabetes

Age	ASCVD or 10-year ASCVD risk >20%	Recommended statin intensity^ and combination treatment*
<40 years	No	None†
	Yes	High ■ In patients with ASCVD, if LDL cholesterol ≥70 mg/dL despite maximally tolerated statin dose, consider adding additional LDL-lowering therapy (such as ezetimibe or PCSK9 inhibitor)#
≥40 years	No	Moderate‡
	Yes	High ■ In patients with ASCVD, if LDL cholesterol ≥70 mg/dL despite maximally tolerated statin dose, consider adding additional LDL-lowering therapy (such as ezetimibe or PCSK9 inhibitor)

ASCVD, atherosclerotic cardiovascular disease; PCSK9, proprotein convertase subtilisin/kexin type 9. *In addition to lifestyle therapy. ^For patients who do not tolerate the intended intensity of statin, the maximally tolerated statin dose should be used. †Moderate-intensity statin may be considered based on risk-benefit profile and presence of ASCVD risk factors. ASCVD risk factors include LDL cholesterol ≥100 mg/dL (2.6 mmol/L), high blood pressure, smoking, chronic kidney disease, albuminuria, and family history of premature ASCVD. ‡High-intensity statin may be considered based on risk-benefit profile and presence of ASCVD risk factors. #Adults aged <40 years with prevalent ASCVD were not well represented in clinical trials of nonstatin–based LDL reduction. Before initiating combination lipid-lowering therapy, consider the potential for further ASCVD risk reduction, drug-specific adverse effects, and patient preferences.

ticipants), the combination of moderate-intensity simvastatin (40 mg) and ezetimibe (10 mg) showed a significant reduction of major adverse cardiovascular events with an absolute risk reduction of 5% (40% vs. 45% cumulative incidence at 7 years) and relative risk reduction of 14% (hazard ratio [HR] 0.86 [95% CI 0.78–0.94]) over moderate-intensity simvastatin (40 mg) alone.[94]

Statins and PCSK9 Inhibitors

Placebo-controlled trials evaluating the addition of the PCSK9 inhibitors evolocumab and alirocumab to maximally tolerated doses of statin therapy in participants who were at high risk for ASCVD demonstrated an average reduction in LDL cholesterol ranging from 36–59%. These agents have been approved as adjunctive therapy for patients with ASCVD or familial hypercholesterolemia who are receiving maximally tolerated statin therapy but require additional lowering of LDL cholesterol.[95,96]

The effects of PCSK9 inhibition on ASCVD outcomes were investigated in the Further Cardiovascular Outcomes Research With PCSK9 Inhibition in Subjects With Elevated Risk (FOURIER) trial, which enrolled 27,564 patients with prior ASCVD and an additional high-risk feature who were receiving their maximally tolerated statin therapy (two-thirds were on high-intensity statin) but who

Table 17.3—High-Intensity and Moderate-Intensity Statin Therapy*

High-intensity statin therapy (lowers LDL cholesterol by ≥50%)	Moderate-intensity statin therapy (lowers LDL cholesterol by 30–50%)
Atorvastatin 40–80 mg	Atorvastatin 10–20 mg
Rosuvastatin 20–40 mg	Rosuvastatin 5–10 mg
	Simvastatin 20–40 mg
	Pravastatin 40–80 mg
	Lovastatin 40 mg
	Fluvastatin XL 80 mg
	Pitavastatin 2–4 mg

*Once-daily dosing. XL, extended release.

still had an LDL cholesterol ≥70 mg/dL or a non-HDL cholesterol ≥100 mg/dL.[93] Patients were randomized to receive subcutaneous injections of evolocumab (either 140 mg every 2 weeks or 420 mg every month based on patient preference) versus placebo. Evolocumab reduced LDL cholesterol by 59% from a median of 92–30 mg/dL in the treatment arm.

During the median follow-up of 2.2 years, the composite outcome of cardiovascular death, MI, stroke, hospitalization for angina, or revascularization occurred in 11.3% vs. 9.8% of the placebo and evolocumab groups, respectively, representing a 15% relative risk reduction ($P < 0.001$). The combined endpoint of cardiovascular death, MI, or stroke was reduced by 20%, from 7.4 to 5.9% ($P < 0.001$). Importantly, similar benefits were seen in a prespecified subgroup of patients with diabetes, comprising 11,031 patients (40% of the trial).[97]

Treatment of Other Lipoprotein Fractions or Targets

Recommendations

10.26 For patients with fasting triglyceride levels ≥500 mg/dL (5.7 mmol/L), evaluate for secondary causes of hypertriglyceridemia and consider medical therapy to reduce the risk of pancreatitis. **C**

10.27 In adults with moderate hypertriglyceridemia (fasting or nonfasting triglycerides 175–499 mg/dL), clinicians should address and treat lifestyle factors (obesity and metabolic syndrome), secondary factors (diabetes, chronic liver or kidney disease and/or nephrotic syndrome, hypothyroidism), and medications that raise triglycerides. **C**

Hypertriglyceridemia should be addressed with dietary and lifestyle changes including weight loss and abstinence from alcohol.[98] Severe hypertriglyceridemia (fasting triglycerides ≥500 mg/dL and especially >1,000 mg/dL) may warrant pharmacologic therapy (fibric acid derivatives and/or fish oil) to reduce the risk of acute pancreatitis. In addition, if 10-year ASCVD risk is ≥7.5%, it is reasonable to initiate moderate-intensity statin therapy or increase statin intensity from moderate to high. In patients with moderate hypertriglyceridemia, lifestyle interventions, treatment of secondary factors, and avoidance of medications that might raise triglycerides are recommended.

Low levels of HDL cholesterol, often associated with elevated triglyceride levels, are the most prevalent pattern of dyslipidemia in individuals with type 2 diabetes. However, the evidence for the use of drugs that target these lipid fractions is substantially less robust than that for statin therapy.[99] In a large trial in patients with diabetes, fenofibrate failed to reduce overall cardiovascular outcomes.[100]

Other Combination Therapy

Recommendations

10.28 Combination therapy (statin/fibrate) has not been shown to improve atherosclerotic cardiovascular disease outcomes and is generally not recommended. **A**

10.29 Combination therapy (statin/niacin) has not been shown to provide additional cardiovascular benefit above statin therapy alone, may increase the risk of stroke with additional side effects, and is generally not recommended. **A**

Statin and Fibrate

Combination therapy (statin and fibrate) is associated with an increased risk for abnormal transaminase levels, myositis, and rhabdomyolysis. The risk of rhabdomyolysis is more common with higher doses of statins and renal insufficiency and appears to be higher when statins are combined with gemfibrozil (compared with fenofibrate).[101]

In the ACCORD study, in patients with type 2 diabetes who were at high risk for ASCVD, the combination of fenofibrate and simvastatin did not reduce the rate of fatal cardiovascular events, nonfatal MI, or nonfatal stroke as compared with simvastatin alone. Prespecified subgroup analyses suggested heterogeneity in treatment effects with possible benefit for men with both a triglyceride level ≥204 mg/dL (2.3 mmol/L) and an HDL cholesterol level ≤34 mg/dL (0.9 mmol/L).[102] A prospective trial of a newer fibrate in this specific population of patients is ongoing.[103]

Statin and Niacin

The Atherothrombosis Intervention in Metabolic Syndrome With Low HDL/High Triglycerides: Impact on Global Health Outcomes (AIM-HIGH) trial randomized over 3,000 patients (about one-third with diabetes) with established ASCVD, low LDL cholesterol levels (<180 mg/dL [4.7 mmol/L]), low HDL cholesterol levels (men <40 mg/dL [1.0 mmol/L] and women <50 mg/dL [1.3 mmol/L]), and triglyceride levels of 150–400 mg/dL (1.7–4.5 mmol/L) to statin therapy plus extended-release niacin or placebo. The trial was halted early due to lack of efficacy on the primary ASCVD outcome (first event of the composite of death from CHD, nonfatal MI, ischemic stroke, hospitalization for an ACS, or symptom-driven coronary or cerebral revascularization) and a possible increase in ischemic stroke in those on combination therapy.[104]

The much larger Heart Protection Study 2–Treatment of HDL to Reduce the Incidence of Vascular Events (HPS2-THRIVE) trial also failed to show a benefit of adding niacin to background statin therapy.[105] A total of 25,673 patients with prior vascular disease were randomized to receive 2 g of extended-release niacin and 40 mg of laropiprant (an antagonist of the prostaglandin D2 receptor DP_1 that has been shown to improve adherence to niacin therapy) versus a matching placebo daily and followed for a median follow-up period of 3.9 years. There was no significant difference in the rate of coronary death, MI, stroke, or coronary revascularization with the addition of niacin–laropiprant versus placebo (13.2% vs. 13.7%; rate ratio 0.96; $P = 0.29$). Niacin–laropiprant was associated with an increased incidence of new-onset diabetes (absolute excess, 1.3 percentage points; $P < 0.001$) and disturbances in diabetes control among those with diabetes. In addition, there was an increase in serious adverse events associated with the gastrointestinal system, musculoskeletal system, skin, and, unexpectedly, infection and bleeding.

Therefore, combination therapy with a statin and niacin is not recommended given the lack of efficacy on major ASCVD outcomes and increased side effects.

Diabetes with Statin Use

Several studies have reported a modestly increased risk of incident diabetes with statin use,[106,107] which may be limited to those with diabetes risk factors. An analysis of one of the initial studies suggested that although statin use was associated with diabetes risk, the cardiovascular event rate reduction with statins far outweighed the risk of incident diabetes even for patients at highest risk for diabetes.[108] The absolute risk increase was small (over 5 years of follow-up, 1.2% of participants on placebo developed diabetes and 1.5% on rosuvastatin developed diabetes).[108] A meta-analysis of 13 randomized statin trials with 91,140 participants showed an odds ratio of 1.09 for a new diagnosis of diabetes, so that (on average) treatment of 255 patients with statins for 4 years resulted in one additional case of diabetes while simultaneously preventing 5.4 vascular events among those 255 patients.[107]

Lipid-Lowering Agents and Cognitive Function

Although this issue has been raised, several lines of evidence point against this association, as detailed in a 2018 European Atherosclerosis Society Consensus Panel statement.[109] First, there are three large randomized trials of statin versus placebo where specific cognitive tests were performed, and no differences were seen between statin and placebo.[110–113] In addition, no change in cognitive function has been reported in studies with the addition of ezetimibe[90] or PCSK9 inhibitors[93,114] to statin therapy, including among patients treated to very low LDL cholesterol levels. In addition, the most recent systematic review of the U.S. Food and Drug Administration's (FDA's) postmarketing surveillance databases, randomized controlled trials, and cohort, case-control, and cross-sectional studies evaluating cognition in patients receiving statins found that published data do not reveal an adverse effect of statins on cognition.[115] Therefore, a concern that statins or other lipid-lowering agents might cause cognitive dysfunction or dementia is not currently supported by evidence and should not deter their use in individuals with diabetes at high risk for ASCVD.[115]

ANTIPLATELET AGENTS

Recommendations

10.30 Use aspirin therapy (75–162 mg/day) as a secondary prevention strategy in those with diabetes and a history of atherosclerotic cardiovascular disease. **A**

10.31 For patients with atherosclerotic cardiovascular disease and documented aspirin allergy, clopidogrel (75 mg/day) should be used. **B**

10.32 Dual antiplatelet therapy (with low-dose aspirin and a P2Y12 inhibitor) is reasonable for a year after an acute coronary syndrome **A** and may have benefits beyond this period. **B**

10.33 Aspirin therapy (75–162 mg/day) may be considered as a primary prevention strategy in those with diabetes who are at increased cardiovascular risk, after a discussion with the patient on the benefits versus increased risk of bleeding. **C**

Risk Reduction

Aspirin has been shown to be effective in reducing cardiovascular morbidity and mortality in high-risk patients with previous MI or stroke (secondary prevention) and is strongly recommended. In primary prevention, however, among patients with no previous cardiovascular events, its net benefit is more controversial.[116,117]

Previous randomized controlled trials of aspirin specifically in patients with diabetes failed to consistently show a significant reduction in overall ASCVD endpoints, raising questions about the efficacy of aspirin for primary prevention in people with diabetes, although some sex differences were suggested.[118–120]

The Antithrombotic Trialists' Collaboration published an individual patient-level meta-analysis[116] of the six large trials of aspirin for primary prevention in the general population. These trials collectively enrolled over 95,000 participants, including almost 4,000 with diabetes. Overall, they found that aspirin reduced the risk of serious vascular events by 12% (RR 0.88 [95% CI 0.82–0.94]). The largest reduction was for nonfatal MI, with little effect on CHD death (RR 0.95 [95% CI 0.78–1.15]) or total stroke.

Most recently, the ASCEND (A Study of Cardiovascular Events iN Diabetes) trial randomized 15,480 patients with diabetes but no evident cardiovascular disease to aspirin 100 mg daily or placebo.[121] The primary efficacy endpoint was vascular death, MI, or stroke or transient ischemic attack. The primary safety outcome was major bleeding (i.e., intracranial hemorrhage, sight-threatening bleeding in the eye, gastrointestinal bleeding, or other serious bleeding). During a mean follow-up of 7.4 years, there was a significant 12% reduction in the primary efficacy endpoint (8.5% vs. 9.6%; $P = 0.01$). In contrast, major bleeding was significantly increased from 3.2 to 4.1% in the aspirin group (rate ratio 1.29; $P = 0.003$), with most of the excess being gastrointestinal bleeding and other extracranial bleeding. There were no significant differences by sex, weight, or duration of diabetes or other baseline factors including ASCVD risk score.

Two other large randomized trials of aspirin for primary prevention, in patients without diabetes (ARRIVE [Aspirin to Reduce Risk of Initial Vascular Events])[122] and in the elderly (ASPREE [Aspirin in Reducing Events in the Elderly]),[123] including 11% with diabetes, found no benefit of aspirin on the primary efficacy endpoint and an increased risk of bleeding. In ARRIVE, with 12,546 patients over a period of 60 months follow-up, the primary endpoint occurred in 4.29% vs. 4.48% of patients in the aspirin versus placebo groups (HR 0.96 [95% CI 0.81–1.13]; $P = 0.60$). Gastrointestinal bleeding events (characterized as mild) occurred in 0.97% of patients in the aspirin group vs. 0.46% in the placebo group (HR 2.11 [95% CI 1.36–3.28]; $P = 0.0007$). In ASPREE, including 19,114 persons, for the rate of cardiovascular disease (fatal CHD, MI, stroke, or hospitalization for heart failure) after a median of 4.7 years of follow-up, the rates per 1,000 person-years were 10.7 vs. 11.3 events in aspirin vs. placebo groups (HR

0.95 [95% CI 0.83–1.08]). The rate of major hemorrhage per 1,000 person-years was 8.6 events vs. 6.2 events, respectively (HR 1.38 [95% CI 1.18–1.62]; $P < 0.001$).

Thus, aspirin appears to have a modest effect on ischemic vascular events, with the absolute decrease in events depending on the underlying ASCVD risk. The main adverse effect is an increased risk of gastrointestinal bleeding. The excess risk may be as high as 5 per 1,000 per year in real-world settings. However, for adults with ASCVD risk >1% per year, the number of ASCVD events prevented will be similar to the number of episodes of bleeding induced, although these complications do not have equal effects on long-term health.[124]

Treatment Considerations

In 2010, a position statement of the ADA, the American Heart Association, and the American College of Cardiology Foundation recommended that low-dose (75–162 mg/day) aspirin for primary prevention is reasonable for adults with diabetes and no previous history of vascular disease who are at increased ASCVD risk and who are not at increased risk for bleeding.[125] These recommendations for using aspirin as primary prevention include both men and women aged ≥50 years with diabetes and at least one additional major risk factor (family history of premature ASCVD, hypertension, dyslipidemia, smoking, or chronic kidney disease/albuminuria) who are not at increased risk of bleeding (e.g., older age, anemia, renal disease).[126–129] Noninvasive imaging techniques such as coronary computed tomography angiography may potentially help further tailor aspirin therapy, particularly in those at low risk,[130] but are not generally recommended. For patients over the age of 70 years (with or without diabetes), the balance appears to have greater risk than benefit.[121,123] Thus, for primary prevention, the use of aspirin needs to be carefully considered and may generally not be recommended. Aspirin may be considered in the context of high cardiovascular risk with low bleeding risk, but generally not in older adults. For patients with documented ASCVD, use of aspirin for secondary prevention has far greater benefit than risk; for this indication, aspirin is still recommended.[116]

Aspirin Use in People <50 Years of Age

Aspirin is not recommended for those at low risk of ASCVD (such as men and women aged <50 years with diabetes with no other major ASCVD risk factors) as the low benefit is likely to be outweighed by the risks of bleeding. Clinical judgment should be used for those at intermediate risk (younger patients with one or more risk factors or older patients with no risk factors) until further research is available. Patients' willingness to undergo long-term aspirin therapy should also be considered.[131] Aspirin use in patients aged <21 years is generally contraindicated due to the associated risk of Reye's syndrome.

Aspirin Dosing

Average daily dosages used in most clinical trials involving patients with diabetes ranged from 50 mg to 650 mg but were mostly in the range of 100–325 mg/day. There is little evidence to support any specific dose, but using the lowest possible dose may help to reduce side effects.[132] In the U.S., the most common low-dose tablet is 81 mg. Although platelets from patients with diabetes have altered function, it is unclear what, if any, effect that finding has on the required dose of aspirin for cardioprotective effects in the patient with diabetes. Many alternate pathways for platelet activation exist that are independent of thromboxane A_2 and thus are not sensitive to the effects of aspirin.[133] "Aspirin resistance" has been described in patients with diabetes when measured by a variety of ex vivo and in vitro methods (platelet aggregometry, measurement of thromboxane B_2),[134] but other studies suggest no impairment in aspirin response among patients with diabetes.[135] A recent trial suggested that more frequent dosing regimens of aspirin may reduce platelet reactivity in individuals with diabetes;[136] however, these observations alone are insufficient to empirically recommend that higher doses of aspirin be used in this group at this time. Another recent meta-analysis raised the hypothesis that low-dose aspirin efficacy is reduced in those weighing more than 70 kg;[137] however, the ASCEND trial found benefit of low-dose aspirin in those in this weight range, which would thus not validate this suggested hypothesis.[121] It appears that 75–162 mg/day is optimal.

Indications for P2Y12 Receptor Antagonist Use

A P2Y12 receptor antagonist in combination with aspirin should be used for at least 1 year in patients following an ACS and may have benefits beyond this period. Evidence supports use of either ticagrelor or clopidogrel if no percutaneous coronary intervention was performed and clopidogrel, ticagrelor, or prasugrel if a percutaneous coronary intervention was performed.[138] In patients with diabetes and prior MI (1–3 years before), adding ticagrelor to aspirin significantly reduces the risk of recurrent ischemic events including cardiovascular and CHD death.[139]

CARDIOVASCULAR DISEASE

RECOMMENDATIONS

Screening

10.34 In asymptomatic patients, routine screening for coronary artery disease is not recommended as it does not improve outcomes as long as atherosclerotic cardiovascular disease risk factors are treated. **A**

10.35 Consider investigations for coronary artery disease in the presence of any of the following: atypical cardiac symptoms (e.g., unexplained dyspnea, chest discomfort); signs or symptoms of associated vascular disease including carotid bruits, transient ischemic attack, stroke, claudication, or peripheral arterial disease; or electrocardiogram abnormalities (e.g., Q waves). **E**

Treatment

10.36 In patients with known atherosclerotic cardiovascular disease, consider ACE inhibitor or angiotensin receptor blocker therapy to reduce the risk of cardiovascular events. **B**

10.37 In patients with prior myocardial infarction, β-blockers should be continued for at least 2 years after the event. **B**

10.38 In patients with type 2 diabetes with stable congestive heart failure, metformin may be used if estimated glomerular filtration rate remains >30 mL/min but should be avoided in unstable or hospitalized patients with congestive heart failure. **B**

10.39 Among patients with type 2 diabetes who have established atherosclerotic cardiovascular disease, sodium–glucose cotransporter 2 inhibitors or glucagon-like peptide 1 receptor agonists with demonstrated cardiovascular disease benefit (Table 9.1 in the *Standards of Medical Care in Diabetes—2019* [DOI:10.2337/dc19-S009]) are recommended as part of the antihyperglycemic regimen. **A**

10.40 Among patients with atherosclerotic cardiovascular disease at high risk of heart failure or in whom heart failure coexists, sodium–glucose cotransporter 2 inhibitors are preferred. **C**

CARDIAC TESTING

Candidates for advanced or invasive cardiac testing include those with 1) typical or atypical cardiac symptoms and 2) an abnormal resting electrocardiogram (ECG). Exercise ECG testing without or with echocardiography may be used as the initial test. In adults with diabetes ≥40 years of age, measurement of coronary artery calcium is also reasonable for cardiovascular risk assessment. Pharmacologic stress echocardiography or nuclear imaging should be considered in individuals with diabetes in whom resting ECG abnormalities preclude exercise stress testing (e.g., left bundle branch block or ST-T abnormalities). In addition, individuals who require stress testing and are unable to exercise should undergo pharmacologic stress echocardiography or nuclear imaging.

SCREENING ASYMPTOMATIC PATIENTS

The screening of asymptomatic patients with high ASCVD risk is not recommended,[140] in part because these high-risk patients should already be receiving intensive medical therapy—an approach that provides similar benefit as invasive revascularization.[141,142] There is also some evidence that silent ischemia may reverse over time, adding to the controversy concerning aggressive screening strategies.[143] In prospective studies, coronary artery calcium has been established as an independent predictor of future ASCVD events in patients with diabetes and is consistently superior to both the UK Prospective Diabetes Study (UKPDS) risk engine and the Framingham Risk Score in predicting risk in this population.[144–146] However, a randomized observational trial demonstrated no clinical benefit to routine screening of asymptomatic patients with type 2 diabetes and normal ECGs.[147] Despite abnormal myocardial perfusion imaging in more than one in five patients, cardiac outcomes were essentially equal (and very low) in screened versus unscreened patients. Accordingly, indiscriminate screening is not considered cost-effective. Studies have found that a risk factor–based approach to the initial diagnostic evaluation and subsequent follow-up for coronary artery disease fails to identify which patients with type 2 diabetes will have silent ischemia on screening tests.[148,149]

Any benefit of newer noninvasive coronary artery disease screening methods, such as computed tomography calcium scoring and computed tomography angiography, to identify patient subgroups for different treatment strategies remains unproven in asymptomatic patients with diabetes, though research is ongoing. Although asymptomatic patients with diabetes with higher coronary disease burden have more future cardiac events,[144,150,151] the role of these tests beyond risk stratification is not clear.

While coronary artery screening methods, such as calcium scoring, may improve cardiovascular risk assessment in people with type 2 diabetes,[152] their routine use leads to radiation exposure and may result in unnecessary invasive testing such as coronary angiography and revascularization procedures. The ultimate balance of benefit, cost, and risks of such an approach in asymptomatic patients remains controversial, particularly in the modern setting of aggressive ASCVD risk factor control.

LIFESTYLE AND PHARMACOLOGIC INTERVENTIONS

Intensive lifestyle intervention focusing on weight loss through decreased caloric intake and increased physical activity as performed in the Action for Health in Diabetes (Look AHEAD) trial may be considered for improving glucose control, fitness, and some ASCVD risk factors.[153] Patients at increased ASCVD risk should receive aspirin and a statin and ACE inhibitor or ARB therapy if the patient has hypertension, unless there are contraindications to a particular drug class. While clear benefit exists for ACE inhibitor or ARB therapy in patients with diabetic kidney disease or hypertension, the benefits in patients with ASCVD in the absence of these conditions are less clear, especially when LDL cholesterol is concomitantly controlled.[154,155] In patients with prior MI, active angina, or HFrEF, β-blockers should be used.[156]

ANTIHYPERGLYCEMIC THERAPIES AND CARDIOVASCULAR OUTCOMES

In 2008, the FDA issued a guidance for industry to perform cardiovascular outcomes trials for all new medications for the treatment for type 2 diabetes amid concerns of increased cardiovascular risk.[157] Previously approved diabetes medications were not subject to the guidance. Recently published cardiovascular outcomes trials have provided additional data on cardiovascular outcomes in patients with type 2 diabetes with cardiovascular disease or at high risk for cardiovascular disease (see Table 17.4). Cardiovascular outcomes trials of dipeptidyl peptidase 4 (DPP-4) inhibitors have all, so far, not shown cardiovascular benefits relative to placebo. However, results from other new agents have provided a mix of results.

The BI 10773 (Empagliflozin) Cardiovascular Outcome Event Trial in Type 2 Diabetes Mellitus Patients (EMPA-REG OUTCOME) trial was a randomized, double-blind trial that assessed the effect of empagliflozin, an SGLT2 inhibitor, versus placebo on cardiovascular outcomes in 7,020 patients with type 2 diabetes and existing cardiovascular disease. Study participants had a mean age of 63 years, 57% had diabetes for more than 10 years, and 99% had established cardiovascular disease. EMPA-REG OUTCOME showed that over a median follow-up of

3.1 years, treatment reduced the composite outcome of MI, stroke, and cardiovascular death by 14% (absolute rate 10.5% vs. 12.1% in the placebo group, HR in the empagliflozin group 0.86 [95% CI 0.74–0.99]; $P = 0.04$ for superiority) and cardiovascular death by 38% (absolute rate 3.7% vs. 5.9%, HR 0.62 [95% CI 0.49–0.77]; $P < 0.001$).[8] The FDA added an indication for empagliflozin to reduce the risk of major adverse cardiovascular death in adults with type 2 diabetes and cardiovascular disease.

A second large cardiovascular outcomes trial program of an SGLT2 inhibitor, canagliflozin, has been reported.[9] The Canagliflozin Cardiovascular Assessment Study (CANVAS) integrated data from two trials, including the CANVAS trial that started in 2009 before the approval of canagliflozin and the CANVAS-Renal (CANVAS-R) trial that started in 2014 after the approval of canagliflozin. Combining both these trials, 10,142 participants with type 2 diabetes (two-thirds with established CVD) were randomized to canagliflozin or placebo and were followed for an average 3.6 years. The mean age of patients was 63 years and 66% had a history of cardiovascular disease. The combined analysis of the two trials found that canagliflozin significantly reduced the composite outcome of cardiovascular death, MI, or stroke versus placebo (occurring in 26.9 vs. 31.5 participants per 1,000 patient-years; HR 0.86 [95% CI 0.75–0.97]; $P < 0.001$ for noninferiority; $P = 0.02$ for superiority). The specific estimates for canagliflozin versus placebo on the primary composite cardiovascular outcome were HR 0.88 (0.75–1.03) for the CANVAS trial and 0.82 (0.66–1.01) for CANVAS-R, with no heterogeneity found between trials. In the combined analysis, there was not a statistically significant difference in cardiovascular death (HR 0.87 [95% CI 0.72–1.06]). The initial CANVAS trial was partially unblinded prior to completion because of the need to file interim cardiovascular outcomes data for regulatory approval of the drug.[158] Of note, there was an increased risk of lower limb amputation with canaglifozin (6.3 vs. 3.4 participants per 1,000 patient-years; HR 1.97 [95% CI 1.41–2.75]).[9]

The Liraglutide Effect and Action in Diabetes: Evaluation of Cardiovascular Outcome Results (LEADER) trial was a randomized, double-blind trial that assessed the effect of liraglutide, a glucagon-like peptide 1 (GLP-1) receptor agonist, versus placebo on cardiovascular outcomes in 9,340 patients with type 2 diabetes at high risk for cardiovascular disease or with cardiovascular disease. Study participants had a mean age of 64 years and a mean duration of diabetes of nearly 13 years. Over 80% of study participants had established cardiovascular disease. After a median follow-up of 3.8 years, LEADER showed that the primary composite outcome (MI, stroke, or cardiovascular death) occurred in fewer participants in the treatment group (13.0%) when compared with the placebo group (14.9%) (HR 0.87 [95% CI 0.78–0.97]; $P < 0.001$ for noninferiority; $P = 0.01$ for superiority). Deaths from cardiovascular causes were significantly reduced in the liraglutide group (4.7%) compared with the placebo group (6.0%) (HR 0.78 [95% CI 0.66–0.93]; $P = 0.007$).[159] The FDA approved the use of liraglutide to reduce the risk of major adverse cardiovascular events, including heart attack, stroke, and cardiovascular death, in adults with type 2 diabetes and established cardiovascular disease.

Results from a moderate-sized trial of another GLP-1 receptor agonist, semaglutide, were consistent with the LEADER trial.[160] Semaglutide is a once-weekly GLP-1 receptor agonist approved by the FDA for the treatment of type 2 diabetes. The Trial to Evaluate Cardiovascular and Other Long-term Outcomes With Semaglutide in Subjects With Type 2 Diabetes (SUSTAIN-6) was the initial randomized trial powered to test noninferiority of semaglutide for the purpose of initial regulatory approval. In this study, 3,297 patients with type 2 diabetes were randomized to receive once-weekly semaglutide (0.5 mg or 1.0 mg) or placebo for 2 years. The primary outcome (the first occurrence of cardiovascular death, nonfatal MI, or nonfatal stroke) occurred in 108 patients (6.6%) in the semaglutide group vs. 146 patients (8.9%) in the placebo group (HR 0.74 [95% CI 0.58–0.95]; $P < 0.001$). More patients discontinued treatment in the semaglutide group because of adverse events, mainly gastrointestinal.

The Evaluation of Lixisenatide in Acute Coronary Syndrome (ELIXA) trial studied the once-daily GLP-1 receptor agonist lixisenatide on cardiovascular outcomes in patients with type 2 diabetes who had had a recent acute coronary event.[161] A total of 6,068 patients with type 2 diabetes with a recent hospitalization for MI or unstable angina within the previous 180 days were randomized to receive lixisenatide or placebo in addition to standard care and were followed for a median of approximately 2.1 years. The primary outcome of cardiovascular death, MI, stroke, or hospitalization for unstable angina occurred in 406 patients (13.4%) in the lixisenatide group vs. 399 (13.2%) in the placebo group (HR 1.2 [95% CI 0.89–1.17]), which demonstrated the noninferiority of lixisenatide to placebo ($P < 0.001$) but did not show superiority ($P = 0.81$).

The Exenatide Study of Cardiovascular Event Lowering (EXSCEL) trial also reported results with the once-weekly GLP-1 receptor agonist extended-release exenatide and found that major adverse cardiovascular events were numerically lower with use of extended-release exenatide compared with placebo, although this difference was not statistically significant.[162] A total of 14,752 patients with type 2 diabetes (of whom 10,782 [73.1%] had previous cardiovascular disease) were randomized to receive extended-release exenatide 2 mg or placebo and followed for a median of 3.2 years. The primary endpoint of cardiovascular death, MI, or stroke occurred in 839 patients (11.4%; 3.7 events per 100 person-years) in the exenatide group and in 905 patients (12.2%; 4.0 events per 100 person-years) in the placebo group (HR 0.91 [95% CI 0.83–1.00]; $P < 0.001$ for noninferiority) but was not superior to placebo with respect to the primary endpoint ($P = 0.06$ for superiority). However, all-cause mortality was lower in the exenatide group (HR 0.86 [95% CI 0.77–0.97]). The incidence of acute pancreatitis, pancreatic cancer, medullary thyroid carcinoma, and serious adverse events did not differ significantly between the two groups.

The Harmony Outcomes trial randomized 9,463 patients with type 2 diabetes and cardiovascular disease to once-weekly subcutaneous albiglutide or matching placebo, in addition to their standard care. Over a median duration of 1.6 years, the GLP-1 receptor agonist reduced the risk of cardiovascular death, MI, or stroke to an incidence rate of 4.6 events per 100 person-years in the albiglutide group vs. 5.9 events in the placebo group (HR 0.78, $P = 0.0006$ for superiority).[163] This agent is not currently available for clinical use.

In summary, there are now several large randomized controlled trials reporting statistically significant reductions in cardiovascular events for two of the FDA-approved SGLT2 inhibitors (empagliflozin and canagliflozin) and three FDA-approved GLP-1 receptor agonists (liraglutide, albiglutide [although that

Table 17.4—Cardiovascular Outcomes Trials of Available Antihyperglycemic Medications Completed After the Issuance of the FDA 2008 Guidelines

	DPP-4 inhibitors			GLP-1 receptor agonists				SGLT2 inhibitors		
	SAVOR-TIMI 53 (168) (n = 16,492)	EXAMINE (175) (n = 5,380)	TECOS (171) (n = 14,671)	ELIXA (161) (n = 6,068)	LEADER (159) (n = 9,340)	SUSTAIN-6 (160)* (n = 3,297)	EXSCEL (162) (n = 14,752)	EMPA-REG OUTCOME (8) (n = 7,020)	CANVAS (9) (n = 4,330)	CANVAS-R (9) (n = 5,812)
Intervention	Saxagliptin/placebo	Alogliptin/placebo	Sitagliptin/placebo	Lixisenatide/placebo	Liraglutide/placebo	Semaglutide/placebo	Exenatide QW/placebo	Empagliflozin/placebo	Canagliflozin/placebo	
Main inclusion criteria	Type 2 diabetes and history of or multiple risk factors for CVD	Type 2 diabetes and ACS within 15–90 days before randomization	Type 2 diabetes and preexisting CVD	Type 2 diabetes and history of ACS (<180 days)	Type 2 diabetes and preexisting CVD, kidney disease, or HF at ≥50 years of age or cardiovascular risk at ≥60 years of age	Type 2 diabetes and preexisting CVD, HF, or CKD at ≥50 years of age or cardiovascular risk at ≥60 years of age	Type 2 diabetes with or without preexisting CVD	Type 2 diabetes and preexisting CVD	Type 2 diabetes and preexisting CVD at ≥30 years of age or >2 cardiovascular risk factors at ≥50 years of age	
A1C inclusion criteria (%)	≥6.5	6.5–11.0	6.5–8.0	5.5–11.0	≥7.0	≥7.0	6.5–10.0	7.0–10.0	7.0–10.5	
Age (years)††	65.1	61.0	65.4	60.3	64.3	64.6	62	63.1	63.3	
Diabetes duration (years)††	10.3	7.1	11.6	9.3	12.8	13.9	12	57% >10	13.5	
Median follow-up (years)	2.1	1.5	3.0	2.1	3.8	2.1	3.2	3.1	5.7	2.1
Statin use (%)	78	91	80	93	72	73	74	77	75	
Metformin use (%)	70	66	82	66	76	73	77	74	77	

(continued)

Table 17.4 (continued)

	DPP-4 inhibitors			GLP-1 receptor agonists				SGLT2 inhibitors		
	SAVOR-TIMI 53 (168) (n = 16,492)	EXAMINE (175) (n = 5,380)	TECOS (171) (n = 14,671)	ELIXA (161) (n = 6,068)	LEADER (159) (n = 9,340)	SUSTAIN-6 (160)* (n = 3,297)	EXSCEL (162) (n = 14,752)	EMPA-REG OUTCOME (8) (n = 7,020)	CANVAS (9) (n = 4,330)	CANVAS-R (9) (n = 5,812)
Prior CVD/CHF (%)	78/13	100/28	74/18	100/22	81/18	60/24	73.1/16.2	99/10	65.6/14.4	
Mean baseline A1C (%)	8.0	8.0	7.2	7.7	8.7	8.7	8.0	8.1	8.2	
Mean difference in A1C between groups at end of treatment (%)	−0.3^	−0.3^	−0.3^	−0.3^	−0.4^	−0.7 or −1.0^†	−0.53^	−0.3^‡	−0.58^	
Year started/reported	2010/2013	2009/2013	2008/2015	2010/2015	2010/2016	2013/2016	2010/2017	2010/2015	2009/2017	
Primary outcome§	3-point MACE 1.00 (0.89–1.12)	3-point MACE 0.96 (95% UL ≤1.16)	4-point MACE 0.98 (0.89–1.08)	4-point MACE 1.02 (0.89–1.17)	3-point MACE 0.87 (0.78–0.97)	3-point MACE 0.74 (0.58–0.95)	3-point MACE 0.91 (0.83–1.00)	3-point MACE 0.86 (0.74–0.99)	3-point MACE 0.86 (0.75–0.97)§	Progression to albumin-uria** 0.73 (0.47–0.77)
Key secondary outcome§	Expanded MACE 1.02 (0.94–1.11)	4-point MACE 0.95 (95% UL ≤1.14)	3-point MACE 0.99 (0.89–1.10)	Expanded MACE 1.00 (0.90–1.11)	Expanded MACE 0.88 (0.81–0.96)	Expanded MACE 0.74 (0.62–0.89)	Individual components of MACE (see below)	4-point MACE 0.89 (0.78–1.01)	All-cause and cardiovascular mortality (see below)	40% reduction in composite eGFR, renal replacement, renal death 0.60 (0.47–0.77)
Cardiovascular death§	1.03 (0.87–1.22)	0.85 (0.66–1.10)	1.03 (0.89–1.19)	0.98 (0.78–1.22)	0.78 (0.66–0.93)	0.98 (0.65–1.48)	0.88 (0.76–1.02)	0.62 (0.49–0.77)	0.96 (0.77–1.18)¶	0.87 (0.72–1.06)#
MI§	0.95 (0.80–1.12)	1.08 (0.88–1.33)	0.95 (0.81–1.11)	1.03 (0.87–1.22)	0.86 (0.73–1.00)	0.74 (0.51–1.08)	0.97 (0.85–1.10)	0.87 (0.70–1.09)	0.85 (0.65–1.11)	0.85 (0.61–1.19)

(continued)

Table 17.4 (continued)

	DPP-4 inhibitors			GLP-1 receptor agonists				SGLT2 inhibitors		
	SAVOR-TIMI 53 (168) (n = 16,492)	EXAMINE (175) (n = 5,380)	TECOS (171) (n = 14,671)	ELIXA (161) (n = 6,068)	LEADER (159) (n = 9,340)	SUSTAIN-6 (160)* (n = 3,297)	EXSCEL (162) (n = 14,752)	EMPA-REG OUTCOME (8) (n = 7,020)	CANVAS (9) (n = 4,330)	CANVAS-R (9) (n = 5,812)
Stroke§	1.11 (0.88–1.39)	0.91 (0.55–1.50)	0.97 (0.79–1.19)	1.12 (0.79–1.58)	0.86 (0.71–1.06)	0.61 (0.38–0.99)	0.85 (0.70–1.03)	1.18 (0.89–1.56)	0.97 (0.70–1.35)	0.82 (0.57–1.18)
HF hospitalization§	1.27 (1.07–1.51)	1.19 (0.90–1.58)	1.00 (0.83–1.20)	0.96 (0.75–1.23)	0.87 (0.73–1.05)	1.11 (0.77–1.61)	0.94 (0.78–1.13)	0.65 (0.50–0.85)	0.77 (0.55–1.08)	0.56 (0.38–0.83)
Unstable angina hospitalizations§	1.19 (0.89–1.60)	0.90 (0.60–1.37)	0.90 (0.70–1.16)	1.11 (0.47–2.62)	0.98 (0.76–1.26)	0.82 (0.47–1.44)	1.05 (0.94–1.18)	0.99 (0.74–1.34)	—	
All-cause mortality§	1.11 (0.96–1.27)	0.88 (0.71–1.09)	1.01 (0.90–1.14)	0.94 (0.78–1.13)	0.85 (0.74–0.97)	1.05 (0.74–1.50)	0.86 (0.77–0.97)	0.68 (0.57–0.82)	0.87 (0.74–1.01)‡‡	0.90 (0.76–1.07)##
Worsening nephropathy§||	1.08 (0.88–1.32)	—	—	—	0.78 (0.67–0.92)	0.64 (0.46–0.88)	—	0.61 (0.53–0.70)	0.60 (0.47–0.77)	

—, not assessed/reported; ACS, acute coronary syndrome; CHF, congestive heart failure; CKD, chronic kidney disease; CVD, cardiovascular disease; DPP-4, dipeptidyl peptidase 4; eGFR, estimated glomerular filtration rate; GLP-1, glucagon-like peptide 1; HF, heart failure; MACE, major adverse cardiac event; MI, myocardial infarction; SGLT2, sodium–glucose cotransporter 2; UL, upper limit. Data from this table was adapted from Cefalu et al.[176] in the January 2018 issue of *Diabetes Care*. *Powered to rule out a hazard ratio of 1.8; superiority hypothesis not prespecified. **On the basis of prespecified outcomes, the renal outcomes are not viewed as statistically significant. ††Age was reported as means in all trials except EXAMINE, which reported medians; diabetes duration was reported as means in all but four trials, with SAVOR-TIMI 58, EXAMINE, and EXSCEL reporting medians and EMPA-REG OUTCOME reporting as percentage of population with diabetes duration >10 years. †A1C change of 0.66% with 0.5 mg- and 1.05% with 1-mg dose of semaglutide. ‡A1C change of 0.30 in EMPA-REG OUTCOME is based on pooled results for both doses (i.e., 0.24% for 10 mg and 0.36% for 25 mg of empagliflozin). §Outcomes reported as hazard ratio (95% CI). ||Worsening nephropathy is defined as the new onset of urine albumin-to-creatinine ratio >300 mg/g creatinine or a doubling of the serum creatinine level and an estimated glomerular filtration rate of <45 mL/min/1.73 m², the need for continuous renal-replacement therapy, or death from renal disease in EMPA-REG OUTCOME, LEADER, and SUSTAIN-6 and as doubling of creatinine level, initiation of dialysis, renal transplantation, or creatinine >6.0 mg/dL (530 mmol/L) in SAVOR-TIMI 53. Worsening nephropathy was a prespecified exploratory adjudicated outcome in SAVOR-TIMI 53, LEADER, and SUSTAIN-6 but not in EMPA-REG OUTCOME. ¶Significant difference in A1C between groups (*P* < 0.05). #Nontruncated data set. ‡‡Truncated integrated data set (refers to pooled data from CANVAS after 20 November 2012 plus CANVAS-R; prespecified in treating hierarchy as the principal data set for analysis for superiority of all-cause mortality and cardiovascular death in the CANVAS Program). ##Nontruncated integrated data (refers to pooled data from CANVAS, including before 20 November 2012 plus CANVAS-R).

agent was removed from the market for business reasons], and semaglutide [lower risk of cardiovascular events in a moderate-sized clinical trial but one not powered as a cardiovascular outcomes trial]). In these trials, the majority, if not all, patients in the trial had ASCVD. The empagliflozin and liraglutide trials further demonstrated significant reductions in cardiovascular death. Once-weekly exenatide did not have statistically significant reductions in major adverse cardiovascular events or cardiovascular mortality but did have a significant reduction in all-cause mortality. In contrast, other GLP-1 receptor agonists have not shown similar reductions in cardiovascular events (Table 17.4). Additional large randomized trials of other agents in these classes are ongoing.

Of note, these studies examined the drugs in combination with metformin (Table 17.4) in the great majority of patients for whom metformin was not contraindicated or was tolerated. For patients with type 2 diabetes who have ASCVD, on lifestyle and metformin therapy, it is recommended to incorporate an agent with strong evidence for cardiovascular risk reduction, especially those with proven reduction of cardiovascular death, after consideration of drug-specific patient factors (Table 9.1). See Figure 9.1 in the *Standards of Medical Care in Diabetes—2019* (DOI:10.2337/dc19-S009) for additional recommendations on antihyperglycemic treatment in adults with type 2 diabetes.

Antihyperglycemic Therapies and Heart Failure

As many as 50% of patients with type 2 diabetes may develop heart failure.[164] Data on the effects of glucose-lowering agents on heart failure outcomes have demonstrated that thiazolidinediones have a strong and consistent relationship with increased risk of heart failure.[165-167] Therefore, thiazolidinedione use should be avoided in patients with symptomatic heart failure.

Recent studies have also examined the relationship between DPP-4 inhibitors and heart failure and have had mixed results. The Saxagliptin Assessment of Vascular Outcomes Recorded in Patients with Diabetes Mellitus – Thrombolysis in Myocardial Infarction 53 (SAVOR-TIMI 53) study showed that patients treated with saxagliptin (a DPP-4 inhibitor) were more likely to be hospitalized for heart failure than those given placebo (3.5% vs. 2.8%, respectively).[168] Two other recent multicenter, randomized, double-blind, noninferiority trials, Examination of Cardiovascular Outcomes with Alogliptin versus Standard of Care (EXAMINE) and Trial Evaluating Cardiovascular Outcomes with Sitagliptin (TECOS), did not show associations between DPP-4 inhibitor use and heart failure. The FDA reported that the hospital admission rate for heart failure in EXAMINE was 3.9% for patients randomly assigned to alogliptin compared with 3.3% for those randomly assigned to placebo.[169] Alogliptin had no effect on the composite endpoint of cardiovascular death and hospital admission for heart failure in the post hoc analysis (HR 1.0 [95% CI 0.82–1.21]).[170] TECOS showed no difference in the rate of heart failure hospitalization for the sitagliptin group (3.1%; 1.07 per 100 person-years) compared with the placebo group (3.1%; 1.09 per 100 person-years).[171]

In four cardiovascular outcome trials of GLP-1 receptor agonists, no evidence for an increased risk of heart failure was found and the agents had a neutral effect on hospitalization for heart failure.[159-162]

A benefit on the incidence of heart failure has been observed with the use of some SGLT2 inhibitors. In EMPA-REG OUTCOME, the addition of empagliflozin to standard care led to a significant 35% reduction in hospitalization for heart failure compared with placebo.[8] Although the majority of patients in the study did not have heart failure at baseline, this benefit was consistent in patients with and without a prior history of heart failure.[172] Similarly, in CANVAS, there was a 33% reduction in hospitalization for heart failure with canagliflozin versus placebo.[9] Although heart failure hospitalizations were prospectively adjudicated in both trials, the type(s) of heart failure events prevented were not characterized. These preliminary findings, which strongly suggest heart failure–related benefits of SGLT2 inhibitors (particularly the prevention of heart failure), are being followed up with new outcomes trials in patients with established heart failure, both with and without diabetes, to determine their efficacy in treatment of heart failure.

REFERENCES

1. American Diabetes Association. Economic costs of diabetes in the U.S. in 2017. *Diabetes Care* 2018;41:917–928

2. Ali MK, Bullard KM, Saaddine JB, Cowie CC, Imperatore G, Gregg EW. Achievement of goals in U.S. diabetes care, 1999–2010. *N Engl J Med* 2013;368:1613–1624

3. Buse JB, Ginsberg HN, Bakris GL, et al.; American Heart Association; American Diabetes Association. Primary prevention of cardiovascular diseases in people with diabetes mellitus: a scientific statement from the American Heart Association and the American Diabetes Association. *Diabetes Care* 2007;30:162–172

4. Gaede P, Lund-Andersen H, Parving H-H, Pedersen O. Effect of a multifactorial intervention on mortality in type 2 diabetes. *N Engl J Med* 2008;358:580–591

5. Cavender MA, Steg PG, Smith SC Jr., et al.; REACH Registry Investigators. Impact of diabetes mellitus on hospitalization for heart failure, cardiovascular events, and death: outcomes at 4 years from the Reduction of Atherothrombosis for Continued Health (REACH) registry. *Circulation* 2015;132:923–931

6. McAllister DA, Read S, Kerssens J, et al. Incidence of hospitalisation for heart failure and case-fatality among 3.25 million people with and without diabetes. *Circulation*. 27 June 2018 [Epub ahead of print]. DOI:10.1161/CIRCULATIONAHA.118.034986

7. Lam CSP, Voors AA, de Boer RA, Solomon SD, van Veldhuisen DJ. Heart failure with preserved ejection fraction: from mechanisms to therapies. *Eur Heart J* 2018;39:2780–2792

8. Zinman B, Wanner C, Lachin JM, et al.; EMPA-REG OUTCOME Investigators. Empagliflozin, cardiovascular outcomes, and mortality in type 2 diabetes. *N Engl J Med* 2015;373:2117–2128

9. Neal B, Perkovic V, Mahaffey KW, et al.; CANVAS Program Collaborative Group. Canagliflozin and cardiovascular and renal events in type 2 diabetes. *N Engl J Med* 2017;377:644–657

10. Fitchett D, Butler J, van de Borne P, et al.; EMPA-REG OUTCOME® trial investigators. Effects of empagliflozin on risk for cardiovascular death and heart failure hospitalization across the spectrum of heart failure risk in the EMPA-REG OUTCOME® trial. *Eur Heart J* 2018;39:363–370

11. Blood Pressure Lowering Treatment Trialists' Collaboration. Blood pressure-lowering treatment based on cardiovascular risk: a meta-analysis of individual patient data. *Lancet* 2014;384:591–598

12. Grundy SM, Stone NJ, Bailey AL, et al. 2018 AHA/ACC/AACVPR/AAPA/ABC/ACPM/ADA/AGS/APhA/ASPC/NLA/PCNA guideline on the management of blood cholesterol: a report of the American College of Cardiology/American Heart Association Task Force on Clinical Practice Guidelines. *J Am Coll Cardiol*. November 2018 [Epub ahead of print]. DOI:10.1016/j.jacc.2018.11.003

13. Muntner P, Colantonio LD, Cushman M, et al. Validation of the atherosclerotic cardiovascular disease Pooled Cohort risk equations. *JAMA* 2014; 311:1406–1415

14. DeFilippis AP, Young R, McEvoy JW, et al. Risk score overestimation: the impact of individual cardiovascular risk factors and preventive therapies on the performance of the American Heart Association-American College of Cardiology-Atherosclerotic Cardiovascular Disease risk score in a modern multi-ethnic cohort. *Eur Heart J* 2017;38:598–608

15. Bohula EA, Morrow DA, Giugliano RP, et al. Atherothrombotic risk stratification and ezetimibe for secondary prevention. *J Am Coll Cardiol* 2017;69:911–921

16. Bohula EA, Bonaca MP, Braunwald E, et al. Atherothrombotic risk stratification and the efficacy and safety of vorapaxar in patients with stable ischemic heart disease and previous myocardial infarction. *Circulation* 2016;134:304–313

17. de Boer IH, Bangalore S, Benetos A, et al. Diabetes and hypertension: a position statement by the American Diabetes Association. *Diabetes Care* 2017;40:1273–1284

18. Bobrie G, Genes N, Vaur L, et al. Is "isolated home" hypertension as opposed to "isolated office" hypertension a sign of greater cardiovascular risk? *Arch Intern Med* 2001;161:2205–2211

19. Sega R, Facchetti R, Bombelli M, et al. Prognostic value of ambulatory and home blood pressures compared with office blood pressure in the general population: follow-up results from the Pressioni Arteriose Monitorate e Loro Associazioni (PAMELA) study. *Circulation* 2005;111:1777–1783

20. Omboni S, Gazzola T, Carabelli G, Parati G. Clinical usefulness and cost effectiveness of home blood pressure telemonitoring: meta-analysis of randomized controlled studies. *J Hypertens* 2013;31:455–467; discussion 467–468

21. Emdin CA, Rahimi K, Neal B, Callender T, Perkovic V, Patel A. Blood pressure lowering in type 2 diabetes: a systematic review and meta-analysis. *JAMA* 2015;313:603–615

22. Arguedas JA, Leiva V, Wright JM. Blood pressure targets for hypertension in people with diabetes mellitus. *Cochrane Database Syst Rev* 2013;10:CD008277

23. Ettehad D, Emdin CA, Kiran A, et al. Blood pressure lowering for prevention of cardiovascular disease and death: a systematic review and meta-analysis. *Lancet* 2016;387:957–967

24. Brunström M, Carlberg B. Effect of antihypertensive treatment at different blood pressure levels in patients with diabetes mellitus: systematic review and meta-analyses. *BMJ* 2016;352:i717

25. Bangalore S, Kumar S, Lobach I, Messerli FH. Blood pressure targets in subjects with type 2 diabetes mellitus/impaired fasting glucose: observations from traditional and Bayesian random-effects meta-analyses of randomized trials. *Circulation* 2011;123:2799–2810

26. Thomopoulos C, Parati G, Zanchetti A. Effects of blood-pressure-lowering treatment on outcome incidence in hypertension: 10 - should blood pressure management differ in hypertensive patients with and without diabetes mellitus? Overview and meta-analyses of randomized trials. *J Hypertens* 2017;35:922–944

27. Xie X, Atkins E, Lv J, et al. Effects of intensive blood pressure lowering on cardiovascular and renal outcomes: updated systematic review and meta-analysis. *Lancet* 2016;387:435–443

28. Cushman WC, Evans GW, Byington RP, et al.; ACCORD Study Group. Effects of intensive blood-pressure control in type 2 diabetes mellitus. *N Engl J Med* 2010;362:1575–1585

29. Patel A, MacMahon S, Chalmers J, et al.; ADVANCE Collaborative Group. Effects of a fixed combination of perindopril and indapamide on macrovascular and microvascular outcomes in patients with type 2 diabetes mellitus (the ADVANCE trial): a randomised controlled trial. *Lancet* 2007;370: 829–840

30. Bakris GL. The implications of blood pressure measurement methods on treatment targets for blood pressure. *Circulation* 2016;134:904–905

31. Margolis KL, O'Connor PJ, Morgan TM, et al. Outcomes of combined cardiovascular risk factor management strategies in type 2 diabetes: the ACCORD randomized trial. *Diabetes Care* 2014;37:1721–1728

32. Buckley LF, Dixon DL, Wohlford GF IV, Wijesinghe DS, Baker WL, Van Tassell BW. Intensive versus standard blood pressure control in SPRINT-eligible participants of ACCORD-BP [published correction appears in *Diabetes Care* 2018;41:2048]. *Diabetes Care* 2017;40:1733–1738

33. Brouwer TF, Vehmeijer JT, Kalkman DN, et al. Intensive blood pressure lowering in patients with and patients without type 2 diabetes: a pooled analysis from two randomized trials. *Diabetes Care* 2018;41:1142–1148

34. Lamprea-Montealegre JA, de Boer IH. Reevaluating the evidence for blood pressure targets in type 2 diabetes. *Diabetes Care* 2018;41:1132–1133

35. de Boer IH, Bakris G, Cannon CP. Individualizing blood pressure targets for people with diabetes and hypertension: comparing the ADA and the ACC/AHA recommendations. *JAMA* 2018;319:1319–1320

36. Basu S, Sussman JB, Rigdon J, Steimle L, Denton BT, Hayward RA. Benefit and harm of intensive blood pressure treatment: derivation and validation of risk models using data from the SPRINT and ACCORD trials. *PLoS Med* 2017;14:e1002410

37. Phillips RA, Xu J, Peterson LE, Arnold RM, Diamond JA, Schussheim AE. Impact of cardiovascular risk on the relative benefit and harm of intensive treatment of hypertension. *J Am Coll Cardiol* 2018;71:1601–1610

38. Whelton PK, Carey RM, Aronow WS, et al. 2017 ACC/AHA/AAPA/ABC/ACPM/AGS/APhA/ASH/ASPC/NMA/PCNA guideline for the prevention, detection, evaluation, and management of high blood pressure in adults: a report of the American College of Cardiology/American Heart Association Task Force on Clinical Practice Guidelines. *J Am Coll Cardiol* 2018;71:e127–e248

39. Wright JT Jr., Williamson JD, Whelton PK, et al.; SPRINT Research Group. A randomized trial of intensive versus standard blood-pressure control. *N Engl J Med* 2015;373:2103–2116

40. Beddhu S, Greene T, Boucher R, et al. Intensive systolic blood pressure control and incident chronic kidney disease in people with and without diabetes mellitus: secondary analyses of two randomised controlled trials. *Lancet Diabetes Endocrinol* 2018;6:555–563

41. Sink KM, Evans GW, Shorr RI, et al. Syncope, hypotension, and falls in the treatment of hypertension: results from the randomized clinical Systolic Blood Pressure Intervention Trial. *J Am Geriatr Soc* 2018;66:679–686

42. American College of Obstetricians and Gynecologists' Task Force on Hypertension in Pregnancy. Hypertension in pregnancy. Report of the American College of Obstetricians and Gynecologists' Task Force on Hypertension in Pregnancy. *Obstet Gynecol* 2013;122:1122–1131

43. Abalos E, Duley L, Steyn DW. Antihypertensive drug therapy for mild to moderate hypertension during pregnancy. *Cochrane Database Syst Rev* 2014;2:CD002252

44. Al-Balas M, Bozzo P, Einarson A. Use of diuretics during pregnancy. *Can Fam Physician* 2009;55:44–45

45. Irgens HU, Reisaeter L, Irgens LM, Lie RT. Long term mortality of mothers and fathers after pre-eclampsia: population based cohort study. *BMJ* 2001;323:1213–1217

46. Sacks FM, Svetkey LP, Vollmer WM, et al.; DASH-Sodium Collaborative Research Group. Effects on blood pressure of reduced dietary sodium and the Dietary Approaches to Stop Hypertension (DASH) diet. *N Engl J Med* 2001;344:3–10

47. James PA, Oparil S, Carter BL, et al. 2014 evidence-based guideline for the management of high blood pressure in adults: report from the panel members appointed to the Eighth Joint National Committee (JNC 8). *JAMA* 2014;311:507–520

48. Bakris GL, Weir MR; Study of Hypertension and the Efficacy of Lotrel in Diabetes (SHIELD) Investigators. Achieving goal blood pressure in patients with type 2 diabetes: conventional versus fixed-dose combination approaches. *J Clin Hypertens* (Greenwich) 2003;5:202–209

49. Feldman RD, Zou GY, Vandervoort MK, Wong CJ, Nelson SAE, Feagan BG. A simplified approach to the treatment of uncomplicated hypertension: a cluster randomized, controlled trial. *Hypertension* 2009;53:646–653

50. Webster R, Salam A, de Silva HA, Selak V, Stepien S, Rajapakse S, et al. Fixed low-dose triple combination antihypertensive medication vs usual care for blood pressure control in patients with mild to moderate hypertension in Sri Lanka: a randomized clinical trial. *JAMA* 2018;320:566–579

51. Bangalore S, Kamalakkannan G, Parkar S, Messerli FH. Fixed-dose combinations improve medication compliance: a meta-analysis. *Am J Med* 2007;120:713–719

52. Catalá-López F, Macías Saint-Gerons D, González-Bermejo D, et al. Cardiovascular and renal outcomes of renin-angiotensin system blockade in adult patients with diabetes mellitus: a systematic review with network meta-analyses. *PLoS Med* 2016;13:e1001971

53. Palmer SC, Mavridis D, Navarese E, et al. Comparative efficacy and safety of blood pressure-lowering agents in adults with diabetes and kidney disease: a network meta-analysis. *Lancet* 2015;385:2047–2056

54. Barzilay JI, Davis BR, Bettencourt J, et al.; ALLHAT Collaborative Research Group. Cardiovascular outcomes using doxazosin vs. chlorthalidone for the treatment of hypertension in older adults with and without glucose disorders: a report from the ALLHAT study. *J Clin Hypertens* (Greenwich) 2004;6:116–125

55. Weber MA, Bakris GL, Jamerson K, et al.; ACCOMPLISH Investigators. Cardiovascular events during differing hypertension therapies in patients with diabetes. *J Am Coll Cardiol* 2010;56:77–85

56. Bangalore S, Fakheri R, Toklu B, Messerli FH. Diabetes mellitus as a compelling indication for use of renin angiotensin system blockers: systematic review and meta-analysis of randomized trials. *BMJ* 2016;352:i438

57. Carlberg B, Samuelsson O, Lindholm LH. Atenolol in hypertension: is it a wise choice? *Lancet* 2004;364:1684–1689

58. Yusuf S, Teo KK, Pogue J, et al.; ONTARGET Investigators. Telmisartan, ramipril, or both in patients at high risk for vascular events. *N Engl J Med* 2008;358:1547–1559

59. Fried LF, Emanuele N, Zhang JH, et al.; VA NEPHRON-D Investigators. Combined angiotensin inhibition for the treatment of diabetic nephropathy. *N Engl J Med* 2013;369:1892–1903

60. Makani H, Bangalore S, Desouza KA, Shah A, Messerli FH. Efficacy and safety of dual blockade of the renin-angiotensin system: meta-analysis of randomised trials. *BMJ* 2013;346:f360

61. Zhao P, Xu P, Wan C, Wang Z. Evening versus morning dosing regimen drug therapy for hypertension. *Cochrane Database Syst Rev* 2011;10:CD004184

62. Hermida RC, Ayala DE, Mojón A, Fernández JR. Influence of time of day of blood pressure-lowering treatment on cardiovascular risk in hypertensive patients with type 2 diabetes. *Diabetes Care* 2011;34:1270–1276

63. Nilsson E, Gasparini A, Ärnlöv J, et al. Incidence and determinants of hyperkalemia and hypokalemia in a large healthcare system. *Int J Cardiol* 2017;245:277–284

64. Bandak G, Sang Y, Gasparini A, et al. Hyperkalemia after initiating renin-angiotensin system blockade: the Stockholm Creatinine Measurements (SCREAM) project. *J Am Heart Assoc* 2017;6:e005428

65. Hughes-Austin JM, Rifkin DE, Beben T, et al. The relation of serum potassium concentration with cardiovascular events and mortality in community-living individuals. *Clin J Am Soc Nephrol* 2017;12:245–252

66. James MT, Grams ME, Woodward M, et al.; CKD Prognosis Consortium. A meta-analysis of the association of estimated GFR, albuminuria, diabetes mellitus, and hypertension with acute kidney injury. *Am J Kidney Dis* 2015;66:602–612

67. Iliescu R, Lohmeier TE, Tudorancea I, Laffin L, Bakris GL. Renal denervation for the treatment of resistant hypertension: review and clinical perspective. *Am J Physiol Renal Physiol* 2015;309:F583–F594

68. Bakris GL, Agarwal R, Chan JC, et al.; Mineralocorticoid Receptor Antagonist Tolerability Study–Diabetic Nephropathy (ARTS-DN) Study Group. Effect of finerenone on albuminuria in patients with diabetic nephropathy: a randomized clinical trial. *JAMA* 2015;314:884–894

69. Williams B, MacDonald TM, Morant S, et al.; British Hypertension Society's PATHWAY Studies Group. Spironolactone versus placebo, bisoprolol, and doxazosin to determine the optimal treatment for drug-resistant hypertension (PATHWAY-2): a randomised, double-blind, crossover trial. *Lancet* 2015;386:2059–2068

70. Filippatos G, Anker SD, Böhm M, et al. A randomized controlled study of finerenone vs. eplerenone in patients with worsening chronic heart failure and diabetes mellitus and/or chronic kidney disease. *Eur Heart J* 2016;37:2105–2114

71. Bomback AS, Klemmer PJ. Mineralocorticoid receptor blockade in chronic kidney disease. *Blood Purif* 2012;33:119–124

72. Jensen MD, Ryan DH, Apovian CM, et al.; American College of Cardiology/American Heart Association Task Force on Practice Guidelines; Obesity Society. 2013 AHA/ACC/TOS guideline for the management of overweight and obesity in adults: a report of the American College of Cardiology/American Heart Association Task Force on Practice Guidelines and The Obesity Society. *J Am Coll Cardiol* 2014;129(25 Suppl. 2):S102–S138

73. Estruch R, Ros E, Salas-Salvadó J, et al.; PREDIMED Study Investigators. Primary prevention of cardiovascular disease with a Mediterranean diet supplemented with extra-virgin olive oil or nuts. *N Engl J Med* 2018;378:e34

74. Eckel RH, Jakicic JM, Ard JD, et al. 2013 AHA/ACC guideline on lifestyle management to reduce cardiovascular risk: a report of the American College of Cardiology/American Heart Association Task Force on Practice Guidelines. *Circulation* 2013;129:S76–S99

75. Chasman DI, Posada D, Subrahmanyan L, Cook NR, Stanton VP Jr., Ridker PM. Pharmacogenetic study of statin therapy and cholesterol reduction. *JAMA* 2004;291:2821–2827

76. Meek C, Wierzbicki AS, Jewkes C, et al. Daily and intermittent rosuvastatin 5 mg therapy in statin intolerant patients: an observational study. *Curr Med Res Opin* 2012;28:371–378

77. Mihaylova B, Emberson J, Blackwell L, et al.; Cholesterol Treatment Trialists' (CTT) Collaborators. The effects of lowering LDL cholesterol with statin therapy in people at low risk of vascular disease: meta-analysis of individual data from 27 randomised trials. *Lancet* 2012;380:581–590

78. Baigent C, Keech A, Kearney PM, et al.; Cholesterol Treatment Trialists' (CTT) Collaborators. Efficacy and safety of cholesterol-lowering treatment: prospective meta-analysis of data from 90,056 participants in 14 randomised trials of statins. *Lancet* 2005;366:1267–1278

79. Pyörälä K, Pedersen TR, Kjekshus J, Faergeman O, Olsson AG, Thorgeirsson G. Cholesterol lowering with simvastatin improves prognosis of diabetic patients with coronary heart disease. A subgroup analysis of the Scandinavian Simvastatin Survival Study (4S). *Diabetes Care* 1997;20:614–620

80. Collins R, Armitage J, Parish S, Sleigh P, Peto R; Heart Protection Study Collaborative Group. MRC/BHF Heart Protection Study of cholesterol-lowering with simvastatin in 5963 people with diabetes: a randomised placebo-controlled trial. *Lancet* 2003;361:2005–2016

81. Goldberg RB, Mellies MJ, Sacks FM, et al.; The Care Investigators. Cardiovascular events and their reduction with pravastatin in diabetic and glucose-intolerant myocardial infarction survivors with average cholesterol levels: subgroup analyses in the Cholesterol and Recurrent Events (CARE) trial. *Circulation* 1998;98:2513–2519

82. Shepherd J, Barter P, Carmena R, et al. Effect of lowering LDL cholesterol substantially below currently recommended levels in patients with coronary heart disease and diabetes: the Treating to New Targets (TNT) study. *Diabetes Care* 2006;29:1220–1226

83. Sever PS, Poulter NR, Dahlöf B, et al. Reduction in cardiovascular events with atorvastatin in 2,532 patients with type 2 diabetes: Anglo-Scandinavian Cardiac Outcomes Trial–lipid-lowering arm (ASCOT-LLA). *Diabetes Care* 2005;28:1151–1157

84. Knopp RH, d'Emden M, Smilde JG, Pocock SJ. Efficacy and safety of atorvastatin in the prevention of cardiovascular end points in subjects with type 2 diabetes: the Atorvastatin Study for Prevention of Coronary Heart Disease Endpoints in Non-Insulin-Dependent Diabetes Mellitus (ASPEN). *Diabetes Care* 2006;29:1478–1485

85. Colhoun HM, Betteridge DJ, Durrington PN, et al.; CARDS investigators. Primary prevention of cardiovascular disease with atorvastatin in type 2 diabetes in the Collaborative Atorvastatin Diabetes Study (CARDS): multicentre randomised placebo-controlled trial. *Lancet* 2004;364:685–696

86. Kearney PM, Blackwell L, Collins R, et al.; Cholesterol Treatment Trialists' (CTT) Collaborators. Efficacy of cholesterol-lowering therapy in 18,686 people with diabetes in 14 randomised trials of statins: a meta-analysis. *Lancet* 2008;371:117–125

87. Taylor F, Huffman MD, Macedo AF, et al. Statins for the primary prevention of cardiovascular disease. *Cochrane Database Syst Rev* 2013;1:CD004816

88. Carter AA, Gomes T, Camacho X, Juurlink DN, Shah BR, Mamdani MM. Risk of incident diabetes among patients treated with statins: population based study [published correction appears in *BMJ* 2013;347:f4356]. *BMJ* 2013;346:f2610

89. Baigent C, Blackwell L, Emberson J, et al.; Cholesterol Treatment Trialists' (CTT) Collaboration. Efficacy and safety of more intensive lowering of LDL cholesterol: a meta-analysis of data from 170,000 participants in 26 randomised trials. *Lancet* 2010;376:1670–1681

90. Cannon CP, Blazing MA, Giugliano RP, et al.; IMPROVE-IT Investigators. Ezetimibe added to statin therapy after acute coronary syndromes. *N Engl J Med* 2015;372:2387–2397

91. de Ferranti SD, de Boer IH, Fonseca V, et al. Type 1 diabetes mellitus and cardiovascular disease: a scientific statement from the American Heart Association and American Diabetes Association. *Circulation* 2014;130:1110–1130

92. Cannon CP, Braunwald E, McCabe CH, et al.; Pravastatin or Atorvastatin Evaluation and Infection Therapy-Thrombolysis in Myocardial Infarction 22 Investigators. Intensive versus moderate lipid lowering with statins after acute coronary syndromes. *N Engl J Med* 2004;350:1495–1504

93. Sabatine MS, Giugliano RP, Keech AC, et al.; FOURIER Steering Committee and Investigators. Evolocumab and clinical outcomes in patients with cardiovascular disease. *N Engl J Med* 2017;376:1713–1722

94. Giugliano RP, Cannon CP, Blazing MA, et al.; IMPROVE-IT (Improved Reduction of Outcomes: Vytorin Efficacy International Trial) Investigators. Benefit of adding ezetimibe to statin therapy on cardiovascular outcomes and safety in patients with versus without diabetes mellitus: results from IMPROVE-IT (Improved Reduction of Outcomes: Vytorin Efficacy International Trial). *Circulation* 2018;137:1571–1582

95. Moriarty PM, Jacobson TA, Bruckert E, et al. Efficacy and safety of alirocumab, a monoclonal antibody to PCSK9, in statin-intolerant patients: design and rationale of ODYSSEY ALTERNATIVE, a randomized phase 3 trial. *J Clin Lipidol* 2014;8:554–561

96. Zhang X-L, Zhu Q-Q, Zhu L, et al. Safety and efficacy of anti-PCSK9 antibodies: a meta-analysis of 25 randomized, controlled trials. *BMC Med* 2015;13:123

97. Sabatine MS, Leiter LA, Wiviott SD, et al. Cardiovascular safety and efficacy of the PCSK9 inhibitor evolocumab in patients with and without diabetes and the effect of evolocumab on glycaemia and risk of new-onset diabetes: a prespecified analysis of the FOURIER randomised controlled trial. *Lancet Diabetes Endocrinol* 2017;5:941–950

98. Berglund L, Brunzell JD, Goldberg AC, et al.; Endocrine Society. Evaluation and treatment of hypertriglyceridemia: an Endocrine Society clinical practice guideline. *J Clin Endocrinol Metab* 2012;97:2969–2989

99. Singh IM, Shishehbor MH, Ansell BJ. High-density lipoprotein as a therapeutic target: a systematic review. *JAMA* 2007;298:786–798

100. Keech A, Simes RJ, Barter P, et al.; FIELDstudy investigators. Effects of long-term fenofibrate therapy on cardiovascular events in 9795 people with type 2 diabetes mellitus (the FIELD study): randomised controlled trial. *Lancet* 2005;366:1849–1861

101. Jones PH, Davidson MH. Reporting rate of rhabdomyolysis with fenofibrate + statin versus gemfibrozil + any statin. *Am J Cardiol* 2005;95:120–122

102. Ginsberg HN, Elam MB, Lovato LC, et al.; ACCORD Study Group. Effects of combination lipid therapy in type 2 diabetes mellitus. *N Engl J Med* 2010;362:1563–1574

103. Kowa Research Institute, Inc. Pemafibrate to Reduce Cardiovascular Out-coMes by Reducing Triglycerides IN patiENts With diabeTes (PROMI-NENT) In: ClinicalTrials.gov [Internet]. Bethesda, MD, National Library of Medicine. Available from https://clinicaltrials.gov/ct2/show/NCT03071692. NLM Identifier: NCT03071692. Accessed 8 October 2018

104. Boden WE, Probstfield JL, Anderson T, et al.; AIM-HIGH Investigators. Niacin in patients with low HDL cholesterol levels receiving intensive statin therapy. *N Engl J Med* 2011;365:2255–2267

105. Landray MJ, Haynes R, Hopewell JC, et al.; HPS2-THRIVE Collaborative Group. Effects of extended-release niacin with laropiprant in high-risk patients. *N Engl J Med* 2014;371:203–212

106. Rajpathak SN, Kumbhani DJ, Crandall J,Barzilai N, Alderman M, Ridker PM. Statin therapy and risk of developing type 2 diabetes: a meta-analysis. *Diabetes Care* 2009;32:1924–1929

107. Sattar N, Preiss D, Murray HM, et al. Statins and risk of incident diabetes: a collaborative meta-analysis of randomised statin trials. *Lancet* 2010;375:735–742

108. Ridker PM, Pradhan A, MacFadyen JG, Libby P, Glynn RJ. Cardiovascular benefits and diabetes risks of statin therapy in primary prevention: an analysis from the JUPITER trial. *Lancet* 2012;380:565–571

109. Mach F, Ray KK, Wiklund O, et al.; European Atherosclerosis Society Consensus Panel. Adverse effects of statin therapy: perception vs. the evidence – focus on glucose homeostasis, cognitive, renal and hepatic function, haemorrhagic stroke and cataract. *Eur Heart J* 2018;39:2526–2539

110. Heart Protection Study Collaborative Group. MRC/BHF Heart Protection Study of cholesterol lowering with simvastatin in 20,536 high-risk individuals: a randomised placebo-controlled trial. *Lancet* 2002;360:7–22

111. Shepherd J, Blauw GJ, Murphy MB, et al.; PROSPER study group. PROspective Study of Pravastatin in the Elderly at Risk. Pravastatin in elderly individuals at risk of vascular disease (PROSPER): a randomised controlled trial. *Lancet* 2002;360:1623–1630

112. Trompet S, van Vliet P, de Craen AJM, et al. Pravastatin and cognitive function in the elderly. Results of the PROSPER study. *J Neurol* 2010;257:85–90

113. Yusuf S, Bosch J, Dagenais G, et al.; HOPE-3 Investigators. Cholesterol lowering in intermediate-risk persons without cardiovascular disease. *N Engl J Med* 2016;374:2021–2031

114. Giugliano RP, Mach F, Zavitz K, et al.; EBBINGHAUS Investigators. Cognitive function in a randomized trial of evolocumab. *N Engl J Med* 2017;377:633–643

115. Richardson K, Schoen M, French B, et al. Statins and cognitive function: a systematic review. *Ann Intern Med* 2013;159:688–697

116. Baigent C, Blackwell L, Collins R, et al.; Antithrombotic Trialists' (ATT) Collaboration. Aspirin in the primary and secondary prevention of vascular disease: collaborative meta-analysis of individual participant data from randomised trials. *Lancet* 2009;373:1849–1860

117. Perk J, De Backer G, Gohlke H, et al.; European Association for Cardiovascular Prevention & Rehabilitation (EACPR); ESC Committee for Practice Guidelines (CPG). European Guidelines on cardiovascular disease prevention in clinical practice (version 2012): The Fifth Joint Task Force of the European Society of Cardiology and Other Societies on Cardiovascular Disease Prevention in Clinical Practice (constituted by representatives of nine societies and by invited experts). *Eur Heart J* 2012;33:1635–1701

118. Belch J, MacCuish A, Campbell I, et al. The prevention of progression of arterial disease and diabetes (POPADAD) trial: factorial randomised placebo controlled trial of aspirin and antioxidants in patients with diabetes and asymptomatic peripheral arterial disease. *BMJ* 2008;337:a1840

119. Zhang C, Sun A, Zhang P, et al. Aspirin for primary prevention of cardiovascular events in patients with diabetes: a meta-analysis. *Diabetes Res Clin Pract* 2010;87:211–218

120. De Berardis G, Sacco M, Strippoli GFM, et al. Aspirin for primary prevention of cardiovascular events in people with diabetes: meta-analysis of randomised controlled trials. *BMJ* 2009;339:b4531

121. ASCEND Study Collaborative Group. Effects of aspirin for primary prevention in persons with diabetes mellitus. *N Engl J Med* 2018;379: 1529–1539

122. Gaziano JM, Brotons C, Coppolecchia R, et al.; ARRIVE Executive Committee. Use of aspirin to reduce risk of initial vascular events in patients at moderate risk of cardiovascular disease (ARRIVE): a randomised, double-blind, placebo-controlled trial. *Lancet* 2018;392:1036–1046

123. McNeil JJ, Wolfe R, Woods RL, et al.; ASPREE Investigator Group. Effect of aspirin on cardiovascular events and bleeding in the healthy elderly. *N Engl J Med* 2018;379:1509–1518

124. Pignone M, Earnshaw S, Tice JA, Pletcher MJ. Aspirin, statins, or both drugs for the primary prevention of coronary heart disease events in men: a cost-utility analysis. *Ann Intern Med* 2006;144:326–336

125. Pignone M, Alberts MJ, Colwell JA, et al.; American Diabetes Association; American Heart Association; American College of Cardiology Foundation. Aspirin for primary prevention of cardiovascular events in people with diabetes: a position statement of the American Diabetes Association, a scientific statement of the American Heart Association, and an expert consensus document of the American College of Cardiology Foundation. *Diabetes Care* 2010;33:1395–1402

126. Huxley RR, Peters SAE, Mishra GD, Woodward M. Risk of all-cause mortality and vascular events in women versus men with type 1 diabetes: a systematic review and meta-analysis. *Lancet Diabetes Endocrinol* 2015;3:198–206

127. Peters SAE, Huxley RR, Woodward M. Diabetes as risk factor for incident coronary heart disease in women compared with men: a systematic review and meta-analysis of 64 cohorts including 858,507 individuals and 28,203 coronary events. *Diabetologia* 2014;57:1542–1551

128. Kalyani RR, Lazo M, Ouyang P, et al. Sex differences in diabetes and risk of incident coronary artery disease in healthy young and middle-aged adults. *Diabetes Care* 2014;37:830–838

129. Peters SAE, Huxley RR, Woodward M. Diabetes as a risk factor for stroke in women compared with men: a systematic review and meta-analysis of 64 cohorts, including 775,385 individuals and 12,539 strokes. *Lancet* 2014;383:1973–1980

130. Dimitriu-Leen AC, Scholte AJHA, van Rosendael AR, et al. Value of coronary computed tomography angiography in tailoring aspirin therapy for primary prevention of atherosclerotic events in patients at high risk with diabetes mellitus. *Am J Cardiol* 2016;117:887–893

131. Mora S, Ames JM, Manson JE. Low-dose aspirin in the primary prevention of cardiovascular disease: shared decision making in clinical practice. *JAMA* 2016;316:709–710

132. Campbell CL, Smyth S, Montalescot G, Steinhubl SR. Aspirin dose for the prevention of cardiovascular disease: a systematic review. *JAMA* 2007;297:2018–2024

133. Davì G, Patrono C. Platelet activation and atherothrombosis. *N Engl J Med* 2007;357:2482–2494

134. Larsen SB, Grove EL, Neergaard-Petersen S, Würtz M, Hvas A-M, Kristensen SD. Determinants of reduced antiplatelet effect of aspirin in patients with stable coronary artery disease. *PLoS One* 2015;10:e0126767

135. Zaccardi F, Rizzi A, Petrucci G, et al. In vivo platelet activation and aspirin responsiveness in type 1 diabetes. *Diabetes* 2016;65:503–509

136. Bethel MA, Harrison P, Sourij H, et al. Randomized controlled trial comparing impact on platelet reactivity of twice-daily with once-daily aspirin in people with type 2 diabetes. *Diabet Med* 2016;33:224–230

137. Rothwell PM, Cook NR, Gaziano JM, et al. Effects of aspirin on risks of vascular events and cancer according to bodyweight and dose: analysis of individual patient data from randomised trials. *Lancet* 2018;392:387–399

138. Vandvik PO, Lincoff AM, Gore JM, et al. Primary and secondary prevention of cardiovascular disease: Antithrombotic Therapy and Prevention of Thrombosis, 9th ed: American College of Chest Physicians Evidence-Based Clinical Practice Guidelines [published correction appears in *Chest* 2012;141:1129]. *Chest* 2012;141(Suppl. 2):e637S–e668S

139. Bhatt DL, Bonaca MP, Bansilal S, et al. Reduction in ischemic events with ticagrelor in diabetic patients with prior myocardial infarction in PEGA-SUS-TIMI 54. *J Am Coll Cardiol* 2016;67:2732–2740

140. Bax JJ, Young LH, Frye RL, Bonow RO, Steinberg HO, Barrett EJ. Screening for coronary artery disease in patients with diabetes. *Diabetes Care* 2007;30:2729–2736

141. Boden WE, O'Rourke RA, Teo KK, et al.; COURAGE Trial Research Group. Optimal medical therapy with or without PCI for stable coronary disease. *N Engl J Med* 2007;356:1503–1516

142. BARI 2D Study Group, Frye RL, August P, et al. A randomized trial of therapies for type 2 diabetes and coronary artery disease. *N Engl J Med* 2009;360:2503–2015

143. Wackers FJT, Chyun DA, Young LH, et al.; Detection of Ischemia in Asymptomatic Diabetics (DIAD) Investigators. Resolution of asymptomatic myocardial ischemia in patients with type 2 diabetes in the Detection of Ischemia in Asymptomatic Diabetics (DIAD) study. *Diabetes Care* 2007;30:2892–2898

144. Elkeles RS, Godsland IF, Feher MD, et al.; PREDICT Study Group. Coronary calcium measurement improves prediction of cardiovascular events in asymptomatic patients with type 2 diabetes: the PREDICT study. *Eur Heart J* 2008;29:2244–2251

145. Raggi P, Shaw LJ, Berman DS, Callister TQ. Prognostic value of coronary artery calcium screening in subjects with and without diabetes. *J Am Coll Cardiol* 2004;43:1663–1669

146. Anand DV, Lim E, Hopkins D, et al. Risk stratification in uncomplicated type 2 diabetes: prospective evaluation of the combined use of coronary artery calcium imaging and selective myocardial perfusion scintigraphy. *Eur Heart J* 2006;27:713–721

147. Young LH, Wackers FJT, Chyun DA, et al.; DIAD Investigators. Cardiac outcomes after screening for asymptomatic coronary artery disease in patients with type 2 diabetes: the DIAD study: a randomized controlled trial. *JAMA* 2009;301:1547–1555

148. Wackers FJT, Young LH, Inzucchi SE, et al.; Detection of Ischemia in Asymptomatic Diabetics Investigators. Detection of silent myocardial ischemia in asymptomatic diabetic subjects: the DIAD study. *Diabetes Care* 2004;27:1954–1961

149. Scognamiglio R, Negut C, Ramondo A, Tiengo A, Avogaro A. Detection of coronary artery disease in asymptomatic patients with type 2 diabetes mellitus. *J Am Coll Cardiol* 2006;47:65–71

150. Hadamitzky M, Hein F, Meyer T, et al. Prognostic value of coronary computed tomographic angiography in diabetic patients without known coronary artery disease. *Diabetes Care* 2010;33:1358–1363

151. Choi E-K, Chun EJ, Choi S-I, et al. Assessment of subclinical coronary atherosclerosis in asymptomatic patients with type 2 diabetes mellitus with single photon emission computed tomography and coronary computed tomography angiography. *Am J Cardiol* 2009;104:890–896

152. Malik S, Zhao Y, Budoff M, et al. Coronary artery calcium score for long-term risk classification in individuals with type 2 diabetes and metabolic syndrome from the Multi-Ethnic Study of Atherosclerosis. *JAMA Cardiol* 2017;2:1332–1340

153. Wing RR, Bolin P, Brancati FL, et al.; Look AHEAD Research Group. Cardiovascular effects of intensive lifestyle intervention in type 2 diabetes. *N Engl J Med* 2013;369:145–154

154. Braunwald E, Domanski MJ, Fowler SE, et al.; PEACE Trial Investigators. Angiotensin-converting-enzyme inhibition in stable coronary artery disease. *N Engl J Med* 2004;351:2058–2068

155. Telmisartan Randomised AssessmeNt Study in ACE iNtolerant subjects with cardiovascular Disease (TRANSCEND) Investigators, Yusuf S, Teo K, et al. Effects of the angiotensin-receptor blocker telmisartan on cardiovascular events in high-risk patients intolerant to angiotensin-converting enzyme inhibitors: a randomised controlled trial. *Lancet* 2008;372:1174–1183

156. Kezerashvili A, Marzo K, De Leon J. Beta blocker use after acute myocardial infarction in the patient with normal systolic function: when is it "ok" to discontinue? *Curr Cardiol Rev* 2012;8:77–84

157. U.S. Food and Drug Administration. Guidance for industry. Diabetes mellitus—evaluating cardiovascular risk in new antidiabetic therapies to treat type 2 diabetes [Internet]. Silver Spring, MD, 2008. Available from http://www.fda.gov/downloads/Drugs/GuidanceComplianceRegulatoryInformation/Guidances/ucm071627.pdf. Accessed 3 November 2017

158. Neal B, Perkovic V, Matthews DR, et al.; CANVAS-R Trial Collaborative Group. Rationale, design and baseline characteristics of the CANagliflozin cardioVascular Assessment Study-Renal (CANVAS-R): a randomized, placebo-controlled trial. *Diabetes Obes Metab* 2017;19:387–393

159. Marso SP, Daniels GH, Brown-Frandsen K, et al.; LEADER Steering Committee; LEADER Trial Investigators. Liraglutide and cardiovascular outcomes in type 2 diabetes. *N Engl J Med* 2016;375:311–322

160. Marso SP, Bain SC, Consoli A, et al.; SUSTAIN-6 Investigators. Semaglutide and cardiovascular outcomes in patients with type 2 diabetes. *N Engl J Med* 2016;375:1834–1844

161. Pfeffer MA, Claggett B, Diaz R, et al.; ELIXA Investigators. Lixisenatide in patients with type 2 diabetes and acute coronary syndrome. *N Engl J Med* 2015;373:2247–2257

162. Holman RR, Bethel MA, Mentz RJ, et al.; EXSCEL Study Group. Effects of once-weekly exenatide on cardiovascular outcomes in type 2 diabetes. *N Engl J Med* 2017;377:1228–1239

163. Hernandez AF, Green JB, Janmohamed S, et al.; Harmony Outcomes committees and investigators. Albiglutide and cardiovascular outcomes in patients with type 2 diabetes and cardiovascular disease (Harmony Outcomes): a double-blind, randomised placebo-controlled trial. *Lancet* 2018;392:1519–1529

164. Kannel WB, Hjortland M, Castelli WP. Role of diabetes in congestive heart failure: the Framingham study. *Am J Cardiol* 1974;34:29–34

165. Dormandy JA, Charbonnel B, Eckland DJA, et al.; PROactive Investigators. Secondary prevention of macrovascular events in patients with type 2 diabetes in the PROactive Study (PROspective pioglitAzone Clinical Trial In macroVascular Events): a randomised controlled trial. *Lancet* 2005;366: 1279–1289

166. Singh S, Loke YK, Furberg CD. Long-term risk of cardiovascular events with rosiglitazone: a meta-analysis. *JAMA* 2007;298:1189–1195

167. Lincoff AM, Wolski K, Nicholls SJ, Nissen SE. Pioglitazone and risk of cardiovascular events in patients with type 2 diabetes mellitus: a meta-analysis of randomized trials. *JAMA* 2007;298:1180–1188

168. Scirica BM, Bhatt DL, Braunwald E, et al.; SAVOR-TIMI 53 Steering Committee and Investigators. Saxagliptin and cardiovascular outcomes in patients with type 2 diabetes mellitus. *N Engl J Med* 2013;369:1317–1326

169. U.S. Food and Drug Administration. FDA Drug Safety Communication: FDA adds warnings about heart failure risk to labels of type 2 diabetes medicines containing saxagliptin and alogliptin [Internet], 2016. Available from http://www.fda.gov/Drugs/DrugSafety/ucm486096.htm. Accessed 24 September 2018

170. Zannad F, Cannon CP, Cushman WC, et al.; EXAMINE Investigators. Heart failure and mortality outcomes in patients with type 2 diabetes taking alogliptin versus placebo in EXAMINE: a multicentre, randomised, double-blind trial. *Lancet* 2015;385:2067–2076

171. Green JB, Bethel MA, Armstrong PW, et al.; TECOS Study Group. Effect of sitagliptin on cardiovascular outcomes in type 2 diabetes. *N Engl J Med* 2015;373:232–242

172. Fitchett D, Butler J, van de Borne P, et al. Effects of empagliflozin on risk for cardiovascular death and heart failure hospitalization across the spectrum of heart failure risk in the EMPA-REG OUTCOME trial. *Eur Heart J* 2017;39:363–370

173. Hansson L, Zanchetti A, Carruthers SG, et al.; HOT Study Group. Effects of intensive blood-pressure lowering and low-dose aspirin in patients with hypertension: principal results of the Hypertension Optimal Treatment (HOT) randomised trial. *Lancet* 1998;351:1755–1762

174. Zoungas S, Chalmers J, Neal B, et al.; ADVANCE-ON Collaborative Group. Follow-up of blood-pressure lowering and glucose control in type 2 diabetes. *N Engl J Med* 2014;371:1392–1406

175. White WB, Cannon CP, Heller SR, et al.; EXAMINE Investigators. Alogliptin after acute coronary syndrome in patients with type 2 diabetes. *N Engl J Med* 2013;369:1327–1335

176. Cefalu WT, Kaul S, Gerstein HC, et al. Cardiovascular outcomes trials in type 2 diabetes: where do we go from here? Reflections from a *Diabetes Care* Editors' Expert Forum. *Diabetes Care* 2018;41:14–31

Chapter 18
Microvascular Complications and Foot Care

The American Diabetes Association (ADA) *Standards of Medical Care in Diabetes* includes ADA's current clinical practice recommendations and is intended to provide the components of diabetes care, general treatment goals and guidelines, and tools to evaluate quality of care. Members of the ADA Professional Practice Committee, a multidisciplinary expert committee, are responsible for updating the *Standards of Care* annually, or more frequently as warranted. For a detailed description of ADA standards, statements, and reports, as well as the evidence-grading system for ADA's clinical practice recommendations, please refer to the Introduction to *Standards of Medical Care in Diabetes*. Readers who wish to comment on the *Standards of Care* are invited to do so at professional.diabetes.org/SOC.

For prevention and management of diabetes complications in children and adolescents, please refer to Section 13 "Children and Adolescents" in the *Standards of Medical Care in Diabetes—2019* (DOI:10.2337/dc19-S013).

CHRONIC KIDNEY DISEASE

RECOMMENDATIONS

Screening
11.1 At least once a year, assess urinary albumin (e.g., spot urinary albumin-to-creatinine ratio) and estimated glomerular filtration rate in patients with type 1 diabetes with duration of ≥5 years, in all patients with type 2 diabetes, and in all patients with comorbid hypertension. **B***

Treatment
11.2 Optimize glucose control to reduce the risk or slow the progression of chronic kidney disease. **A**
11.3 For patients with type 2 diabetes and chronic kidney disease, consider use of a sodium–glucose cotransporter 2 inhibitor or glucagon-like peptide 1

Chapter 18 is an excerpt from American Diabetes Association, 11. Microvascular Complications and Foot Care: *Standards of Medical Care in Diabetes—2019*. *Diabetes Care* 2019; 42(Suppl. 1):S103–S123. DOI:doi.org/10.2337/dc19-S011.

* See Table 1.1 (p. 4) for an explanation of the American Diabetes Association evidence-grading system for *Standards of Medical Care in Diabetes*.

receptor agonist shown to reduce risk of chronic kidney disease progression, cardiovascular events, or both (Table 9.1 in the *Standards of Medical Care in Diabetes—2019* [DOI:10.2337/dc19-S009]). **C**

11.4 Optimize blood pressure control to reduce the risk or slow the progression of chronic kidney disease. **A**

11.5 For people with non-dialysis-dependent chronic kidney disease, dietary protein intake should be approximately 0.8 g/kg body weight per day (the recommended daily allowance). For patients on dialysis, higher levels of dietary protein intake should be considered. **B**

11.6 In nonpregnant patients with diabetes and hypertension, either an ACE inhibitor or an angiotensin receptor blocker is recommended for those with modestly elevated urinary albumin-to-creatinine ratio (30–299 mg/g creatinine) **B** and is strongly recommended for those with urinary albumin-to-creatinine ratio ≥300 mg/g creatinine and/or estimated glomerular filtration rate <60 mL/min/1.73 m^2. **A**

11.7 Periodically monitor serum creatinine and potassium levels for the development of increased creatinine or changes in potassium when ACE inhibitors, angiotensin receptor blockers, or diuretics are used. **B**

11.8 Continued monitoring of urinary albumin-to-creatinine ratio in patients with albuminuria treated with an ACE inhibitor or an angiotensin receptor blocker is reasonable to assess the response to treatment and progression of chronic kidney disease. **E**

11.9 An ACE inhibitor or an angiotensin receptor blocker is not recommended for the primary prevention of chronic kidney disease in patients with diabetes who have normal blood pressure, normal urinary albumin-to-creatinine ratio (<30 mg/g creatinine), and normal estimated glomerular filtration rate. **B**

11.10 When estimated glomerular filtration rate is <60 mL/min/1.73 m^2, evaluate and manage potential complications of chronic kidney disease. **E**

11.11 Patients should be referred for evaluation for renal replacement treatment if they have an estimated glomerular filtration rate <30 mL/min/1.73 m^2. **A**

11.12 Promptly refer to a physician experienced in the care of kidney disease for uncertainty about the etiology of kidney disease, difficult management issues, and rapidly progressing kidney disease. **B**

Epidemiology of Diabetes and Chronic Kidney Disease

Chronic kidney disease (CKD) is diagnosed by the persistent presence of elevated urinary albumin excretion (albuminuria), low estimated glomerular filtration rate (eGFR), or other manifestations of kidney damage.[1,2] In this section, the focus will be on CKD attributed to diabetes (diabetic kidney disease), which occurs in 20–40% of patients with diabetes.[1,3–5] CKD typically develops after diabetes duration of 10 years in type 1 diabetes but may be present at diagnosis of type 2 diabetes. CKD can progress to end-stage renal disease (ESRD) requiring dialysis or kidney transplantation and is the leading cause of ESRD in the U.S.[6] In addition, among people with type 1 or 2 diabetes, the presence of CKD markedly increases cardiovascular risk and healthcare costs.[7]

Assessment of Albuminuria and Estimated Glomerular Filtration Rate

Screening for albuminuria can be most easily performed by urinary albumin-to-creatinine ratio (ACR) in a random spot urine collection.[1,2] Timed or 24-h collections are more burdensome and add little to prediction or accuracy. Measurement of a spot urine sample for albumin alone (whether by immunoassay or by using a sensitive dipstick test specific for albuminuria) without simultaneously measuring urine creatinine (Cr) is less expensive but susceptible to false-negative and false-positive determinations as a result of variation in urine concentration due to hydration.

Normal urinary ACR is generally defined as <30 mg/g Cr, and increased urinary albumin excretion is defined as ≥30 mg/g Cr. However, urinary ACR is a continuous measurement, and differences within the normal and abnormal ranges are associated with renal and cardiovascular outcomes.[7-9] Furthermore, because of biological variability in urinary albumin excretion, two of three specimens of urinary ACR collected within a 3- to 6-month period should be abnormal before considering a patient to have albuminuria. Exercise within 24 h, infection, fever, congestive heart failure, marked hyperglycemia, menstruation, and marked hypertension may elevate urinary ACR independently of kidney damage.

eGFR should be calculated from serum Cr using a validated formula. The Chronic Kidney Disease Epidemiology Collaboration (CKD-EPI) equation is generally preferred.[2] eGFR is routinely reported by laboratories with serum Cr, and eGFR calculators are available from www.nkdep.nih.gov. An eGFR <60 mL/min/1.73 m^2 is generally considered abnormal, though optimal thresholds for clinical diagnosis are debated.[10]

Urinary albumin excretion and eGFR each vary within people over time, and abnormal results should be confirmed to stage CKD.[1,2]

Diagnosis of Diabetic Kidney Disease

Diabetic kidney disease is usually a clinical diagnosis made based on the presence of albuminuria and/or reduced eGFR in the absence of signs or symptoms of other primary causes of kidney damage. The typical presentation of diabetic kidney disease is considered to include a long-standing duration of diabetes, retinopathy, albuminuria without hematuria, and gradually progressive loss of eGFR. However, signs of CKD may be present at diagnosis or without retinopathy in type 2 diabetes, and reduced eGFR without albuminuria has been frequently reported in type 1 and type 2 diabetes and is becoming more common over time as the prevalence of diabetes increases in the U.S.[3,4,11,12]

An active urinary sediment (containing red or white blood cells or cellular casts), rapidly increasing albuminuria or nephrotic syndrome, rapidly decreasing eGFR, or the absence of retinopathy (in type 1 diabetes) may suggest alternative or additional causes of kidney disease. For patients with these features, referral to a nephrologist for further diagnosis, including the possibility of kidney biopsy, should be considered. It is rare for patients with type 1 diabetes to develop kidney disease without retinopathy. In type 2 diabetes, retinopathy is only moderately sensitive and specific for CKD caused by diabetes, as confirmed by kidney biopsy.[13]

Staging of Chronic Kidney Disease

Stages 1–2 CKD have been defined by evidence of kidney damage (usually albuminuria) with eGFR ≥60 mL/min/1.73 m², while stages 3–5 CKD have been defined by progressively lower ranges of eGFR[14] (Table 18.1). At any eGFR, the degree of albuminuria is associated with risk of CKD progression, cardiovascular disease (CVD), and mortality.[7] Therefore, Kidney Disease: Improving Global Outcomes (KDIGO) recommends a more comprehensive CKD staging that incorporates albuminuria at all stages of eGFR; this system is more closely associated with risk but is also more complex and does not translate directly to treatment decisions.[2] Regardless of classification scheme, both eGFR and albuminuria should be quantified to guide treatment decisions: CKD complications (Table 18.2) correlate with eGFR, many drugs are limited to acceptable eGFR ranges, and the degree of albuminuria may influence choice of antihypertensive (see Section 10 "Cardiovascular Disease and Risk Management" in the *Standards of Medical Care*

Table 18.1 — CKD Stages and Corresponding Focus of Kidney-Related Care

CKD stage†			Focus of kidney-related care			
Stage	eGFR (mL/min/1.73 m²)	Evidence of kidney damage*	Diagnose cause of kidney injury	Evaluate and treat risk factors for CKD progression**	Evaluate and treat CKD complications***	Prepare for renal replacement therapy
No clinical evidence of CKD	≥60	–				
1	≥90	+	✓	✓		
2	60–89	+	✓	✓		
3	30–59	+/–	✓	✓	✓	
4	15–29	+/–		✓	✓	✓
5	<15	+/–			✓	✓

CKD, chronic kidney disease; eGFR, estimated glomerular filtration rate. †CKD stages 1 and 2 are defined by evidence of kidney damage (+), while CKD stages 3–5 are defined by reduced eGFR with or without evidence of kidney damage (+/–). At any stage of CKD, the degree of albuminuria, observed history of eGFR loss, and cause of kidney damage (including possible causes other than diabetes) may also be used to characterize CKD, gauge prognosis, and guide treatment decisions. *Kidney damage is most often manifest as albuminuria (UACR ≥30 mg/g Cr) but can also include glomerular hematuria, other abnormalities of the urinary sediment, radiographic abnormalities, and other presentations. **Risk factors for CKD progression include elevated blood pressure, hyperglycemia, and albuminuria. ***See Table 18.2.

in Diabetes—2019 [DOI:10.2337/dc19-S010]) or glucose-lowering medications. Observed history of eGFR loss (which is also associated with risk of CKD progression and other adverse health outcomes) and cause of kidney damage (including possible causes other than diabetes) may also affect these decisions.[15]

Acute Kidney Injury

Acute kidney injury (AKI) is usually diagnosed by a rapid increase in serum Cr, which is also reflected as a rapid decrease in eGFR, over a relatively short period of time. People with diabetes are at higher risk of AKI than those without diabetes.[16] Other risk factors for AKI include preexisting CKD, the use of medications that cause kidney injury (e.g., nonsteroidal anti-inflammatory drugs), and the use of medications that alter renal blood flow and intrarenal hemodynamics. In particular, many antihypertensive medications (e.g., diuretics, ACE inhibitors, and angiotensin receptor blockers [ARBs]) can reduce intravascular volume, renal blood flow, and/or glomerular filtration. There is a concern that sodium–glucose cotransporter 2 (SGLT2) inhibitors may promote AKI through volume depletion, particularly when combined with diuretics or other medications that reduce glomerular filtration. However, existing evidence from clinical trials and observational studies suggests that SGLT2 inhibitors do not significantly increase AKI.[17–19] Timely identification and treatment of AKI are important because AKI is associated with increased risks of progressive CKD and other poor health outcomes.[20]

Surveillance

Albuminuria and eGFR should be monitored regularly to enable timely diagnosis of CKD, monitor progression of CKD, detect superimposed kidney diseases including AKI, assess risk of CKD complications, dose drugs appropriately, and determine whether nephrology referral is needed. Among people with existing kidney disease, albuminuria and eGFR may change due to progression of CKD, development of a separate superimposed cause of kidney disease, AKI, or other effects of medications, as noted above. Serum potassium should also be monitored for patients treated with ACE inhibitors, ARBs, and diuretics because these medications can cause hyperkalemia or hypokalemia, which are associated with cardiovascular risk and mortality.[21–23] For patients with eGFR <60 mL/min/1.73 m^2, appropriate medication dosing should be verified, exposure to nephrotoxins (e.g., nonsteroidal anti-inflammatory drugs and iodinated contrast) should be minimized, and potential CKD complications should be evaluated (Table 18.2).

The need for annual quantitative assessment of albumin excretion after diagnosis of albuminuria, institution of ACE inhibitors or ARB therapy, and achieving blood pressure control is a subject of debate. Continued surveillance can assess both response to therapy and disease progression and may aid in assessing adherence to ACE inhibitor or ARB therapy. In addition, in clinical trials of ACE inhibitors or ARB therapy in type 2 diabetes, reducing albuminuria from levels ≥300 mg/g Cr has been associated with improved renal and cardiovascular outcomes, leading some to suggest that medications should be titrated to minimize urinary ACR. However, this approach has not been formally evaluated in prospective trials. In type 1 diabetes, remission of albuminuria may occur spontaneously

Table 18.2—Selected Complications of CKD

Complication	Medical and laboratory evaluation
Elevated blood pressure	Blood pressure, weight
Volume overload	History, physical examination, weight
Electrolyte abnormalities	Serum electrolytes
Metabolic acidosis	Serum electrolytes
Anemia	Hemoglobin; iron testing if indicated
Metabolic bone disease	Serum calcium, phosphate, PTH, vitamin 25(OH)D

Complications of chronic kidney disease (CKD) generally become prevalent when estimated glomerular filtration rate falls below 60mL/min/1.73 m² (stage 3 CKD or greater) and become more common and severe as CKD progresses. Evaluation of elevated blood pressure and volume overload should occur at every clinical contact possible; laboratory evaluations are generally indicated every 6–12 months for stage 3 CKD, every 3–5 months for stage 4 CKD, and every 1–3 months for stage 5 CKD, or as indicated to evaluate symptoms or changes in therapy. PTH, parathyroid hormone; 25(OH)D, 25-hydroxyvitamin D.

and cohort studies evaluating associations of change in albuminuria with clinical outcomes have reported inconsistent results.[24,25]

The prevalence of CKD complications correlates with eGFR.[25a] When eGFR is <60 mL/min/1.73 m², screening for complications of CKD is indicated (Table 18.2). Early vaccination against hepatitis B virus is indicated in patients likely to progress to ESRD (see Section 4 "Comprehensive Medical Evaluation and Assessment of Comorbidities" in the *Standards of Medical Care in Diabetes—2019* [DOI:10.2337/dc19-S004]) for further information on immunization).

Interventions

Nutrition

For people with non-dialysis-dependent CKD, dietary protein intake should be approximately 0.8 g/kg body weight per day (the recommended daily allowance).[1] Compared with higher levels of dietary protein intake, this level slowed GFR decline with evidence of a greater effect over time. Higher levels of dietary protein intake (>20% of daily calories from protein or >1.3 g/kg/day) have been associated with increased albuminuria, more rapid kidney function loss, and CVD mortality and therefore should be avoided. Reducing the amount of dietary protein below the recommended daily allowance of 0.8 g/kg/day is not recommended because it does not alter glycemic measures, cardiovascular risk measures, or the course of GFR decline.

Restriction of dietary sodium (to <2,300 mg/day) may be useful to control blood pressure and reduce cardiovascular risk,[26] and restriction of dietary potassium may be necessary to control serum potassium concentration.[16,21–23] These interventions may be most important for patients with reduced eGFR, for whom urinary excretion of sodium and potassium may be impaired. Recommendations for dietary sodium and potassium intake should be individualized on the basis of comorbid conditions, medication use, blood pressure, and laboratory data.

Glycemic Targets

Intensive glycemic control with the goal of achieving near-normoglycemia has been shown in large prospective randomized studies to delay the onset and progression of albuminuria and reduced eGFR in patients with type 1 diabetes[27,28] and type 2 diabetes.[1,29–34] Insulin alone was used to lower blood glucose in the Diabetes Control and Complications Trial (DCCT)/Epidemiology of Diabetes Interventions and Complications (EDIC) study of type 1 diabetes, while a variety of agents were used in clinical trials of type 2 diabetes, supporting the conclusion that glycemic control itself helps prevent CKD and its progression. The effects of glucose-lowering therapies on CKD have helped define A1C targets (see Table 6.2 in the *Standards of Medical Care in Diabetes—2019* [DOI:10.2337/dc19-S006]).

The presence of CKD affects the risks and benefits of intensive glycemic control and a number of specific glucose-lowering medications. In the Action to Control Cardiovascular Risk in Diabetes (ACCORD) trial of type 2 diabetes, adverse effects of intensive glycemic control (hypoglycemia and mortality) were increased among patients with kidney disease at baseline.[35,36] Moreover, there is a lag time of at least 2 years in type 2 diabetes to over 10 years in type 1 diabetes for the effects of intensive glucose control to manifest as improved eGFR outcomes.[33,37,38] Therefore, in some patients with prevalent CKD and substantial comorbidity, target A1C levels may be less intensive.[1,39]

Direct Renal Effects of Glucose-Lowering Medications

Some glucose-lowering medications also have effects on the kidney that are direct, i.e., not mediated through glycemia. For example, SGLT2 inhibitors reduce renal tubular glucose reabsorption, weight, systemic blood pressure, intraglomerular pressure, and albuminuria and slow GFR loss through mechanisms that appear independent of glycemia.[18,40–43] Glucagon-like peptide 1 receptor agonists (GLP-1 RA) also have direct effects on the kidney and have been reported to improve renal outcomes compared with placebo.[44–47] Renal effects should be considered when selecting antihyperglycemia agents (see Section 9 "Pharmacologic Approaches to Glycemic Treatment" in the *Standards of Medical Care in Diabetes—2019* [DOI:10.2337/dc19-S009]).

Selection of Glucose-Lowering Medications for Patients with Chronic Kidney Disease

For patients with type 2 diabetes and established CKD, special considerations for the selection of glucose-lowering medications include limitations to available medications when eGFR is diminished and a desire to mitigate high risks of CKD progression, CVD, and hypoglycemia.[48,49] Drug dosing may require modification with eGFR <60 mL/min/1.73 m^2.[1]

The U.S. Food and Drug Administration (FDA) revised its guidance for the use of metformin in CKD in 2016,[50] recommending use of eGFR instead of serum Cr to guide treatment and expanding the pool of patients with kidney disease for whom metformin treatment should be considered. The revised FDA guidance states that metformin is contraindicated in patients with an eGFR <30 mL/min/1.73 m^2, eGFR should be monitored while taking metformin, the benefits and risks of continuing treatment should be reassessed when eGFR falls <45 mL/min/1.73 m^2, metformin should not be initiated for patients with an eGFR <45 mL/min/1.73 m^2, and metformin should be temporarily discontinued at the time of or before iodinated contrast imaging procedures in patients with eGFR 30–60 mL/min/1.73 m². Within these constraints, metformin should be considered the first-line treatment for all patients with type 2 diabetes, including those with CKD.

SGLT2 inhibitors and GLP-1 RAs should be considered for patients with type 2 diabetes and CKD who require another drug added to metformin to attain target A1C or cannot use or tolerate metformin. SGLT2 inhibitors and GLP-1 RA are suggested because they appear to reduce risks of CKD progression, CVD events, and hypoglycemia.

A number of large cardiovascular outcomes trials in patients with type 2 diabetes at high risk for CVD or with existing CVD examined kidney effects as secondary outcomes. These trials include EMPA-REG OUTCOME (BI 10773 [Empagliflozin] Cardiovascular Outcome Event Trial in Type 2 Diabetes Mellitus Patients), CANVAS (Canagliflozin Cardiovascular Assessment Study), LEADER (Liraglutide Effect and Action in Diabetes: Evaluation of Cardiovascular Outcome Results), and SUSTAIN-6 (Trial to Evaluate Cardiovascular and Other Long-term Outcomes With Semaglutide in Subjects With Type 2 Diabetes).[42,44,47,51] Specifically, compared with placebo, empagliflozin reduced the risk of incident or worsening nephropathy (a composite of progression to urinary ACR >300 mg/g Cr, doubling of serum Cr, ESRD, or death from ESRD) by 39% and the risk of doubling of serum Cr accompanied by eGFR ≤45 mL/min/1.73 m² by 44%; canagliflozin reduced the risk of progression of albuminuria by 27% and the risk of reduction in eGFR, ESRD, or death from ESRD by 40%; liraglutide reduced the risk of new or worsening nephropathy (a composite of persistent macroalbuminuria, doubling of serum Cr, ESRD, or death from ESRD) by 22%; and semaglutide reduced the risk of new or worsening nephropathy (a composite of persistent urinary ACR >300 mg/g Cr, doubling of serum Cr, or ESRD) by 36% (each $P < 0.01$).

These analyses were limited by evaluation of study populations not selected primarily for CKD and examination of renal effects as secondary outcomes. However, all of these trials included large numbers of people with kidney disease (for example, the baseline prevalence of albuminuria in EMPA-REG OUTCOME was 53%), and some of the cardiovascular outcomes trials (CANVAS and LEADER) were enriched with patients with kidney disease through eligibility criteria based on albuminuria or reduced eGFR. In addition, subgroup analyses of CANVAS and LEADER suggested that the renal benefits of canagliflozin and liraglutide were as great or greater for participants with CKD at baseline[19,46] and in CANVAS were similar for participants with or without atherosclerotic cardiovascular disease (ASCVD) at baseline.[52] Smaller, shorter-term trials also demonstrate favorable renal effects of medications in these classes.[53,53a] Together, these consistent results suggest likely renal benefits of both drug classes.

Several large clinical trials of SGLT2 inhibitors focused on patients with CKD, and assessment of primary renal outcomes are completed or ongoing. Canagliflozin and Renal Endpoints in Diabetes with Established Nephropathy Clinical Evaluation (CREDENCE), a placebo-controlled trial of canagliflozin among 4,401 adults with type 2 diabetes, urinary ACR ≥300 mg/g, and eGFR 30–90 mL/min/1.73 m², has a primary composite endpoint of ESRD, doubling of serum Cr, or renal or cardiovascular death.[54] It was stopped early due to positive efficacy, with detailed results expected in 2019.

In addition to renal effects, some SGLT2 inhibitors and GLP-1 RA have demonstrated cardiovascular benefits. Namely, in EMPA-REG OUTCOME, CANVAS, and LEADER, empagliflozin, canagliflozin, and liraglutide, respectively, each reduced cardiovascular events, evaluated as primary outcomes, compared with placebo (see Section 10 "Cardiovascular Disease and Risk Management" for further discussion in the *Standards of Medical Care in Diabetes—2019* [DOI: 10.2337/dc19-S010]). The glucose-lowering effects of SGLT2 inhibitors are blunted with eGFR.[18,51] However, the cardiovascular benefits of empagliflozin, canagliflozin, and liraglutide were similar among participants with and without kidney disease at baseline.[42,44,51,55] Most participants with CKD in these trials also had diagnosed ASCVD at baseline, though approximately 28% of CANVAS participants with CKD did not have diagnosed ASCVD.[19]

Important caveats limit the strength of evidence supporting the recommendation of SGLT2 inhibitors and GLP-1 RA in patients with type 2 diabetes and CKD. As noted above, published data address a limited group of CKD patients, mostly with coexisting ASCVD. Renal events have been examined primarily as secondary outcomes in published large trials. Also, adverse event profiles of these agents must be considered. Please refer to Table 9.1 in the *Standards of Medical Care in Diabetes—2019* (DOI:10.2337/dc19-S009) for drug-specific factors, including adverse event information, for these agents. Therefore, additional clinical trials are needed to more rigorously assess the benefits and risks of these classes of drugs among people with CKD.

For patients with type 2 diabetes and CKD, the selection of specific agents may depend on comorbidity and CKD stage. SGLT2 inhibitors may be more useful for patients at high risk of CKD progression (i.e., with albuminuria or a history of documented eGFR loss) (Figure 9.1 in the *Standards of Medical Care in Diabetes—2019* [DOI:10.2337/dc19-S009]) because they appear to have large beneficial effects on CKD incidence. Empagliflozin and canagliflozin are only approved by the FDA for use with eGFR ≥45 mL/min/1.73 m² (though pivotal trials for each included participants with eGFR ≥30 mL/min/1.73 m² and demonstrated benefit in subgroups with low eGFR).[18,19] and dapagliflozin is only approved for eGFR ≥60 mL/min/1.73 m². Some GLP-1 RA may be used with lower eGFR and may have greater benefits for reduction of ASCVD than for CKD progression or HF.

Cardiovascular Disease and Blood Pressure

Hypertension is a strong risk factor for the development and progression of CKD.[56] Antihypertensive therapy reduces the risk of albuminuria,[57–60] and among patients with type 1 or 2 diabetes with established CKD (eGFR <60 mL/min/1.73 m² and urinary ACR ≥300 mg/g Cr), ACE inhibitor or ARB therapy reduces the risk of progression to ESRD.[61–63] Moreover, antihypertensive therapy reduces risks of cardiovascular events.[57]

Blood pressure levels <140/90 mmHg are generally recommended to reduce CVD mortality and slow CKD progression among people with diabetes.[60] Lower blood pressure targets (e.g., <130/80 mmHg) may be considered for patients based on individual anticipated benefits and risks. Patients with CKD are at increased risk of CKD progression (particularly those with albuminuria) and CVD and therefore may be suitable in some cases for lower blood pressure targets.

ACE inhibitors or ARBs are the preferred first-line agent for blood pressure treatment among patients with diabetes, hypertension, eGFR <60 mL/min/1.73 m², and urinary ACR ≥300 mg/g Cr because of their proven benefits for prevention of CKD progression.[61–64] In general, ACE inhibitors and ARBs are considered to have similar benefits[65,66] and risks. In the setting of lower levels of albuminuria (30–299 mg/g Cr), ACE inhibitor or ARB therapy has been demonstrated to reduce progression to more advanced albuminuria (≥300 mg/g Cr) and cardiovascular events but not progression to ESRD.[64,67] While ACE inhibitors or ARBs are often prescribed for albuminuria without hypertension, clinical trials have not been performed in this setting to determine whether this improves renal outcomes.

Absent kidney disease, ACE inhibitors or ARBs are useful to control blood pressure but may not be superior to alternative proven classes of antihypertensive therapy, including thiazide-like diuretics and dihydropyridine calcium channel blockers.[68] In a trial of people with type 2 diabetes and normal urine albumin excretion, an ARB reduced or suppressed the development of albuminuria but increased the rate of cardiovascular events.[69] In a trial of people with type 1 diabetes exhibiting neither albuminuria nor hypertension, ACE inhibitors or ARBs did not prevent the development of diabetic glomerulopathy assessed by kidney biopsy.[70] *Therefore, ACE inhibitors or ARBs are not recommended for patients without hypertension to prevent the development of CKD.*

Two clinical trials studied the combinations of ACE inhibitors and ARBs and found no benefits on CVD or CKD, and the drug combination had higher adverse event rates (hyperkalemia and/or AKI).[71,72] *Therefore, the combined use of ACE inhibitors and ARBs should be avoided.*

Mineralocorticoid receptor antagonists (spironolactone, eplerenone, and finerenone) in combination with ACE inhibitors or ARBs remain an area of great interest. Mineralocorticoid receptor antagonists are effective for management of resistant hypertension, have been shown to reduce albuminuria in short-term studies of CKD, and may have additional cardiovascular benefits.[73–75] There has been, however, an increase in hyperkalemic episodes in those on dual therapy, and larger, longer trials with clinical outcomes are needed before recommending such therapy.

Referral to a Nephrologist

Consider referral to a physician experienced in the care of kidney disease when there is uncertainty about the etiology of kidney disease, difficult management issues (anemia, secondary hyperparathyroidism, metabolic bone disease, resistant hypertension, or electrolyte disturbances), or advanced kidney disease (eGFR <30 mL/min/1.73 m²) requiring discussion of renal replacement therapy for ESRD. The threshold for referral may vary depending on the frequency with which a provider encounters patients with diabetes and kidney disease. Consultation with a nephrologist when stage 4 CKD develops (eGFR <30 mL/min/1.73 m²) has been found to reduce cost, improve quality of care, and delay dialysis.[76] However, other specialists and providers should also educate their patients about the progressive nature of CKD, the kidney preservation benefits of proactive treatment of blood pressure and blood glucose, and the potential need for renal replacement therapy.

DIABETIC RETINOPATHY

RECOMMENDATIONS

11.13 Optimize glycemic control to reduce the risk or slow the progression of diabetic retinopathy. **A**

11.14 Optimize blood pressure and serum lipid control to reduce the risk or slow the progression of diabetic retinopathy. **A**

Screening

11.15 Adults with type 1 diabetes should have an initial dilated and comprehensive eye examination by an ophthalmologist or optometrist within 5 years after the onset of diabetes. **B**

11.16 Patients with type 2 diabetes should have an initial dilated and comprehensive eye examination by an ophthalmologist or optometrist at the time of the diabetes diagnosis. **B**

11.17 If there is no evidence of retinopathy for one or more annual eye exam and glycemia is well controlled, then exams every 1–2 years may be considered. If any level of diabetic retinopathy is present, subsequent dilated retinal examinations should be repeated at least annually by an ophthalmologist or optometrist. If retinopathy is progressing or sight-threatening, then examinations will be required more frequently. **B**

11.18 Telemedicine programs that use validated retinal photography with remote reading by an ophthalmologist or optometrist and timely referral for a comprehensive eye examination when indicated can be an appropriate screening strategy for diabetic retinopathy. **B**

11.19 Women with preexisting type 1 or type 2 diabetes who are planning pregnancy or who are pregnant should be counseled on the risk of development and/or progression of diabetic retinopathy. **B**

11.20 Eye examinations should occur before pregnancy or in the first trimester in patients with preexisting type 1 or type 2 diabetes, and then patients should be monitored every trimester and for 1 year postpartum as indicated by the degree of retinopathy. **B**

Treatment

11.21 Promptly refer patients with any level of macular edema, severe nonproliferative diabetic retinopathy (a precursor of proliferative diabetic retinopathy), or any proliferative diabetic retinopathy to an ophthalmologist who is knowledgeable and experienced in the management of diabetic retinopathy. **A**

11.22 The traditional standard treatment, panretinal laser photocoagulation therapy, is indicated to reduce the risk of vision loss in patients with high-risk proliferative diabetic retinopathy and, in some cases, severe nonproliferative diabetic retinopathy. **A**

11.23 Intravitreous injections of anti-vascular endothelial growth factor ranibizumab are not inferior to traditional panretinal laser photocoagulation and are also indicated to reduce the risk of vision loss in patients with proliferative diabetic retinopathy. **A**

11.24 Intravitreous injections of anti-vascular endothelial growth factor are indicated for central-involved diabetic macular edema, which occurs beneath the foveal center and may threaten reading vision. **A**

11.25 The presence of retinopathy is not a contraindication to aspirin therapy for cardioprotection, as aspirin does not increase the risk of retinal hemorrhage. **A**

Diabetic retinopathy is a highly specific vascular complication of both type 1 and type 2 diabetes, with prevalence strongly related to both the duration of diabetes and the level of glycemic control.[77] Diabetic retinopathy is the most frequent cause of new cases of blindness among adults aged 20–74 years in developed countries. Glaucoma, cataracts, and other disorders of the eye occur earlier and more frequently in people with diabetes.

In addition to diabetes duration, factors that increase the risk of, or are associated with, retinopathy include chronic hyperglycemia,[78] nephropathy,[79] hypertension,[80] and dyslipidemia.[81] Intensive diabetes management with the goal of achieving near-normoglycemia has been shown in large prospective randomized studies to prevent and/or delay the onset and progression of diabetic retinopathy and potentially improve patient-reported visual function.[30,82–84]

Several case series and a controlled prospective study suggest that pregnancy in patients with type 1 diabetes may aggravate retinopathy and threaten vision, especially when glycemic control is poor at the time of conception.[85,86] Laser photocoagulation surgery can minimize the risk of vision loss.[86]

SCREENING

The preventive effects of therapy and the fact that patients with proliferative diabetic retinopathy (PDR) or macular edema may be asymptomatic provide strong support for screening to detect diabetic retinopathy.

An ophthalmologist or optometrist who is knowledgeable and experienced in diagnosing diabetic retinopathy should perform the examinations. Youth with type 1 or type 2 diabetes are also at risk for complications and need to be screened for diabetic retinopathy.[87] If diabetic retinopathy is present, prompt referral to an ophthalmologist is recommended. Subsequent examinations for patients with type 1 or type 2 diabetes are generally repeated annually for patients with minimal to no retinopathy. Exams every 1–2 years may be cost effective after one or more normal eye exams, and in a population with well controlled type 2 diabetes, there was essentially no risk of development of significant retinopathy with a 3-year interval after a normal examination.[88] Less frequent intervals have been found in simulated modeling to be potentially effective in screening for diabetic retinopathy in patients without diabetic retinopathy.[89] More frequent examinations by the ophthalmologist will be required if retinopathy is progressing.

Retinal photography with remote reading by experts has great potential to provide screening services in areas where qualified eye care professionals are not readily available.[82,83] High-quality fundus photographs can detect most clinically significant diabetic retinopathy. Interpretation of the images should be performed by a trained eye care provider. Retinal photography may also enhance efficiency and reduce costs when the expertise of ophthalmologists can be used for more complex examinations and for therapy.[90,91] In-person exams are still necessary when the retinal photos are of unacceptable quality and for follow-up if abnormalities are detected. Retinal photos are not a substitute for comprehensive eye exams, which should be performed at least initially and at intervals thereafter as recommended by an eye care professional. Results of eye examinations should be documented and transmitted to the referring healthcare professional.

Type 1 Diabetes

Because retinopathy is estimated to take at least 5 years to develop after the onset of hyperglycemia, patients with type 1 diabetes should have an initial dilated and comprehensive eye examination within 5 years after the diagnosis of diabetes.[92]

Type 2 Diabetes

Patients with type 2 diabetes who may have had years of undiagnosed diabetes and have a significant risk of prevalent diabetic retinopathy at the time of diagnosis should have an initial dilated and comprehensive eye examination at the time of diagnosis.

Pregnancy

Pregnancy is associated with a rapid progression of diabetic retinopathy.[93,94] Women with preexisting type 1 or type 2 diabetes who are planning pregnancy or who have become pregnant should be counseled on the risk of development and/or progression of diabetic retinopathy. In addition, rapid implementation of intensive glycemic management in the setting of retinopathy is associated with early worsening of retinopathy.[86] Women who develop gestational diabetes mellitus do not require eye examinations during pregnancy and do not appear to be at increased risk of developing diabetic retinopathy during pregnancy.[95]

TREATMENT

Two of the main motivations for screening for diabetic retinopathy are to prevent loss of vision and to intervene with treatment when vision loss can be prevented or reversed.

Photocoagulation Surgery

Two large trials, the Diabetic Retinopathy Study (DRS) in patients with PDR and the Early Treatment Diabetic Retinopathy Study (ETDRS) in patients with macular edema, provide the strongest support for the therapeutic benefits of photocoagulation surgery. The DRS[96] showed in 1978 that panretinal photocoagulation surgery reduced the risk of severe vision loss from PDR from 15.9% in untreated eyes to 6.4% in treated eyes with the greatest benefit ratio in those with more advanced baseline disease (disc neovascularization or vitreous hemorrhage).

In 1985, the ETDRS also verified the benefits of panretinal photocoagulation for high-risk PDR and in older-onset patients with severe nonproliferative diabetic retinopathy or less-than-high-risk PDR. Panretinal laser photocoagulation is still commonly used to manage complications of diabetic retinopathy that involve retinal neovascularization and its complications.

Anti-Vascular Endothelial Growth Factor Treatment

Recent data from the Diabetic Retinopathy Clinical Research Network and others demonstrate that intravitreal injections of anti-vascular endothelial growth factor (anti-VEGF) agent, specifically ranibizumab, resulted in visual acuity outcomes that were not inferior to those observed in patients treated with panretinal laser at 2 years of follow-up.[97] In addition, it was observed that patients treated with ranibizumab tended to have less peripheral visual field loss, fewer vitrectomy surgeries for secondary complications from their proliferative disease, and a lower risk of developing diabetic macular edema. However, a potential drawback in using anti-VEGF therapy to manage proliferative disease is that patients were required to have a greater number of visits and received a greater number of treatments than is typically required for management with panretinal laser, which may not be optimal for some patients. Other emerging therapies for retinopathy that may use sustained intravitreal delivery of pharmacologic agents are currently under investigation. The FDA approved ranibizumab for the treatment of diabetic retinopathy in 2017.

While the ETDRS[98] established the benefit of focal laser photocoagulation surgery in eyes with clinically significant macular edema (defined as retinal edema located at or within 500 μm of the center of the macula), current data from well-designed clinical trials demonstrate that intravitreal anti-VEGF agents provide a more effective treatment regimen for central-involved diabetic macular edema than monotherapy or even combination therapy with laser.[99–101] There are currently three anti-VEGF agents commonly used to treat eyes with central-involved diabetic macular edema—bevacizumab, ranibizumab, and aflibercept.[77]

In both the DRS and the ETDRS, laser photocoagulation surgery was beneficial in reducing the risk of further visual loss in affected patients but generally not beneficial in reversing already diminished acuity. Anti-VEGF therapy improves vision and has replaced the need for laser photocoagulation in the vast majority of patients with diabetic macular edema.[102] Most patients require near-monthly administration of intravitreal therapy with anti-VEGF agents during the first 12 months of treatment, with fewer injections needed in subsequent years to maintain remission from central-involved diabetic macular edema.

Adjunctive Therapy

Lowering blood pressure has been shown to decrease retinopathy progression, although tight targets (systolic blood pressure <120 mmHg) do not impart additional benefit.[83] ACE inhibitors and ARBs are both effective treatments in diabetic retinopathy.[103] In patients with dyslipidemia, retinopathy progression may be slowed by the addition of fenofibrate, particularly with very mild nonproliferative diabetic retinopathy at baseline.[81,104]

RECOMMENDATIONS

Screening

11.26 All patients should be assessed for diabetic peripheral neuropathy starting at diagnosis of type 2 diabetes and 5 years after the diagnosis of type 1 diabetes and at least annually thereafter. **B**

11.27 Assessment for distal symmetric polyneuropathy should include a careful history and assessment of either temperature or pinprick sensation (small-fiber function) and vibration sensation using a 128-Hz tuning fork (for large-fiber function). All patients should have annual 10-g monofilament testing to identify feet at risk for ulceration and amputation. **B**

11.28 Symptoms and signs of autonomic neuropathy should be assessed in patients with microvascular complications. **E**

Treatment

11.29 Optimize glucose control to prevent or delay the development of neuropathy in patients with type 1 diabetes **A** and to slow the progression of neuropathy in patients with type 2 diabetes. **B**

11.30 Assess and treat patients to reduce pain related to diabetic peripheral neuropathy **B** and symptoms of autonomic neuropathy and to improve quality of life. **E**

11.31 Pregabalin, duloxetine, or gabapentin are recommended as initial pharmacologic treatments for neuropathic pain in diabetes. **A**

The diabetic neuropathies are a heterogeneous group of disorders with diverse clinical manifestations. The early recognition and appropriate management of neuropathy in the patient with diabetes is important.

1. Diabetic neuropathy is a diagnosis of exclusion. Nondiabetic neuropathies may be present in patients with diabetes and may be treatable.
2. Numerous treatment options exist for symptomatic diabetic neuropathy.
3. Up to 50% of diabetic peripheral neuropathy (DPN) may be asymptomatic. If not recognized and if preventive foot care is not implemented, patients are at risk for injuries to their insensate feet.
4. Recognition and treatment of autonomic neuropathy may improve symptoms, reduce sequelae, and improve quality of life.

Specific treatment for the underlying nerve damage, other than improved glycemic control, is currently not available. Glycemic control can effectively prevent DPN and cardiac autonomic neuropathy (CAN) in type 1 diabetes[105,106] and may modestly slow their progression in type 2 diabetes,[32] but does not reverse neuronal loss. Therapeutic strategies (pharmacologic and nonpharmacologic) for the relief of painful DPN and symptoms of autonomic neuropathy can potentially reduce pain[107] and improve quality of life.

DIAGNOSIS

Diabetic Peripheral Neuropathy

Patients with type 1 diabetes for 5 or more years and all patients with type 2 diabetes should be assessed annually for DPN using the medical history and simple clinical tests. Symptoms vary according to the class of sensory fibers involved. The most common early symptoms are induced by the involvement of small fibers and include pain and dysesthesia (unpleasant sensations of burning and tingling). The involvement of large fibers may cause numbness and loss of protective sensation (LOPS). LOPS indicates the presence of distal sensorimotor polyneuropathy and is a risk factor for diabetic foot ulceration. The following clinical tests may be used to assess small- and large-fiber function and protective sensation:

1. Small-fiber function: pinprick and temperature sensation
2. Large-fiber function: vibration perception and 10-g monofilament
3. Protective sensation: 10-g monofilament

These tests not only screen for the presence of dysfunction but also predict future risk of complications. Electrophysiological testing or referral to a neurologist is rarely needed, except in situations where the clinical features are atypical or the diagnosis is unclear.

In all patients with diabetes and DPN, causes of neuropathy other than diabetes should be considered, including toxins (e.g., alcohol), neurotoxic medications (e.g., chemotherapy), vitamin B_{12} deficiency, hypothyroidism, renal disease, malignancies (e.g., multiple myeloma, bronchogenic carcinoma), infections (e.g., HIV), chronic inflammatory demyelinating neuropathy, inherited neuropathies, and vasculitis.[108] See the American Diabetes Association position statement "Diabetic Neuropathy" for more details.[107]

Diabetic Autonomic Neuropathy

The symptoms and signs of autonomic neuropathy should be elicited carefully during the history and physical examination. Major clinical manifestations of diabetic autonomic neuropathy include hypoglycemia unawareness, resting tachycardia, orthostatic hypotension, gastroparesis, constipation, diarrhea, fecal incontinence, ED, neurogenic bladder, and sudomotor dysfunction with either increased or decreased sweating.

Cardiac Autonomic Neuropathy

CAN is associated with mortality independently of other cardiovascular risk factors.[109,110] In its early stages, CAN may be completely asymptomatic and detected only by decreased heart rate variability with deep breathing. Advanced disease may be associated with resting tachycardia (>100 bpm) and orthostatic hypotension (a fall in systolic or diastolic blood pressure by >20 mmHg or >10 mmHg, respectively, upon standing without an appropriate increase in heart rate). CAN treatment is generally focused on alleviating symptoms.

Gastrointestinal Neuropathies

Gastrointestinal neuropathies may involve any portion of the gastrointestinal tract with manifestations including esophageal dysmotility, gastroparesis, constipation, diarrhea, and fecal incontinence. Gastroparesis should be suspected in individuals with erratic glycemic control or with upper gastrointestinal symptoms without another identified cause. Exclusion of organic causes of gastric outlet obstruction or peptic ulcer disease (with esophagogastroduodenoscopy or a barium study of the stomach) is needed before considering a diagnosis of or specialized testing for gastroparesis. The diagnostic gold standard for gastroparesis is the measurement of gastric emptying with scintigraphy of digestible solids at 15-min intervals for 4 h after food intake. The use of ^{13}C octanoic acid breath test is emerging as a viable alternative.

Genitourinary Disturbances

Diabetic autonomic neuropathy may also cause genitourinary disturbances, including sexual dysfunction and bladder dysfunction. In men, diabetic autonomic neuropathy may cause ED and/or retrograde ejaculation.[107] Female sexual dysfunction occurs more frequently in those with diabetes and presents as decreased sexual desire, increased pain during intercourse, decreased sexual arousal, and inadequate lubrication.[111] Lower urinary tract symptoms manifest as urinary incontinence and bladder dysfunction (nocturia, frequent urination, urination urgency, and weak urinary stream). Evaluation of bladder function should be performed for individuals with diabetes who have recurrent urinary tract infections, pyelonephritis, incontinence, or a palpable bladder.

TREATMENT

Glycemic Control

Near-normal glycemic control, implemented early in the course of diabetes, has been shown to effectively delay or prevent the development of DPN and CAN in patients with type 1 diabetes.[112-115] Although the evidence for the benefit of near-normal glycemic control is not as strong for type 2 diabetes, some studies have demonstrated a modest slowing of progression without reversal of neuronal loss.[32,116] Specific glucose-lowering strategies may have different effects. In a post hoc analysis, participants, particularly men, in the Bypass Angioplasty Revascularization Investigation in Type 2 Diabetes (BARI 2D) trial treated with insulin sensitizers had a lower incidence of distal symmetric polyneuropathy over 4 years than those treated with insulin/sulfonylurea.[117]

Neuropathic Pain

Neuropathic pain can be severe and can impact quality of life, limit mobility, and contribute to depression and social dysfunction.[118] No compelling evidence exists in support of glycemic control or lifestyle management as therapies for neuropathic pain in diabetes or prediabetes, which leaves only pharmaceutical interventions.[119]

Pregabalin and duloxetine have received regulatory approval by the FDA, Health Canada, and the European Medicines Agency for the treatment of neuropathic pain in diabetes. The opioid tapentadol has regulatory approval in the U.S. and Canada, but the evidence of its use is weaker.[120] Comparative effectiveness studies and trials that include quality-of-life outcomes are rare, so treatment decisions must consider each patient's presentation and comorbidities and often follow a trial-and-error approach. Given the range of partially effective treatment options, a tailored and stepwise pharmacologic strategy with careful attention to relative symptom improvement, medication adherence, and medication side effects is recommended to achieve pain reduction and improve quality of life.[121–123]

Pregabalin, a calcium channel α2-δ subunit ligand, is the most extensively studied drug for DPN. The majority of studies testing pregabalin have reported favorable effects on the proportion of participants with at least 30–50% improvement in pain.[120,122,124–127] However, not all trials with pregabalin have been positive,[120,122,128,129] especially when treating patients with advanced refractory DPN.[126] Adverse effects may be more severe in older patients[130] and may be attenuated by lower starting doses and more gradual titration. The related drug, *gabapentin*, has also shown efficacy for pain control in diabetic neuropathy and may be less expensive, although it is not FDA approved for this indication.[131]

Duloxetine is a selective norepinephrine and serotonin reuptake inhibitor. Doses of 60 and 120 mg/day showed efficacy in the treatment of pain associated with DPN in multicenter randomized trials, although some of these had high drop-out rates.[120,122,127,129] Duloxetine also appeared to improve neuropathy-related quality of life.[132] In longer-term studies, a small increase in A1C was reported in people with diabetes treated with duloxetine compared with placebo.[133] Adverse events may be more severe in older people but may be attenuated with lower doses and slower titrations of duloxetine.

Tapentadol is a centrally acting opioid analgesic that exerts its analgesic effects through both µ-opioid receptor agonism and noradrenaline reuptake inhibition. Extended-release tapentadol was approved by the FDA for the treatment of neuropathic pain associated with diabetes based on data from two multicenter clinical trials in which participants titrated to an optimal dose of tapentadol were randomly assigned to continue that dose or switch to placebo.[134,135] However, both used a design enriched for patients who responded to tapentadol and therefore their results are not generalizable. A recent systematic review and meta-analysis by the Special Interest Group on Neuropathic Pain of the International Association for the Study of Pain found the evidence supporting the effectiveness of tapentadol in reducing neuropathic pain to be inconclusive.[120] Therefore, given the high risk for addiction and safety concerns compared with the relatively modest pain reduction, the use of extended-release tapentadol is not generally recommended as a first- or second-line therapy. The use of any opioids for management of chronic neuropathic pain carries the risk of addiction and should be avoided.

Tricyclic antidepressants, venlafaxine, carbamazepine, and topical capsaicin, although not approved for the treatment of painful DPN, may be effective and considered for the treatment of painful DPN.[107,120,122]

Orthostatic Hypotension

Treating orthostatic hypotension is challenging. The therapeutic goal is to minimize postural symptoms rather than to restore normotension. Most patients require both nonpharmacologic measures (e.g., ensuring adequate salt intake, avoiding medications that aggravate hypotension, or using compressive garments over the legs and abdomen) and pharmacologic measures. Physical activity and exercise should be encouraged to avoid deconditioning, which is known to exacerbate orthostatic intolerance, and volume repletion with fluids and salt is critical.

Midodrine and droxidopa are approved by the FDA for the treatment of orthostatic hypotension.

Gastroparesis

Treatment for diabetic gastroparesis may be very challenging. A low-fiber, low-fat eating plan provided in small frequent meals with a greater proportion of liquid calories may be useful.[136-138] In addition, foods with small particle size may improve key symptoms.[139] Withdrawing drugs with adverse effects on gastrointestinal motility including opioids, anticholinergics, tricyclic antidepressants, GLP-1 RA, pramlintide, and possibly dipeptidyl peptidase 4 inhibitors may also improve intestinal motility.[136,140] In cases of severe gastroparesis, pharmacologic interventions are needed. Only metoclopramide, a prokinetic agent, is approved by the FDA for the treatment of gastroparesis. However, the level of evidence regarding the benefits of metoclopramide for the management of gastroparesis is weak, and given the risk for serious adverse effects (extrapyramidal signs such as acute dystonic reactions, drug-induced parkinsonism, akathisia, and tardive dyskinesia), its use in the treatment of gastroparesis beyond 12 weeks is no longer recommended by the FDA or the European Medicines Agency. It should be reserved for severe cases that are unresponsive to other therapies.[140] Other treatment options include domperidone (available outside of the U.S.) and erythromycin, which is only effective for short-term use due to tachyphylaxis.[141,142] Gastric electrical stimulation using a surgically implantable device has received approval from the FDA, although its efficacy is variable and use is limited to patients with severe symptoms that are refractory to other treatments.[143]

Erectile Dysfunction

In addition to treatment of hypogonadism if present, treatments for ED may include phosphodiesterase type 5 inhibitors, intracorporeal or intraurethral prostaglandins, vacuum devices, or penile prostheses. As with DPN treatments, these interventions do not change the underlying pathology and natural history of the disease process but may improve the patient's quality of life.

FOOT CARE

RECOMMENDATIONS

11.32 Perform a comprehensive foot evaluation at least annually to identify risk factors for ulcers and amputations. **B**

11.33 Patients with evidence of sensory loss or prior ulceration or amputation should have their feet inspected at every visit. **C**

11.34 Obtain a prior history of ulceration, amputation, Charcot foot, angioplasty or vascular surgery, cigarette smoking, retinopathy, and renal disease and assess current symptoms of neuropathy (pain, burning, numbness) and vascular disease (leg fatigue, claudication). **B**

11.35 The examination should include inspection of the skin, assessment of foot deformities, neurological assessment (10-g monofilament testing with at least one other assessment: pinprick, temperature, vibration), and vascular assessment including pulses in the legs and feet. **B**

11.36 Patients with symptoms of claudication or decreased or absent pedal pulses should be referred for ankle-brachial index and for further vascular assessment as appropriate. **C**

11.37 A multidisciplinary approach is recommended for individuals with foot ulcers and high-risk feet (e.g., dialysis patients and those with Charcot foot or prior ulcers or amputation). **B**

11.38 Refer patients who smoke or who have histories of prior lower-extremity complications, loss of protective sensation, structural abnormalities, or peripheral arterial disease to foot care specialists for ongoing preventive care and lifelong surveillance. **C**

11.39 Provide general preventive foot self-care education to all patients with diabetes. **B**

11.40 The use of specialized therapeutic footwear is recommended for high-risk patients with diabetes including those with severe neuropathy, foot deformities, or history of amputation. **B**

Foot ulcers and amputation, which are consequences of diabetic neuropathy and/or PAD, are common and represent major causes of morbidity and mortality in people with diabetes. Early recognition and treatment of patients with diabetes and feet at risk for ulcers and amputations can delay or prevent adverse outcomes.

The risk of ulcers or amputations is increased in people who have the following risk factors:

- Poor glycemic control
- Peripheral neuropathy with LOPS
- Cigarette smoking
- Foot deformities
- Preulcerative callus or corn
- PAD
- History of foot ulcer
- Amputation
- Visual impairment
- CKD (especially patients on dialysis)

Clinicians are encouraged to review ADA screening recommendations for further details and practical descriptions of how to perform components of the comprehensive foot examination.[144]

EVALUATION FOR LOSS OF PROTECTIVE SENSATION

All adults with diabetes should undergo a comprehensive foot evaluation at least annually. Detailed foot assessments may occur more frequently in patients with histories of ulcers or amputations, foot deformities, insensate feet, and PAD.[145] To assess risk, clinicians should ask about history of foot ulcers or amputation, neuropathic and peripheral vascular symptoms, impaired vision, renal disease, tobacco use, and foot care practices. A general inspection of skin integrity and musculoskeletal deformities should be performed. Vascular assessment should include inspection and palpation of pedal pulses.

The neurological exam performed as part of the foot examination is designed to identify LOPS rather than early neuropathy. The 10-g monofilament is the most useful test to diagnose LOPS. Ideally, the 10-g monofilament test should be performed with at least one other assessment (pinprick, temperature or vibration sensation using a 128-Hz tuning fork, or ankle reflexes). Absent monofilament sensation suggests LOPS, while at least two normal tests (and no abnormal test) rules out LOPS.

EVALUATION FOR PERIPHERAL ARTERIAL DISEASE

Initial screening for PAD should include a history of decreased walking speed, leg fatigue, claudication, and an assessment of the pedal pulses. Ankle-brachial index testing should be performed in patients with symptoms or signs of PAD.

PATIENT EDUCATION

All patients with diabetes and particularly those with high-risk foot conditions (history of ulcer or amputation, deformity, LOPS, or PAD) and their families should be provided general education about risk factors and appropriate management.[146] Patients at risk should understand the implications of foot deformities, LOPS, and PAD; the proper care of the foot, including nail and skin care; and the importance of foot monitoring on a daily basis. Patients with LOPS should be educated on ways to substitute other sensory modalities (palpation or visual inspection using an unbreakable mirror) for surveillance of early foot problems.

The selection of appropriate footwear and footwear behaviors at home should also be discussed. Patients' understanding of these issues and their physical ability to conduct proper foot surveillance and care should be assessed. Patients with visual difficulties, physical constraints preventing movement, or cognitive problems that impair their ability to assess the condition of the foot and to institute appropriate responses will need other people, such as family members, to assist with their care.

TREATMENT

People with neuropathy or evidence of increased plantar pressures (e.g., erythema, warmth, or calluses) may be adequately managed with well-fitted walking shoes or athletic shoes that cushion the feet and redistribute pressure. People with bony deformities (e.g., hammertoes, prominent metatarsal heads, bunions) may need extra wide or deep shoes. People with bony deformities, including Charcot foot, who cannot be accommodated with commercial therapeutic footwear, will require custom-molded shoes. Special consideration and a thorough workup should be performed when patients with neuropathy present with the acute onset of a red, hot, swollen foot or ankle, and Charcot neuroarthropathy should be excluded. Early diagnosis and treatment of Charcot neuroarthropathy is the best way to prevent deformities that increase the risk of ulceration and amputation. The routine prescription of therapeutic footwear is not generally recommended. However, patients should be provided adequate information to aid in selection of appropriate footwear. General footwear recommendations include a broad and square toe box, laces with three or four eyes per side, padded tongue, quality lightweight materials, and sufficient size to accommodate a cushioned insole. Use of custom therapeutic footwear can help reduce the risk of future foot ulcers in high-risk patients.[145,147]

Most diabetic foot infections are polymicrobial, with aerobic gram-positive cocci. Staphylococci and streptococci are the most common causative organisms. Wounds without evidence of soft tissue or bone infection do not require antibiotic therapy. Empiric antibiotic therapy can be narrowly targeted at gram-positive cocci in many patients with acute infections, but those at risk for infection with antibiotic-resistant organisms or with chronic, previously treated, or severe infections require broader-spectrum regimens and should be referred to specialized care centers.[148] Foot ulcers and wound care may require care by a podiatrist, orthopedic or vascular surgeon, or rehabilitation specialist experienced in the management of individuals with diabetes.[148]

Hyperbaric oxygen therapy (HBOT) in patients with diabetic foot ulcers has mixed evidence supporting its use as an adjunctive treatment to enhance wound healing and prevent amputation.[149-151] In a relatively high-quality double-blind study of patients with chronic diabetic foot ulcers, hyperbaric oxygen as an adjunctive therapy resulted in significantly more complete healing of the index ulcer in patients treated with HBOT compared with placebo at 1 year of follow-up.[152] However, multiple subsequently published studies have either failed to demonstrate a benefit of HBOT or have been relatively small with potential flaws in study design.[150] A well-conducted randomized controlled study performed in 103 patients found that HBOT did not reduce the indication for amputation or facilitate wound healing compared with comprehensive wound care in patients with chronic diabetic foot ulcers.[153] A systematic review by the International Working Group on the Diabetic Foot of interventions to improve the healing of chronic diabetic foot ulcers concluded that analysis of the evidence continues to present methodological challenges as randomized controlled studies remain few, with a majority being of poor quality.[150] HBOT also does not seem to have a significant effect on health-related quality of life in patients with diabetic foot ulcers.[154,155] A recent review concluded that the evidence to date remains inconclusive regarding the clinical and cost-effectiveness of HBOT as an adjunctive treatment to standard wound care for diabetic foot ulcers.[156] Results from the recently published Dutch DAMOCLES (Does Applying More Oxygen Cure Lower Extremity Sores?) trial demonstrated that HBOT in patients with diabetes and ischemic wounds did not significantly improve complete wound healing and limb salvage.[157] The Centers for Medicare & Medicaid Services currently covers HBOT for diabetic foot ulcers that have failed a standard course of wound therapy when there are no measurable signs of healing for at least 30 consecutive days.[158] HBOT should be a topic of shared decision making before treatment is considered for selected patients with diabetic foot ulcers.[158]

REFERENCES

1. Tuttle KR, Bakris GL, Bilous RW, et al. Diabetic kidney disease: a report from an ADA Consensus Conference. *Diabetes Care* 2014;37:2864–2883

2. National Kidney Foundation. KDIGO 2012 clinical practice guideline for the evaluation and management of chronic kidney disease. *Kidney Int Suppl* 2013;3:1–150

3. Afkarian M, Zelnick LR, Hall YN, et al. Clinical manifestations of kidney disease among US adults with diabetes, 1988–2014. *JAMA* 2016;316: 602–610

4. de Boer IH, Rue TC, Hall YN, Heagerty PJ, Weiss NS, Himmelfarb J. Temporal trends in the prevalence of diabetic kidney disease in the United States. *JAMA* 2011;305:2532–2539

5. de Boer IH; DCCT/EDIC Research Group. Kidney disease and related findings in the Diabetes Control and Complications Trial/Epidemiology of Diabetes Interventions and Complications study. *Diabetes Care* 2014;37: 24–30

6. United States Renal Data System. *Annual Data Report: Epidemiology of Kidney Disease in the United States*. Bethesda, MD, National Institutes of Health, National Institute of Diabetes and Digestive and Kidney Diseases, 2016

7. Fox CS, Matsushita K, Woodward M, et al.; Chronic Kidney Disease Prognosis Consortium. Associations of kidney disease measures with mortality and end-stage renal disease in individuals with and without diabetes: a meta-analysis. *Lancet* 2012;380:1662–1673

8. Afkarian M, Sachs MC, Kestenbaum B, et al. Kidney disease and increased mortality risk in type 2 diabetes. *J Am Soc Nephrol* 2013;24:302–308

9. Groop P-H, Thomas MC, Moran JL, et al.; FinnDiane Study Group. The presence and severity of chronic kidney disease predicts all-cause mortality in type 1 diabetes. *Diabetes* 2009;58:1651–1658

10. Delanaye P, Glassock RJ, Pottel H, Rule AD. An age-calibrated definition of chronic kidney disease: rationale and benefits. *Clin Biochem Rev* 2016;37: 17–26

11. Kramer HJ, Nguyen QD, Curhan G, Hsu C-Y. Renal insufficiency in the absence of albuminuria and retinopathy among adults with type 2 diabetes mellitus. *JAMA* 2003;289:3273–3277

12. Molitch ME, Steffes M, Sun W, et al.; Epidemiology of Diabetes Interventions and Complications Study Group. Development and progression of renal insufficiency with and without albuminuria in adults with type 1 diabetes in the Diabetes Control and Complications Trial and the Epidemiology of Diabetes Interventions and Complications study. *Diabetes Care* 2010;33:1536–1543

13. He F, Xia X, Wu XF, Yu XQ, Huang FX. Diabetic retinopathy in predicting diabetic nephropathy in patients with type 2 diabetes and renal disease: a meta-analysis. *Diabetologia* 2013;56:457–466

14. Levey AS, Coresh J, Balk E, et al.; National Kidney Foundation. National Kidney Foundation practice guidelines for chronic kidney disease: evaluation, classification, and stratification. *Ann Intern Med* 2003;139:137–147

15. Coresh J, Turin TC, Matsushita K, et al. Decline in estimated glomerular filtration rate and subsequent risk of end-stage renal disease and mortality. *JAMA* 2014;311:2518–2531

16. James MT, Grams ME, Woodward M, et al.; CKD Prognosis Consortium. A meta-analysis of the association of estimated GFR, albuminuria, diabetes mellitus, and hypertension with acute kidney injury. *Am J Kidney Dis* 2015;66:602–612

17. Nadkarni GN, Ferrandino R, Chang A, et al. Acute kidney injury in patients on SGLT2 inhibitors: a propensity-matched analysis. *Diabetes Care* 2017;40:1479–1485

18. Wanner C, Inzucchi SE, Lachin JM, et al.; EMPA-REG OUTCOME Investigators. Empagliflozin and progression of kidney disease in type 2 diabetes. *N Engl J Med* 2016;375:323–334

19. Neuen BL, Ohkuma T, Neal B, et al. Cardiovascular and renal outcomes with canagliflozin according to baseline kidney function: data from the CANVAS Program. *Circulation* 2018;138:1537–1550

20. Thakar CV, Christianson A, Himmelfarb J, Leonard AC. Acute kidney injury episodes and chronic kidney disease risk in diabetes mellitus. *Clin J Am Soc Nephrol* 2011;6:2567–2572

21. Hughes-Austin JM, Rifkin DE, Beben T, et al. The relation of serum potassium concentration with cardiovascular events and mortality in community-living individuals. *Clin J Am Soc Nephrol* 2017;12:245–252

22. Bandak G, Sang Y, Gasparini A, et al. Hyperkalemia after initiating renin-angiotensin system blockade: the Stockholm Creatinine Measurements (SCREAM) Project. *J Am Heart Assoc* 2017;6:e005428

23. Nilsson E, Gasparini A, Ärnlöv J, et al. Incidence and determinants of hyperkalemia and hypokalemia in a large healthcare system. *Int J Cardiol* 2017;245:277–284

24. de Boer IH, Gao X, Cleary PA, et al.; Diabetes Control and Complications Trial/Epidemiology of Diabetes Interventions and Complications (DCCT/EDIC) Research Group. Albuminuria changes and cardiovascular and renal outcomes in type 1 diabetes: the DCCT/EDIC study. *Clin J Am Soc Nephrol* 2016;11:1969–1977

25. Sumida K, Molnar MZ, Potukuchi PK, et al. Changes in albuminuria and subsequent risk of incident kidney disease. *Clin J Am Soc Nephrol* 2017; 12:1941–1949

25a. Inker LA, Grams ME, Levey AS, et al.; CKD Prognosis Consortium. Relationship of estimated GFR and albuminuria to concurrent laboratory abnormalities: an individual participant data meta-analysis in a global consortium. *Am J Kidney Dis* 19 October 2018 [Epub ahead of print]. DOI: 10.1053/j.ajkd.2018.08.013

26. Mills KT, Chen J, Yang W, et al.; Chronic Renal Insufficiency Cohort (CRIC) Study Investigators. Sodium excretion and the risk of cardiovascular disease in patients with chronic kidney disease. *JAMA* 2016;315:2200–2210

27. DCCT/EDIC Research Group. Effect of intensive diabetes treatment on albuminuria in type 1 diabetes: long-term follow-up of the Diabetes Control and Complications Trial and Epidemiology of Diabetes Interventions and Complications study. *Lancet Diabetes Endocrinol* 2014;2:793–800

28. de Boer IH, Sun W, Cleary PA, et al.; DCCT/EDIC Research Group. Intensive diabetes therapy and glomerular filtration rate in type 1 diabetes. *N Engl J Med* 2011;365:2366–2376

29. UK Prospective Diabetes Study (UKPDS) Group. Effect of intensive blood-glucose control with metformin on complications in overweight patients with type 2 diabetes (UKPDS 34). *Lancet* 1998;352:854–865

30. UK Prospective Diabetes Study (UKPDS) Group. Intensive blood-glucose control with sulphonylureas or insulin compared with conventional treatment and risk of complications in patients with type 2 diabetes (UKPDS 33). *Lancet* 1998;352:837–853

31. Patel A, MacMahon S, Chalmers J, et al.; ADVANCE Collaborative Group. Intensive blood glucose control and vascular outcomes in patients with type 2 diabetes. *N Engl J Med* 2008;358:2560–2572

32. Ismail-Beigi F, Craven T, Banerji MA, et al.; ACCORD trial group. Effect of intensive treatment of hyperglycaemia on microvascular outcomes in type 2 diabetes: an analysis of the ACCORD randomised trial. *Lancet* 2010;376:419–430

33. Zoungas S, Chalmers J, Neal B, et al.; ADVANCE-ON Collaborative Group. Follow-up of blood-pressure lowering and glucose control in type 2 diabetes. *N Engl J Med* 2014;371:1392–1406

34. Zoungas S, Arima H, Gerstein HC, et al.; Collaborators on Trials of Lowering Glucose (CONTROL) group. Effects of intensive glucose control on microvascular outcomes in patients with type 2 diabetes: a meta-analysis of individual participant data from randomised controlled trials. *Lancet Diabetes Endocrinol* 2017;5:431–437

35. Miller ME, Bonds DE, Gerstein HC, et al.; ACCORD Investigators. The effects of baseline characteristics, glycaemia treatment approach, and glycated haemoglobin concentration on the risk of severe hypoglycaemia: post hoc epidemiological analysis of the ACCORD study. *BMJ* 2010;340:b5444

36. Papademetriou V, Lovato L, Doumas M, et al.; ACCORD Study Group. Chronic kidney disease and intensive glycemic control increase cardiovascular risk in patients with type 2 diabetes. *Kidney Int* 2015;87:649–659

37. Perkovic V, Heerspink HL, Chalmers J, et al.; ADVANCE Collaborative Group. Intensive glucose control improves kidney outcomes in patients with type 2 diabetes. *Kidney Int* 2013;83:517–523

38. Wong MG, Perkovic V, Chalmers J, et al.; ADVANCE-ON Collaborative Group. Long-term benefits of intensive glucose control for preventing end-stage kidney disease: ADVANCE-ON. *Diabetes Care* 2016;39:694–700

39. National Kidney Foundation. KDOQI clinical practice guideline for diabetes and CKD: 2012 update. *Am J Kidney Dis* 2012;60:850–886

40. Cherney DZI, Perkins BA, Soleymanlou N, et al. Renal hemodynamic effect of sodium-glucose cotransporter 2 inhibition in patients with type 1 diabetes mellitus. *Circulation* 2014;129:587–597

41. Heerspink HJL, Desai M, Jardine M, Balis D, Meininger G, Perkovic V. Canagliflozin slows progression of renal function decline independently of glycemic effects. *J Am Soc Nephrol* 2017;28:368–375 PubMed

42. Neal B, Perkovic V, Mahaffey KW, et al.; CANVAS Program Collaborative Group. Canagliflozin and cardiovascular and renal events in type 2 diabetes. *N Engl J Med* 2017;377:644–657

43. Zelniker TA, Braunwald E. Cardiac and renal effects of sodium-glucose cotransporter 2 inhibitors in diabetes: JACC state-of-the-art review. *J Am Coll Cardiol* 2018;72:1845–1855

44. Marso SP, Daniels GH, Brown-Frandsen K, et al.; LEADER Steering Committee; LEADER Trial Investigators. Liraglutide and cardiovascular outcomes in type 2 diabetes. *N Engl J Med* 2016;375:311–322

45. Cooper ME, Perkovic V, McGill JB, et al. Kidney disease end points in a pooled analysis of individual patient-level data from a large clinical trials program of the dipeptidyl peptidase 4 inhibitor linagliptin in type 2 diabetes. *Am J Kidney Dis* 2015;66:441–449

46. Mann JFE, Ørsted DD, Brown-Frandsen K, et al.; LEADER Steering Committee and Investigators. Liraglutide and renal outcomes in type 2 diabetes. *N Engl J Med* 2017;377:839–848

47. Marso SP, Bain SC, Consoli A, et al.; SUSTAIN 6 Investigators. Semaglutide and cardiovascular outcomes in patients with type 2 diabetes. *N Engl J Med* 2016;375:1834–1844

48. Karter AJ, Warton EM, Lipska KJ, et al. Development and validation of a tool to identify patients with type 2 diabetes at high risk of hypoglycemia-related emergency department or hospital use. *JAMA Intern Med* 2017;177:1461–1470

49. Moen MF, Zhan M, Hsu VD, et al. Frequency of hypoglycemia and its significance in chronic kidney disease. *Clin J Am Soc Nephrol* 2009;4:1121–1127

50. U.S. Food and Drug Administration. FDA drug safety communication: FDA revises warnings regarding use of the diabetes medicine metformin in certain patients with reduced kidney function [Internet], 2016. Available from http://www.fda.gov/Drugs/DrugSafety/ucm493244.htm. Accessed 14 October 2016

51. Zinman B, Wanner C, Lachin JM, et al.; EMPA-REG OUTCOME Investigators. Empagliflozin, cardiovascular outcomes, and mortality in type 2 diabetes. *N Engl J Med* 2015;373:2117–2128

52. Mahaffey KW, Neal B, Perkovic V, et al.; CANVAS Program Collaborative Group. Canagliflozin for primary and secondary prevention of cardiovascular events: results from the CANVAS Program (Canagliflozin Cardiovascular Assessment Study). *Circulation* 2018;137:323–334

53. Tuttle KR, Lakshmanan MC, Rayner B, et al. Dulaglutide versus insulin glargine in patients with type 2 diabetes and moderate-to-severe chronic kidney disease (AWARD-7): a multicentre, open-label, randomised trial. *Lancet Diabetes Endocrinol* 2018;6:605–617

53a. Lambers-Heerspink HJ, Desai M, Jardine M, et al. Canagliflozin slows progression of renal function decline independent of glycemic effects. *J Am Soc Nephrol* 2017;28:368–375

54. Jardine MJ, Mahaffey KW, Neal B, et al.; CREDENCE study investigators. The Canagliflozin and Renal Endpoints in Diabetes with Established Nephropathy Clinical Evaluation (CREDENCE) study rationale, design, and baseline characteristics. *Am J Nephrol* 2017;46:462–472

55. Wanner C, Lachin JM, Inzucchi SE, et al.; EMPA-REG OUTCOME Investigators. Empagliflozin and clinical outcomes in patients with type 2 diabetes, established cardiovascular disease and chronic kidney disease. *Circulation* 2018;137:119–129

56. Leehey DJ, Zhang JH, Emanuele NV, et al.; VANEPHRON-D Study Group. BP and renal outcomes in diabetic kidney disease: the Veterans Affairs Nephropathy in Diabetes Trial. *Clin J Am Soc Nephrol* 2015;10:2159–2169

57. Emdin CA, Rahimi K, Neal B, Callender T, Perkovic V, Patel A. Blood pressure lowering in type 2 diabetes: a systematic review and meta-analysis. *JAMA* 2015;313:603–615

58. Cushman WC, Evans GW, Byington RP, et al.; ACCORD Study Group. Effects of intensive blood-pressure control in type 2 diabetes mellitus. *N Engl J Med* 2010;362:1575–1585

59. UK Prospective Diabetes Study Group. Tight blood pressure control and risk of macrovascular and microvascular complications in type 2 diabetes: UKPDS 38. *BMJ* 1998;317:703–713

60. de Boer IH, Bangalore S, Benetos A, et al. Diabetes and hypertension: a position statement by the American Diabetes Association. *Diabetes Care* 2017;40:1273–1284

61. Brenner BM, Cooper ME, de Zeeuw D, et al.; RENAAL Study Investigators. Effects of losartan on renal and cardiovascular outcomes in patients with type 2 diabetes and nephropathy. *N Engl J Med* 2001;345:861–869

62. Lewis EJ, Hunsicker LG, Bain RP, Rohde RD; The Collaborative Study Group. The effect of angiotensin-converting-enzyme inhibition on diabetic nephropathy. *N Engl J Med* 1993;329:1456–1462

63. Lewis EJ, Hunsicker LG, Clarke WR, et al.; Collaborative Study Group. Renoprotective effect of the angiotensin-receptor antagonist irbesartan in patients with nephropathy due to type 2 diabetes. *N Engl J Med* 2001;345:851–860

64. Heart Outcomes Prevention Evaluation Study Investigators. Effects of ramipril on cardiovascular and microvascular outcomes in people with diabetes mellitus: results of the HOPE study and MICRO-HOPE substudy. *Lancet* 2000;355:253–259

65. Barnett AH, Bain SC, Bouter P, et al.; Diabetics Exposed to Telmisartan and Enalapril Study Group. Angiotensin-receptor blockade versus converting-enzyme inhibition in type 2 diabetes and nephropathy. *N Engl J Med* 2004;351:1952–1961

66. Wu H-Y, Peng C-L, Chen P-C, et al. Comparative effectiveness of angiotensin-converting enzyme inhibitors versus angiotensin II receptor blockers for major renal outcomes in patients with diabetes: a 15-year cohort study. *PLoS One* 2017;12:e0177654

67. Parving HH, Lehnert H, Bröchner-Mortensen J, Gomis R, Andersen S, Arner P; Irbesartan in Patients with Type 2 Diabetes and Microalbuminuria Study Group. The effect of irbesartan on the development of diabetic nephropathy in patients with type 2 diabetes. *N Engl J Med* 2001;345: 870–878

68. Bangalore S, Fakheri R, Toklu B, Messerli FH. Diabetes mellitus as a compelling indication for use of renin angiotensin system blockers: systematic review and meta-analysis of randomized trials. *BMJ* 2016;352:i438

69. Haller H, Ito S, Izzo JL Jr., et al.; ROADMAP Trial Investigators. Olmesartan for the delay or prevention of microalbuminuria in type 2 diabetes. *N Engl J Med* 2011;364:907–917

70. Mauer M, Zinman B, Gardiner R, et al. Renal and retinal effects of enalapril and losartan in type 1 diabetes. *N Engl J Med* 2009;361:40–51

71. Yusuf S, Teo KK, Pogue J, et al.; ONTARGET Investigators. Telmisartan, ramipril, or both in patients at high risk for vascular events. *N Engl J Med* 2008;358:1547–1559

72. Fried LF, Emanuele N, Zhang JH, et al.; VA NEPHRON-D Investigators. Combined angiotensin inhibition for the treatment of diabetic nephropathy. *N Engl J Med* 2013;369:1892–1903

73. Bakris GL, Agarwal R, Chan JC, et al.; Mineralocorticoid Receptor Antagonist Tolerability Study–Diabetic Nephropathy (ARTS-DN) Study Group. Effect of finerenone on albuminuria in patients with diabetic nephropathy: a randomized clinical trial. *JAMA* 2015;314:884–894

74. Williams B, MacDonald TM, Morant S, et al.; British Hypertension Society's PATHWAY Studies Group. Spironolactone versus placebo, bisoprolol, and doxazosin to determine the optimal treatment for drug-resistant hypertension (PATHWAY-2): a randomised, double-blind, crossover trial. *Lancet* 2015;386:2059–2068

75. Filippatos G, Anker SD, Böhm M, et al. A randomized controlled study of finerenone vs. eplerenone in patients with worsening chronic heart failure and diabetes mellitus and/or chronic kidney disease. *Eur Heart J* 2016;37: 2105–2114

76. Smart NA, Dieberg G, Ladhani M, Titus T. Early referral to specialist nephrology services for preventing the progression to end-stage kidney disease. *Cochrane Database Syst Rev* 2014;6:CD007333

77. Solomon SD, Chew E, Duh EJ, et al. Diabetic retinopathy: a position statement by the American Diabetes Association. *Diabetes Care* 2017;40:412–418

78. Klein R. Hyperglycemia and microvascular and macrovascular disease in diabetes. *Diabetes Care* 1995;18:258–268

79. Estacio RO, McFarling E, Biggerstaff S, Jeffers BW, Johnson D, Schrier RW. Overt albuminuria predicts diabetic retinopathy in Hispanics with NIDDM. *Am J Kidney Dis* 1998;31:947–953

80. Leske MC, Wu S-Y, Hennis A, et al.; Barbados Eye Study Group. Hyperglycemia, blood pressure, and the 9-year incidence of diabetic retinopathy: the Barbados Eye Studies. *Ophthalmology* 2005;112:799–805

81. Chew EY, Davis MD, Danis RP, et al.; Action to Control Cardiovascular Risk in Diabetes Eye Study Research Group. The effects of medical management on the progression of diabetic retinopathy in persons with type 2 diabetes: the Action to Control Cardiovascular Risk in Diabetes (ACCORD) Eye Study. *Ophthalmology* 2014;121:2443–2451

82. Nathan DM, Genuth S, Lachin J, et al.; Diabetes Control and Complications Trial Research Group. The effect of intensive treatment of diabetes on the development and progression of long-term complications in insulin-dependent diabetes mellitus. *N Engl J Med* 1993;329:977–986

83. Chew EY, Ambrosius WT, Davis MD, et al.; ACCORD Study Group; ACCORD Eye Study Group. Effects of medical therapies on retinopathy progression in type 2 diabetes. *N Engl J Med* 2010;363:233–244

84. Gubitosi-Klug RA, Sun W, Cleary PA, et al.; Writing Team for the DCCT/ EDIC Research Group. Effects of prior intensive insulin therapy and risk factors on patient-reported visual function outcomes in the Diabetes Control and Complications Trial/Epidemiology of Diabetes Interventions and Complications (DCCT/EDIC) cohort. *JAMA Ophthalmol* 2016;134: 137–145

85. Fong DS, Aiello LP, Ferris FL 3rd, Klein R. Diabetic retinopathy. *Diabetes Care* 2004;27:2540–2553

86. Diabetes Control and Complications Trial Research Group. Effect of pregnancy on microvascular complications in the diabetes control and complications trial. *Diabetes Care* 2000;23:1084–1091

87. Dabelea D, Stafford JM, Mayer-Davis EJ, et al.; SEARCH for Diabetes in Youth Research Group. Association of type 1 diabetes vs type 2 diabetes diagnosed during childhood and adolescence with complications during teenage years and young adulthood. *JAMA* 2017;317:825–835

88. Agardh E, Tababat-Khani P. Adopting 3-year screening intervals for sight-threatening retinal vascular lesions in type 2 diabetic subjects without retinopathy. *Diabetes Care* 2011;34:1318–1319

89. Nathan DM, Bebu I, Hainsworth D, et al.; DCCT/EDIC Research Group. Frequency of evidence-based screening for retinopathy in type 1 diabetes. *N Engl J Med* 2017;376:1507–1516

90. Daskivich LP, Vasquez C, Martinez C Jr., Tseng C-H, Mangione CM. Implementation and evaluation of a large-scale teleretinal diabetic retinopathy screening program in the Los Angeles County Department of Health Services. *JAMA Intern Med* 2017;177:642–649

91. Sim DA, Mitry D, Alexander P, et al. The evolution of teleophthalmology programs in the United Kingdom: beyond diabetic retinopathy screening. *J Diabetes Sci Technol* 2016;10:308–317

92. Hooper P, Boucher MC, Cruess A, et al. Canadian Ophthalmological Society evidence-based clinical practice guidelines for the management of diabetic retinopathy. *Can J Ophthalmol* 2012;47(Suppl. 1):S1–S30

93. Axer-Siegel R, Hod M, Fink-Cohen S, et al. Diabetic retinopathy during pregnancy. *Ophthalmology* 1996;103:1815–1819

94. Best RM, Chakravarthy U. Diabetic retinopathy in pregnancy. *Br J Ophthalmol* 1997;81:249–251

95. Gunderson EP, Lewis CE, Tsai A-L, et al. A 20-year prospective study of childbearing and incidence of diabetes in young women, controlling for glycemia before conception: the Coronary Artery Risk Development in Young Adults (CARDIA) Study. *Diabetes* 2007;56:2990–2996

96. The Diabetic Retinopathy Study Research Group. Preliminary report on effects of photocoagulation therapy. *Am J Ophthalmol* 1976;81:383–396

97. Gross JG, Glassman AR, Jampol LM, et al.; Writing Committee for the Diabetic Retinopathy Clinical Research Network. Panretinal photocoagulation vs intravitreous ranibizumab for proliferative diabetic retinopathy: a randomized clinical trial. *JAMA* 2015;314:2137–2146

98. Early Treatment Diabetic Retinopathy Study Research Group. Photocoagulation for diabetic macular edema. Early Treatment Diabetic Retinopathy Study report number 1. *Arch Ophthalmol* 1985;103:1796–1806

99. Elman MJ, Aiello LP, Beck RW, et al.; Diabetic Retinopathy Clinical Research Network. Randomized trial evaluating ranibizumab plus prompt or deferred laser or triamcinolone plus prompt laser for diabetic macular edema. *Ophthalmology* 2010;117:1064–1077.e35

100. Mitchell P, Bandello F, Schmidt-Erfurth U, et al.; RESTORE study group. The RESTORE study: ranibizumab monotherapy or combined with laser versus laser monotherapy for diabetic macular edema. *Ophthalmology* 2011;118:615–625

101. Elman MJ, Bressler NM, Qin H, et al.; Diabetic Retinopathy Clinical Research Network. Expanded 2-year follow-up of ranibizumab plus prompt or deferred laser or triamcinolone plus prompt laser for diabetic macular edema. *Ophthalmology* 2011;118:609–614

102. Nguyen QD, Brown DM, Marcus DM, et al.; RISE and RIDE Research Group. Ranibizumab for diabetic macular edema: results from 2 phase III randomized trials: RISE and RIDE. *Ophthalmology* 2012;119:789–801

103. Shih C-J, Chen H-T, Kuo S-C, et al. Comparative effectiveness of angiotensin-converting enzyme inhibitors and angiotensin II receptor blockers in patients with type 2 diabetes and retinopathy. *CMAJ* 2016;188:E148–E157

104. Shi R, Zhao L, Wang F, et al. Effects of lipid-lowering agents on diabetic retinopathy: a meta-analysis and systematic review. *Int J Ophthalmol* 2018;11:287–295

105. Ang L, Jaiswal M, Martin C, Pop-Busui R. Glucose control and diabetic neuropathy: lessons from recent large clinical trials. *Curr Diab Rep* 2014;14:528

106. Martin CL, Albers JW, Pop-Busui R; DCCT/EDIC Research Group. Neuropathy and related findings in the Diabetes Control and Complications Trial/Epidemiology of Diabetes Interventions and Complications study. *Diabetes Care* 2014;37:31–38

107. Pop-Busui R, Boulton AJM, Feldman EL, et al. Diabetic neuropathy: a position statement by the American Diabetes Association. *Diabetes Care* 2017;40:136–154

108. Freeman R. Not all neuropathy in diabetesis of diabetic etiology: differential diagnosis of diabetic neuropathy. *Curr Diab Rep* 2009;9:423–431

109. Pop-Busui R, Evans GW, Gerstein HC, et al.; Action to Control Cardiovascular Risk in Diabetes Study Group. Effects of cardiac autonomic dysfunction on mortality risk in the Action to Control Cardiovascular Risk in Diabetes (ACCORD) trial. *Diabetes Care* 2010;33:1578–1584

110. Pop-Busui R, Cleary PA, Braffett BH, et al.; DCCT/EDIC Research Group. Association between cardiovascular autonomic neuropathy and left ventricular dysfunction: DCCT/EDIC study (Diabetes Control and Complications Trial/Epidemiology of Diabetes Interventions and Complications). *J Am Coll Cardiol* 2013;61:447–454

111. Smith AG, Lessard M, Reyna S, Doudova M, Singleton JR. The diagnostic utility of Sudoscan for distal symmetric peripheral neuropathy. *J Diabetes Complications* 2014;28:511–516

112. Diabetes Control and Complications Trial (DCCT) Research Group. Effect of intensive diabetes treatment on nerve conduction in the Diabetes Control and Complications Trial. *Ann Neurol* 1995;38:869–880

113. CDC Study Group. The effect of intensive diabetes therapy on measures of autonomic nervous system function in the Diabetes Control and Complications Trial (DCCT). *Diabetologia* 1998;41:416–423

114. Albers JW, Herman WH, Pop-Busui R, et al.; Diabetes Control and Complications Trial/Epidemiology of Diabetes Interventions and Complications Research Group. Effect of prior intensive insulin treatment during the Diabetes Control and Complications Trial (DCCT) on peripheral neuropathy in type 1 diabetes during the Epidemiology of Diabetes Interventions and Complications (EDIC) study. *Diabetes Care* 2010;33:1090–1096

115. Pop-Busui R, Low PA, Waberski BH, et al.; DCCT/EDIC Research Group. Effects of prior intensive insulin therapy on cardiac autonomic nervous system function in type 1 diabetes mellitus: the Diabetes Control and Complications Trial/Epidemiology of Diabetes Interventions and Complications study (DCCT/EDIC). *Circulation* 2009;119:2886–2893

116. Callaghan BC, Little AA, Feldman EL, Hughes RAC. Enhanced glucose control for preventing and treating diabetic neuropathy. *Cochrane Database Syst Rev* 2012;6:CD007543

117. Pop-Busui R, Lu J, Brooks MM, et al.; BARI 2D Study Group. Impact of glycemic control strategies on the progression of diabetic peripheral neuropathy in the Bypass Angioplasty Revascularization Investigation 2 Diabetes (BARI 2D) cohort. *Diabetes Care* 2013;36:3208–3215

118. Sadosky A, Schaefer C, Mann R, et al. Burden of illness associated with painful diabetic peripheral neuropathy among adults seeking treatment in the US: results from a retrospective chart review and cross-sectional survey. *Diabetes Metab Syndr Obes* 2013;6:79–92

119. Waldfogel JM, Nesbit SA, Dy SM, et al. Pharmacotherapy for diabetic peripheral neuropathy pain and quality of life: a systematic review. *Neurology* 2017;88:1958–1967

120. Finnerup NB, Attal N, Haroutounian S, et al. Pharmacotherapy for neuro-pathic pain in adults: a systematic review and meta-analysis. *Lancet Neurol* 2015;14:162–173

121. Bril V, England J, Franklin GM, et al.; American Academy of Neurology; American Association of Neuromuscular and Electrodiagnostic Medicine; American Academy of Physical Medicine and Rehabilitation. Evidence-based guideline: treatment of painful diabetic neuropathy: report of the American Academy of Neurology, the American Association of Neuromus-cular and Electrodiagnostic Medicine, and the American Academy of Phys-ical Medicine and Rehabilitation [published correction appears in Neurology 2011;77:603]. *Neurology* 2011;76:1758–1765

122. Griebeler ML, Morey-Vargas OL, Brito JP, et al. Pharmacologic interven-tions for painful diabetic neuropathy: an umbrella systematic review and comparative effectiveness network meta-analysis. *Ann Intern Med* 2014;161:639–649

123. Ziegler D, Fonseca V. From guideline to patient: a review of recent recom-mendations for pharmacotherapy of painful diabetic neuropathy. *J Diabetes Complications* 2015;29:146–156

124. Freeman R, Durso-Decruz E, Emir B. Efficacy, safety, and tolerability of pregabalin treatment for painful diabetic peripheral neuropathy: findings from seven randomized, controlled trials across a range of doses. *Diabetes Care* 2008;31:1448–1454

125. Moore RA, Straube S, Wiffen PJ, Derry S, McQuay HJ. Pregabalin for acute and chronic pain in adults. *Cochrane Database Syst Rev* 2009;3: CD007076

126. Raskin P, Huffman C, Toth C, et al. Pregabalin in patients with inadequately treated painful diabetic peripheral neuropathy: a randomized withdrawal trial. *Clin J Pain* 2014;30:379–390

127. Tesfaye S, Wilhelm S, Lledo A, et al. Duloxetine and pregabalin: high-dose monotherapy or their combination? The "COMBO-DN study"– a multina-tional, randomized, double-blind, parallel-group study in patients with dia-betic peripheral neuropathic pain. *Pain* 2013;154:2616–2625

128. Ziegler D, Duan WR, An G, Thomas JW, Nothaft W. A randomized dou-ble-blind, placebo-, and active-controlled study of T-type calcium channel blocker ABT-639 in patients with diabetic peripheral neuropathic pain. *Pain* 2015;156:2013–2020

129. Quilici S, Chancellor J, Löthgren M, et al. Meta-analysis of duloxetine vs. pregabalin and gabapentin in the treatment of diabetic peripheral neuro-pathic pain. *BMC Neurol* 2009;9:6

130. Dworkin RH, Jensen MP, Gammaitoni AR, Olaleye DO, Galer BS. Symp-tom profiles differ in patients with neuropathic versus non-neuropathic pain. *J Pain* 2007;8:118–126

131. Wiffen PJ, Derry S, Bell RF, et al. Gabapentin for chronic neuropathic pain in adults. *Cochrane Database Syst Rev* 2017;6:CD007938

132. Wernicke JF, Pritchett YL, D'Souza DN, et al. A randomized controlled trial of duloxetine in diabetic peripheral neuropathic pain. *Neurology* 2006;67:1411–1420

133. Hardy T, Sachson R, Shen S, Armbruster M, Boulton AJM. Does treatment with duloxetine for neuropathic pain impact glycemic control? *Diabetes Care* 2007;30:21–26

134. Schwartz S, Etropolski M, Shapiro DY, et al. Safety and efficacy of tapentadol ER in patients with painful diabetic peripheral neuropathy: results of a randomized-withdrawal, placebo-controlled trial. *Curr Med Res Opin* 2011;27:151–162

135. Vinik AI, Shapiro DY, Rauschkolb C, et al. A randomized withdrawal, placebo-controlled study evaluating the efficacy and tolerability of tapentadol extended release in patients with chronic painful diabetic peripheral neuropathy. *Diabetes Care* 2014;37:2302–2309

136. Camilleri M, Parkman HP, Shafi MA, Abell TL, Gerson L; American College of Gastroenterology. Clinical guideline: management of gastroparesis. *Am J Gastroenterol* 2013;108:18–37; quiz 38

137. Parrish CR, Pastors JG. Nutritional management of gastroparesis in people with diabetes. *Diabetes Spectr* 2007;20:231–234

138. Parkman HP, Yates KP, Hasler WL, et al.; NIDDK Gastroparesis Clinical Research Consortium. Dietary intake and nutritional deficiencies in patients with diabetic or idiopathic gastroparesis. *Gastroenterology* 2011;141:486–498,498.e1–7

139. Olausson EA, Störsrud S, Grundin H, Isaksson M, Attvall S, Simrén M. A small particle size diet reduces upper gastrointestinal symptoms in patients with diabetic gastroparesis: a randomized controlled trial. *Am J Gastroenterol* 2014;109:375–385

140. Umpierrez GE, Ed. *Therapy for Diabetes Mellitus and Related Disorders.* 6th ed. Alexandria, VA, American Diabetes Association, 2014

141. Sugumar A, Singh A, Pasricha PJ. A systematic review of the efficacy of domperidone for the treatment of diabetic gastroparesis. *Clin Gastroenterol Hepatol* 2008;6:726–733

142. Maganti K, Onyemere K, Jones MP. Oral erythromycin and symptomatic relief of gastroparesis: a systematic review. *Am J Gastroenterol* 2003;98:259–263

143. McCallum RW, Snape W, Brody F, Wo J, Parkman HP, Nowak T. Gastric electrical stimulation with Enterra therapy improves symptoms from diabetic gastroparesis in a prospective study. *Clin Gastroenterol Hepatol* 2010;8:947–954; quiz e116

144. Boulton AJM, Armstrong DG, Albert SF, et al.; American Diabetes Association; American Association of Clinical Endocrinologists. Comprehensive foot examination and risk assessment: a report of the Task Force of the Foot Care Interest Group of the American Diabetes Association, with endorsement by the American Association of Clinical Endocrinologists. *Diabetes Care* 2008;31:1679–1685

145. Hingorani A, LaMuraglia GM, Henke P, et al. The management of diabetic foot: a clinical practice guideline by the Society for Vascular Surgery in collaboration with the American Podiatric Medical Association and the Society for Vascular Medicine. *J Vasc Surg* 2016;63(Suppl. 2):3S–21S

146. Bonner T, Foster M, Spears-Lanoix E. Type 2 diabetes-related foot care knowledge and foot self-care practice interventions in the United States: a systematic review of the literature. *Diabet Foot Ankle* 2016;7:29758

147. Rizzo L, Tedeschi A, Fallani E, et al. Custom-made orthesis and shoes in a structured follow-up program reduces the incidence of neuropathic ulcers in high-risk diabetic foot patients. *Int J Low Extrem Wounds* 2012;11:59–64

148. Lipsky BA, Berendt AR, Cornia PB, et al.; Infectious Diseases Society of America. 2012 Infectious Diseases Society of America clinical practice guideline for the diagnosis and treatment of diabetic foot infections. *Clin Infect Dis* 2012;54:e132–e173

149. Elraiyah T, Tsapas A, Prutsky G, et al. A systematic review and meta-analysis of adjunctive therapies in diabetic foot ulcers. *J Vasc Surg* 2016; 63(2 Suppl.):46S–58S.e1–2

150. Game FL, Apelqvist J, Attinger C, et al.; International Working Group on the Diabetic Foot. Effectiveness of interventions to enhance healing of chronic ulcers of the foot in diabetes: a systematic review. *Diabetes Metab Res Rev* 2016;32(Suppl. 1):154–168

151. Kranke P, Bennett MH, Martyn-St James M, Schnabel A, Debus SE, Weibel S. Hyperbaric oxygen therapy for chronic wounds. *Cochrane Database Syst Rev* 2015;6:CD004123

152. Löndahl M, Katzman P, Nilsson A, Hammarlund C. Hyperbaric oxygen therapy facilitates healing of chronic foot ulcers in patients with diabetes. *Diabetes Care* 2010;33:998–1003

153. Fedorko L, Bowen JM, Jones W, et al. Hyperbaric oxygen therapy does not reduce indications for amputation in patients with diabetes with nonhealing ulcers of the lower limb: a prospective, double-blind, randomized controlled clinical trial. *Diabetes Care* 2016;39:392–399

154. Li G, Hopkins RB, Levine MAH, et al. Relationship between hyperbaric oxygen therapy and quality of life in participants with chronic diabetic foot ulcers: data from a randomized controlled trial. *Acta Diabetol* 2017;54: 823–831

155. Boulton AJM. The Diabetic Foot [Internet], 2000. South Dartmouth, MA, MDText.com, Inc. Available from http://www.ncbi.nlm.nih.gov/books/NBK409609/. Accessed 5 October 2017

156. Health Quality Ontario. Hyperbaric oxygen therapy for the treatment of diabetic foot ulcers: a health technology assessment. *Ont Health Technol Assess Ser* 2017;17:1–142

157. Stoekenbroek RM, Santema TB, Koelemay MJ, et al. Is additional hyperbaric oxygen therapy cost-effective for treating ischemic diabetic ulcers? Study protocol for the Dutch DAMOCLES multicenter randomized clinical trial? *J Diabetes* 2015;7:125–132

158. Huang ET, Mansouri J, Murad MH, et al.; UHMS CPG Oversight Committee. A clinical practice guideline for the use of hyperbaric oxygen therapy in the treatment of diabetic foot ulcers. *Undersea Hyperb Med* 2015;42:205–247

Chapter 19
Hypertension

CHEYENNE NEWSOME, PHARMD, PHC, BCACP

INTRODUCTION

Hypertension, defined as a sustained blood pressure >140/90 mmHg, is common among patients with diabetes.[1] It is estimated that over half of U.S. patients with diabetes also have hypertension; of these patients with hypertension, less than half are achieving blood pressure goals. Hypertension is a well-established risk factor for CVD, HF, and microvascular complications. The prevalence of hypertension increases with aging as do other CVD risk factors.[1] CVD is the most prevalent cause of mortality and morbidity for patients with diabetes, and thus it is imperative to address these risk factors.[2]

Antihypertensive therapy reduces cardiovascular events, HF, and microvascular complications in patients with diabetes.[3-7] In addition to pharmacologic therapy, lifestyle modifications are an important consideration for hypertension. Effective lifestyle modifications to lower blood pressure include reducing excess body weight through caloric restriction, restricting sodium intake to less than 2,300 mg/day, increasing consumption of fruits and vegetables and low-fat dairy products, avoiding excessive alcohol consumption, smoking cessation, reducing sedentary time, and increasing physical activity levels to 150 min per week.[8-10]

Because of the high prevalence of hypertension and the availability of effective treatments to positively impact patient outcomes, it is recommended that patients' blood pressure be measured at every routine clinical visit.[11] This helps provide early diagnoses for patients and identifies patients who are not achieving blood pressure goals and who would benefit from therapy intensification. Blood pressure should be measured by a trained individual and should follow the guidelines established for the general population: measurement in the seated position, with feet on the floor and arm supported at heart level, after 5 min of rest. Cuff size should be appropriate for the upper-arm circumference. Orthostatic blood pressure measurements should be checked on initial visit and as indicated. Patients with "white coat hypertension" experience feelings of anxiety in medical environments, which causes a higher reading than the patient's normal reading when blood pressure is measured in a medical setting. Patients with "masked hypertension" have normal blood pressure when they are in medical settings but elevated blood pressure readings outside of medical settings. Home blood pressure self-monitoring and 24 h ambulatory blood pressure monitoring may provide evidence of white coat hypertension, masked hypertension, or other discrepancies between office and "true" blood pressure.[11] In addition to confirming or refuting a diagnosis of hypertension, home blood pressure assessment may be useful to monitor antihypertensive treatment. Moreover, home blood pressures may improve patient medication adherence and thus help reduce cardiovascular risk.[12]

GOALS OF TREATMENT

Although there is strong evidence showing elevated blood pressure is associated with negative outcomes, there is controversy around the optimal blood pressure goal for patients with diabetes. Multiple randomized controlled trials have shown that treatment to a blood pressure of less than 140/90 mmHg reduces cardiovascular events as well as microvascular complications.[3-7,13,14] There is consensus that blood pressure goal should not be higher than 140/90 mmHg, but there are some instances when even lower blood pressure targets may be appropriate. Intensification of antihypertensive therapy to target blood pressures of <130/80 mmHg or <120/80 mmHg may be beneficial for selected patients with diabetes, such as those with a high risk of CVD. Factors that can guide treatment targets may include risks of treatment (hypotension or adverse drug event), patient life expectancy, comorbidities, patient attitude, overall treatment burden, absolute risk of cardiovascular events, and risk of progressive kidney disease as reflected by albuminuria.[14,15] Patients who have higher risk of cardiovascular events (particularly stroke) or albuminuria (urine albumin-to-creatinine ratio >30 mg/g) and who can attain intensive blood pressure control relatively easily and without substantial adverse effects may be best suited to intensive blood pressure control. In contrast, patients with conditions more common in older adults, such as functional limitations, polypharmacy, and multiple comorbidities, may be best suited to less intensive blood pressure control.[11] It is recommended that patients and clinicians participate in shared decision-making to determine individual blood pressure goals for patients.[16] Blood pressure goals should be re-evaluated as patients' circumstances and risk factors change.

OVERVIEW OF MEDICATIONS AND RATIONALE FOR USE

Antihypertensive medications do not cure high blood pressure; they reduce blood pressure only when taken and must be taken indefinitely to keep blood pressure at goal if no significant lifestyle modifications to reduce blood pressure are adopted. Many antihypertensive classes and medications are available; however, only a few have been shown to have clinical benefits, and some have significant adverse effects. It is recommended that the initial antihypertensive medication be from a drug class that has demonstrated reduction in cardiovascular events in patients with diabetes. These classes are *1)* ACE inhibitors,[17,18] *2)* ARBs,[17,18] *3)* thiazide-like diuretics,[19] or *4)* dihydropyridine calcium channel blockers.[20] The general recommendations for initial therapy should be re-evaluated in patients with medical conditions in whom specific agents might offer benefits independent of blood pressure control.

Table 19.1 — Medication Overview by Class

Medication class	Medication	Mechanism of action	Adverse effects	Considerations
Thiazide and Thiazide-type Diuretic	■ Chlorthalidone ■ Hydrochlorothia-zide	■ Increases excretion of sodium and chloride in equal amounts at the distal renal tubule of the kidney nephron	■ Phototoxicity ■ Hyponatremia ■ Hypercalcemia ■ Hypokalemia ■ Hypophosphatemia ■ Hypomagnesemia ■ Hyperuricemia ■ Male sexual dysfunction	■ Chlorthalidone may be preferred over hydro-chlorothiazide as it has shown a superior reduction in cardiovascular events[38] ■ Monitor serum electrolytes and creatinine within the first 1–2 weeks of therapy ■ Can exacerbate gout by increasing serum uric acid
Calcium Channel Blockers, Dihydro-pyridine	■ Amlodipine ■ Felodipine	■ Lowers blood pressure by caus-ing a direct vasodilation in the peripheral arteries of the vascu-lar smooth muscle; also blocks the influx of calcium ions into cardiac and vascular smooth muscles	■ Peripheral edema ■ Dizziness ■ Flushing ■ Headache ■ Nausea ■ Fatigue ■ Palpitations	■ Peripheral edema is dose dependent, and dose reduction may resolve edema ■ Also indicated for angina and Raynaud's phe-nomenon ■ Significant drug-drug interactions with clopido-grel, simvastatin, cyclosporine and tacrolimus
Calcium Channel Blockers, Non-dihydropyridine	■ Diltiazem SR ■ Verapamil SR	■ Blocks calcium ion influx dur-ing depolarization of cardiac and vascular smooth muscle; decreases peripheral vascular resistance and causes relaxation of the vascular smooth muscle, resulting in a decrease of both systolic and diastolic blood pressure	■ Bradyarrhythmia ■ Peripheral edema ■ Dizziness ■ Headache ■ Fatigue ■ Constipation ■ Heart failure	■ Avoid with β-blockers due to risk of bradycar-dia or heart block ■ Both are CYP3A4 liver enzyme substrates and also a moderate CYP3A4 inhibitor; therefore they have many drug-drug interactions

(continued)

Table 19.1 (continued)

Medication class	Medication	Mechanism of action	Adverse effects	Considerations
ACE Inhibitor	■ Enalapril ■ Lisinopril ■ Ramipril	■ ACE inhibition prevents the conversion of angiotensin I to angiotensin II, which is a potent vasoconstrictor; decreased angiotensin II leads to decreased vasopressor activity and decreased aldosterone secretion	■ Angioedema ■ Cough ■ Syncope ■ Dizziness ■ Headache ■ Hyperkalemia ■ Renal impairment	■ Because of constriction of the efferent renal arteriole, increase in serum creatinine within a week of initiation is frequently observed; if serum creatinine stabilizes, it is appropriate to continue the ACE inhibitor ■ Monitor serum potassium and creatinine within the first 1–2 weeks of therapy ■ Dose titration can occur every 1–2 weeks ■ Teratogenic
ARB	■ Candesartan ■ Olmesartan ■ Losartan	■ Blocks the vasoconstrictor effects of angiotensin II by selectively blocking the binding of angiotensin II to the angiotensin II receptor type 1 in vascular smooth muscle, which decreases vasoconstriction, synthesis and release of aldosterone, and renal absorption of sodium	■ Angioedema ■ Dizziness ■ Renal impairment ■ Upper respiratory tract infections	■ Because of constriction of the efferent renal arteriole, increase in serum creatinine within a week of initiation is frequently observed; if serum creatinine stabilizes, it is appropriate to continue the ARB ■ Monitor serum potassium and creatinine within the first 1–2 weeks of therapy ■ Losartan increases urine excretion of uric acid and can be beneficial for patients with gout ■ Dose titration can occur every 1–2 weeks ■ Teratogenic
Aldosterone Antagonist	■ Spironolactone ■ Eplerenone	■ Inhibits the effect of aldosterone by competing for the aldosterone-dependent sodium–potassium exchange site in the distal tubule cells; this increases the secretion of water and sodium, while decreasing the excretion of potassium	■ Hyperkalemia ■ ED* ■ Irregular menses* ■ Gynecomastia* *Eplerenone does not cause gynecomastia or menses disruption, and causes less ED	■ Drug of choice for resistant hypertension ■ Monitor serum potassium and creatinine within the first 1–2 weeks of therapy ■ 4 weeks to full effect and between dose titrations

(continued)

Table 19.1 (continued)

Medication class	Medication	Mechanism of action	Adverse effects	Considerations
β-adrenergic Blockers— β-1-selective/ Cardioselective	■ Atenolol ■ Bisoprolol ■ Metoprolol ■ Nebivolol	■ Blocks the binding of epinephrine and norepinephrine, decreases contractility of cardiac muscles, reduces cardiac output, suppresses renin production	■ Bradyarrhythmia ■ Pruritus ■ Dyspnea ■ Dizziness ■ Fatigue ■ Depression ■ Diarrhea	■ β-2 adrenergic receptors are responsible for respiratory dilation ■ Avoid nonselective β-adrenergic blockers in patients with reactive airway disease β-1-selective adrenergic blockers preferred for reactive airway disease ■ α-1 and nonselective β-blockers may be more effective at blood pressure control because they reduce cardiac contractility and cause peripheral vasodilation ■ Mask symptoms of hypoglycemia—patient may only experience sweating ■ Taper off to avoid rebound tachycardia
β-adrenergic Blockers— β-Nonselective	■ Nadolol ■ Propranolol	■ Blocks the binding of epinephrine and norepinephrine, decreases contractility of cardiac muscles, reduces cardiac output, suppresses renin production	■ ED ■ Hyperglycemia	
β-Blockers—α-1 and Nonselective β-Blockers	■ Carvedilol ■ Labetalol	■ Blocks the binding of epinephrine and norepinephrine, decreases contractility of cardiac muscles, reduces cardiac output, suppresses renin production ■ The α-1 adrenergic blocking activity blunts the pressor effect of phenylephrine, causes vasodilation, and reduces peripheral vascular resistance.		
Loop Diuretics	■ Bumetanide ■ Furosemide ■ Torsemide	■ Inhibits the reabsorption of sodium and chloride in the ascending limb of the loop of Henle causing an increase in urine output, reducing plasma and extracellular fluid volume; cardiac output also decreases. Eventually, cardiac output returns to normal with an accompanying decrease in peripheral resistance.	■ Hyperuricemia ■ Hypomagnesemia ■ Hypochloremia ■ Hypokalemia	■ Beneficial in patients with edema or symptomatic congestive heart failure ■ More potent diuretic effect than thiazide in patients with eGFR <30 mL/min

(continued)

Table 19.1 (continued)

Medication class	Medication	Mechanism of action	Adverse effects	Considerations
Direct Vasodilators	▪ Hydralazine	▪ Decreases blood pressure by exhibiting a peripheral-vaso-dilating effect through a direct relaxation of vascular smooth muscle; also indirectly increases renin secretion, ultimately leading to sodium reabsorption, as a response to reflex sympathetic discharge	▪ Palpitations ▪ Tachycardia ▪ Edema ▪ Angina ▪ Headache	▪ Short half-life, dosed four times a day, difficult for patients to adhere to regimen
Centrally Acting α-2 Adrenergic Agonist	▪ Clonidine	▪ Stimulates α-2 adrenergic receptors in the brain, resulting in reduced sympathetic outflow from the CNS and decreased peripheral resistance, renal vascular resistance, heart rate, and blood pressure	▪ Somnolence ▪ Xerostomia ▪ Fatigue ▪ Orthostatic hypotension	▪ When discontinuing therapy, gradually decrease the dose over 2–4 days to reduce the risk of withdrawal symptoms and rebound hypertension ▪ Avoid alcohol and other CNS depressants ▪ Available as an oral tablet and a transdermal patch applied once weekly
Diuretics—Potassium Sparing	▪ Triamterene ▪ Amiloride	▪ Inhibits the reabsorption of sodium in exchange for potassium and hydrogen ions by exerting a direct effect on the distal renal tubule	▪ Hypercalcemia ▪ Hyperuricemia ▪ Orthostatic hypotension	▪ Minimally effective as monotherapy; can be used in combination with thiazide-type diuretic to overcome hypokalemia
▪ α-1 Adrenergic Antagonists	▪ Doxazosin ▪ Terazosin	▪ Directly relaxes vascular smooth muscle and causes vasodilation by inhibiting α-1 adrenergic receptors	▪ Orthostatic hypotension ▪ Palpitations ▪ Asthenia ▪ Dizziness ▪ Headache ▪ Lethargy ▪ Somnolence ▪ First dose effect of somnolence or hypotension	▪ Not recommended for monotherapy because increased risk of heart failure[39] ▪ Initiate at low doses at bedtime to reduce orthostatic hypotension ▪ Taper off medication slowly to avoid rebound hypertension ▪ Also indicated for benign prostatic hypertrophy

There are certain patient characteristics that make ACE inhibitors or ARBs optimal therapy, and other factors that make ACE inhibitors and ARBs a less favorable prospect. For patients with albuminuria (urine albumin-to-creatinine ratio >30 mg/g), initial treatment should include an ACE inhibitor or ARB in order to reduce the risk of progressive kidney disease.[11] However, in the absence of albuminuria, risk of progressive kidney disease is low, and ACE inhibitors and ARBs have not been found to provide superior cardioprotection when compared to thiazide-like diuretics or dihydropyridine calcium channel blockers.[21] ACE inhibitors or ARBs are also first line in patients who have HF or have had an ST-segment elevation myocardial infarction (STEMI).[10] ACE inhibitors and ARBs are teratogenic and should be avoided in pregnancy. ACE inhibitors and ARBs are not recommended as initial monotherapy in black patients because they have shown inferior efficacy in major cardiovascular outcomes compared to calcium channel blockers.[22-25] If patients experience a cough with an ACE inhibitor, they can be switched to an ARB, as ARBs have much lower incidence of cough than ACE inhibitors.[26] ACE inhibitors and ARBs should be avoided in combination except in rare circumstances.

Previously, β-blockers were also considered appropriate initial antihypertensive therapy, but they are no longer preferred for patients unless there are specific comorbidities.[10,11,27] Compared to other antihypertensive medications in the primary treatment of hypertension, β-blockers may be associated with inferior protection against stroke risk.[27-29] β-Blockers may be used for the rate-control treatment in atrial fibrillation, prior MI, active angina, or HF, but have not been shown to reduce mortality as blood pressure-lowering agents in the absence of these conditions.[4] Therefore, β-blockers should not be recommended for antihypertensive therapy routinely unless there is a compelling indication.

There is some evidence that there may be a benefit of evening versus morning dosing of antihypertensive medications with regard to blood pressure control and reduction of cardiovascular outcomes.[30,31] The mechanism underlying this benefit is not well understood. Switching to bedtime dosing can also be a beneficial way to reduce symptoms of hypotension, but should be recommended cautiously in patients who routinely have to get up at night to urinate.[11]

Resistant hypertension is defined as blood pressure >140/90 mmHg despite a therapeutic strategy that includes appropriate lifestyle management plus a diuretic and two other antihypertensive drugs belonging to different classes at adequate doses.[16] Prior to diagnosing resistant hypertension, a number of other conditions should be excluded, including medication nonadherence, white coat hypertension, and secondary hypertension. Mineralocorticoid receptor antagonists are effective for management of resistant hypertension in patients with T2D when added to existing treatment with an ACE inhibitor or ARB, thiazide-like diuretic, and dihydropyridine calcium channel blocker.[32] Mineralocorticoid receptor antagonists also reduce albuminuria and reduce the risk of morbidity and mortality in some patients who have HF with reduced ejection fraction.[15,16,33,34]

An important side effect to monitor for antihypertensive medications is orthostatic hypotension. The definition of orthostatic hypotension is a decrease in systolic blood pressure of 20 mmHg or a decrease in diastolic blood pressure of 10 mmHg within 3 min of standing when compared with blood pressure from the sitting or supine position.[35] Orthostatic hypotension can be caused by volume depletion or diabetic autonomic neuropathy, and can be further exacerbated by antihypertensive medications.[36] Orthostatic hypotension is common in people with T2D and hypertension and is associated with an increased risk of mortality and HF.[37] It is important to re-evaluate blood pressure goals when new information about patients' risks for events or side effects arises.

A BRIEF OVERVIEW OF EACH CLASS OF MEDICATION

See Table 19.1.

A BRIEF OVERVIEW OF COMBINATION THERAPY

Most patients will require multiple antihypertensive medications to achieve goal blood pressure.[40] When initiating therapy, how far patients are above their goal blood pressure should be considered. If patients have blood pressure between 140/90 mmHg and 159/99 mmHg, pharmacologic therapy can be initiated with a single medication. For patients with blood pressure ≥160/100 mmHg, it is recommended to start with two antihypertensive medications.[16,41] Other patients may achieve goal blood pressure with monotherapy initially, but with aging, the elasticity of vessels reduces as does the body's ability to process sodium, which leads to increasing blood pressure. Therefore, patients may need to add on additional antihypertensive therapy as they age. There is consensus that the amount of blood pressure reduction is the major determinant in reduction of cardiovascular risk in patients with hypertension, not the choice of antihypertensive drug (assuming that the patient does not have an indication for a particular drug).[42-45] When selecting how to optimize hypertensive medications, it may be advantageous to add an agent rather than titrating to the maximum dose of an agent. Using maximum doses of blood pressure medications generally produces a lesser blood pressure response and more toxicity than adding an additional blood pressure medication at a low dose.[46-48] Although many patients will require multiple blood pressure medications, combination pills can lessen pill burden by reducing the number of pills a patient takes. Additionally, fixed-dose combination preparations may improve patient adherence and blood pressure control.[49,50]

There are many blood pressure medications with different mechanisms of action that can be taken together; however, there are some combinations to avoid or to be cautious of using. Multiple diuretics are efficacious for hypertension, but have the risk of combined dehydration, hypovolemia, hypoperfusion, and renal injury. Patients should maintain adequate hydration, and their renal function should be monitored if combination diuretics are needed. Mineralocorticoid receptor antagonists are often added for patients with resistant hypertension who are already taking three or more medications, but may increase the risk of hyperkalemia when combined with an ACE inhibitor or ARB, emphasizing the importance of regular monitoring of serum creatinine and potassium in these patients.[16] ACE inhibitors and ARBs should not routinely be combined. The dual blockade of the renin-angiotensin-aldosterone system, which may increase the risk of adverse events such as hyperkalemia, hypotension, and renal failure, argues against the use of this combination.[51] With the exception of combining ACE inhibitors and ARBs, all other combinations of first-line medication classes (i.e., thiazide-like diuretics, calcium channel blockers, ACE inhibitors, and ARBs) are considered safe.

Table 19.2—Doses and Dose Adjustments for the Most Prominent Antihypertensives

Class	Medication	Dose	Dose adjustment
ACE Inhibitors	Benazepril	10–40 mg once daily or in 2 divided doses	■ eGFR <30 mL/min/1.73 m²: initial dose is 5 mg daily
	Enalapril	5–40 mg once daily or in 2 divided doses	■ CrCl <30 mL/min: initial dose is 2.5 mg daily
	Fosinopril	10–80 mg once daily or in 2 divided doses	
	Lisinopril	10–40 mg once daily or in 2 divided doses	■ CrCl 10–30 mL/min: initial dose is 5 mg daily ■ CrCl <10 mL/min or hemodialysis: initial dose is 2.5 mg daily ■ Combination with diuretic: initial dose is 5 mg daily

	Quinapril	10–80 mg once daily or in 2 divided doses	■ Combination with diuretic: initial dose is 5 mg daily
			■ Renal impairment:
			  – CrCl 30–60 mL/min: initial dose is 5 mg daily
			  – CrCl 10–30 mL/min: initial dose is 2.5 mg daily

	Ramipril	2.5–20 mg once daily or in 2 divided doses	■ CrCl <60 mL/min: initial dose is 1.25 mg once daily, max dose is 5 mg daily
ARBs	Irbesartan	150–300 mg once daily	■ Volume- or salt-depleted (e.g., vigorous diuretic therapy, hemodialysis): initial dose is 75 mg orally once daily
	Losartan	50–100 mg once daily	■ Renal impairment in volume-depleted patients: initiate at 25 mg daily; depending on blood pressure response, a 25-mg dose given twice daily may be needed ■ Hepatic impairment (mild to moderate): initial dose 25 mg orally once daily ■ Intravascular depletion: initiate at 25 mg orally once daily
	Olmesartan	20–40 mg once daily	
	Telmisartan	20–80 mg once daily	
	Valsartan	40–320 mg once daily	
Thiazide and Thiazide-Type Diuretics	Chlorthalidone	12.5–100 mg once daily	■ Anuria: use is contraindicated
	Hydrochlorothiazide	12.5–50 mg once daily or in 2 divided doses	■ Anuria: use is contraindicated ■ Geriatric: initial doses, 12.5–25 mg, with slower titration than with younger patients

(continued)

Table 19.2 (continued)

Class	Medication	Dose	Dose adjustment
Calcium Channel Blockers—Non-dihydro-pyridine	Diltiazem	120–540 mg once daily	■ Geriatric: initiate at low end of dosing range
	Verapamil	Immediate release: 80–120 mg three times daily Sustained release: 180–480 mg once daily	■ Hepatic impairment (severe): Use 30% of dose given to patients with normal hepatic function ■ Low-weight patients: 40 mg orally three times daily for immediate-release tablets, 120 mg once daily for sustained release
Calcium Channel Blockers—Dihydro-pyridine	Amlodipine	2.5–10 mg once daily	
	Felodipine	2.5–10 mg once daily	
Aldo-sterone Antagonist	Spironolac-tone	50–200 mg once daily or in divided doses	■ Renal impairment: – eGFR ≥50 mL/min/1.73 m²: initial dose is 12.5–25 mg once a day; maintenance dose, may increase to 25 mg once or twice a day after 4 weeks – eGFR 30–49 mL/min 1.73 m²: initial dose is 12.5 mg orally once daily or every other day; maintenance dose, may increase to 12.5–25 mg once a day after 4 weeks
	Eplerenone	50 mg once daily	■ CrCl ≤50 mL/min: contraindicated ■ Concomitant moderate CYP3A inhibitor (e.g., erythromycin, saquinavir, verapamil, fluconazole): initial dose is 25 mg orally once daily; may increase to a maximum of 25 mg twice daily if blood pressure response is inadequate
β-Blockers	Bisoprolol	2.5–20 mg once daily	■ Liver disease: initial dose is 2.5 mg once daily, maximum dose is 10 mg once daily ■ Renal impairment: initial dose is 2.5 mg once daily, maximum dose is 10 mg once daily
	Nebivolol	5–40 mg once daily	■ Liver disease (moderate): initial dose is 2.5 mg daily, titrate dose cautiously ■ Renal impairment (CrCl <30 mL/min): initial dose is 2.5 mg per day, titrate dose cautiously
	Carvedilol	6.25–25 mg twice daily	■ Hepatic impairment (severe): use is contraindicated ■ Hepatic impairment (liver cirrhosis): initial dosage, consider reduction of approximately 20%
	Labetalol	100–800 mg twice daily	■ Hepatic impairment: average required dose is 50% of usual dosing ■ Geriatric: maximum dose is 200 mg b.i.d.
Loop Diuretics	Furosemide	40 mg twice daily	■ Concomitant medication: reduce dosage of other antihypertensive agents by at least 50% when furosemide is added to a regimen, further reduction in dosage or discontinuation of other agents may be necessary

DIURETIC COMBINATIONS

- HCTZ/Spironolactone: 25 mg/25 mg
- HCTZ/Triamterene: 25 mg/37.5 mg, 25 mg/50 mg, 50 mg/75 mg

ACE INHIBITORS AND DIURETICS

- Benazepril/HCTZ: 5 mg/6.25 mg, 10 mg/12.5 mg, 20 mg/12.5 mg, 20 mg/25 mg
- Enalapril/HCTZ: 5 mg/12.5 mg, 10 mg/25 mg
- Lisinopril/HCTZ: 10 mg/12.5 mg, 20 mg/12.5 mg, 20 mg/25 mg

ARBs AND DIURETICS

- Losartan/HCTZ: 50 mg/12.5 mg, 100 mg/12.5 mg, 100 mg/25 mg
- Valsartan/HCTZ: 80 mg/12.5 mg, 160 mg/12.5 mg, 320 mg/12.5 mg, 160 mg/25 mg, 320 mg/25 mg

CALCIUM CHANNEL BLOCKERS AND ACE INHIBITORS

- Amlodipine/Benazepril: 2.5 mg/10 mg, 5 mg/10 mg, 5 mg/20 mg, 5 mg/40 mg, 10 mg/20 mg, 10 mg/40 mg

ACE INHIBITORS

Benazepril (Lotensin): https://dailymed.nlm.nih.gov/dailymed/drugInfo.cfm?setid=60f0fb82-d870-4f07-82af-e4aeb79ed023

Enalapril (Vasotec): https://dailymed.nlm.nih.gov/dailymed/drugInfo.cfm?setid=ac0289a6-9533-4f8c-b46c-506dce1b90b5

Lisinopril (Prinivil, Zestril): https://dailymed.nlm.nih.gov/dailymed/drugInfo.cfm?setid=27ccb2f4-abf8-4825-9b05-0bb367b4ac07

Ramipril (Altace): https://dailymed.nlm.nih.gov/dailymed/drugInfo.cfm?setid=8b59207a-ea5c-4697-a8b6-94c3015a00de

ARBs

Losartan (Cozaar): https://dailymed.nlm.nih.gov/dailymed/drugInfo.
cfm?setid=5ac32c20-169d-475a-fc8a-934f758d6ab0

Olmesartan (Benicar): https://dailymed.nlm.nih.gov/dailymed/drugInfo.
cfm?setid=d5658d8a-f8e9-454d-89a9-34884e753001

DIURETICS

Chlorthalidone (Thalitone): https://dailymed.nlm.nih.gov/dailymed/drugInfo.
cfm?setid=193c85ba-43c2-4be2-82cf-7b394a83390e

Furosemide (Lasix): https://dailymed.nlm.nih.gov/dailymed/drugInfo.
cfm?setid=a15d7845-5827-481d-ba3f-e4883489a5ef

Hydrochlorothiazide (Microzide): https://dailymed.nlm.nih.gov/dailymed/drugInfo.cfm?setid=7b38ac8a-4540-4eb2-aedd-9aa966d22190

Spironolactone (Aldactone): https://dailymed.nlm.nih.gov/dailymed/drugInfo.
cfm?setid=8a96e2c9-049a-43ab-abf3-21baedeb736f

CALCIUM CHANNEL BLOCKERS

Amlodipine (Norvasc): https://dailymed.nlm.nih.gov/dailymed/drugInfo.
cfm?setid=b52e2905-f906-4c46-bb24-2c7754c5d75b

Diltiazem (Cardizem): https://dailymed.nlm.nih.gov/dailymed/drugInfo.
cfm?setid=5e39be50-ea17-4077-a2dc-668267049f6a

Verapamil (Calan, Isoptin): https://dailymed.nlm.nih.gov/dailymed/drugInfo.
cfm?setid=0742cf97-601b-4c13-a6c3-1a6a616ed292

β-BLOCKERS

Carvedilol (Coreg): https://dailymed.nlm.nih.gov/dailymed/drugInfo.
cfm?setid=7d485d38-5d43-4a54-bc63-82734035c66a

REFERENCES

1. Keenan NL, Rosendorf KA; Centers for Disease Control and Prevention. Prevalence of hypertension and controlled hypertension—United States 2005–2008. *Morbidity and Mortality Weekly Report (MMWR)* Suppl. 2011;60(1):94–97. Available from www.cdc.gov/mmwr/preview/mmwrhtml/su6001a21.htm

2. Matheus AS, Tannus LR, Cobas RA, et al. Impact of diabetes on cardiovascular disease: an update. *Int J Hypertens* 2013:653789

3. Emdin CA, Rahimi K, Neal B, et al. Blood pressure lowering in type 2 diabetes: a systematic review and meta-analysis. *JAMA* 2015;313(6):603–615

4. Ettehad D, Emdin CA, Kiran A, et al. Blood pressure lowering for prevention of cardiovascular disease and death: a systematic review and meta-analysis. *Lancet* 2016;387:957–967

5. Brunström M, Carlberg B. Effect of antihypertensive treatment at different blood pressure levels in patients with diabetes mellitus: systematic review and meta-analyses. *BMJ* 2016;352:i717

6. Bangalore S, Kumar S, Lobach I, Messerli FH. Blood pressure targets in subjects with type 2 diabetes mellitus/impaired fasting glucose: observations from traditional and Bayesian random-effects meta-analyses of randomized trials. *Circulation* 2011;123:2799–2810

7. Thomopoulos C, Parati G, Zanchetti A. Effects of blood-pressure-lowering treatment on outcome incidence in hypertension: 10—Should blood pressure management differ in hypertensive patients with and without diabetes mellitus? Overview and meta-analyses of randomized trials. *J Hypertens* 2017;35:922–944

8. Sacks FM, Svetkey LP, Vollmer WM, et al.; DASH-Sodium Collaborative Research Group. Effects on blood pressure of reduced dietary sodium and the Dietary Approaches to Stop Hypertension (DASH) diet. *N Engl J Med* 2001;344:3–10

9. Young DR, Hivert MF, Alhassan S, et al.; Endorsed by the Obesity Society; Physical Activity Committee of the Council on Lifestyle and Cardiometabolic Health; Council on Clinical Cardiology; Council on Epidemiology and Prevention; Council on Functional Genomics and Translational Biology; and Stroke Council. Sedentary behavior and cardiovascular morbidity and mortality: a science advisory from the American Heart Association. *Circulation* 2016;134:e262–e279

10. James PA, Oparil S, Carter BL, et al. 2014 evidence-based guideline for the management of high blood pressure in adults: report from the panel members appointed to the Eighth Joint National Committee (JNC 8). *JAMA* 2014;311:507–520

11. de Boer IH, Bangalore S, Benetos A, et al. Diabetes and hypertension: a position statement by the American Diabetes Association. *Diabetes Care* 2017;40:1273–1284

12. Omboni S, Gazzola T, Carabelli G, Parati G. Clinical usefulness and cost effectiveness of home blood pressure telemonitoring: meta-analysis of randomized controlled studies. *J Hypertens* 2013;31:455–467; discussion 467–468

13. Arguedas JA, Leiva V, Wright JM. Blood pressure targets for hypertension in people with diabetes mellitus. *Cochrane Database Syst Rev* 2013;10:CD008277

14. Xie X, Atkins E, Lv J, et al. Effects of intensive blood pressure lowering on cardiovascular and renal outcomes: updated systematic review and meta-analysis. *Lancet* 2016;387:435–443

15. Sundström J, Arima H, Woodward M, et al.; Blood Pressure Lowering Treatment Trialists' Collaboration. Blood pressure-lowering treatment based on cardiovascular risk: a meta-analysis of individual patient data. *Lancet* 2014;384:591–598

16. American Diabetes Association. *Standards of Medical Care in Diabetes—2018. Diabetes Care* 2018;41(Suppl. 1):S86–S91

17. Catalá-López F, Macías Saint-Gerons D, González-Bermejo D, et al. Cardiovascular and renal outcomes of renin-angiotensin system blockade in adult patients with diabetes mellitus: a systematic review with network meta-analyses. *PLoS Med* 2016;13:e1001971

18. Palmer SC, Mavridis D, Navarese E, et al. Comparative efficacy and safety of blood pressure-lowering agents in adults with diabetes and kidney disease: a network meta-analysis. *Lancet* 2015;385:2047–2056

19. Barzilay JI, Davis BR, Bettencourt J, et al.; ALLHAT Collaborative Research Group. Cardiovascular outcomes using doxazosin vs. chlorthalidone for the treatment of hypertension in older adults with and without glucose disorders: a report from the ALLHAT study. *J Clin Hypertens* (Greenwich) 2004;6:116–125

20. Weber MA, Bakris GL, Jamerson K, et al.; ACCOMPLISH Investigators. Cardiovascular events during differing hypertension therapies in patients with diabetes. *J Am Coll Cardiol* 2010;56:77–85

21. Bangalore S, Fakheri R, Toklu B, Messerli FH. Diabetes mellitus as a compelling indication for use of renin angiotensin system blockers: systematic review and meta-analysis of randomized trials. *BMJ* 2016;352:i438

22. Flack JM, Sica DA, Bakris G, et al.; International Society on Hypertension in Blacks. Management of high blood pressure in Blacks: an update of the International Society on Hypertension in Blacks consensus statement. *Hypertension* 2010;56(5):780–800

23. Julius S, Alderman MH, Beevers G, et al. Cardiovascular risk reduction in hypertensive black patients with left ventricular hypertrophy: the LIFE study. *J Am Coll Cardiol* 2004;43(6):1047–1055

24. ALLHAT Officers and Coordinators for the ALLHAT Collaborative Research Group. Major outcomes in high-risk hypertensive patients randomized to angiotensin-converting enzyme inhibitor or calcium channel blocker vs diuretic: the Antihypertensive and Lipid-Lowering Treatment to Prevent Heart Attack Trial (ALLHAT). *JAMA* 2002;288:2981–2997

25. Wright JT Jr., Dunn JK, Cutler JA, et al. Outcomes in hypertensive black and nonblack patients treated with chlorthalidone, amlodipine, and lisinopril. *JAMA* 2005;293:1595–1608

26. ONTARGET Investigators, Yusuf S, Teo KK, Pogue J, et al. Telmisartan, ramipril, or both in patients at high risk for vascular events. *N Engl J Med* 2008;358(15):1547–1559

27. Medical Research Council trial of treatment of hypertension in older adults: principal results. MRC Working Party. *BMJ* 1992;304(6824):405–412

28. Lindholm LH, Carlberg B, Samuelsson O. Should beta blockers remain first choice in the treatment of primary hypertension? A meta-analysis. *Lancet* 2005;366(9496):1545–1553

29. Wiysonge CS, Bradley HA, Volmink J, et al. Beta-blockers for hypertension. *Cochrane Database Syst Rev* 2012;11:CD002003

30. Zhao P, Xu P, Wan C, Wang Z. Evening versus morning dosing regimen drug therapy for hypertension. *Cochrane Database Syst Rev* 2011;(10): CD004184

31. Hermida RC, Ayala DE, Mojón A, Fernández JR. Influence of time of day of blood pressure-lowering treatment on cardiovascular risk in hypertensive patients with type 2 diabetes. *Diabetes Care* 2011;34:1270–1276

32. Zoungas S, de Galan BE, Ninomiya T, et al.; ADVANCE Collaborative Group. Combined effects of routine blood pressure lowering and intensive glucose control on macrovascular and microvascular outcomes in patients with type 2 diabetes: new results from the ADVANCE trial. *Diabetes Care* 2009;32:2068–2074

33. Margolis KL, O'Connor PJ, Morgan TM, et al. Outcomes of combined cardiovascular risk factor management strategies in type 2 diabetes: the ACCORD randomized trial. *Diabetes Care* 2014;37:1721–1728

34. Patel A, MacMahon S, Chalmers J, et al.; ADVANCE Collaborative Group. Effects of a fixed combination of perindopril and indapamide on macrovascular and microvascular outcomes in patients with type 2 diabetes mellitus (the ADVANCE trial): a randomised controlled trial. *Lancet* 2007;370: 829–840

35. Freeman R, Wieling W, Axelrod FB, et al. Consensus statement on the definition of orthostatic hypotension, neurally mediated syncope and the postural tachycardia syndrome. *Auton Neurosci* 2011;161:46–48

36. Pop-Busui R, Boulton AJM, Feldman EL, et al. Diabetic neuropathy: a position statement by the American Diabetes Association. *Diabetes Care* 2017;40:136–154

37. Fleg JL, Evans GW, Margolis KL, et al. Orthostatic hypotension in the ACCORD (Action to Control Cardiovascular Risk in Diabetes) blood pressure trial: prevalence, incidence, and prognostic significance. *Hypertension* 2016;68:888–895

38. Dorsch MP, Gillespie BW, Erickson SR, et al. Chlorthalidone reduces cardiovascular events compared with hydrochlorothiazide: a retrospective cohort analysis. *Hypertension* 2011;57(4):689–694

39. ALLHAT Collaborative Research Group. Major cardiovascular events in hypertensive patients randomized to doxazosin vs chlorthalidone: the antihypertensive and lipid-lowering treatment to prevent heart attack trial (ALLHAT) [erratum, *JAMA* 2000;283(23):2976]. *JAMA* 2000;283(15):1967–1975

40. Mancia G. Effects of intensive blood pressure control in the management of patients with type 2 diabetes mellitus in the Action to Control Cardiovascular Risk in Diabetes (ACCORD) trial. *Circulation* 2010;122(8):847–849

41. Bakris GL, Weir MR; Study of Hypertension and the Efficacy of Lotrel in Diabetes (SHIELD) Investigators. Achieving goal blood pressure in patients with type 2 diabetes: conventional versus fixed-dose combination approaches. *J Clin Hypertens* (Greenwich) 2003;5:202–209

42. Blood Pressure Lowering Treatment Trialists' Collaboration, Turnbull F, Neal B, et al. Effects of different regimens to lower blood pressure on major cardiovascular events in older and younger adults: meta-analysis of randomised trials. *BMJ* 2008;336:1121

43. Law MR, Morris JK, Wald NJ. Use of blood pressure lowering drugs in the prevention of cardiovascular disease: meta-analysis of 147 randomised trials in the context of expectations from prospective epidemiological studies. *BMJ* 2009;338:b1665

44. Rosendorff C, Black HR, Cannon CP, et al. Treatment of hypertension in the prevention and management of ischemic heart disease: a scientific statement from the American Heart Association Council for High Blood Pressure Research and the Councils on Clinical Cardiology and Epidemiology and Prevention. *Circulation* 2007;115:2761–2788

45. Mancia G, Fagard R, Narkiewicz K, et al. 2013 ESH/ESC guidelines for the management of arterial hypertension: the task force for the management of arterial hypertension of the European Society of Hypertension (ESH) and of the European Society of Cardiology (ESC). *J Hypertens* 2013;31:1281–1357

46. Materson BJ, Reda DJ, Cushman WC, et al. Single-drug therapy for hypertension in men. A comparison of six antihypertensive agents with placebo. The Department of Veterans Affairs Cooperative Study Group on Antihypertensive Agents [erratum, *N Engl J Med* 1994;330(23):1689]. *N Engl J Med* 1993;328(13):914–921

47. Epstein M, Bakris G. Newer approaches to antihypertensive therapy. Use of fixed-dose combination therapy. *Arch Intern Med* 1996;156(17):1969–1978

48. Bakris GL. Maximizing cardiorenal benefit in the management of hypertension: achieve blood pressure goals. *J Clin Hypertens* (Greenwich) 1999;1(2):141–147

49. Brixner DI, Jackson KC 2nd, Sheng X, et al. Assessment of adherence, persistence, and costs among valsartan and hydrochlorothiazide retrospective cohorts in free- and fixed-dose combinations. *Curr Med Res Opin* 2008;24(9):2597–2607

50. Bangalore S, Kamalakkannan G, Parkar S, Messerli FH. Fixed-dose combinations improve medication compliance: a meta-analysis. *Am J Med* 2007;120(8):713–719

51. Lotensin (oral tablets) [product information], 2014; Micardis (oral tablets) [product information], 2014

Chapter 20
Lipids

Cheyenne Newsome, PharmD, PhC, BCACP

INTRODUCTION

Arteriosclerosis is a thickening, hardening, and loss of elasticity of the walls of the arteries. Atherosclerosis is a specific type of arteriosclerosis, but the terms are sometimes used interchangeably. Atherosclerosis refers to when the buildup of fats, cholesterol, and other substances in and on the artery walls leads to narrowing of the vessel lumen and restricts blood flow. Abnormalities of plasma lipoproteins result in a predisposition to ASCVD.[1] ASCVD is defined as ACS, MI, angina, coronary or other arterial revascularization, stroke, transient ischemic attack, or PAD. Premature coronary arteriosclerosis is the most common and significant consequence of dyslipidemia. Patients with T2D have an increased prevalence of lipid abnormalities, contributing to their high risk of ASCVD.[2] Treatments for patients who are at risk but who have not yet experienced their first cardiovascular or cerebrovascular event are termed primary prevention, whereas those for patients who already have manifestations of vascular disease are termed secondary prevention.

Lipids are essential substrates for cell membrane formation and hormone synthesis, and provide a source of free fatty acids for cellular functions. Cholesterol, triglycerides, and phospholipids are the major lipids in the body and are known as lipoproteins. The three major classes of lipoproteins are low-density lipoproteins (LDL), high-density lipoproteins (HDL), and very-low-density lipoproteins (VLDL). HDL transports excess cholesterol from peripheral tissue (called reverse cholesterol transport) to the liver and has been shown to be cardioprotective for the occurrence of ASCVD.[3] Although HDL is beneficial, LDL is a major contributor to ASCVD. Atherosclerotic lesions are thought to arise from transport and retention of plasma LDL cholesterol in the epithelial cell wall. Once in the artery, LDL undergoes oxidation, which leads to decreased LDL-receptor expression and increased levels of coagulation promoters and vasoactive substances, with a reduction in vasodilator and antiplatelets. The effect of this is massive accumulation of cholesterol on the arterial walls. An imbalance between plaque synthesis and degradation can lead to a weakened plaque prone to rupture. LDL is catabolized through interaction with cell surface receptors on liver, adrenal, and smooth muscle cells. Increased intracellular cholesterol resulting from LDL catabolism inhibits the activity of 3-hydroxy-3-methylglutaryl coenzyme A reductase (HMG-CoA reductase), the rate-limiting enzyme for intracellular cholesterol biosynthesis. Increased intracellular cholesterol also causes reduced synthesis of LDL receptors, which limits subsequent cholesterol uptake from the plasma.[1] Triglycerides are also an important component of lipids, as hypertriglyceridemia has been associated with ASCVD independent of other lipid abnormalities.[4] Obesity and insulin resistance are common causes of a high concentration of triglycerides, and thus hypertriglyceridemia is common in patients with T2D.[2] Patients with hypertriglyceridemia are also at increased risk of developing acute pancreatitis.

Lifestyle modification focusing on weight loss (if indicated); reducing intake of saturated fat, trans fat, and cholesterol; increasing intake of dietary n-3 fatty acids, viscous fiber, and plant sterols; and increasing physical activity should be recommended to improve the lipid profile, specifically HDL, in patients with diabetes. Glycemic control may also beneficially modify plasma lipid levels, particularly in patients with very high triglycerides and poor glycemic control. Abstinence from alcohol may also reduce triglycerides.[2]

GOALS OF TREATMENT

Previously, strategies for using drug therapy to reduce ASCVD events focused on treating to specific cholesterol targets based on risk stratification. These included LDL goals of less than 100 mg/dL for all patients with diabetes, and stricter goals of <70 mg/dL or <55 mg/dL for patients with diabetes who had additional risk factors.[5] While targets for various lipid parameters exist, the only approach that has been evaluated in multiple randomized controlled trials is the use of fixed doses of cholesterol-lowering drugs to reduce ASCVD risk.[6] Because of this, the American Diabetes Association no longer employs only LDL goals as the primary endpoint to achieve ASCVD reduction.[2] Instead, statin therapy is recommended with different intensities for patients with varying levels of ASCVD risk. It is recommended that patients with elevated triglycerides receive additional intervention. This is not to reduce ASCVD, but instead to reduce the risk of pancreatitis. It is preferred for fasting triglycerides to be less than 500 mg/dL. In patients with triglycerides >1,000 mg/dL, initiating pharmacotherapy should be considered.[2]

OVERVIEW OF MEDICATIONS AND RATIONALE FOR USE

Statins are the cornerstone for ASCVD reduction for patients with diabetes. Multiple clinical trials have demonstrated the beneficial effects of statin therapy on ASCVD outcomes in subjects with and without preexisting heart disease.[7,8] Specific trials in patients with diabetes showed significant primary and secondary prevention of ASCVD events and death from cardiovascular causes in patients with diabetes.[9,10] Meta-analyses, including data from over 18,000 patients with diabetes from trials of statin therapy, demonstrate clinically significant reduction in all-cause mortality and vascular mortality.[11] Accordingly, statins are the drugs of choice for LDL cholesterol lowering and cardioprotection, and the only class recommended as initial therapy for ASCVD reduction.

For primary prevention, moderate-dose statin therapy is recommended for those 40 years and older, though high-intensity therapy may be considered on an individual basis when additional ASCVD risk factors are present. The evidence of benefit is strong for patients with diabetes aged 40–75 years, an age-group well represented in statin trials. Patients with diabetes between the age of 40 and 75 years are recommended to receive statin therapy. At minimum, these patients should receive moderate-intensity statin therapy, but high-intensity statin therapy could be considered if they have significant ASCVD risk factors.

The evidence of statins for primary prevention is lower for patients aged >75 years; relatively few older patients with diabetes have been enrolled in primary prevention trials. However, heterogeneity by age has not been seen in the relative benefit of lipid-lowering therapy in trials that included older participants; because older age confers higher risk, the absolute benefits are actually greater.[8,12] Moderate-intensity statin therapy is recommended in patients with diabetes who are 75 years or older. However, the risk-benefit profile should be routinely evaluated in this population, with downward titration of dose performed as needed for tolerability.[2] In adults with diabetes mellitus who are <40 or >75 years of age, it is reasonable to evaluate the potential for ASCVD benefits, adverse effects, and drug-drug interactions, and to consider patient preferences when deciding to initiate, continue, or intensify statin therapy.

High-intensity statin therapy is recommended for all patients with diabetes and ASCVD. This recommendation is based on the Cholesterol Treatment Trialists' Collaboration involving 26 statin trials, of which 5 compared high-intensity to moderate-intensity statins. Together, they found reductions in nonfatal cardiovascular events with more intensive therapy in patients with and without diabetes.[8,12,13]

Table 20.1 shows the recommended lipid-lowering strategies, and Table 20.2 shows the two statin-dosing intensities that are recommended for use in clinical practice. High-intensity statin therapy will achieve approximately 50% reduction in LDL cholesterol, and moderate-intensity statin regimens achieve 30–50% reductions in LDL cholesterol. Low-dose statin therapy is generally not recommended in patients with diabetes but is sometimes the only dose of statin that a patient can tolerate. For patients who do not tolerate the intended intensity of statin, the maximally tolerated statin dose should be used; even a less-than-daily statin dosing (i.e., once or twice a week) may be beneficial.[14] Mild myalgia and arthralgia are common side effects of statins. However, rhabdomyolysis may occur. Rhabdomyolysis is a rare but serious adverse reaction that causes muscle cells to break down as well as complications of kidney failure. If patients receiving statin therapy express they are experiencing muscle pain, tenderness, stiffness, cramping, weakness, or fatigue, a thorough history should be conducted to identify alternative causes to avoid unnecessary discontinuation of statins. If rhabdomyolysis is suspected, a serum creatinine kinase level can be drawn for diagnosis.

OVERVIEW OF COMBINATION THERAPY

Over the past few years, there have been multiple large randomized trials investigating the benefits of adding nonstatin agents to statin therapy, including two that evaluated further lowering of LDL cholesterol with ezetimibe[12] or PCSK9 inhibitors.[13] Both trials found a significant benefit in the reduction of ASCVD events that was directly related to the degree of further LDL cholesterol lowering. Approximately one-third of participants in these trials had diabetes. For patients

Table 20.1 — Recommendations for Statin and Combination Treatment in Adults with Diabetes

Age	ASCVD	Recommended statin intensity^ and combination treatment*
<40 years	No	None†
	Yes	High
		■ If LDL cholesterol ≥70 mg/dL despite maximally tolerated statin dose, consider adding additional LDL-lowering therapy (such as ezetimibe or PCSK9 inhibitor)#
≥40 years	No	Moderate‡
	Yes	High
		■ If LDL cholesterol ≥70 mg/dL despite maximally tolerated statin dose, consider adding additional LDL-lowering therapy (such as ezetimibe or PCSK9 inhibitor)

*In addition to lifestyle therapy. ^For patients who do not tolerate the intended intensity of statin, the maximally tolerated statin dose should be used. †Moderate-intensity statin may be considered based on risk-benefit profile and presence of ASCVD risk factors. ASCVD risk factors include LDL cholesterol ≥100 mg/dL (2.6 mmol/L), high blood pressure, smoking, CKD, albuminuria, and family history of premature ASCVD. ‡High-intensity statin may be considered based on risk-benefit profile and presence of ASCVD risk factors. #Adults aged <40 years with prevalent ASCVD were not well represented in clinical trials of non-statin-based LDL reduction. Before initiating combination lipid-lowering therapy, consider the potential for further ASCVD risk reduction, drug-specific adverse effects, and patient preferences.

with ASCVD who are on high-intensity (and maximally tolerated) statin therapy and have an LDL cholesterol >70 mg/dL, the addition of nonstatin LDL-lowering therapy is recommended after considering the potential for further ASCVD risk reduction, drug-specific adverse effects, and patient preference. There are no other available medications that have been shown to be effective at reducing the risk of ASCVD in patients.

STATINS AND EZETIMIBE

IMPROVE-IT was a randomized controlled trial with 18,144 patients, comparing the addition of ezetimibe to simvastatin therapy versus simvastatin alone. Individuals were ≥50 years of age, had been hospitalized for ACS (not marking going forward) within 10 days of therapy initiation, and were treated for an average of 6 years. Overall, the addition of ezetimibe led to a 6.4% relative benefit and a 2% absolute reduction in major adverse cardiovascular events. The degree of benefit was directly proportional to the change in LDL cholesterol, which was 70 mg/dL in the statin group on average and 54 mg/dL in the combination group. In those with diabetes (27% of participants), the combination of moderate-intensity simvastatin (40 mg) and ezetimibe (10 mg) showed a significant reduc-

Table 20.2—High-Intensity and Moderate-Intensity Statin Therapy*

High-intensity statin therapy (lowers LDL cholesterol by ≥50%)	Moderate-intensity statin therapy (lowers LDL cholesterol by 30–50%)
Atorvastatin 40–80 mg	Atorvastatin 10–20 mg
Rosuvastatin 20–40 mg	Rosuvastatin 5–10 mg
	Simvastatin 20–40 mg
	Pravastatin 40–80 mg
	Lovastatin 40 mg
	Fluvastatin XL 80 mg
	Pitavastatin 2–4 mg

*Once-daily dosing. XL, extended release.

tion of major adverse cardiovascular events, with an absolute risk reduction of 5% (40% vs. 45%) and relative risk reduction of 14% (RR 0.86 [95% CI 0.78–0.94]) over moderate-intensity simvastatin (40 mg) alone.[12]

STATINS AND PCSK9 INHIBITORS

Placebo-controlled trials evaluating the addition of the PCSK9 inhibitors evolocumab and alirocumab to maximally tolerated doses of statin therapy in participants who were at high risk for ASCVD demonstrated an average reduction in LDL cholesterol ranging from 36–59%. These agents have been approved as adjunctive therapy for patients with ASCVD or familial hypercholesterolemia who are receiving maximally tolerated statin therapy but require additional lowering of LDL cholesterol.[15,16]

The effects of PCSK9 inhibition on ASCVD outcomes were investigated in the FOURIER trial, which enrolled 27,564 patients with prior ASCVD and an additional high-risk feature who were receiving their maximally tolerated statin therapy (two-thirds were on high-intensity statin) but who still had an LDL cholesterol >70 mg/dL or a non-HDL cholesterol >100 mg/dL.[17] Patients were randomized to receive subcutaneous injections of evolocumab (either 140 mg every 2 weeks or 420 mg every month based on patient preference) versus placebo. Evolocumab reduced LDL cholesterol by 59% from a median of 92–30 mg/dL in the treatment arm.

During the median follow-up of 2.2 years, the composite outcome of cardiovascular death, MI, stroke, hospitalization for angina, or revascularization occurred in 11.3% vs. 9.8% of the placebo and evolocumab groups, respectively, representing a 15% relative risk reduction (*P* = 0.001). The combined endpoint of cardiovascular death, MI, or stroke was reduced by 20%, from 7.4% to 5.9% (*P* = 0.001). Importantly, similar benefits were seen in a prespecified subgroup of patients with diabetes, comprising 11,031 patients (40% of the enrolled participants).[18]

Table 20.3—Overview of Each Class of Medication

Medication class	Medication	Mechanism of action	Adverse effects	Considerations
HMG-CoA Reductase Inhibitors (Statins)	Rosuvastatin Atorvastatin Lovastatin Pitavastatin Fluvastatin Pravastatin Simvastatin	Selectively and competitively inhibits HMG-CoA reductase, a rate-limiting enzyme in cholesterol synthesis	Myalgia Arthralgia Constipation, nausea, diarrhea Stomach pain/cramps	■ Monitor liver function and lipid panel at baseline and as clinically warranted ■ Creatinine kinase should be measured in individuals with muscle symptoms ■ Hepatic function should be measured if symptoms suggesting hepatotoxicity arise (abdominal pain, dark-colored urine, or yellowing of the skin or sclera) ■ Patients on simvastatin and lovastatin should not eat large amounts of grapefruit or drink more than 1 L/day of grapefruit juice
PCSK9 Inhibitors	Alirocumab Evolocumab	Inhibits the binding of PCSK9 to LDL receptors on hepatocytes, thus reducing degradation of the LDL receptors. Increased LDL receptors are then available to clear LDL from circulation and lower LDL levels	Neurocognitive Swelling, pain, or bruising at injection site Back pain Influenza Nasopharyngitis	■ Monitoring: LDL at baseline and within 4–8 weeks of treatment initiation or dosage increase ■ If dose is missed, take as soon as possible if there are at least 7 days before the next scheduled dose. If less than 7 days remain, skip the missed dose ■ Requires injection ■ Very high cost relative to other agents
Cholesterol Absorption Inhibitors	Ezetimibe	Reduces blood cholesterol by acting at the brush border of the small intestine to inhibit the absorption of cholesterol, leading to a decrease in the delivery of intestinal cholesterol to the liver. This reduces hepatic cholesterol stores and increases the clearance of cholesterol from the blood	Stomach pain Fatigue Myalgia Arthralgia Diarrhea	
Omega-3 Fatty Acids	Omega-3 Acid Ethyl Esters Omega-3 Carboxylic Acids Icosapent ethyl	Not fully known; may increase hepatic mitochondrial and peroxisomal β-oxidation to reduce hepatic synthesis of triglycerides or increase plasma lipoprotein lipase activity	Belching Fishy taste Indigestion	■ Potential for increased bleeding when combined with antiplatelet or anticoagulant ■ Can cause significant increase in LDL (up to 50%)

(continued)

Table 20.3 (continued)

Medication class	Medication	Mechanism of action	Adverse effects	Considerations
Bile Acid Sequestrants	Colesevelam Cholestyramine Colestipol	Binds to bile acids to prevent reabsorption in the intestine. Serum bile acids are depleted, which activates conversion of cholesterol into bile acids. Demand for cholesterol in liver is increased, and there is an increase in LDL receptors, which increases clearance of LDL from the blood	Constipation Bloating Indigestion Nausea Flatulence	■ Must be taken with a meal ■ Bile acid sequestrants can reduce absorption of medications and vitamins. Administer medications with a narrow therapeutic window (warfarin, levothyroxine) 4 h before or after administration of a bile acid sequestrant ■ Contraindicated in patients with triglycerides >500 mg/dL
Niacin	Niacin	Not fully known; may reduce esterification of hepatic triglycerides, decrease release of free fatty acids from adipose tissue, and enhance the removal of triglycerides from plasma	Facial and neck flushing Nausea, vomiting, diarrhea Increased uric acid Increased glucose Peptic ulcers	■ To reduce flushing, patients can take aspirin or eat a low-fat snack 30–60 min prior to administration of niacin ■ Monitor liver function, A1C, uric acid
Fibric Acid Derivatives	Fenofibrate Gemfibrozil	Stimulates peroxisome proliferator activated receptor α (PPAR-α), which leads to 1) VLDL catabolism, 2) fatty acid oxidation, and 3) elimination of triglyceride-rich particles	Abdominal pain Gallstones Increased liver function tests Increased serum creatinine Indigestion Nausea Stomach pain	■ Monitoring: liver function, renal function ■ Significant reduction in triglycerides

HMG-CoA, 3-hydroxy-3-methylglutaryl coenzyme A reductase; VLDL, very-low-density lipoproteins.

STATINS AND FIBRATES

Fibrate-statin combinations produce significant additional decreases in tri-glycerides (30–50%) and increases in HDL cholesterol (10–20%) in comparison with statin monotherapy. The combination of a statin and fibrate is associated with an increased risk for abnormal transaminase levels, myositis, and rhabdomy-olysis. The risk of rhabdomyolysis is more common with higher doses of statins and renal insufficiency and appears to be higher when statins are combined with gemfibrozil (compared with fenofibrate).[19] For this reason, statins are contraindi-cated with gemfibrozil, and statins should be dose reduced if combined with feno-fibrate. In the ACCORD study, in patients with T2D who were at high risk for ASCVD, the combination of fenofibrate and simvastatin did not reduce the rate of fatal cardiovascular events, nonfatal MI, or nonfatal stroke compared with sim-vastatin alone. Prespecified subgroup analyses suggested heterogeneity in treat-ment effects, with possible benefit for men with both a triglyceride level of ≥204 mg/dL and an HDL cholesterol level of ≤34 mg/dL.[20]

STATINS AND NIACIN

In combination with statins, niacin further reduces LDL cholesterol (10–20%), non-HDL cholesterol, and triglycerides (10–30%), and increases HDL cholesterol (20–40%). The AIM-HIGH trial randomized over 3,000 patients (about one-third with diabetes) with established ASCVD, LDL cholesterol levels <180 mg/dL, low HDL cholesterol levels (men <40 mg/dL and women <50 mg/dL), and triglyceride levels of 150–400 mg/dL to statin therapy plus extended-release niacin or placebo. The trial was halted early due to lack of effi-cacy on the primary ASCVD outcome (first event of the composite of death from CHD, nonfatal MI, ischemic stroke, hospitalization for ACS, or symptom-driven coronary or cerebral revascularization) and a possible increase in ischemic stroke in those on combination therapy.[21]

The much larger HPS2-THRIVE trial also failed to show a benefit of adding niacin to background statin therapy.[22] A total of 25,673 patients with prior vascular disease were randomized to receive 2 g of extended-release niacin and 40 mg of laropiprant (an antagonist of the prostaglandin D2 receptor DP1 that has been shown to improve adherence to niacin therapy) versus a matching placebo daily and followed for a median follow-up period of 3.9 years. There was no significant difference in the rate of coronary death, MI, stroke, or coronary revascularization with the addition of niacin–laropiprant versus placebo (13.2% vs. 13.7%; rate ratio 0.96; $P = 0.29$). Niacin–laropiprant was associated with an increased inci-dence of new onset diabetes (absolute excess, 1.3 percentage points; $P < 0.001$) and disturbances in diabetes control among those with diabetes. In addition, there was an increase in serious adverse events associated with the gastrointestinal system, musculoskeletal system, skin, and, unexpectedly, infection and bleeding. There-fore, combination therapy with a statin and niacin is not recommended, given the lack of efficacy on major ASCVD outcomes and the side effects, including worsen-ing of diabetes.

STATINS AND OMEGA-3 FATTY ACIDS

The main lipid parameter benefit of omega-3 fatty acids is reduction in triglycerides. The Combination of Prescription Omega-3 With Simvastatin (COMBOS) study evaluated the change in lipid parameters of prescription omega-3 fatty acids when added to stable moderate-intensity statin therapy in patients with persistent hypertriglyceridemia. This study randomized 254 patients who were on stable therapy of simvastatin 40 mg daily and had fasting triglycerides between 200 and 499 mg/dL. Patients then received 4 g per day of prescription omega-3 fatty acids in addition to their simvastatin therapy. The addition of prescription omega-3 fatty acids reduced triglyceride levels by 29.5% ($P < 0.001$).[23] LDL was relatively unchanged in this study, while other studies of omega-3 fatty acids have shown increases in LDL of 5–10%.[24] Omega-3 fatty acids eicosapentaenoic acid (EPA) and docosahexaenoic acid (DHA) are responsible for the decrease in triglycerides. DHA-containing omega-3 fatty acids are more associated with LDL increase than EPA-only prescription omega-3 fatty acids.[25,26] A prescription fatty acid containing EPA only became available in the U.S. in 2012 and may be preferred since it has not been associated with increased LDL levels. No clinical trials have shown clinical benefit for prescription omega-3 fatty acids for reduction in ASCVD or prevention of pancreatitis.

STATINS AND BILE ACID SEQUESTRANTS

In combination with moderate-intensity statins, bile acid sequestrants can reduce LDL cholesterol by an additional 10–25% and may slightly increase triglycerides and HDL.[27–29] In addition to LDL lowering, colesevelam, a second-generation bile acid sequestrant, is approved as an adjunct to antidiabetes therapy for improving glycemic control in adults with T2D. A reduction in A1C of 0.32–0.41% was observed when colesevelam was added to monotherapy or combination therapy with metformin, sulfonylureas, or insulin.[30–32] However, there are not any clinical outcomes data for bile acid sequestrants in combination with statins, which limits the support of combining them with statins for the goal of ASCVD reduction.

IMPORTANT COMBINATION PRODUCTS

- Simcor: simvastatin and niacin
- Advicor: niacin and lovastatin
- Vytorin: simvastatin and ezetimibe

Table 20.4—Doses and Dose Adjustments for Prominent Medications in the Chapter

Medication	Dose	Dose adjustment
HMG-CoA Reductase Inhibitors		
Rosuvastatin	5–40 mg once daily	▪ CrCl less than 30 mL/min: 5 mg orally once daily; maximum 10 mg orally once daily ▪ Contraindicated in patients with active liver disease ▪ Concomitant gemfibrozil: avoid if possible; if concomitant use is required, initiate at 5 mg orally once daily, maximum 10 mg/day ▪ Rosuvastatin is a CYP3A4 substrate, and CYP3A4 inhibitors will increase the concentrations: reduce to 5–10 mg once daily ▪ Asian descent: initial, consider 5 mg orally once daily
Atorvastatin	10–80 mg once daily	▪ Avoid or reduce dose with CYP3A4 enzyme inhibitors ▪ No adjustment needed for renal impairment or dialysis ▪ Contraindicated in patients with active liver disease ▪ Avoid use with gemfibrozil
Lovastatin, Immediate Release	10–80 mg once daily or in divided doses	▪ Lovastatin is a CYP3A4 substrate, and CYP3A4 inhibitors will increase the concentrations: reduce dose or do not use ▪ Avoid use with gemfibrozil
Lovastatin, Extended Release	20–60 mg once daily	▪ Renal insufficiency: initial, 20 mg orally once daily ▪ Geriatric: initial, 20 mg orally once daily in the evening at bedtime ▪ Avoid use with gemfibrozil ▪ Lovastatin is a CYP3A4 substrate, and CYP3A4 inhibitors will increase the concentrations: reduce dose or do not use
Pitavastatin	1–4 mg once daily	▪ Renal impairment (moderate, eGFR 30–59 mL/min/1.73 m²): initial, 1 mg orally once daily; maximum 2 mg/day ▪ Renal impairment (severe, eGFR 15–29 mL/min/1.73 m², not receiving hemodialysis): initial, 1 mg orally once daily; maximum 2 mg/day ▪ Active liver disease (including unexplained persistent elevations of hepatic transaminases): use is contraindicated ▪ Hemodialysis: initial, 1 mg orally once daily; maximum 2 mg/day ▪ Avoid use with gemfibrozil
Fluvastatin, Immediate Release	20–40 mg once or twice daily	▪ Fluvastatin is a CYP3A4, CYP2C8, and CYP2C9 substrate. CYP3A4, CYP2C8, and CYP2C9 inhibitors will increase the concentrations: reduce dose or do not use ▪ Avoid use with gemfibrozil
Fluvastatin, Extended Release	80 mg daily	

(continued)

Table 20.4 (continued)

Medication	Dose	Dose adjustment
Pravastatin	40–80 mg daily	■ Renal impairment (severe): initial, 10 mg orally once daily ■ Hepatic impairment (active liver disease or unexplained, persistent elevations of serum transaminases): use is contraindicated ■ Pravastatin is a CYP3A4 substrate, and CYP3A4 inhibitors will increase the concentrations: dose reduction may be needed ■ Avoid use with gemfibrozil
Simvastatin	5–40 mg daily	■ Renal impairment (mild or moderate): no adjustment necessary ■ Renal impairment (severe): initial, 5 mg orally once daily ■ Simvastatin is a CYP3A4 substrate, and CYP3A4 inhibitors will increase the concentrations: reduce dose or do not use ■ Avoid use with gemfibrozil
		PCSK9 Inhibitors
Alirocumab	75–150 mg subcutaneously once every 2 weeks or 300 mg subcutaneously once every 4 weeks	■ Renal impairment (mild or moderate): no adjustment necessary ■ Hepatic impairment (mild or moderate): no adjustment necessary
Evolocumab	140 mg subcutaneously every 2 weeks or 420 mg subcutaneously monthly	■ Renal impairment (mild or moderate): no adjustment necessary ■ Hepatic impairment (mild or moderate): no adjustment necessary
		Cholesterol Absorption Inhibitors
Ezetimibe	10 mg once daily	■ Hepatic impairment (moderate to severe, Child-Pugh score 7–15): use not recommended
		Fibric Acid Derivatives
Fenofibrate	120–160 mg daily	■ Renal impairment (mild to moderate): 40–54 mg daily ■ Renal impairment (severe) or hemodialysis: contraindicated ■ Active liver disease, primary biliary cirrhosis, or unexplained persistent liver function abnormalities: contraindicated
Gemfibrozil	600 mg orally twice daily 30 min before the morning and evening meal	■ Severe renal impairment: avoid use
Colesevelam	3,750 mg orally once daily or in two divided doses	
Cholestyramine	4–24 g per day, in divided doses if over 8 g	

(continued)

Table 20.4 (continued)

Medication	Dose	Dose adjustment
Colestipol	2–16 g per day	
Niacin, Extended Release	500–2,000 mg once daily at bedtime	Hepatic impairment, active liver disease, unexplained transaminase elevations, and significant or unexplained hepatic dysfunction: contraindicated
Niacin, Immediate Release	250–6,000 mg, in divided doses if >1,500 mg per day	
Omega-3 Acid Ethyl Esters	4 g daily, may be given once daily or divided into two doses	

MONOGRAPHS (COMBINATION PRODUCTS EXCLUDED)

HMG-CoA REDUCTASE INHIBITORS

Atorvastatin (Lipitor): https://dailymed.nlm.nih.gov/dailymed/drugInfo.cfm?setid=c6e131fe-e7df-4876-83f7-9156fc4e8228

Rosuvastatin (Crestor): https://dailymed.nlm.nih.gov/dailymed/drugInfo.cfm?setid=bb0f3b5e-4bc6-41c9-66b9-6257e2513512

Simvastatin (Zocor): https://dailymed.nlm.nih.gov/dailymed/drugInfo.cfm?setid=fdbfe194-b845-42c5-bb87-a48118bc72e7

Pitavastatin (Livalo): https://dailymed.nlm.nih.gov/dailymed/drugInfo.cfm?setid=44dcbf97-99ec-427c-ba50-207e0069d6d2

Pravastatin (Pravachol): https://dailymed.nlm.nih.gov/dailymed/drugInfo.cfm?setid=897ad8b7-921d-eb02-a61c-3419e662a2da

Fluvastatin (Lescol): https://dailymed.nlm.nih.gov/dailymed/drugInfo.cfm?setid=e38126a5-9d6a-422f-812c-a01610108162

Lovastatin (Mevacor): https://dailymed.nlm.nih.gov/dailymed/drugInfo.cfm?setid=10a557fe-6620-4b15-862a-d3ff5dece612

OMEGA-3 FATTY ACIDS

Omega-3 Acid Ethyl Esters (Lovaza): https://dailymed.nlm.nih.gov/dailymed/drugInfo.cfm?setid=5ada82f0-a5fd-46c9-aecc-f106f614c9f0

Icosapent Ethyl Capsule (Vascepa): https://dailymed.nlm.nih.gov/dailymed/drugInfo.cfm?setid=9c1a2828-1583-4414-ab22-a60480e8e508

CHOLESTEROL ABSORPTION INHIBITORS

Ezetimibe (Zetia): https://dailymed.nlm.nih.gov/dailymed/drugInfo.
cfm?setid=a773b0b2-d31c-4ff4-b9e8-1eb2d3a4d62a

NIACIN

Niacin (Niaspan): https://dailymed.nlm.nih.gov/dailymed/drugInfo.
cfm?setid=35433c7b-556c-49a0-bfb5-0d498359925b

FIBRIC ACID DERIVATIVES

Fenofibrate (Tricor): https://dailymed.nlm.nih.gov/dailymed/drugInfo.
cfm?setid=b693e68d-f812-4993-54b6-852e3517c344

Gemfibrozil (Lopid): https://dailymed.nlm.nih.gov/dailymed/drugInfo.
cfm?setid=c48855b7-215e-453b-b3b1-a0f9dee7221f

PCSK9 INHIBITORS

Alirocumab (Praluent): https://dailymed.nlm.nih.gov/dailymed/drugInfo.
cfm?setid=446f6b5c-0dd4-44ff-9bc2-c2b41f2806b4

Evolocumab (Repatha): https://dailymed.nlm.nih.gov/dailymed/drugInfo.
cfm?setid=709338ae-ab8f-44a9-b7d5-abaabec3493a

BILE ACID SEQUESTRANTS

Cholestyramine (Questran): https://dailymed.nlm.nih.gov/dailymed/search.cfm?l
abeltype=all&query=questran&pagesize=20&page=1

Colesevelam (Welchol): https://dailymed.nlm.nih.gov/dailymed/drugInfo.
cfm?setid=4a06d3b2-7229-4398-baba-5d0a72f63821

REFERENCES

1. Talbert RL. Hyperlipidemia. In *Pharmacotherapy: A Pathophysiologic Approach*, 9th ed. DiPiro JT, Talbert RL, Yee GC, et al., Eds. New York, McGraw-Hill, 2014, p. 291–317

2. American Diabetes Association. *Standards of Medical Care in Diabetes—2018. Diabetes Care* 2018;41(Suppl. 1):S4–S159

3. Rader DL. Mechanisms of disease: HDL metabolism as a target for novel therapies. *Nat Clin Pract Cardiovasc Med* 2007;4:102–109

4. McBride P. Triglycerides and risk for coronary artery disease. *Curr Atheroscler Rep* 2008;10(5):386–390

5. Jellinger PS, Handelsman Y, Rosenblit PD, et al. American Association of Clinical Endocrinologists and American College of Endocrinology guidelines for the management of dyslipidemia and prevention of cardiovascular disease. *Endocr Pract* 2017;23:1–87

6. Stone NJ, Robinson J, Lichtenstein AH, et al. 2013 ACC/AHA guideline on the treatment of blood cholesterol to reduce atherosclerotic cardiovascular risk in adults: a report of the American College of Cardiology/American Heart Association Task Force on Practice Guidelines. *Circulation* 2014; (25 Suppl. 2):S1–S45

7. Mihaylova B, Emberson J, Blackwell L, et al.; Cholesterol Treatment Trialists' (CTT) Collaborators. The effects of lowering LDL cholesterol with statin therapy in people at low risk of vascular disease: meta-analysis of individual data from 27 randomised trials. *Lancet* 2012;380:581–590

8. Baigent C, Keech A, Kearney PM, et al.; Cholesterol Treatment Trialists' (CTT) Collaborators. Efficacy and safety of cholesterol-lowering treatment: prospective meta-analysis of data from 90,056 participants in 14 randomised trials of statins. *Lancet* 2005;366:1267–1278

9. Knopp RH, d'Emden M, Smilde JG, Pocock SJ. Efficacy and safety of atorvastatin in the prevention of cardiovascular end points in subjects with type 2 diabetes: the Atorvastatin Study for Prevention of Coronary Heart Disease Endpoints in Non-Insulin-Dependent Diabetes Mellitus (ASPEN). *Diabetes Care* 2006;29:1478–1485

10. Colhoun HM, Betteridge DJ, Durrington PN, et al.; CARDS investigators. Primary prevention of cardiovascular disease with atorvastatin in type 2 diabetes in the Collaborative Atorvastatin Diabetes Study (CARDS): multicentre randomised placebo-controlled trial. *Lancet* 2004;364:685–696

11. Kearney PM, Blackwell L, Collins R, et al.; Cholesterol Treatment Trialists' (CTT) Collaborators. Efficacy of cholesterol-lowering therapy in 18,686 people with diabetes in 14 randomised trials of statins: a meta-analysis. *Lancet* 2008;371:117–125

12. Cannon CP, Blazing MA, Giugliano RP, et al.; IMPROVE-IT Investigators. Ezetimibe added to statin therapy after acute coronary syndromes. *N Engl J Med* 2015;372:2387–2397

13. Shepherd J, Barter P, Carmena R, et al. Effect of lowering LDL cholesterol substantially below currently recommended levels in patients with coronary heart disease and diabetes: the Treating to New Targets (TNT) study. *Diabetes Care* 2006;29:1220–1226

14. Meek C, Wierzbicki AS, Jewkes C, et al. Daily and intermittent rosuvastatin 5 mg therapy in statin intolerant patients: an observational study. *Curr Med Res Opin* 2012;28:371–378

15. Moriarty PM, Jacobson TA, Bruckert E, et al. Efficacy and safety of alirocumab, a monoclonal antibody to PCSK9, in statin-intolerant patients: design and rationale of ODYSSEY ALTERNATIVE, a randomized phase 3 trial. *J Clin Lipidol* 2014;8:554–561

16. Zhang X-L, Zhu Q-Q, Zhu L, et al. Safety and efficacy of anti-PCSK9 antibodies: a meta-analysis of 25 randomized, controlled trials. *BMC Med* 2015;13:123

17. Sabatine MS, Giugliano RP, Keech AC, et al.; FOURIER Steering Committee and Investigators. Evolocumab and clinical outcomes in patients with cardiovascular disease. *N Engl J Med* 2017;376:1713–1722

18. Sabatine MS, Leiter LA, Wiviott SD, et al. Cardiovascular safety and efficacy of the PCSK9 inhibitor evolocumab in patients with and without diabetes and the effect of evolocumab on glycaemia and risk of new-onset diabetes: a prespecified analysis of the FOURIER randomised controlled trial [article online], 2017. *Lancet Diabetes Endocrinol.* Available from https://www.thelancet.com/journals/landia/article/PIIS2213-8587(17)30313-3/fulltext. Accessed 28 September 2017

19. Jones PH, Davidson MH. Reporting rate of rhabdomyolysis with fenofibrate + statin versus gemfibrozil + any statin. *Am J Cardiol* 2005;95:120–122

20. Ginsberg HN, Elam MB, Lovato LC, et al.; ACCORD Study Group. Effects of combination lipid therapy in type 2 diabetes mellitus. *N Engl J Med* 2010;362:1563–1574

21. Boden WE, Probstfield JL, Anderson T, et al.; AIM-HIGH Investigators. Niacin in patients with low HDL cholesterol levels receiving intensive statin therapy. *N Engl J Med* 2011;365:2255–2267

22. Landray MJ, Haynes R, Hopewell JC, et al.; HPS2-THRIVE Collaborative Group. Effects of extended-release niacin with laropiprant in high-risk patients. *N Engl J Med* 2014;371:203–212

23. Davidson MH, Stein EA, Bays HE, et al.; COMBination of prescription Omega-3 with Simvastatin (COMBOS) Investigators. Efficacy and tolerability of adding prescription omega-3 fatty acids 4 g/d to simvastatin 40 mg/d in hypertriglyceridemic patients: an 8-week, randomized, double-blind, placebo-controlled study. *Clin Ther* 2007;29(7):1354–1367

24. Harris WS. N-3 fatty acids and serum lipoproteins: human studies. *Am J Clin Nutr* 1997;65:1645S–1654S

25. Mori TA, Burke V, Puddey IB, et al. Purified eicosapentaenoic and docosahexaenoic acids have differential effects on serum lipids and lipoproteins, LDL particle size, glucose, and insulin in mildly hyperlipidemic men. *Am J Clin Nutr* 2000;71:1085–1094

26. Wei MY, Jacobson TA. Effects of eicosapentaenoic acid versus docosahexaenoic acid on serum lipids: a systematic review and meta-analysis. *Curr Atheroscler Rep* 2011;13:474–483

27. Davidson MH, Toth P, Weiss S, et al. Low-dose combination therapy with colesevelam hydrochloride and lovastatin effectively decreases low-density lipoprotein cholesterol in patients with primary hypercholesterolemia. *Clin Cardiol* 2001;24(6):467–474

28. Hunninghake D, Insull W Jr., Toth P, et al. Coadministration of colesevelam hydrochloride with atorvastatin lowers LDL cholesterol additively. *Athero-sclerosis* 2001;158(2):407–416

29. Knapp HH, Schrott H, Ma P, et al. Efficacy and safety of combination simvastatin and colesevelam in patients with primary hypercholesterolemia. *Am J Med* 2001;110(5):352–360

30. Bays HE, Goldberg RB, Truitt KE, Jones MR. Colesevelam hydrochloride therapy in patients with type 2 diabetes mellitus treated with metformin: glucose and lipid effects. *Arch Intern Med* 2008;168:1975–1983

31. Fonseca VA, Rosenstock J, Wang AC, et al. Colesevelam HCl improves glycemic control and reduces LDL cholesterol in patients with inadequately controlled type 2 diabetes on sulfonylurea-based therapy. *Diabetes Care* 2008;31:1479–1484

32. Goldberg RB, Fonseca VA, Truitt KE, Jones MR. Efficacy and safety of colesevelam in patients with type 2 diabetes mellitus and inadequate glycemic control receiving insulin-based therapy. *Arch Intern Med* 2008;168:1531–1540

Chapter 21
Antiplatelets
Megan Willson, PharmD, BCPS
Kimberly C. McKeirnan, PharmD, BCACP

INTRODUCTION

Platelets play an integral role in homeostasis and coagulation. Thrombosis occurs through the process of platelet activation, adhesion, and aggregation because of tissue injury.[1] Although platelets are critical in homeostasis with injury to prevent hemorrhage, the platelet cascade and formation of clots in CVD lead to significant morbidity and mortality. CVD comprises CHD, including acute MI; cerebrovascular disease, including stroke; PAD; and atherosclerosis. Therapy that modulates platelet activity is an important component of the treatment and prevention of these diseases.

The staggering statistics reported in the 2018 Heart Disease and Stroke Statistics Update illustrate the importance of treating heart disease. Heart disease remained the leading cause of death in 2018, with stroke the fifth-leading cause of death. It is estimated that 1 in 3 deaths in the U.S. are due to CVD, or approximately 2,300 deaths per day. Stroke statistics are similarly frightening, with 1 in 19 deaths due to stroke; stroke remains the leading cause of long-term disability. Prevention and treatment of heart disease and stroke are important targets for improving health in the U.S. and are reflected in the American Heart Association (AHA) goals. Although rates of CVD and stroke are decreasing with lifestyle modifications and medical advancement, the prevalence remains high.[2]

CVD significantly impacts morbidity and mortality and can also cause significant economic burden. Costs include the direct costs of caring for individuals with heart disease, as well as the indirect costs of the loss of affected individuals' productivity. It is estimated that both direct and indirect costs for heart disease (including stroke) are approximately $330 billion annually.[2]

Risk factors for CVD include hypertension, dyslipidemia, smoking, diabetes mellitus, family history of premature CHD, obesity, and CKD.[3] Diabetes mellitus alone is thought to increase the risk of CVD twofold.[4] Control of risk factors is extremely important to modifying long-term outcomes and risk for patients. The American Diabetes Association recommends that patients are assessed for risk yearly to guide therapy and risk-reduction strategies for CVD. As in the general population, CVD is the leading cause of death for patients with diabetes.[5] Not only do diabetes and elevated blood glucose increase risk of events, but patients who experience cardiovascular events have worse outcomes, with more complicated hospital stays and more cardiovascular event reoccurrences.[4,6,7]

Atherosclerosis and thrombosis both contribute to CVD in patients with diabetes. Atherosclerosis leads to a blockage of a vessel, which then leads to platelet aggregation, activation, and adhesion. Platelet function is altered in diabetes with increased propensity toward thrombosis. Diabetes enhances platelet aggregation, adhesion, and thrombin generation. Specific changes in lipid membrane fluidity have led to hyperreactivity of platelets. Increasing production of thromboxane A2 may increase the sensitivity of platelets to stimuli. Alterations in nitric oxide production and increased expression of activation adhesion molecules glycoprotein IIb-IIIa and P-selection may also be contributing to platelet dysfunction. Other changes affecting platelet activity are alterations of intracellular calcium and magnesium levels, increased arachidonic acid metabolism, decreased prostacyclin production, and decreased antioxidant levels.[4]

This chapter will discuss the following antiplatelet therapies commonly used today: aspirin, prasugrel, clopidogrel, ticagrelor, dipyridamole/aspirin, and cilostazol. Many trials have been conducted for primary and secondary prevention of cardiovascular events. The data from some of the trials will be summarized here. Many of the trials had high subsets of patients with diabetes mellitus.

GOALS OF THERAPY

Table 21.1—Goals of Therapy

- Reduce morbidity and mortality from CVD
- Prevent primary and secondary occurrence of CVD events including stroke and MI
- Control risk factors to decrease cardiovascular risk
  - Hypertension
  - Dyslipidemia
  - Smoking
  - Family history of premature coronary disease
  - Chronic kidney disease
  - Albuminuria
- Reduce risk of bleeding and other adverse effects of antiplatelet therapy
- Reduce symptoms of atherosclerotic disease
  - Chest pain or angina
  - Leg pain
  - Numbness

Source: American Diabetes Association.[8]

ANTIPLATELET THERAPY

ASPIRIN

Aspirin reduces platelet aggregation by irreversibly inhibiting prostaglandin cyclooxygenase-1 (COX-1).[9] Aspirin has greater potency for inhibiting platelet aggregation than any other salicylic acid derivative.[9] Aspirin is indicated to reduce the risk of death and nonfatal stroke for patients who have had an ischemic stroke or transient ischemia of the brain; to reduce the risk of vascular mortality in patients with a suspected acute MI; to reduce the risk of death or nonfatal MI in patients with a previous MI or unstable angina pectoris; to reduce the risk of MI and death in patients with chronic stable angina pectoris; and specifically in patients who have undergone revascularization procedures or for patients who had a preexisting indication for aspirin.[9]

The manufacturers recommend aspirin dosing as shown in Table 21.2.

Table 21.2—Aspirin Dosing

Indication	Dose
Ischemic Stroke and Transient Ischemic Attack	50–325 mg once daily to be continued indefinitely
Suspected Acute MI	Initial dose of 160–162.5 mg as soon as MI is suspected, with an ongoing maintenance dose of 160–162.5 mg once daily for 30 days post-infarction. Ongoing therapy should be considered for prevention of recurrent MI
Prevention of Recurrent MI	75–325 mg once daily to be continued indefinitely
Unstable Angina Pectoris	75–325 mg once daily to be continued indefinitely
Chronic Stable Angina Pectoris	75–325 mg once daily to be continued indefinitely
Coronary Artery Bypass Graft (CABG)	325 mg daily starting 6 h post-procedure, to be continued for 1 year post-procedure
Percutaneous Transluminal Coronary Angioplasty	Initial dose of 325 mg given 2 h pre-surgery, followed by a maintenance dose of 160–325 mg daily to be continued indefinitely

Aspirin is available in a multitude of doses and combination products. Doses should be administered with a full glass of water to minimize gastrointestinal distress. Aspirin is not recommended for patients under the age of 12 years due to the risk for Reye's syndrome.[10] The manufacturer also warns against stomach bleeding as an important side effect.[10] The risk of stomach bleeding is increased in patients who are over 60 years of age, take aspirin at a higher dose or for longer than recommended, take additional blood-thinning medications or corticosteroids, drink three or more alcoholic beverages per day, have a history of stomach ulcers or bleeding problems, or take prescription or nonprescription NSAIDs.[10]

PRASUGREL

Prasugrel, a thienopyridine, inhibits platelet activation and aggregation by irreversibly binding to the $P2Y_{12}$ class of adenosine diphosphate (ADP) receptors on platelets. This medication is indicated for use in patients with unstable angina or non-ST-elevated myocardial infarction (NSTEMI) and patients with STEMI when managing with percutaneous coronary intervention (PCI).[11]

Doses are available as a yellow 5-mg tablet and a beige 10-mg tablet.[11] Initial dosing should begin with a single 60-mg oral loading dose on day 1, followed by a 10-mg dose thereafter administered orally once a day, with or without food. Patients taking prasugrel should also take 75–325 mg of aspirin daily. After receiving a 60-mg loading dose, 90% of patients achieved 50% inhibition of platelet aggregation within 1 h.[11] Average steady-state platelet aggregation inhibition was approximately 70% and occurred after 3–5 days of receiving a 10-mg daily dose following the single 60-mg loading dose. The elimination half-life is approximately 7 h.

Prasugrel carries a black box warning of increased bleeding risk and is contraindicated for patients who have an active pathological bleed (i.e. peptic ulcer, intracranial hemorrhage), those who have had a prior transient ischemic attack or stroke, and those allergic to any component of the product. Because of the increased risk of bleeding, caution should be used in patients over the age of 75, those with an increased likelihood of bleeding such as from recent trauma or surgery, and those taking medications that may cause bleeding, such as NSAIDs or other oral anticoagulants.

Prasugrel is converted into an active metabolite primarily by CYP3A4 and CYP2B6, although CYP2C9 and CYP2C19 are involved to a lesser extent. However, medications that potentially inhibit or induce these enzymes, such as ketoconazole and rifampin, do not appear to have a clinically significant impact on pharmacokinetics or platelet aggregation when used in combination with prasugrel. This can be beneficial for patients with a complex medication regimen.

Prasugrel is categorized as pregnancy category B, although there are no adequate studies in pregnant women. Reproductive studies in rats and rabbits receiving doses up to 30 times the recommended human dose showed no evidence of fetal harm. However, prasugrel should be recommended for pregnant women only if the benefits outweigh the potential fetal risk.

Dose adjustments are not necessary for patients with mild to moderate hepatic impairment, although severe hepatic disease has been associated with an increased bleeding risk. Prasugrel has not been studied in these patients. Renal impairment does not require dose adjustment either, but there are limited data for patients with ESRD.[11]

CLOPIDOGREL

Clopidogrel, another medication in the thienopyridine class, is indicated for patients with unstable angina (UA), NSTEMI, STEMI, and those who have suffered from a recent stroke, recent MI, or with established PAD. Contraindications for use of clopidogrel include active bleeding and hypersensitivity to components of the medication.[12]

Clopidogrel is supplied as a 75-mg pink tablet. An additional 300-mg pink tablet is also available for the loading dose. Dosing for patients with UA/NSTEMI includes a 300-mg loading dose followed by a 75-mg once-daily dose.[12] Initiate aspirin (75–325 mg once daily) and continue in combination with clopidogrel.[12] For patients with STEMI, the dosing is the same, except the 300-mg loading dose is optional. For patients with a recent MI, recent stroke, or established PAD, the dose is also 75 mg daily with or without food, but the loading dose is not recommended.[12]

Clopidogrel must be activated to an active metabolite by CYP2C19. Clopidogrel carries a black box warning due to diminished antiplatelet effect in patients who are poor metabolizers of CYP2C19. Although a higher dosage regimen could be considered, there are not currently recommended dosing guidelines for this patient population. In cases where the patient is suspected to be a poor metabolizer, genetic testing or choosing an alternative product is recommended.[12] Because some proton pump inhibitors (PPIs), such as omeprazole, are moderate inhibitors of CYP2C19, coadministration is not recommended. An alternate PPI or different class of acid-reducing medication may be preferred.

Although clopidogrel does not have the black box warning for bleeding that prasugrel carries, bleeding is still a concern due to the nature of this medication. Although clopidogrel has a relatively short half-life, only 6 h, the inhibitory effect on platelet aggregation exists for the lifetime of the platelet, approximately 7–10 days after exposure. For patients who are undergoing surgery, clopidogrel should be discontinued for at least 5 days prior to surgery. In an emergency, hemostasis may be restored by administering exogenous platelets, although even this may not be effective within 4 h of the 300-mg loading dose or 2 h of the 75-mg maintenance dose. Taking NSAIDs, warfarin, and aspirin with clopidogrel increases the risk of bleeding and should be given only when benefits outweigh the risk.

Like prasugrel, clopidogrel is pregnancy category B because animal studies did not reveal any evidence of impairment, but well-controlled studies in humans do not exist. Dose adjustment is not necessary for geriatric patients or those with hepatic impairment. In patients with severe (CrCl 5–15 mL/min) or moderate renal impairment (CrCl 30–60 mL/min), taking clopidogrel resulted in low inhibition of aggregation of 25%.[12] Dosing guidelines for patients with renal impairment are not provided by the manufacturer, but choosing an alternative medication in this class may be preferred.

TICAGRELOR

Like the other thienopyridines, ticagrelor is a $P2Y_{12}$ platelet inhibitor used to reduce the risk of cardiovascular death, MI, and stroke in patients with ACS. For the first 12 months following ACS, ticagrelor has been shown to be superior to clopidogrel.[13] Unlike clopidogrel, ticagrelor doses exhibit low inhibition of aggregation in patients with impaired renal function. To initiate ticagrelor, administer a 180-mg loading dose followed by a 90-mg dose twice daily for the first year after an ACS event. After the first year, the dose should be decreased to 60 mg twice daily. Ticagrelor is available in a round, yellow 90-mg tablet and a round, pink 60-mg tablet. Patients taking ticagrelor should also be taking a daily aspirin dose of 75–100 mg.[13]

Ticagrelor is contraindicated in patients who have a history of intracranial hemorrhage, hypersensitivity to any of the medication components, or any active bleeding. Ticagrelor has two boxed warnings: one because of the risk of fatal bleeding associated with the mechanism of action of this medication, and the other to warn about the concomitant use with aspirin doses >100 mg daily. Higher aspirin doses do not have an established benefit in the ACS setting, and there is a strong suggestion from the Platelet Inhibition and Patient Outcomes (PLATO) trial that use of such doses reduces the effectiveness of ticagrelor.[13] During clinical trials, 14% of patients taking ticagrelor reported experiencing dyspnea, although pulmonary function tests did not detect any abnormalities. For patients who have a preexisting pulmonary condition, an alternative thienopyridine may be preferred.[13]

CYP3A4 is the primary enzyme responsible for metabolizing ticagrelor and forming the major active metabolite. Strong inhibitors of CYP3A4, such as ketoconazole and clarithromycin, substantially increase the effects of ticagrelor and increase patient risk of experiencing an adverse bleeding event. Strong inducers of CYP3A4 have the opposite effect and reduce the potency of ticagrelor. Ticagrelor may also increase serum concentrations of medications metabolized by CYP3A4, such as simvastatin and lovastatin.

Unlike clopidogrel and prasugrel, ticagrelor is classified as pregnancy category C. Animal studies showed structural abnormalities at maternal doses five to seven times the maximum recommended human dose. If a patient is of childbearing age, an alternative thienopyridine may be a better option. Additionally, ticagrelor does not require dose adjustment in patients with renal impairment, making it a better choice for these patients than clopidogrel. Since ticagrelor is metabolized by the liver, use should be avoided for patients with severe hepatic impairment and caution should be used in patients with moderate hepatic impairment.

DIPYRIDAMOLE/ASPIRIN

Another antiplatelet option is the combination of dipyridamole and aspirin. This combination product is used to reduce the risk of stroke for patients who have had an ischemic stroke or transient ischemia of the brain. Dipyridamole inhibits platelet aggregation by reducing the uptake of adenosine into platelets, which results in an increased concentration of local adenosine, stimulating platelet adenylate cyclase and increasing cAMP levels. Aspirin inhibits platelet aggregation by irreversibly inhibiting cyclooxygenase, inhibiting generation of thromboxane A2, and reducing induction of aggregation.[14]

This combination product is supplied as a red and ivory capsule with 25 mg of aspirin and 200 mg of extended-release dipyridamole. The recommended dosing is one capsule given with or without food twice daily. Some patients report experiencing intolerable headaches when first taking this medication. If this is the case, the manufacturer recommends starting with one capsule at bedtime and a low-dose aspirin in the morning. When the headache is reduced, patients can return to the usual dose.[14]

Dipyridamole/aspirin is contraindicated for patients with an allergy to aspirin or any other component of the product. Use should be avoided in children and teenagers due to the risk of Reye's syndrome. Aspirin/dipyridamole is classified as pregnancy category D due to the teratogenic effects. Adverse serious events associated with this combination include increased bleeding risk, elevated hepatic enzymes, and hepatic failure. Hypotension and chest pain may also occur due to the vasodilatory effect. Because it contains aspirin, this medication should also be avoided in patients with renal failure (eGFR <10 mL/min/1.73 m²).[14]

There are many drug interactions to be aware of that could be concerning for patients with diabetes. The most concerning is the risk for increased potency of oral hypoglycemics. Moderate doses of aspirin may increase the effectiveness of oral medications used to lower blood glucose and may lead to hypoglycemia. Other notable drug interactions include ACE inhibitors, other anticoagulants, anticonvulsants, β-blockers, diuretics, methotrexate, and NSAIDs.[14]

CILOSTAZOL

Cilostazol has yet another mechanism of action for inhibiting platelet aggregation. Cilostazol inhibits platelet aggregation by suppressing cAMP degradation, leading to an increase in cAMP in platelets and blood vessels. This medication is indicated for reducing symptoms of intermittent claudication. The recommended dose is 100 mg twice daily. Cilostazol should be taken at least half an hour before or 2 h after breakfast and dinner. Patients should be counseled that medication may work within 2–4 weeks, but may take up to 12 weeks before the full effect is seen. Cilostazol is available as 50-mg triangular and 100-mg round tablets.[15]

Cilostazol is contraindicated for patients with HF due to the inhibition of phosphodiesterase III, a mechanism that has been shown to decrease survival in patients will class III and IV HF. Tachycardia may occur with cilostazol, so it should be used with caution for patients who have a history of heart disease. White blood cell counts should also be monitored because of the risk of agranulocytosis. Other common side effects include headache (27%), infection (14%), diarrhea (12%), abnormal stool (12%), and rhinitis (12%).[15]

Cilostazol has shown teratogenicity in rats at high doses and is pregnancy category C. No significant differences have been observed for geriatric populations, so dose adjustment with age is not necessary. Dose adjustments are also not required for patients with renal impairment or mild hepatic impairment.[15]

The effect of cilostazol is seen as early as 3 h after dosing and lasts for 12 h following a single dose. Cilostazol and the active metabolite have half-lives of 11 h and 13 h, respectively. Metabolism occurs predominantly through CYP3A4 and CYP2C19, leading to the need for a dose reduction to 50 mg twice daily when administered in combination with strong or moderate inhibitors of either CYP3A4 or CYP2C19.[15]

VORAPAXAR

Vorapaxar is another antiplatelet agent with a unique mechanism of action. It works by acting as a protease-activated receptor-1 (PAR-1) antagonist, which inhibits thrombin-induced and thrombin receptor agonist peptide–induced platelet aggregation. It is currently indicated for the reduction of thrombotic cardiovascular events in patients with a history of MI or with PAD. The dose of vorapaxar is 2.08 mg by mouth. It can be taken with or without food. This medication has only been studied either in combination with either aspirin or clopidogrel. Study outcomes demonstrated a reduction in composite endpoint of cardiovascular death, MI, stroke, and urgent revascularization.[16]

Vorapaxar is contraindicated in patients with a history of stroke, transient ischemic attack, or intracranial hemorrhage due to the increased risk of intracranial hemorrhage and active pathological bleeding. A major side effect is bleeding, which was significantly increased. It is recommended to avoid the use of vorapaxar with anticoagulants, such as warfarin. Currently, there is no reversal agent for vorapaxar. Other side effects that occurred included anemia, depression, rash, and diplopia or ocular motor disturbances.[16]

Vorapaxar is a pregnancy category B medication. Currently, there is no controlled information from pregnant individuals, but animal data show no teratogenic effects at normal human levels. It is known to cross into the breast milk of rats and should be used with caution when breast-feeding. It is currently unknown if vorapaxar is excreted into human breast milk. There is no contraindication or dosing adjustment in the geriatric population, but bleeding risk should be evaluated prior to initiating therapy. No dosage adjustments are needed for renal dysfunction or for mild to moderate hepatic dysfunction. It is not recommended to be used in patients who have severe hepatic dysfunction due to increased risk of bleeding.[16]

Eighty percent or more of the antiplatelet effect is achieved at approximately 1 week and steady state is achieved at 21 days. The terminal half-life is 8 days, which can yield a continued antiplatelet effect of approximately 50% at 4 weeks after discontinuation of the medication. Metabolism occurs through CYP3A4 and CYP2J2. Vorapaxar should be avoided in patients who are receiving strong inducers or inhibitors of CYP3A.[16]

COMBINATION THERAPY

CORONARY HEART DISEASE AND MYOCARDIAL INFARCTION

Combination use of antiplatelet therapy has long been established for secondary prevention of MI. Currently, dual antiplatelet therapy is recommended for management of patients who received either medical management, PCI, or CABG.[17,18] The Clopidogrel in Unstable Angina to Prevent Recurrent Events (CURE) trial and Clopidogrel for the Reduction of Events During Observation (CREDO) trial established that dual antiplatelet therapy with clopidogrel and aspirin is better than aspirin for patients experiencing ACS with regard to death from cardiovascular causes, nonfatal MI, and refractory ischemia.[19] The

CREDO trial demonstrated that the combination of clopidogrel and aspirin prior to elective PCI reduced death, MI, and need for urgent revascularization.[20] The TRial to assess Improvement in Therapeutic Outcomes by optimizing platelet InhibitioN with prasugrel Thrombolysis In Myocardial Infarction 38 (TRITON-TIMI 38) trial demonstrates that prasugrel for treatment of ACS with scheduled PCI is superior to clopidogrel in the reduction of the combined cardiovascular outcome of death from cardiovascular causes, nonfatal MI, and nonfatal stroke. However, patients in the prasugrel group had increased rates of bleeding. Based on post hoc analysis, prasugrel should not be used in patients aged 75 years or older, patients who weigh ≤60 kg, and patients who have had prior TIA or stroke, due to increased rates of bleeding.[21] Subgroup analysis was conducted to further elucidate the benefits of prasugrel versus clopidogrel. The major benefit appears to be from the reduction of MIs. Specifically, looking at the subpopulation of patients with diabetes mellitus demonstrated a significant net clinical benefit with prasugrel compared to clopidogrel (14.6% vs 19.2%, $P = 0.001$). Subgroup analysis data suggest benefits in patients with diabetes outweigh safety risks.[22] Ticagrelor was also compared to clopidogrel in patients experiencing ACS. Ticagrelor demonstrated improved rates of the composite outcome of death from vascular causes, MI, or stroke, while showing no difference in rates of major bleeding.[23]

The recommended duration of dual antiplatelet therapy is continuing to evolve with new evidence. Current guideline recommendations are outlined in Table 21.3.[24]

Dual antiplatelet therapy has been studied up to 18–36 months. Prasugrel and clopidogrel combined with aspirin have demonstrated improved efficacy compared to aspirin alone but had increased rates of moderate and severe bleeding.[23] Ticagrelor taken with aspirin showed improved composite efficacy endpoint at 3 years compared to aspirin alone, but the combination had increased risk of major bleeding.[25]

STROKE

Dual antiplatelet therapy is not as well defined in stroke prevention as it is in prevention of MI. Current stroke guidelines recommend use of dual antiplatelet therapy (clopidogrel and aspirin) for 21 days for minor strokes or TIAs.[26] This recommendation is based on the Clopidogrel in High-risk patients with Acute Nondisabling Cerebrovascular Events (CHANCE) trial, which demonstrated a reduction in ischemic stroke with no increase in hemorrhagic strokes at 90 days.[27] The trial was conducted in China, potentially limiting the external validity of the trial.[28] The Platelet-Oriented Inhibition in New TIA and minor ischemic stroke (POINT) trial demonstrated similar results in an expanded population. Ischemic stroke was significantly reduced when clopidogrel was added to aspirin for a total of 90 days in patients with minor stroke or TIA when initiated within 12 h of stroke symptom onset. However, major hemorrhage was increased in the dual antiplatelet therapy arm. Approximately 25% of patients in both trial arms had diabetes.[29] Currently, dual antiplatelet therapy is limited to minor stroke and TIA for a short duration after the event. Data are unavailable to support dual antiplatelet therapy for moderate and severe stroke or long-term therapy.

Table 21.3—Duration of Dual Antiplatelet Therapy[24]

Indication	Intervention	Duration (medication)	Additional notes
Stable Ischemic Heart Disease	BMS	1 month (clopidogrel)	May be reasonable for > 1 month in those with low risk of bleeding
	DES	6 months (clopidogrel)	May be reasonable for > 1 month in those with low risk of bleeding
	CABG	May be reasonable for 12 months of therapy (clopidogrel)	
Recent ACS	Medical Therapy	At least 12 months (clopidogrel, ticagrelor)	Not high risk of bleeding or no significant bleeding on DAPT >12 months may be reasonable
	Lytic (STEMI)	Minimum 14 days and ideally 12 months (clopidogrel)	Not high risk of bleeding or no significant bleeding on DAPT >12 months may be reasonable
	PCI (BMS or DES)	At least 12 months (clopidogrel, prasugrel, ticagrelor)	Not high risk of bleeding or no significant bleeding on DAPT >12 months may be reasonable
	CABG	Resume DAPT to complete 1 year	

BMS, bare metal stent; CABG, coronary artery bypass graft; DAPT, dual antiplatelet therapy; DES, drug eluting stent.

PERIPHERAL ARTERIAL DISEASE

Aspirin, clopidogrel, ticagrelor, and cilostazol alone are all effective in treating PAD. No data are available for treatment of PAD using these therapies in combination. Limited data are available looking at dual antiplatelet therapy in patients who have undergone endovascular procedures. A meta-analysis reviewed dual antiplatelet therapy compared to mono antiplatelet therapy after endovascular arterial revascularization procedures. Nine trials were included in the analysis, with only one trial conducted in the peripheral arteries. Conclusions of the meta-analysis found no difference in efficacy comparing dual antiplatelets to a single agent, as well as no difference in rates of bleeding.[30]

Table 21.4—Dose and Dose Adjustments for Commonly Used Medications

Drug	Usual dose	Dose adjustments
Aspirin	■ Prevention of MI: 81 mg p.o. daily[29] ■ Stroke prevention: 160–300 mg daily[25] ■ Acute treatment of MI: 162–325 mg chewed as soon as possible[17,18] ■ PAD: 75–325 mg p.o. daily[31]	■ Must use doses <100 mg daily in combination with ticagrelor[20]
Prasugrel[11]	■ ACS: 60-mg loading dose followed by 10 mg once daily	■ Consider reducing dose to 5 mg daily in patients who weigh less than 60 kg ■ Use in combination with aspirin
Clopidogrel[12]	■ ACS: 300-mg load followed by 75 mg daily ■ Recent MI, stroke, or PAD: 75 mg daily	■ Avoid use with CYP2C19 inhibitors
Ticagrelor[13]	■ ACS: 180-mg loading dose followed by 90 mg twice daily for the first year. After 1 year of therapy, lower dose to 60 mg twice daily	■ Use in combination with aspirin at doses <100 mg daily
Aspirin/Dipyridamole[14]	■ Stroke and TIA: 1 (25-mg/200-mg) capsule twice daily with or without food	■ For intolerable headaches, consider reducing dose to bedtime and aspirin 81 mg daily in the morning
Cilostazol[15]	■ Intermittent claudication: 100 mg twice daily	■ Reduce dose to 50 mg twice daily when used in combination with CYP2C19 inhibitors and strong or moderate CYP3A4 inhibitors
Vorapaxar[16]	■ Prevention of cardiovascular events in patients with history of MI or PAD: 2.08 mg once daily	■ Avoid with inducers or inhibitors of CYP3A

MONOGRAPHS

Aspirin: https://dailymed.nlm.nih.gov/dailymed/drugInfo.cfm?setid=9829f56f-723c-473f-89ee-4cb2efb3b8bc

Aspirin/extended-release dipyridamole (Aggrenox): https://dailymed.nlm.nih.gov/dailymed/drugInfo.cfm?setid=938ab0b5-8377-404a-8f61-5c630bda5932

Cilostazol: https://dailymed.nlm.nih.gov/dailymed/drugInfo.cfm?setid=ceac1ae3-c343-28ca-c083-b748d21a15e6

Clopidogrel (Plavix): https://dailymed.nlm.nih.gov/dailymed/drugInfo.cfm?setid=01b14603-8f29-4fa3-8d7e-9d523f802e0b

Prasugrel: https://dailymed.nlm.nih.gov/dailymed/drugInfo.cfm?setid=cd6bf899-06b7-4f52-96c5-ffc94a7288ff

Ticagrelor (Brilinta): https://dailymed.nlm.nih.gov/dailymed/drugInfo.cfm?setid=f7b3f443-e83d-4bf2-0e96-023448fed9a8

Vorapaxar (Zontivity): https://dailymed.nlm.nih.gov/dailymed/drugInfo.cfm?setid=f001f406-8cf1-40a4-bbf5-1775fe020122#S12.2

REFERENCES

1. Periayah MH, Halim AS, Saad AZM. Mechanism action of platelets and crucial blood coagulation pathways in hemostasis. *Int J Hematol Oncol Stem Cell Res* 2017;11(4):319–327

2. Benjamin EJ, Virani SS, Callaway CW, et al.; on behalf of the American Heart Association Council on Epidemiology and Prevention Statistics Committee and Stroke Statistics Subcommittee. Heart disease and stroke statistics—2018 update: a report from the American Heart Association. *Circulation* 2018;137:e67–e492

3. Goff DC Jr., Lloyd-Jones DM, Bennett G, et al. 2013 ACC/AHA guideline on the assessment of cardiovascular risk: a report of the American College of Cardiology/American Heart Association Task Force on Practice Guidelines. *Circulation* 2014;129(Suppl. 2):S49–S73

4. Colwell JA, Nesto RW. The platelet in diabetes: focus on prevention of ischemic events. *Diabetes Care* 2003;26:2181–2188

5. Chamberlain JJ, Johnson EL, Leal S, et al. Cardiovascular disease and risk management: review of the American Diabetes Association *Standards of Medical Care in Diabetes—2018*. *Ann Intern Med* 2018;168:640–650

6. Hammoud T, Tanguay JF, Bourassa MG. Management of coronary artery disease: therapeutic options in patients with diabetes. *J Am Coll Cardiol* 2000;36(2):355–365

7. Sharma A, Garg A, Elmariah S, et al. Duration of dual antiplatelet therapy following drug-eluting stent implantation in diabetic and non-diabetic patients: a systematic review and meta-analysis of randomized controlled trials. *Progress Cardiovasc Dis* 2018;60:500–507

8. American Diabetes Association. 9. Cardiovascular disease and risk management: *Standards of Medical Care in Diabetes—2018*. *Diabetes Care* 2018;41(Suppl.1):S86–S104

9. Bayer Aspirin: The Wonder Drug. Available from https://www.bayeraspirinhcp.com/static/documents/Bayer_Aspirin_Wonder_Drug.pdf. Accessed 3 August 2018

10. Adult Aspirin Regimen Low Dose [package information]. Available from https://dailymed.nlm.nih.gov/dailymed/drugInfo.cfm?setid=9829f56f-723c-473f-89ee-4cb2efb3b8bc. Accessed 3 August 2018

11. Effient (prasugrel) [prescribing information]. Indianapolis, IN, Eli Lilly and Company, 2011. Available from https://www.accessdata.fda.gov/drugsatfda_docs/label/2011/022307s003lbl.pdf

12. Plavix (clopidogrel) [prescribing information]. Bridgewater, NJ, Bristol-Myer Squibb/Sanofi Pharmaceuticals Partnership, 2010. Available from https://www.accessdata.fda.gov/drugsatfda_docs/label/2010/020839s048lbl.pdf

13. Brilinta (ticagrelor) [prescribing information]. Wilmington, DE, AstraZeneca Pharmaceuticals LP, 2016. Available from https://www.accessdata.fda.gov/drugsatfda_docs/label/2016/022433s020lbl.pdf

14. Aggrenox (aspirin/extended-release dipyridamole) [prescribing information]. Ridgefield, CT, Boehringer Ingelheim Pharmaceuticals, Inc., 2015. Available from https://www.accessdata.fda.gov/drugsatfda_docs/label/2012/020884s030lbl.pdf

15. Pletal (cilostazol) [prescribing information]. Rockville, MD, Otsuka America Pharmaceuticals Inc., 2017. Available from https://www.accessdata.fda.gov/drugsatfda_docs/label/2017/020863s024lbl.pdf

16. Zontivity (vorapaxar) [prescribing information]. Princeton, NJ, Aralez Pharmaceuticals US Inc., 2017. Available from https://dailymed.nlm.nih.gov/dailymed/drugInfo.cfm?setid=f001f406-8cf1-40a4-bbf5-1775fe020122#S12.2

17. O'Gara PT, Kushner FG, Ascheim DD, et al. 2013 ACCF/AHA guideline for the management of ST-elevation myocardial infarction: a report of the American College of Cardiology Foundation/American Heart Association Task Force on Practice Guidelines. *J Am Coll Cardiol* 2013;61:e78–e140

18. Amsterdam EA, Wenger NK, Brindis RG, et al. 2014 ACC/AHA guideline for the management of patients with non-ST elevation acute coronary syndromes: a report of the American College of Cardiology/American Heart

Association Task Force on Practice Guidelines. *Circulation* 2014;130:e344–e426

19. Yusuf S, Zhao F, Mehta SR, et al. the Clopidogrel in Unstable Angina to Prevent Recurrent Events (CURE) Trial Investigators. Effects of clopidogrel in addition to aspirin in patients with acute coronary syndromes without ST-segment elevation. *N Engl J Med* 2001;345:494–502

20. Steinhubl SR, Berger PB, Mann JT 3rd, et al. Early and sustained dual oral antiplatelet therapy following percutaneous coronary intervention: a randomized controlled trial. *JAMA* 2002;288(19):2411–2420

21. Wiviott SD, Braunwald E, McCabe CH, et al. Prasugrel versus clopidogrel in patients with acute coronary syndromes. *N Engl J Med* 2007;357(20):2001–2015

22. Montalescot G. Benefits for specific subpopulations in TRITON-TIMI 38. *Eur Heart J Supplements* 2009;11(Suppl. G):G18–G24

23. Wallentin L, Becker RC, Budaj A, et al.; PLATO Investigators. Ticagrelor versus clopidogrel in patients with acute coronary syndromes. *N Engl J Med* 2009;361(11):1045–1057

24. Levine GN, Bates ER, Bittl JA, et al.; 2016 ACC/AHA guideline focused update on duration of dual antiplatelet therapy in patients with coronary artery disease: a report of the American College of Cardiology/American Heart Association Task Force on Clinical Practice Guidelines: an update of the 2011 ACCF/AHA/SCAI guideline for percutaneous coronary intervention, 2011 ACCF/AHA guideline for coronary artery bypass graft surgery, 2012 ACC/AHA/ACP/AATS/PCNA/SCAI/STS guideline for the diagnosis and management of patients with stable ischemic heart disease, 2013 ACCF/AHA guideline for the management of ST-elevation myocardial infarction, 2014 ACC/AHA guideline for the management of patients with non–ST-elevation acute coronary syndromes, and 2014 ACC/AHA guideline on perioperative cardiovascular evaluation and management of patients undergoing noncardiac surgery. *Circulation* 2016;134:e123–e155. DOI: 10.1161/CIR.0000000000000404

25. Bonaca MP, Bhatt DL, Cohen M, et al. Long-term use of ticagrelor in patients with prior myocardial infarction. *N Engl J Med* 2015;372(19):1791–1800

26. Powers WJ, Rabinstein AA, Ackerson T, et al.; on behalf of the American Heart Association Stroke Council. 2018 guidelines for the early management of patients with acute ischemic stroke: a guideline for healthcare professionals from the American Heart Association/American Stroke Association. *Stroke* 2018;49:e46–e99

27. Wang Y, Wang Y, Zhao X, et al.; CHANCE Investigators. Clopidogrel with aspirin in acute minor stroke or transient ischemic attack. *N Engl J Med* 2013;369(1):11–19

28. Johnston SC, Easton JD, Farrant M, et al. Clopidogrel and aspirin in acute ischemic stroke and high-risk TIA. *N Engl J Med* 2018;379:215–225

29. Peeters Weem SM, van Haelst ST, den Ruijter HM, et al. Lack of evidence for dual antiplatelet therapy after endovascular arterial procedures: a meta-analysis. *Eur J Vasc Endovasc Surg* 2016;52:253–262

30. Mehta SR, Bassand JP, Chrolavicius S, et al.; CURRENT-OASIS 7 Investigators. Dose comparisons of clopidogrel and aspirin in acute coronary syndromes. *N Engl J Med* 2010;363(10):930–942

31. Gerhard-Herman MD, Gornik HL, Barrett C, et al. 2016 AHA/ACC guideline on the management of patients with lower extremity peripheral artery disease: executive summary: a report of the American College of Cardiology/American Heart Association Task Force on Clinical Practice Guidelines. *Circulation* 2017;135:e686–e725

Chapter 22
Medications for Smoking Cessation
Anne P. Kim, PharmD, MPH, MIT

INTRODUCTION

Nicotine is an addictive compound that can be delivered in a number of ways—cigarettes, smokeless tobacco (e.g., oral snuff, chewing tobacco), electronic cigarettes (e-cigarettes), and heat-not-burn (HNB) products.[1] For adults, the most commonly used tobacco product is cigarettes; for youth, the most commonly used is e-cigarettes.[2,3] Although the prevalence of cigarette smoking in adults has declined over the years (prevalence in 2005 was 20.9% and in 2016 was 15.5% or 37.8 million), the prevalence of e-cigarette smoking in youth has rapidly increased (high school students—from 1.5% in 2011 to 11.3%, or 1.73 million, in 2017; middle school students—from 0.6% in 2011 to 3.3%, or 0.39 million, in 2017).[2,3] There is concern that this marked increase in e-cigarette use by youth will lead to quicker, early initiation of cigarette smoking by acting as a gateway device.[4,5] A survey showed, however, that the majority of youth using e-cigarettes were vaping only the flavoring, followed distantly by vaping of nicotine.[6]

Cigarette smoking continues to be the leading cause of preventable disease (e.g., cancer, COPD, CVD, and diabetes) and premature death. Cigarettes are the most commonly used tobacco product, leading to an estimated 480,000 smoking-related deaths per year.[2,7]

The 2014 U.S. Surgeon General's report indicates that new research data have expanded the list of diseases caused by smoking cigarettes, including diabetes mellitus.[7,8] Active smokers have a 30–40% increased risk of developing T2D, in a dose-dependent manner, compared to nonsmokers.[7]

It is well established that cigarette smoking is associated with increased risk of cardiovascular morbidity and mortality and that diabetes also is associated with increased risk of cardiovascular morbidity and mortality. The Multiple Risk Factor Intervention Trial (MRFIT), the prospective study of women in Finland, and the Paris Prospective Study showed that cigarette smoking is a significant risk factor for increased risk of cardiovascular events.[9–11] A meta-analysis that included 89 prospective cohort studies demonstrated active cigarette smoking significantly increases the risk of cardiovascular mortality, total CVD, CHD, and stroke in patients with diabetes.[12]

The American Diabetes Association states that smoking cessation is one intervention of few that is safe and cost-effective for all patients who smoke.[13] Smoking cessation has been shown to decrease cardiovascular events. A meta-analysis of 46 prospective cohort or nested case-controlled studies on patients with diabetes reported lower risks of cardiovascular outcomes (e.g., stroke, MI) in those who quit smoking cigarettes compared to those who actively smoke cigarettes.[14] Unfortunately, as few as 20% of patients are counseled on smoking cessation, with a common barrier being time limitations of healthcare providers.[15]

Goals of smoking cessation counseling and pharmacotherapy include:

- Prevention/mitigation of symptoms of nicotine withdrawal.
- Cessation of tobacco use (or decreased use) and maintained abstinence.
- Decreased risk of morbidity and mortality from smoking-related diseases (including diabetes).

The American Diabetes Association recommendations for smoking cessation and prevention are provided in Table 22.1.

Table 22.1 — Recommendations Regarding Diabetes and Smoking

Assessment of smoking status and history
■ Systematic documentation of a history of tobacco use must be obtained from all adolescent and adult individuals with diabetes.
Counseling on smoking prevention and cessation

■ All healthcare providers should advise individuals with diabetes not to initiate smoking. This advice should be consistently repeated to prevent smoking and other tobacco use among children and adolescents with diabetes under age 21 years.
■ Among smokers, cessation counseling must be completed as a routine component of diabetes care.
■ Every smoker should be urged to quit in a clear, strong, and personalized manner that describes the added risks of smoking and diabetes.
■ Every diabetic smoker should be asked if he or she is willing to quit at this time.
  – If no, initiate brief and motivational discussion regarding need to stop using tobacco, risks of continued use, and encouragement to quit as well as support when ready.
  – If yes, assess preference for and initiate either minimal, brief, or intensive cessation counseling and offer pharmacological supplements as appropriate.

Effective systems for delivery of smoking cessation
■ Training of all diabetes healthcare providers in the Public Health Service guidelines regarding smoking should be implemented. ■ Follow-up procedures designed to assess and promote quitting status must be arranged for all diabetic smokers.

Source: American Diabetes Association.[13]

The U.S. Department of Health and Human Services created the "5 A's" model for healthcare providers to use as a tool to promote smoking cessation.[16] Table 22.2 lists the steps of the "5 A's" model.

The American College of Cardiology recently published the "Pathway for Tobacco Cessation Treatment" that builds on the "5 A's" model (Figure 22.1).[1]

Studies have shown the individual efficacy of counseling and pharmacotherapy, but the combination of counseling and pharmacotherapy is better than either

Table 22.2—The "5 A's" Model for Treating Tobacco Use and Dependence

Ask about tobacco use.	Identify and document tobacco use status for every patient at every visit.
Advise to quit.	In a clear, strong, and personalized manner, urge every tobacco user to quit.
Assess willingness to make a quit attempt.	Is the tobacco user willing to make a quit attempt at this time?
Assess in quit attempt.	For patients willing to make a quit attempt, offer medication and provide or refer for counseling or additional treatment to help quit. For patients unwilling to quit at the time, provide interventions designed to increase future quit attempts.
Arrange for follow-up.	For patients willing to make a quit attempt, arrange for follow-up contacts, beginning within the first week after the quit date. For patients unwilling to make a quit attempt at the time, address tobacco dependence and willingness to quit at next clinic visit.

Source: Fiore.[16]

alone in smoking cessation rates.[16–18] Thus, it is recommended that both are provided to all patients, if feasible and appropriate.[16]

The intent of pharmacotherapy interventions is to prevent or reduce any symptoms of nicotine withdrawal and thus assist the patient in achieving smoking cessation. Common symptoms of nicotine withdrawal include irritability, anxiety, depression, difficulty concentrating, headaches, difficulty sleeping, increased appetite, and restlessness.[19,20] First-line pharmacotherapies that are FDA approved for smoking cessation include nicotine replacement therapy (NRT), varenicline, and bupropion sustained release (SR). Second-line, non-FDA-approved medications include nortriptyline and clonidine. Other options have been assessed to have little to no proven clinical benefit in increasing smoking cessation rates (e.g., selective serotonin reuptake inhibitors, electronic nicotine delivery systems [ENDS]).[16,18] The medications detailed below are those that have sufficient evidence to support their use in clinical practice.

FIRST-LINE MEDICATIONS FOR SMOKING CESSATION

- Nicotine Replacement Therapy
- Long-acting Nicotine Replacement Therapy
- Short-acting Nicotine Replacement Therapy
- Varenicline
- Bupropion SR

NICOTINE REPLACEMENT THERAPY

NRT is an FDA-approved, first-line intervention for smoking cessation.[16] NRT is available in a variety of formulations: transdermal patch, gum, lozenge, inhaler, and nasal spray. The transdermal patch formulation is long-acting, and the others are short-acting formulations of NRT. NRT patches, lozenges, and gum are available over the counter (OTC). A meta-analysis of 150 randomized trials concluded that all NRT formulations are efficacious in achieving smoking cessation.[21] Any of the NRT products may be administered, depending on a number of factors such as patient preference, cost, and side effects.[22]

Mechanism of Action

NRT partially replaces the nicotine that was previously supplied from cigarettes or other forms of tobacco at the site of nicotine receptors. Stimulated nicotine receptors in the peripheral and central nervous systems diminish the severity of nicotine withdrawal symptoms, including nicotine craving, associated with smoking cessation.[22]

Because of the different NRT formulations, specific drug administration instructions, pharmacokinetic parameters, efficacy data, and adverse events will be discussed under each product below, after the following sections on common adverse events/warnings and precautions and drug interactions. Dosages are outlined in Table 22.3 (see page 388).

Adverse Events/Warnings and Precautions

Adverse events associated with NRT include gastrointestinal effects (e.g., nausea, vomiting), insomnia, and increased heart rate.[18,23]

NRT should be used with caution in those who have acute CVD (e.g., recent MI, unstable angina pectoris) because of nicotine's sympathomimetic effect, which can increase heart rate and contractility and constrict blood vessels. Benefits may outweigh risk in patients with CVD who continue to smoke, as clinical studies have not shown increased risk of adverse cardiovascular events with use of NRT.[22,24]

NRT has not been intentionally studied in pregnant smokers, and the insufficient evidence available is limited and conflicting.[18] Nicotine is suspected to cause reproductive toxicity, including fetal neuro-teratogenicity.[23] It is recommended that pregnant smokers be encouraged to quit smoking without the aid of medications.[16]

Adolescents who smoke may be prone to poisoning (in some cases, fatal poisoning) from NRT. Symptoms of NRT overdose in adolescents include nausea, vomiting, diarrhea, increased salivation, pallor, sweating, headache, dizziness, mental confusion, marked weakness, tremor, respiratory failure, and auditory or visual disturbance. These symptoms may be followed by hypotension, breathing difficulties, circulatory collapse, and convulsions with higher levels of unwanted NRT exposure.[23]

Drug Interactions

The sympathomimetic nature of NRT products may cause the following effects:[16]

- Decrease in the sedative effects of benzodiazepines.
- Decrease in subcutaneous absorption of insulin.
- Decrease in the capacity of β-blockers to decrease blood pressure and heart rate.
- Decrease in the analgesic effect of opioids.

It may be necessary to adjust these medications when NRT therapy is discontinued.[16]

LONG-ACTING NRT

Nicotine transdermal patches provide nicotine at a continuous rate over a long duration and can be worn for up to 24 h. Patients may wear the 16-h patch

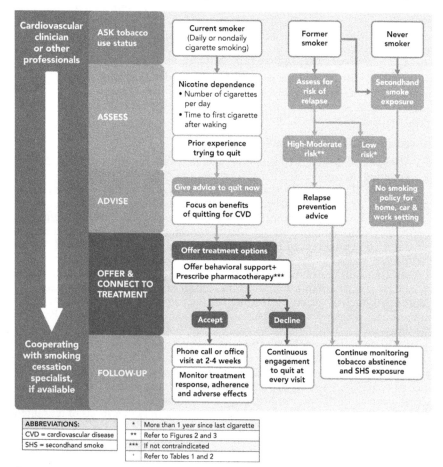

Figure 22.1—Pathway for Tobacco Cessation Treatment. *Source*: Reprinted with permission from Barua.[1]

if they are having trouble sleeping.[16,22] The pharmacokinetics of nicotine vary, depending on the NRT formulation administered. Nicotine transdermal patches are manufactured in a variety of delivery designs, which results in differing pharmacokinetic parameters. In general, the maximum rate of nicotine absorption is reached after 6–12 h of patch administration. Peak blood levels are reached after 16–24 h. Absolute bioavailability is about 82%.[25] Compared to placebo, use of the transdermal patch increased the likelihood of long-term smoking cessation by nearly twofold (OR 1.9 [95% CI 1.7–2.2]) in a meta-analysis of 25 clinical trials. A longer duration of therapy (>14 weeks) with the patch was similarly effective (OR 1.9 [95% CI 1.7–2.3]) and did not increase the rate of smoking cessation.[16] Despite rotating administration sites, NRT transdermal patches may produce local skin reactions that tend to be mild and self-limiting. Skin reactions may be treated with topical hydrocortisone cream or triamcinolone cream. If skin reactions are intolerable, patient should discontinue nicotine patch therapy.[16]

SHORT-ACTING NRT

Nicotine gum is available in several flavors and in the original flavor. There is a specific chewing technique ("chew and park") that optimizes nicotine release from the gum. Gum should be chewed until a taste emerges, then park the gum between the cheek and upper or lower gums until the taste disappears. This should be repeated for 30 min or until there is no more taste released upon chewing, which indicates all the nicotine has been released.[16] Buccal absorption of nicotine may be disrupted by acidic beverages (e.g., coffee). Patients should be advised to only consume water 15 min before and during chewing.[16] Nicotine gum is formulated so that one piece of gum provides NRT for 1–2 h each. Because the rate of nicotine release depends on the patient's chewing speed, another piece of gum may be needed within the hour to appease strong cravings.[25] Compared to placebo, use of nicotine gum increased the likelihood of long-term smoking cessation by about 50% (OR 1.5 [95% CI 1.2–1.7]) in a meta-analysis of nine clinical trials. However, many patients do not administer the gum as frequently as needed. They should be advised to chew the gum on a fixed schedule to achieve optimal benefit.[16] Nicotine gum is associated with mild, transient side effects such as mouth soreness, hiccups, dyspepsia, headache, and jaw pain, especially if not using proper chewing technique.[16,25]

Nicotine lozenges release nicotine as they slowly dissolve in the mouth. They are not to be chewed or swallowed. Similar to nicotine gum, lozenges are affected by acidic beverages, which should be avoided 15 min before and during administration.[16] Compared to placebo, the lower, 2-mg dose doubled and the higher, 4-mg dose nearly tripled the odds of achieving smoking cessation. Many patients do not use enough as-needed nicotine lozenges to achieve maximal benefit. They should be advised to administer lozenges per the schedule detailed in Table 22.3.[16] Lozenge-specific side effects include mouth/throat irritation, nausea, hiccups, and heartburn. The higher-dose lozenge is also associated with headache and coughing.[16,22]

Nicotine inhalers consist of a cartridge and mouthpiece that resemble a cigarette.[25] They deposit nicotine in the oropharynx, allowing nicotine to be absorbed through the buccal mucosa rather than the pulmonary route.[16,25] An advantage of the inhaler formulation is potentially addressing the hand-to-mouth behaviors and sensory cues reminiscent of cigarette smoking.[23] Cold temperatures (below around 40°F) decrease the amount of nicotine delivered from the inhaler (poor absorption and bioavailability). It is recommended that the inhaler/cartridge be kept in a warm area (e.g., inside pocket).[16,25] Compared to placebo, use of the nicotine inhaler increased the likelihood of long-term smoking cessation by about twofold (OR 2.1 [95% CI 1.5–2.9]) in a meta-analysis of six clinical trials.[16] As another as-needed NRT product, many patients do not use inhalers as often as needed for optimal benefit. Patients should be advised on appropriate frequency and duration of inhaler administration.[16] Nicotine inhalers are associated with mild, transient mouth/throat irritation, coughing, and rhinitis.[16]

Nicotine nasal spray (Nicotrol) delivers nicotine at higher levels than the other NRT formulations, which has raised concerns for dependence potential. Patients have reported using nicotine nasal sprays longer than the recommended 6–12 months of therapy, and some have reported using the product at a dose higher than recommended.[16] Blood nicotine levels peak after 5–10 min of administration. Nicotine is delivered faster with the nasal spray than with gum or the inhaler, but it is still slower than the delivery of nicotine from smoking cigarettes.[25] The nasal spray should be administered with the head slightly tilted back, without sniffing, swallowing, or inhaling through the nose at time of administration to avoid increased side effects.[16] Compared to placebo, nasal spray administration more than doubled (OR 2.3 [95% CI 1.7–3.0]) the likelihood of achieving smoking cessation in a meta-analysis of four clinical trials.[16] Nicotine nasal spray is associated with persistent nasal/throat irritation, rhinitis/nasal congestion, coughing, and transient changes in taste and smell.[16,22] Patients with severe reactive airway disease should use another NRT formulation besides the nasal spray.[16,22]

VARENICLINE (CHANTIX)

Varenicline is a nicotine receptor partial agonist—a non-nicotine medication—that is approved by the FDA as a first-line intervention for smoking cessation.[16]

Mechanism of Action

Varenicline is an analog of cytisine, which comes from a plant called *Cytisus laburnum* (false tobacco).[25] Varenicline is a selective partial agonist at the α4β2 neuronal nicotinic acetylcholine receptor (nAchR), which is central to the development of nicotine addiction. Because it is selective, varenicline does not bind to other nicotine or non-nicotine receptors/transporters.[25] As a partial agonist, varenicline promotes the release of a lower amount of dopamine than triggered by nicotine from tobacco products, but enough to minimize nicotine withdrawal symptoms and cravings. In addition to exerting agonistic effects, varenicline competitively inhibits the binding of nicotine and thus prevents full stimulation and release of dopamine to activate the mesolimbic region of the CNS (associated with reinforcement and reward).[22,26] Studies show that patients who concomitantly take varenicline and smoke cigarettes experience a lower level of satisfaction.[27,28] Figure 22.2 illustrates the effects of varenicline.

Dosage and Administration

Varenicline should be initiated 1 week prior to the quit date with the following recommended titration schedule:[16,26]

- 0.5 mg once daily for 3 days, then
- 0.5 mg twice daily for 4 days, and then
- 1 mg twice daily for 3 months (may be extended to 6 months).

On day 8 (quit date), when the dosage is first increased to 1 mg twice daily, patients should be instructed to quit smoking.[16,26] If they are unwilling or unable to quit on day 8, patients may gradually approach cessation with varenicline therapy by decreasing smoking by 50% every 4 weeks with the goal of quitting smoking by the end of 12 weeks.[26] After successfully achieving smoking cessation at 12 weeks of therapy, an additional 12 weeks of therapy is recommended, for all patients, to maintain smoking abstinence.[26]

There is no need to adjust the dose for patients with mild to moderate renal impairment. For those with severe renal impairment (CrCl <30 mL/min), the starting dose is the same (0.5 mg once daily) but it can only be titrated, as needed, to a maximum dose of 0.5 mg twice daily.[26]

Varenicline should be taken with food to reduce nausea, and the second dose of the day may be taken with dinner rather than at bedtime to reduce insomnia.[16,26]

Figure 22.2—Pharmacological effects of varenicline in smoking cessation. Courtesy of JJ Neumiller.

Pharmacokinetics

Within 3–4 h of oral administration, maximum plasma concentration of varenicline is reached, and steady-state concentrations are reached after approximately 4 days of therapy. Varenicline follows linear pharmacokinetics. The oral bioavailability of about 90% is not affected by food or time of dosing. Varenicline is ≤20% bound to plasma proteins.[26]

Varenicline is primarily excreted unchanged in the urine (92%), with a half-life of about 24 h.[26]

Clinical Efficacy

Compared to placebo, use of varenicline increased the likelihood of long-term smoking cessation by about twofold (OR 2.1 [95% CI 1.5–3.0]) with the lower 1 mg dose and by about threefold (OR 3.1 [95% CI 2.5–3.8]) with the higher 2-mg dose in meta-analyses of two clinical trials and of four clinical trials, respectively. These findings suggest that 1 mg per day could be used in patients who experience intolerable side effects from the 2-mg dosage regimen.[16] Head-to-head trials against bupropion SR (and placebo) showed varenicline had higher rates of smoking cessation than bupropion SR. (Varenicline and bupropion SR were each better than placebo.)[26–28] The likelihood of long-term smoking cessation was greater with 24 weeks of varenicline therapy than with the standard 12 weeks.[26] Varenicline therapy for extended periods of time (up to 1 year) has been shown to reduce relapse rates.[11]

Choosing a quit date beyond day 8 but within 5 weeks of initiating varenicline was successful in achieving smoking cessation compared to placebo.[26] Another study showed that varenicline therapy and a gradual reduction in smoking for 12 weeks before quitting resulted in improved smoking cessation rates compared to concomitant placebo therapy. Upon quitting smoking at week 12, patients continued varenicline or placebo therapy for an additional 12 weeks.[26]

Compared to placebo, varenicline increased the rate of smoking cessation in patients who had failed previous attempts to quit smoking with varenicline therapy.[26]

Varenicline has been studied as a smoking cessation aid in patients with CVD, COPD, or major depressive disorder (MDD). Varenicline was found to be superior to placebo in achieving smoking cessation in all three patient populations. In addition, a postmarketing trial on neuropsychiatric safety outcomes demonstrated that varenicline is better than placebo at attaining smoking cessation and that exposure to varenicline does not increase the risk of neuropsychiatric adverse events in either patients with a history of psychiatric disorder or patients without. There were, however, neuropsychiatric adverse events that occurred during varenicline therapy, so it remains in the warning and precautions section of the prescribing information document.[26,29]

Adverse Events/Warnings and Precautions

Common adverse events associated with exposure to varenicline include nausea, vomiting, constipation, difficulty sleeping, and abnormal vivid dreams.[16,26]

The FDA issued a black box warning in July 2009 regarding observed serious neuropsychiatric events (e.g., depression, agitation, suicidal ideation and behavior) in adult patients who received varenicline therapy, but it was removed in December 2016 after new study data presented lower-than-suspected rates of serious neuropsychiatric events.[26,30] It is important to note, however, that the risk still remains, particularly for those with a history of mental illnesses such as depression, anxiety disorders, or schizophrenia.[31] Healthcare providers should gather a complete psychiatric history prior to initiating varenicline and monitor patients for any evidence of neuropsychiatric adverse events. Patients who are already taking varenicline should stop therapy and contact their healthcare providers if they experience any changes in mood, thoughts, or behavior so that the healthcare provider may weigh the benefits against the risks and consider the following options: dose reduction, continued treatment with close monitoring, or discontinuing therapy.[16,26]

Varenicline may increase the risk for nonfatal cardiovascular events (e.g., nonfatal MI, nonfatal stroke, hospitalization for angina pectoris). Even though these events were not statistically significant, they were consistent in occurrence; thus, healthcare providers should weigh the benefits and risks of prescribing varenicline therapy to smokers with CVD.[26]

Varenicline has been associated with seizures. The benefits and risks should be assessed before initiating varenicline in patients with a history of seizures or lowered seizure threshold. Patients should immediately stop therapy and contact their healthcare providers if they experience a seizure.[26]

There are insufficient data on varenicline in pregnant smokers. It is not known whether the benefits of using varenicline to quit smoking outweigh the unknown maternal and fetal risks of harm from varenicline exposure.[26] It is recommended that pregnant smokers be encouraged to quit smoking without the aid of medications.[16]

Exposure to varenicline therapy has been associated with postmarketing reports of hypersensitivity reactions (e.g., angioedema) and serious skin reactions (e.g., Stevens-Johnson syndrome). Varenicline should be discontinued immediately upon any signs of hypersensitivity or skin rash.[26]

Increased intoxicating effects of alcohol with concomitant administration of varenicline have been reported postmarketing. It is recommended that patients decrease alcohol consumption until they assess how varenicline affects their ability to tolerate alcohol.[26]

Somnambulism or sleepwalking has been associated with exposure to varenicline therapy. Some cases report harmful behavior to self, other people, or property. Patients should discontinue varenicline and contact their healthcare providers if somnambulism occurs.[26]

Varenicline has also been reported to cause somnolence, dizziness, or difficulty concentrating while driving, which have led to traffic accidents. It is recommended that patients use caution when driving until they assess how varenicline affects them.[26]

Drug Interactions

Because varenicline is mainly eliminated via the kidneys, there are no metabolic interactions.[16] Medications that inhibit varenicline renal excretion, such as cimetidine, may increase the levels of varenicline, but this potential interaction is considered to be not clinically significant. Thus, there are no significant drug interactions with varenicline.[16]

BUPROPION SUSTAINED RELEASE (ZYBAN)

Bupropion SR is an atypical antidepressant that is an FDA-approved medication for smoking cessation. The U.S. Department of Health and Human Services recommends bupropion SR as another first-line intervention available for aiding in smoking cessation, and it may be used in combination with NRT products.[16]

Mechanism of Action

The mechanism of action for facilitating smoking cessation is not fully understood, but bupropion SR's efficacy in smoking cessation is thought to be related to its noradrenergic and/or dopaminergic activity (i.e., its weak inhibition of the synaptic reuptake of norepinephrine and dopamine in the CNS). Bupropion SR has also been shown to act as a nicotine receptor antagonist, which would contribute to its utility in smoking cessation.[25,26]

Dosage and Administration

Bupropion SR should be initiated 1–2 weeks prior to the quit date with the following recommended titration schedule to minimize seizure risk:[16,32]

- 150 mg once daily for 3 days and then
- 150 mg twice daily (at least 8 h apart) for 7–12 weeks (may be extended to 6 months)

Dosages for smoking cessation should not exceed the maximum dose of 300 mg per day. Bupropion SR may be taken with or without food, but it is not to be split, crushed, or chewed. Bupropion SR must be swallowed as a whole tablet to be delivered at the rate intended.[32]

Based on limited data, it is recommended that bupropion SR is used with caution in patients with renal impairment (CrCl <90 mL/min). Healthcare providers may consider a reduction in dose and/or frequency of administration in this population.[32] The same considerations (lower dose and/or frequency) should be applied to patients with mild hepatic impairment (Child-Pugh score of 5 or 6). Patients with moderate to severe hepatic impairment (Child-Pugh score of 7–15) should not exceed a maximum dose of 150 mg every other day.[32]

The second bupropion SR dose of the day may be taken earlier in the afternoon, but at least 8 h after the first dose, instead of in the evening to reduce major changes in sleep pattern (i.e., insomnia).[16]

Pharmacokinetics

Within 3 h of oral administration, maximum plasma concentration of bupropion SR is reached, and steady-state concentrations are reached after approximately 8 days of therapy. Bupropion SR follows linear pharmacokinetics. Based on preclinical animal study data, the bioavailability of orally administered bupropion SR ranges from 5 to 20%, and it is not significantly increased with food intake. Bupropion SR is 84% bound to plasma proteins.[32]

Bupropion SR is mainly metabolized in the liver to many metabolites (three of which are active). Only 0.5% of bupropion SR is excreted as unchanged parent drug. Bupropion SR and the metabolites have long half-lives. Bupropion SR has a half-life of about 21 h, and metabolites have half-lives that range from about 20–37 h.[32]

Clinical Efficacy

Compared to placebo, bupropion SR increased the likelihood of long-term smoking cessation by approximately twofold (OR 2.0 [95% CI 1.8–2.2]) in a meta-analysis of 24 clinical trials.[16] Similar to varenicline, bupropion SR was investigated in patients with COPD, and postmarketing data on neuropsychiatric safety outcomes were analyzed. Bupropion SR demonstrated superiority over placebo in achieving smoking cessation in smoking patients with COPD and in patients with or without a history of a psychiatric disorder. The postmarketing trial also concluded that bupropion SR does not have an increased risk of neuropsychiatric adverse events compared to placebo. Due to the small but consistent occurrence of neuropsychiatric adverse events in adults, however, it remains in the prescribing document under the warnings and precautions section.[32]

Contraindications

Bupropion SR is contraindicated in patients with a history of seizures or eating disorders (bulimia or anorexia nervosa) because of a dose-dependent risk of seizures with bupropion SR exposure. There is increased risk of seizures at dosages higher than 300 mg per day, so doses should not exceed the maximum of 300 mg per day. If patients experience a seizure, bupropion SR should be discontinued and not reinitiated.[32]

Bupropion SR is contraindicated in patients who are taking monoamine oxidase inhibitors (MAOIs) (e.g., linezolid, methylene blue) or have been treated with an MAOI within 14 days, due to increased risk of hypertensive reactions. Bupropion SR alone is associated with increased blood pressure. The risk of hypertension is increased with concomitant administration of MAOIs.[32]

Bupropion SR is also contraindicated in patients who are abruptly discontinuing the use of alcohol, benzodiazepines, barbiturates, and antiepileptic medications.[32]

Adverse Events/Warnings and Precautions

Adverse events associated with bupropion SR therapy include insomnia and dry mouth. Decreasing the dose may help provide relief.[32]

Despite Zyban being used as a smoking-cessation agent, it contains the same active ingredient as the antidepressant Wellbutrin. Thus, bupropion SR has a black box warning regarding suicidal thoughts and behaviors because of short-term trial data that showed increased risk of suicidal thinking and behavior in children, adolescents, and young adults.[32] It is recommended that all patients taking antidepressant therapy be closely monitored for any occurrence or worsening of suicidal thoughts and behaviors. Those who are close in relation to the patient (e.g., family members, caregivers) should be advised about the daily need to observe and communicate any concerns with the healthcare provider.[32]

Antidepressant therapy is known to trigger manic, mixed, or hypomanic episodes in patients with bipolar disorder. Bupropion SR should not be used to treat bipolar depression.[32]

Similar to varenicline, the FDA issued a black box warning in July 2009 regarding observed serious neuropsychiatric events (e.g., depression, agitation, suicidal ideation and behavior) in adult patients who received bupropion SR therapy, but it was removed in May 2017 after new study data presented lower than suspected rates of serious neuropsychiatric events.[30,32] It is important to note, however, that the risk still remains, particularly for those with a history of mental illnesses such as depression, anxiety disorders, or schizophrenia.[31] Healthcare providers should gather a complete psychiatric history prior to initiating bupropion SR and monitor patients for any evidence of neuropsychiatric adverse events. Patients who are already taking bupropion SR should stop therapy and contact their healthcare providers if they experience any changes in mood, thoughts, or behavior so that the healthcare provider may weigh the benefits against the risks and consider the following options: dose reduction, continued treatment with close monitoring, or discontinuing therapy.[32]

Bupropion SR therapy may precipitate angle-closure glaucoma in patients with anatomically narrow angles without a patent iridectomy by dilating pupils.[32]

There are epidemiological study data available that show that bupropion SR is not associated with increased risk of congenital malformations in the first trimester of pregnancy, but there are no data regarding its effectiveness in this population.[16,32] It is recommended that pregnant smokers be encouraged to quit smoking without the aid of medications, and only use bupropion SR when potential benefits clearly justify potential risks of fetal harm.[16,32]

Drug Interactions

As mentioned earlier, bupropion SR should not be administered with MAOIs. Bupropion SR may be initiated after waiting a minimum of 14 days from discontinuing MAOI therapy.[32]

Because bupropion SR can lower seizure threshold, caution should be used when coadministering with other medications that lower seizure threshold.[16]

Bupropion SR is primarily metabolized by CYP2B6, so drugs that inhibit CYP2B6 activity (e.g., ticlopidine, clopidogrel) will increase bupropion SR concentrations. Conversely, drugs that induce the CYP2B6 enzyme (e.g., ritonavir, lopinavir, efavirenz) will decrease bupropion SR levels. Additionally, drugs that are known to be strong inducers (e.g., carbamazepine, phenobarbital, phenytoin) will decrease bupropion SR concentrations, while strong inhibitors (e.g., valproate, cimetidine) will increase bupropion SR concentrations because bupropion SR is extensively metabolized by the liver.[16,32]

Bupropion SR and its metabolites inhibit CYP2D6. Coadministration of bupropion SR may lead to increased concentrations of drugs that are metabolized by CYP2D6 (e.g., tricyclic antidepressants, antipsychotics, β-blockers). Bupropion SR may also lower the efficacy of drugs that are activated by CYP2D6, such as tamoxifen. Higher doses may be needed to reach normal therapeutic benefit of these drugs when administered with bupropion SR.[32]

Digoxin levels may decrease when coadministered with bupropion SR. It is recommended that digoxin levels are monitored with this combination.[32]

SECOND-LINE MEDICATIONS FOR SMOKING CESSATION

- Clonidine
- Nortriptyline

CLONIDINE

Clonidine is a centrally acting α_2 adrenergic receptor agonist that is FDA approved to treat hypertension and is not approved for smoking cessation, but it may be used off-label as a second-line intervention for smoking cessation.[16] It is also used off-label for a variety of other conditions (e.g., chronic pain syndromes, Tourette syndrome, menopausal flushing).[25] Clonidine may be used when first-line therapies are contraindicated or when their use is unsuccessful in achieving smoking cessation.[16]

Mechanism of Action

Clonidine's efficacy in smoking cessation is thought to be related to its effects on the CNS, which likely mitigate symptoms of nicotine withdrawal, including craving.[22] As an α_2 adrenergic receptor agonist, clonidine decreases sympathetic outflow from the CNS.[33]

Dosage and Administration

Clonidine is available as an oral tablet and as a transdermal patch. It should be initiated up to 3 days prior to the quit date.[16] Although there is no specific dosing regimen established for using clonidine as a smoking cessation aid, the recommended/common initial dose is 0.1 mg twice daily for the oral tablet and 0.1 mg once daily for the transdermal patch.[16,34] The dose may be increased by 0.1 mg/day in weekly intervals to a maximum of approximately 0.4 mg per day, if necessary.[16,34] The duration of clonidine therapy ranged from 3–10 weeks in clinical trials, but some recommend that clonidine treatment be given for a maximum of 3–4 weeks for smoking cessation.[16,25] Due to the risk of rebound hypertension (i.e., rapid increase in blood pressure, agitation, headache, confusion, and/or tremor) upon abrupt discontinuation, clonidine should be slowly tapered down over 2–4 days (or longer).[16,33,34]

For the transdermal patch, patients should be counseled to place a new patch on skin that is relatively hairless between the neck and waist, once a week.[16]

Pharmacokinetics

Within 1–3 h of oral administration, maximum plasma concentration of clonidine is reached.[33] Oral bioavailability ranges from 70–80% and transdermal bioavailability is about 60%.[33,35] Clonidine is metabolized by the liver (~50%) and renally excreted as unchanged drug (40–60%), with a half-life of 12–16 h (up to 41 h with severe renal impairment).[33] The transdermal patch formulation releases clonidine at a constant rate over 7 days and, once the patch is removed, clonidine plasma levels slowly decline with a half-life of 20 h.[35]

Clinical Efficacy

Compared to placebo, clonidine increased the likelihood of long-term smoking cessation by approximately twofold (OR 2.1 [95% CI 1.2–3.7]) in a meta-analysis of three clinical trials.[16] Another meta-analysis showed that clonidine was better than placebo in successfully quitting smoking but that many experienced side effects from clonidine therapy. Thus, the therapeutic benefits of clonidine must be weighed against the side-effect profile of this drug, which may limit its usefulness as an intervention for smoking cessation.[34]

Adverse Events/Warnings and Precautions

Adverse events associated with clonidine therapy are mainly due to the anticholinergic properties of clonidine, commonly presenting with dry mouth, dizziness, sedation, and constipation.[33] The transdermal patch may cause some local skin irritation, but in terms of the anticholinergic adverse events listed above, patients may experience them to a lesser degree because of the more constant release of clonidine with the patch.[35]

As clonidine is used to treat hypertension, it may lower blood pressure and cause orthostatic hypotension.[34] Blood pressure should be monitored while on clonidine for smoking cessation, particularly for those who are older (>65 years) as fall risk is a concern in older adults.

The efficacy and safety of clonidine have not been adequately studied in pregnant smokers.[33] It is recommended that pregnant smokers be encouraged to quit smoking without the aid of medications.[16]

Clonidine can cause sedation, so patients should be careful when driving or operating large machinery.[16,33]

Drug Interactions

Clonidine in combination with alcohol, barbiturates, or other sedating medications may enhance CNS depression.[33] Patients should avoid this combination.

Risk of hypotension is increased when clonidine is coadministered with other antihypertensive agents or an antipsychotic agent.[33] Older adults in particular should be monitored for orthostatic hypotension and fall risk.

Caution should be used when administering clonidine with drugs that slow heart rate (e.g., β-blockers, calcium-channel blockers). There have been cases of sinus bradycardia due to this interaction.[33]

NORTRIPTYLINE

Nortriptyline is a tricyclic antidepressant that is FDA approved to treat depression and may be used off-label as a second-line intervention for smoking cessation.[16,36] Second-line therapies, such as nortriptyline, may be used when first-line therapies are contraindicated or when their use is unsuccessful in achieving smoking cessation.[16]

Mechanism of Action

The mechanism of action for assisting in smoking cessation is unknown, as nortriptyline has not been formally studied for this indication in preclinical or clinical trials. It is known that nortriptyline inhibits the reuptake of norepinephrine and serotonin, which may contribute to its efficacy in smoking cessation. Some proposed rationales are briefly described below:[37]

- Smoking cessation causes depression, and depression increases need for smoking or relapse. Nortriptyline is an antidepressant that can prevent depression while quitting smoking.
- The noradrenergic effects of nicotine are replaced with the noradrenergic effects of nortriptyline. This modulation of the noradrenergic receptor systems decreases withdrawal symptoms, including craving.
- Nortriptyline is a weak nicotine receptor antagonist (i.e., having anticholinergic properties), which causes dry mouth and altered taste perception and thus decreases craving.

Dosage and Administration

Nortriptyline should be initiated at 25 mg per day and gradually increased over a period of 10 days to 5 weeks until reaching the target dose of 75–100 mg per day. Therapy should begin 10–28 days prior to the quit date to reach steady-state concentrations by the time target dose is reached. The duration of nortriptyline therapy is 12 weeks, but it may be extended up to 6 months.[16,37] Nortriptyline should be slowly tapered off when discontinuing therapy to avoid withdrawal symptoms (e.g., nausea, headache, malaise).[36]

Therapeutic drug monitoring levels have not been established for the efficacy of nortriptyline in smoking cessation; however, nortriptyline plasma levels may be monitored for patients with depression and/or monitored as needed to prevent toxicity.[16,37]

Pharmacokinetics

Nortriptyline is rapidly absorbed following oral administration, with maximum plasma concentrations achieved within 4–9 h.[38] Oral bioavailability ranges from 46–70%.[39] There is high interindividual variability in time to steady-state concentrations; it may take 6–15 days to reach steady state. Nortriptyline is highly bound to plasma proteins.[38]

Nortriptyline is metabolized in the liver by CYP2D6 to produce primarily the major active metabolite 10-hydroxynortriptyline, which has the potential to accumulate in older adults.[39,40] Additionally, the half-life of nortriptyline is longer in older adults than in younger patients. Nortriptyline half-life ranges from 14–79 h: 14–51 h, with an average of 26 h, for younger patients; 23.5–79 h, with an average of 45 h, for older adults.[41] Thus, lower doses may be warranted for older adults than younger patients. Nortriptyline is mainly excreted as metabolites in the urine (>80%).[38]

Clinical Efficacy

Although nortriptyline has not been evaluated in as many smokers as NRT and bupropion SR have been, nortriptyline appears to be efficacious in quitting smoking.[22] Compared to placebo, nortriptyline about doubled (OR 1.8 [95% CI 1.3–2.6]) the likelihood of achieving smoking cessation in a meta-analysis of four clinical trials.[16] Nortriptyline is recommended as second-line therapy because it is associated with serious side effects that the healthcare provider and patient must weigh against the benefits of using a non-FDA-approved medication for smoking cessation.[16]

Contraindications

Coadministration with MAOIs is contraindicated due to increased risk of developing serotonin syndrome. A minimum of 14 days must pass from time of discontinuing nortriptyline and initiating an MAOI, and vice versa.[36]

Nortriptyline is contraindicated in patients who are recovering from an acute MI episode because nortriptyline is associated with increased risk of arrhythmias and impaired myocardial contractility.[16,36]

Adverse Events/Warnings and Precautions

Common adverse events associated with exposure to nortriptyline include dry mouth, sedation, constipation, urinary retention, blurred vision, dizziness, and tremors.[16,36] Patients should be advised to use caution while driving or operating large machinery since nortriptyline can cause sedation and impair mental/physical abilities.[16,36] Nortriptyline has been associated with risk of both hyperglycemia and hypoglycemia.[36] Patients with diabetes should be able to recognize signs and symptoms of having low and high blood glucose levels and monitor their glucose levels more closely while on nortriptyline.

Similar to bupropion SR, because nortriptyline is an antidepressant, it has a black box warning regarding suicidal thoughts and behaviors in children, adolescents, and young adults. Patients should be closely monitored for suicidality or changes in behavior, and families/caregivers should be advised to keep close observation and to communicate concerns with the healthcare providers.[36]

Consider the risk of overdose prior to initiating nortriptyline in patients because ingestion of an excessive amount of nortriptyline can result in seizures, coma, and/or severe, life-threatening cardiovascular toxicity (death included).[16,36]

Nortriptyline may trigger mania in patients with bipolar disorder and thus should not be used to treat bipolar depression.[36]

Nortriptyline, which dilates pupils, may precipitate angle-closure glaucoma in patients with anatomically narrow angles without a patent iridectomy.[36]

The efficacy and safety of nortriptyline have not been adequately studied in pregnant smokers.[36] It is recommended that pregnant smokers be encouraged to quit smoking without the aid of medications.[16]

Drug Interactions

As mentioned above, nortriptyline should not be coadministered with MAOIs. Serotonin syndrome may also be precipitated by the concomitant use of serotonergic drugs such as triptans, buspirone, and St. John's Wort. Patients should be monitored for symptoms of serotonin syndrome (e.g., agitation, coma, tachycardia, hyperthermia, rigidity, seizures, vomiting, diarrhea).[36]

There are a number of drugs that may interact with nortriptyline. In general, the following should be used with caution when administered with nortriptyline: other tricyclic antidepressants, other anticholinergic drugs, other sympathomimetic drugs, and alcohol. Patients should be monitored for amplified side-effect profiles of either interacting drug.[36]

Nortriptyline is metabolized by CYP2D6. Drugs that inhibit this enzyme (e.g., quinidine, cimetidine, antidepressants, flecainide) will increase nortriptyline levels. Changes in nortriptyline doses may be necessary during times of drug initiation or discontinuation.[36]

COMBINATION THERAPY FOR SMOKING CESSATION

Studies have demonstrated that combination therapy prevents nicotine withdrawal symptoms better than a single intervention alone, but selection of treatments will heavily depend on patient preference (e.g., tolerability of side effects, cost of product).[16]

The U.S. Department of Health and Human Services recognizes combination therapies comprising first-line medications as first-line combination therapies and those combinations mixed with a second-line medication as second-line combination therapies.[16]

A few recent studies have shown promising results with varenicline plus nicotine transdermal patch and varenicline plus bupropion SR;[16] however, more robust studies with longer follow-up data may be needed to support widespread use of combination therapy with varenicline.[42,43]

- First-line combination therapy
  - Nicotine transdermal patch + bupropion SR
  - Nicotine transdermal patch + nicotine inhaler
  - Nicotine transdermal patch + nicotine gum/nasal spray

- Second-line combination therapy
  - Nicotine transdermal patch + nortriptyline
  - Nicotine transdermal patch + second-generation antidepressants

NICOTINE TRANSDERMAL PATCH + BUPROPION SR

A meta-analysis of three clinical trials showed that the combination of nicotine transdermal patch and bupropion SR at recommended doses and treatment duration was superior to placebo in maintaining long-term smoking cessation (OR 2.5 [95% CI 1.9–3.4]).[16]

NICOTINE TRANSDERMAL PATCH + NICOTINE INHALER

A meta-analysis of two clinical trials that studied the efficacy of nicotine patch (15 mg) plus nicotine inhaler compared to placebo determined that the NRT combination was better at achieving long-term smoking cessation (OR 2.2 [95% CI 1.3–3.6]).[16]

Table 22.3—Medications for Smoking Cessation

Medication	Dosage
First-Line Medications	
Nicotine Transdermal Patch[16,44]	■ >10 cigarettes per day: Initially 21 mg/24 h for 6–8 weeks; then 14 mg/24 h for 2–4 weeks; then 7 mg/24 h for 2–4 weeks ■ ≤10 cigarettes per day: Initially 14 mg/24 h for 6 weeks; then 7 mg/24 h for 2–4 weeks ■ There are single-dose patches for lighter smokers: 22 mg/24 h and 11 mg/24 h
Nicotine Gum[16]	■ ≥25 cigarettes per day: 4 mg ■ <25 cigarettes per day: 2 mg ■ Initially 1 piece every 1–2 h for 6 weeks; then 1 piece every 2–4 h for 3 weeks; then 1 piece every 4–8 h for 3 weeks ■ Maximum of 24 pieces per day
Nicotine Lozenge[16]	■ First cigarette within 30 min of waking: 4 mg ■ First cigarette more than 30 min after waking: 2 mg ■ Initially at least 9 lozenges per day for 6 weeks; continue use for up to 12 weeks ■ Maximum of 20 lozenges per day
Nicotine Inhalers[16]	■ One dose is equal to 1 inhalation; each cartridge delivers >80 inhalations or 4 mg total ■ Initially 6–16 cartridges per day for up to 6 months ■ Gradually reduce dose for last 3 months of therapy
Nicotine Nasal Spray[16]	■ 1 dose is equal to 1 spray; each spray delivers 0.5 mg (1 spray in each nostril equals 1 mg total); each bottle delivers ~100 doses ■ Initially 1–2 doses per hour, increase as needed for symptom relief; continue use for 3–6 months ■ Recommended minimum of 8 doses per day ■ Maximum of 40 doses per day (i.e., 5 doses per hour)
Varenicline[6,26]	■ Begin 1 week before quit date ■ Initially 0.5 mg once daily for 3 days; then 0.5 mg twice daily for 4 days; then on day 8 (quit day) 1 mg twice daily for 3 months or up to 6 months ■ Dose adjustment for severe renal impairment: maximum of 0.5 mg twice daily
Bupropion SR[16,32]	■ Begin 1–2 weeks before quit date ■ Initially 150 mg once daily for 3 days; then 150 mg twice daily (at least 8 h apart) for 7–12 weeks or up to 6 months (post-quit day) ■ Maximum of 300 mg per day ■ Dose adjustment for moderate to severe hepatic impairment: maximum of 150 mg every other day
Second-Line Medications	
Clonidine[16]	■ Begin up to 3 days before quit date ■ Oral tablet: initially 0.1 mg twice daily ■ Transdermal patch: initially 0.1 mg once daily ■ Increase by 0.1 mg/day every week, as needed; continue use for 3–10 weeks ■ Maximum ~0.4 mg per day ■ Gradually reduce dose over 2–4 days at end of therapy
Nortriptyline[16]	■ Begin 10–28 days before quit date ■ Initially 25 mg per day; gradually increase over 10 days to 5 weeks until at target dose of 75–100 mg per day; continue use for 12 weeks or up to 6 months ■ Gradually reduce dose at end of therapy

NICOTINE TRANSDERMAL PATCH + NICOTINE GUM/NASAL SPRAY

A meta-analysis of three clinical trials concluded that chronic nicotine transdermal patch therapy (>14 weeks; ranging from 18–24 weeks) plus ad libitum short-acting NRT (gum or nasal spray) was better than placebo for long-term smoking cessation (OR 3.6 [95% CI 2.5–5.2]).[16]

NICOTINE TRANSDERMAL PATCH + NORTRIPTYLINE

A meta-analysis of two clinical trials that compared the efficacy of nicotine transdermal patch plus nortriptyline to that of placebo showed that combination therapy was superior for achieving long-term smoking cessation (OR 2.3 [95% CI 1.3–4.2]).[16]

NICOTINE TRANSDERMAL PATCH + SECOND-GENERATION ANTIDEPRESSANTS

A meta-analysis of three clinical trials determined that the combination of nicotine transdermal patch (highest dose being 21 or 22 mg) and second-generation antidepressants (paroxetine 20 mg or venlafaxine 22 mg) was better than placebo in maintaining long-term smoking cessation (OR 2.0 [95% CI 1.2–3.4]).[16]

Table 22.4—Combination Therapy for Smoking Cessation

- First-line combination therapy options
  - Nicotine transdermal patch + bupropion SR
  - Nicotine transdermal patch + nicotine inhaler
  - Nicotine transdermal patch + nicotine gum
  - Nicotine transdermal patch + nicotine nasal spray
- Second-line combination therapy options
  - Nicotine transdermal patch + nortriptyline
  - Nicotine transdermal patch + second-generation antidepressants

MONOGRAPHS

Bupropion SR (Zyban): https://dailymed.nlm.nih.gov/dailymed/drugInfo.cfm?setid=a3327c31-d987-40ec-b3b5-097bbf2f4f8c

Clonidine (Catapres-TTS): https://dailymed.nlm.nih.gov/dailymed/drugInfo.cfm?setid=a842ab83-3531-44dd-a8a8-64dd89e87026 and https://dailymed.nlm.nih.gov/dailymed/drugInfo.cfm?setid=fe0f5dcb-65dd-4d31-80d6-8b97eb040063

Nicotine gum: https://dailymed.nlm.nih.gov/dailymed/drugInfo.cfm?setid=3872c622-1a30-459c-b878-61648bb30627

Nicotine inhaler (Nicotrol): https://dailymed.nlm.nih.gov/dailymed/drugInfo.cfm?setid=62245d7d-b50d-48d9-9f03-071c61620ccf

Nicotine lozenge (Nicorette): https://dailymed.nlm.nih.gov/dailymed/drugInfo.cfm?setid=fdee1637-8049-4bc5-b196-b6d854c9f9f3

Nicotine nasal spray (Nicotrol): https://dailymed.nlm.nih.gov/dailymed/drugInfo.cfm?setid=acb7d02d-249b-4645-ac1b-8ff9a56dd244

Nicotine transdermal patch: https://dailymed.nlm.nih.gov/dailymed/drugInfo.cfm?setid=8a5c7835-3ab1-b3f8-e9db-e5d0cb42b59e

Nortriptyline: https://dailymed.nlm.nih.gov/dailymed/drugInfo.cfm?setid=b58d473a-b19f-4d2a-b1ae-dd398d7a29e1

Varenicline (Chantix): https://dailymed.nlm.nih.gov/dailymed/drugInfo.cfm?setid=f0ff4f27-5185-4881-a749-c6b7a0ca5696

REFERENCES

1. Barua RS, Rigotti NA, Benowitz NL, et al. 2018 ACC expert consensus decision pathway on tobacco cessation treatment. *J Am Coll Cardiol* 2018;72(25):3332–3365. DOI:10.1016/j.jacc.2018.10.027

2. Jamal A, Phillips E, Gentzke AS, et al. Current cigarette smoking among adults—United States, 2016. *Morbidity and Mortality Weekly Report (MMWR)* 2018;67:53–59. DOI:http://dx.doi.org/10.15585/mmwr.mm6702a1

3. Wang TW, Gentzke A, Sharapova S, et al. Tobacco product use among middle and high school students—United States, 2011–2017. *Morbidity and Mortality Weekly Report (MMWR)* 2018;67(22):629–633

4. Glantz SA, Bareham DW. E-cigarettes: use, effects on smoking, risks, and policy implications. *Annu Rev Public Health* 2018;39:215–235

5. Miech R, Patrick ME, O'Malley PM, Johnston LD. E-cigarette use as a predictor of cigarette smoking: results from a 1-year follow-up of a national sample of 12th grade students. *Tob Control* 2017;26(e2):e106–e111

6. Miech R, Patrick ME, O'Malley PM, Johnston LD. What are kids vaping? Results from a national survey of US adolescents. *Tob Control* 2017;26(4): 386–391

7. U.S. Department of Health and Human Services. *The health consequences of smoking—50 years of progress: a report of the surgeon general.* Atlanta, Centers for Disease Control and Prevention, Coordinating Center for Health Promotion, National Center for Chronic Disease Prevention and Health Pro-

motion, Office on Smoking and Health, 2014. Available from http://www. surgeongeneral.gov/library/reports/50-years-of-progress/full-report.pdf

8. Foy CG, Bell RA, Farmer DF, et al. Smoking and incidence of diabetes among U.S. adults: findings from the Insulin Resistance Atherosclerosis Study. *Diabetes Care* 2005;28(10):2501–2507

9. Multiple Risk Factor Intervention Trial Research Group. Multiple risk factor intervention trial: risk factor changes and mortality results. *JAMA* 1982;248(12):1465–1477

10. Jousilahti P, Vartiainen E, Tuomilehto J, Puska P. Sex, age, cardiovascular risk factors, and coronary heart disease: a prospective follow-up study of 14,786 middle-aged men and women in Finland. *Circulation* 1999;99(9): 1165–1172

11. Richard JL, Ducimetiere P, Cambien F. [Tobacco, mortality and morbidity of atherosclerotic cardiovascular diseases: a prospective study in Paris]. In French. *Bull Schwiez Akad Med Wiss* 1979;35(1–3):51–69

12. Pan A, Wang Y, Talaei M, Hu FB. Relation of smoking with total mortality and cardiovascular events among patients with diabetes: a meta-analysis and systematic review. *Circulation* 2015;132(19):1795–1804

13. American Diabetes Association. Smoking and diabetes. *Diabetes Care* 2004;27(Suppl. 1):S74–S75

14. Qin R, Chen T, Lou Q, Yu D. Excess risk of mortality and cardiovascular events associated with smoking among patients with diabetes: meta-analysis of observational prospective studies. *Int J Cardiol* 2013;167(2):342–350

15. Thorndike AN, Regan S, Rigotti NA. The treatment of smoking by US physicians during ambulatory visits: 1994–2003. *Am J Public Health* 2007; 97(10):1878–1883

16. Fiore MC, Jaen CR, Baker TB, et al. *Treating tobacco use and dependence: 2008 update. Clinical Practice Guideline.* Rockville, MD, Agency for Healthcare Research and Quality, May 2008. Available from https://www.ahrq.gov/professionals/clinicians-providers/guidelines-recommendations/tobacco/clinicians/update/index.html. Accessed 15 May 2018

17. Stead LF, Loilpillai P, Fanshawe T, Lancaster T. Combined pharmacotherapy and behavioural interventions for smoking cessation. *Cochrane Database Syst Rev* 2016;3:CD008286. DOI:10.1002/14651858.CD008286.pub3

18. Siu AL; U.S. Preventive Services Task Force. Behavioral and pharmacotherapy interventions for tobacco smoking cessation in adults, including pregnant women: U.S. Preventive Services Task Force recommendation statement. *Ann Intern Med* 2015;163(8):622–634

19. Hughes JR, Hatsukami D. Signs and symptoms of tobacco withdrawal. *Arch Gen Psychiatry* 1986;43(3):289–294

20. Hughes JR. Tobacco withdrawal in self-quitters. *J Consult Clin Psychol* 1992;60(5):689–697

21. Stead LF, Perera R, Bullen C, et al. Nicotine replacement therapy for smoking cessation. *Cochrane Database Syst Rev* 2012;11:CD000146. DOI:10.1002/14651858.CD000146.pub4

22. Nides M. Update on pharmacologic options for smoking cessation treatment. *Am J Med* 2008;121(4A):S20–S31

23. Drug and Therapeutics Bulletin. Republished: nicotine and health. *BMJ* 2014;349:2014.7.0264rep. DOI:10.1136/bmj.2014.7.0264rep

24. Woolf KJ, Zabad MN, Post JM, et al. Effect of nicotine replacement therapy on cardiovascular outcomes after acute coronary syndromes. *Am J Cardiol* 2012;110(7):968–970

25. Frishman WH. Smoking cessation pharmacotherapy: nicotine and non-nicotine preparations. *Prev Cardio* 2007;10(2 Suppl. 1):10–22

26. Chantix (varenicline) [prescribing information]. New York, Pfizer Labs—Division of Pfizer, Inc., December 2016. Available from https://dailymed.nlm.nih.gov/dailymed/drugInfo.cfm?setid=f0ff4f27-5185-4881-a749-c6b7a0ca5696

27. Gonzales D, Rennard SI, Nides M, et al. Varenicline, an alpha4beta2 nicotinic acetylcholine receptor partial agonist, vs sustained-release bupropion and placebo for smoking cessation: a randomized controlled trial. *JAMA* 2006;296(1):47–55

28. Jorenby DE, Hays JT, Rigotti NA, et al. Efficacy of varenicline, an alpha-4beta2 nicotinic acetylcholine receptor partial agonist, vs placebo or sustained-release bupropion for smoking cessation: a randomized controlled trial. *JAMA* 2006;296(1):56–63

29. Anthenelli RM, Benowitz NL, West R, et al. Neuropsychiatric safety and efficacy of varenicline, bupropion, and nicotine patch in smokers with and without psychiatric disorders (EAGLES): a double-blind, randomised, placebo-controlled clinical trial. *Lancet* 2016;387(10037):2507–2520

30. U.S. Food and Drug Administration. Information for healthcare professionals: varenicline (marketed as Chantix) and bupropion (marketed as Zyban, Wellbutrin, and generics). Published 1 July 2009. Available from http://wayback.archive-it.org/7993/20170112032419/http://www.fda.gov/Drugs/DrugSafety/PostmarketDrugSafetyInformationforPatientsandProviders/DrugSafetyInformationforHeathcareProfessionals/ucm169986.htm. Accessed 27 April 2018

31. FDA Drug Safety Communication. FDA revises description of mental health side effects of the stop-smoking medicines Chantix (varenicline) and Zyban (bupropion) to reflect clinical trial findings. Published 16 December

2016. Available from https://www.fda.gov/Drugs/DrugSafety/ucm532221. htm. Accessed 27 April 2018

32. Zyban (bupropion hydrochloride) [prescribing information]. Research Triangle Park, NC, GlaxoSmithKline, May 2017. Available from https://dailymed.nlm.nih.gov/dailymed/drugInfo.cfm?setid=a3327c31-d987 -40ec-b3b5-097bbf2f4f8c

33. Catapres (clonidine hydrochloride) [prescribing information]. Ridgefield, CT, Boehringer Ingelheim Pharmaceuticals, Inc., September 2016. Available from https://dailymed.nlm.nih.gov/dailymed/drugInfo. cfm?setid=d7f569dc-6bed-42dc-9bec-940a9e6b090d

34. Gourlay SG, Stead LF, Benowitz N. Clonidine for smoking cessation. *Cochrane Database Syst Rev* 2004;3:CD000058. DOI:10.1002/14651858. CD000058.pub2

35. Catapres-TTS (clonidine) [prescribing information]. Ridgefield, CT, Boehringer Ingelheim Pharmaceuticals, Inc., August 2016. Available from https:// dailymed.nlm.nih.gov/dailymed/drugInfo.cfm?setid=fe0f5dcb-65dd-4d31- 80d6-8b97eb040063

36. Pamelor (nortriptyline hydrochloride) [prescribing information]. North Wales, PA, TEVA Pharmaceuticals USA, Inc., June 2016. Available from https://dailymed.nlm.nih.gov/dailymed/drugInfo.cfm?setid=b58d473a- b19f-4d2a-b1ae-dd398d7a29e1

37. Hughes JR, Stead LF, Lancaster T. Nortriptyline for smoking cessation: a review. *Nicotine Tob Res* 2005;7(4):491–499

38. Alexanderson B. Pharmacokinetics of nortriptyline in man after single and multiple oral doses: the predictability of steady-state plasma concentrations from single-dose plasma-level data. *Eur J Clin Pharmacol* 1972;4(2):82–91

39. Rubin EH, Biggs JT, Preskorn SH. Nortriptyline pharmacokinetics and plasma levels: implications for clinical practice. *J Clin Psychiatry* 1985;46(10):418–424

40. Venkatakrishnan K, von Moltke LL, Greenblatt DJ. Nortriptyline E-10-hydroxylation in vitro is mediated by human CYP2D6 (high affinity) and CYP3A4 (low affinity): implications for interactions with enzyme-inducing drugs. *J Clin Pharmacol* 1999;39(6):567–577

41. Dawling S, Crome P, Braithwaite R. Pharmacokinetics of single oral doses of nortriptyline in depressed elderly hospital patients and young healthy volunteers. *Clin Pharmacokinet* 1980;5(4):394–401

42. Chang PH, Chiang CH, Ho WC, et al. Combination therapy of varenicline with nicotine replacement therapy is better than varenicline alone: a systematic review and meta-analysis of randomized controlled trials. *BMC Public Health* 2015;15:689

43. Vogeler T, McClain C, Evoy KE. Combination bupropion SR and vareni-cline for smoking cessation: a systematic review. *Am J Drug Alcohol Abuse* 2016;42(2):129–139

44. NicoDerm CQ (nicotine patch, extended release) [prescribing information]. Moon Township, PA, GlaxoSmithKline, May 2016. Available from https://dailymed.nlm.nih.gov/dailymed/drugInfo.cfm?setid=93b2d1b9-83c1-40b5-b6af-90c38c8d6cef

Chapter 23
Medications for the Management of Neuropathy

Damianne Brand-Eubanks, PharmD
Anne P. Kim, PharmD, MPH, MIT

OVERVIEW

Neuropathy, a disease or dysfunction of one or more nerves, is most commonly linked to metabolic, vascular, and/or immune origins, and is one of the leading complications associated with T1D and T2D. There are three primary types of neuropathy found in diabetic patients: diabetic polyneuropathy, autonomic neuropathy, and focal neuropathy (see Table 23.1). The two most common types of diabetic-induced neuropathy are diabetic polyneuropathy, also known as distal symmetric sensorimotor polyneuropathy (DSPN), and diabetic autonomic neuropathy (DAN).

DSPN is a chronic, nerve-length-dependent, sensorimotor neuropathy that affects at least one-third of those with T1D or T2D and up to one-quarter of those with impaired glucose tolerance.[1] Progression of DSPN differs between T1D and T2D. With T2D, there is a milder functional defect early on that can progress to structural degenerative changes, eventually resulting in nerve fiber loss. In comparison, the late structural phase of DSPN affects people with T1D more severely.[2] People with DSPN often have length-dependent symptoms—which usually affect the feet first, as they are the longest nerves in the body—with these symptoms progressing proximally.[3,4] The symptoms begin as sensory and are categorized as either "positive," due to excess or inappropriate nerve activity, or "negative," due to reduced nerve activity (see Table 23.2).[1] Although positive symptoms can lead to the need for pharmacological modulation of varied levels of pain, negative symptoms, such as decreased sensation, can increase risk of painless foot ulcers or both proprioceptive impairment and loss of balance, leading to falls. Negative symptoms are usually not treated; rather, there is an attempt to avoid further damage through better glycemic control.

Chronic hyperglycemia, resulting in microvascular and neuronal damage, is the main mechanism by which DSPN is theorized to develop. Nerve biopsies of diabetic patients diagnosed with DSPN have shown a thickening of the basement membranes of vessels feeding damaged neurons and a greater variation overall of vessel lumen thickness. Damaged blood vessels display a poor vasodilatory response to nitric oxide, and ischemia is prominent in the microvasculature. Following this cascade, hypoxia will eventually result, leading to neuronal starvation and death. Increased influx of glucose and other sugar molecules may increase basement membrane thickening through the polyol flux pathway.[5] This pathway may also be responsible for the destruction of neuronal supporting cells, perpetuating eventual axonal changes. These changes may include an increase of intra-

Table 23.1 — Primary Types of Diabetic-Induced Neuropathy

Origin	Common presentations
Peripheral Polyneuropathy	
Distal Symmetrical	■ Most common in T2D ■ Glove/stocking loss of sensation (pain, vibration, temperature, proprioception) ■ Loss of motor nerve function with clawed toes and small muscle wasting in hands and flexor muscles ■ Charcot joints (loss of sensation results in joint and ligament degeneration, particularly in the foot, causing deterioration of weight-bearing joints in foot and ankle) ■ Acute painful neuropathy with burning pain in legs and feet
Autonomic Neuropathy	
Gastrointestinal	■ Constipation ■ Gastroparesis ■ Diarrhea (hallmark nocturnal)
Cardiac	■ Resting tachycardia ■ Exercise intolerance ■ Orthostatic hypotension (sleep in sitting or semirecumbent position due to risk of silent MI or cardiac death)
Urogenital	■ Loss of bladder tone ■ Urinary retention ■ Risk for bladder infection ■ Decreased sensation of bladder fullness/urge ■ Overflow incontinence ■ ED ■ Female sexual dysfunction
Sweat Glands	■ Anhidrosis: sudomotor dysfunction ■ Gustatory sweating (usually after eating)
Focal Neuropathy	
Amyotrophic	■ Uncommon (occur more often in elderly with poor glycemic control) ■ Proximal thigh muscle pain and weakness ■ Wrist or foot drop

Source: Triplitt.[8]

neuronal sodium, which slows nerve conduction in both sensory and motor neurons. Oxidative stress in tandem with the polyol pathway is another mechanism by which neuronal damage and ultimately DSPN is theorized to occur, with free radicals damaging neuronal tissue.[6] Antioxidant levels in the diabetic patient are depleted, allowing formation of free radicals through the oxidation of glucose and other cellular mechanisms. Free radicals form, and the damage produced can ultimately lead to neuronal cell death.[7]

DAN is the most diverse form of neuropathy affecting patients with diabetes, as this can involve the cardiovascular, gastrointestinal, and genitourinary systems (see Table 23.1). Autonomic neuropathy does not primarily involve large nerve

Table 23.2—Positive and Negative Symptoms of Polyneuropathy

Common symptoms of peripheral neuropathy		
	Sensory Symptoms	Motor Symptoms
Positive	■ Paresthesia ■ Pain: burning, squeezing or tightness, electric shock-like, hypersensitivity	■ Fasciculation ■ Cramps
Negative	■ Numbness ■ Reduced or absent sensation ■ Postural instability	■ Weakness ■ Atrophy

Source: Triplitt.[8]

fibers, as previously described for DSPN. Cardiovascular complications associated with DAN can lead to hypotensive episodes, irregular heartbeat, instability related to anesthetic administration, and an increased risk for both MI and sudden death. Gastrointestinal neuropathy can involve the gastrointestinal tract as a whole and is commonly identified by gastroparesis and esophageal difficulties. Genitourinary neuropathy occurs through loss of coordination of smooth muscle and often results in urinary incontinence issues and sexual dysfunction in both men and women with diabetes. Therapies are available to treat all forms of DAN, although most include intensive glucose control coupled with medications addressing the symptoms associated with the affected organ system.

Previously investigated pharmacological interventions for pain associated with diabetic neuropathy include pregabalin, gabapentin, certain tricyclic antidepressants (TCAs), opioids, antidepressants, and other anticonvulsants.

ANTICONVULSANTS

GABA ANALOGS

The GABA analogs, gabapentin and pregabalin, are structurally related to the neurotransmitter γ-aminobutyric acid (GABA), but do not influence GABA receptors or use this pathway as a mechanism of action. These agents bind to the α_2-δ subunit of neural presynaptic voltage-gated calcium channels, which decrease calcium flux.[9] Subsequently, decreased neurotransmitter release from these neurons occurs, thus limiting neuronal excitation. This mechanism is theorized to account for the analgesic effect and decrease in neuropathic pain.[10]

Gabapentin was initially introduced for treatment of seizures and was later found to have use in diabetic-induced neuropathic pain, though it still does not

Table 23.3 — Recommended Dose and Dose Adjustment of First-, Second-, and Third-Line Medications for Diabetic-Induced Neuropathy

Class	Agent	Initial dose	Maximum dose	Dose adjustment
Anticonvulsants	Pregabalin	25–75 mg 1–3 times daily	600 mg/day	Renal: ■ CrCl 30–60 mL/min: 300 mg maximum ■ CrCl 15–29 mL/min: 150 mg maximum ■ CrCl <15 mL/min: 75 mg maximum
	Gabapentin	100–300 mg/day	3,600 mg/day	Renal: ■ CrCl 30–60 mL/min: 1,500 mg maximum ■ CrCl 16–29 mL/min: 700 mg maximum ■ CrCl 15 mL/min: 300 mg maximum
Antidepressants (Serotonin-Norepinephrine Reuptake Inhibitors)	Duloxetine	20–30 mg/day	120 mg/day	Renal: ■ CrCl <30 mL/min or hepatic cirrhosis: avoid use
	Venlafaxine	37.5 mg/day	225 mg/day	Renal: ■ CrCl 10–50 mL/min or mild-moderate hepatic impairment: decrease dose by 50%
Tricyclic Antidepressants	Amitriptyline	10–25 mg/day	100 mg/day	■ N/A
Topical Medications (Adjunct)	Lidocaine 5% patch	1 patch/day	3 patches/day	■ Small treatment areas advised
	Capsaicin 0.075%	4 times daily		■ N/A
	Isosorbide dinitrate spray	30 mg daily at bedtime to bottom of feet		■ N/A

First-line therapies	Second-line therapies	Adjunct therapies

Source: Vinik[3] and Griebeler.[19]

have FDA approval for this indication. Oral gabapentin has a nonlinear kinetic profile. For instance, the bioavailability of oral gabapentin is reduced from 60 to 33% as the dose increases from 900 to 3,200 mg/day. In addition, administering gabapentin with food increases bioavailability by 10%, without a change in time to maximum concentration (T_{max}). This is considered to be a slight change, so gabapentin may be administered with or without food. Although gabapentin does have a manufacturer-approved maximum dose of 3,600 mg/day, it has been studied at higher doses with similarly successful response.[10]

Pregabalin was approved for use by the FDA for DSPN in 2004. Pregabalin displays linear kinetics, with peak concentrations achieved 1.5 h after administration and steady-state concentrations achieved after 1–2 days of continuous dosing. Pregabalin dosing is recommended to not exceed 300 mg/day in order to mitigate side effects that are observed at higher doses, even though greater response has been observed at doses of up to 600 mg/day.[11,12,13]

Tolerance may develop with continued gabapentin use, while tolerance to pregabalin has not been reported to develop. Continued monitoring to assure successful therapy is still recommended for pregabalin therapy.[11] Common side effects of the GABA analogs include sedation, dizziness, CNS depression, blurred vision, balance issues, tremors, and confusion.

Both gabapentin and pregabalin are primarily cleared by the renal system. Dosing adjustments based on renal impairment may be required. It is important to note that both agents are dialyzable. The half-lives for these agents are 5–7 h, which may be increased in patients with impaired renal function. GABA analogs have not been adequately studied in patients who are pregnant or breast-feeding. They should only be used when the benefit of therapy outweighs the potential risk of maternal/fetal harm.[14] Administration of GABA analogs with other CNS depressants may increase risk of sedation and other similar side effects. Also, caution should be exercised if administering pregabalin with TZDs (e.g., pioglitazone and rosiglitazone), as this combination may increase the risk of weight gain and edema. Discontinuation of either gabapentin or pregabalin should be performed in a downward titration, as withdrawal-like symptoms including sweating, dizziness, sleep disturbances, and muscle pain may occur with abrupt discontinuation of therapy.[11]

OTHER ANTICONVULSANTS

Carbamazepine and valproic acid and its sodium salt (sodium valproate) are other anticonvulsants used off-label to treat DSPN, though more studies are needed to prove both effectiveness in pain treatment and safety for this indication. The mechanism of action for carbamazepine is related to its ability to block voltage-dependent sodium channels, thus reducing ectopic nerve discharge and stabilizing neural membranes while minimizing the effect of normal nerve conductance. Although chemically related to the TCAs, carbamazepine is not considered to have a mechanistic effect on neural transmitters. Carbamazepine has shown to be effective in the treatment of trigeminal neuralgia, but may be used for treating DSPN if patients are refractory to other treatments, due to its difficult-to-manage dosage and side-effect profile.[15]

Valproic acid, in addition to its inhibition of glutamate/N-methyl-D-aspartate (NMDA) receptor-mediated neuronal excitation, has been shown to be a potent inhibitor of histone deacetylase (HDAC) enzymes. HDAC regulation is a possible new approach in the treatment of T2D to modify the metabolism of glucose and fatty acid and the secondarily associated neuronal damage. HDAC is thought to promote the development, proliferation, differentiation, and function of pancreatic β-cells and ameliorate microvascular complications in later stages of the disease.[16] Valproic acid (potentially teratogenic) and carbamazepine should be avoided in women of childbearing age with diabetes.[16]

ANTIDEPRESSANTS

DULOXETINE

Duloxetine is FDA approved for the treatment of DSPN as a dose-dependent, dual-acting selective serotonin-norepinephrine reuptake inhibitor (SNRI). Its effects on serotonin (5-HT) and norepinephrine are considered to be responsible for the analgesic effect of duloxetine.[17] Serotonin and norepinephrine elicit neurogenic transmission in the brainstem and spinal column, and are theorized to minimize pain transmission from the periphery to the CNS via these transmission pathways. Duloxetine is extensively metabolized in the liver and is a substrate of the enzymes CYP2D6 and CYP1A2. It is also a moderate inhibitor of both enzymes, so care should be taken to avoid drug-drug interactions when given concurrently. Common side effects with duloxetine may include nausea/vomiting, dizziness, fatigue, and somnolence. These side effects can occur within the first 8 weeks of treatment or at times of dosage increase, but they typically dissipate with time. Duloxetine has been shown in multiple studies to be well tolerated with slow titration in elderly patients. Dose adjustments for hepatic and renally impaired patients are not necessary.[12,18]

OTHER ANTIDEPRESSANTS: SELECTIVE SEROTONIN-NOREPINEPHRINE REUPTAKE INHIBITORS

Venlafaxine and desvenlafaxine have similar mechanisms of action to those of duloxetine, but little evidence is available to support their effectiveness in DSPN. They are usually considered second-line DSPN treatment medications. These SNRIs are often better tolerated and have fewer drug interactions when compared to TCAs (e.g., amitriptyline), but have shown comparatively less effectiveness in treatment outcomes.[18] Dosing adjustments may be necessary for both renal and hepatic impairment. Though there are no controlled studies in pregnant women, there are reported concerns associated with other SNRIs used in the third trimester, resulting in a pregnancy category C designation. Avoidance in breast-feeding is suggested, due to excretion into breast milk.[19]

TRICYCLIC ANTIDEPRESSANTS

TCAs were the first medication class used in placebo-controlled trials for neuropathic pain, yet there is still not an FDA-approved TCA for treatment of such pain. The primary mechanism of action of TCAs occurs through inhibition of serotonin and norepinephrine reuptake. The analgesic effect is considered to be independent of the primary antidepressant effect and is theorized to be related to a secondary mechanism, such as α-adrenergic, H_1-histaminergic, and muscarinic receptor blockade; sodium-channel blockade; or possibly NMDA blockade. Dopamine is not directly affected by this class of medications, although dopamine reuptake may fluctuate through indirect effects on adrenergic receptors. Similar to other antidepressants, peak plasma levels may occur within 24 h, but the peak effect may not be seen until 2–4 weeks. TCAs are also highly protein bound, particularly to albumin, and interactions with other protein-bound medications (e.g., warfarin) need to be monitored. Hypothetically, TCAs can displace other protein-bound medications from their binding sites. This displacement could lead to increased serum levels, and in the case of warfarin, increased anticoagulation. Close monitoring of labs, including the INR and especially of narrow therapeutic medications like warfarin, should be done if given concurrently.[19] TCAs can be separated into two categories: secondary amines (e.g., amitriptyline, imipramine) and tertiary amines (e.g., nortriptyline, desipramine). Secondary amines are relatively norepinephrine-selective and have been shown to produce a markedly lower incidence of adverse effects. As such, they are considered more favorable for the treatment of neuropathic disorders than are tertiary amines.[19,20] The dose of TCAs for neuropathic pain is usually only half that required for depression. An example of this dosing variance would be amitriptyline, which has been proven effective in neuropathic pain at doses of 25–75 mg daily, while the recommended dose for use in depression is 150–300 mg daily.[18] Caution is advised for using any TCA during pregnancy, especially in the third trimester, due to the concern of possible unknown risks of neonatal withdrawal symptoms. There is currently no known risk of infant harm in breast-feeding, based on limited human data and drug properties. Patients already taking antidepressant therapy must be monitored for the possibility of serotonin syndrome when started on a TCA, as this can potentiate serotonin levels on their current medications.

TOPICAL MEDICATIONS

LIDOCAINE

Topical 5% lidocaine patches have been clinically studied for use in the treatment of localized DSPN. The mechanism of action for lidocaine functions through inhibition of voltage-gated sodium channels, which are theorized to activate spontaneously in damaged neurons. Lidocaine has been shown to decrease perceived pain levels, as well as increase patient quality of life through reduction of the negative impact neuropathy may have on activities of daily living. Topical lidocaine reaches systemic levels equal to one-tenth the level necessary to treat cardiac arrhythmias and is not considered to have a significant effect on the cardiovascular system. Distribution of topical lidocaine is negligible. Metabolism of lidocaine occurs primarily in the liver, with excretion occurring primarily through the kidneys. Lidocaine patches can be used as an adjunct to oral therapy and are not considered a primary agent for pain control in widespread neuropathic damage. When comparing lidocaine and pregabalin for use with localized pain, comparable pain relief (30–50% response) to that of pregabalin has been shown, with fewer adverse effects (primarily dermatological) and higher quality-of-life scores for localized pain.[12]

CAPSAICIN

Capsaicin, an active component of chili peppers, is thought to produce analgesia by selectively stimulating unmyelinated C-fiber afferent neurons causing release and depletion of substance P. Capsaicin binds to the sensory vanilloid transient receptor potential cation channel (TRPV1), which is part of the communication pathway for painful stimuli. Treatment with 0.075% capsaicin cream was studied at a dosing interval of every 6 h, not to exceed four times per day. It showed significant pain relief of 50% from the patient's baseline level, but adverse effects, such as burning at the site of application, led to early subject withdrawal from the study.[19,20] Pain relief with capsaicin may begin to be observed as soon as 2 weeks after initiation with continual administration, but can take up to 6–8 weeks to reach maximal desired effect.[19]

ISOSORBIDE DINITRATE SPRAY

Impaired nitric oxide synthesis or release is thought to contribute to the pathogenesis of diabetic neuropathy and hyperalgesia. Isosorbide dinitrate is a nitric oxide donor, vasodilator, and smooth muscle relaxant that theoretically modulates impaired nitric oxide synthesis or release.[21] There was a reported decrease in pain scores when isosorbide dinitrate was applied on affected areas, but more studies are needed to show consistency in treatment and side-effect profile over a longer duration of treatment.[22]

COMBINATION THERAPY

There was some evidence to support superiority to placebo for the combination of gabapentin and morphine or nortriptyline, and no significant difference when the combination of duloxetine and pregabalin at moderate doses were compared against monotherapy at high doses.[12]

DIABETIC GASTROPARESIS

Gastroparesis is a delay in gastric emptying without an obstruction of the stomach. It occurs in 30–50% of patients with T1D or T2D. Chronically elevated blood glucose and A1C levels are associated with an increased risk of gastroparesis, but the severity of clinical symptoms does not always correspond with the rate of gastric emptying. The mechanism by which diabetic gastroparesis occurs is mainly associated with central autonomic neuropathy affecting the vagus nerve and a decrease in the number of inhibitory neurons associated with gastrointestinal motor control. High blood glucose causes chemical changes in the nerves and damages the blood vessels feeding those nerves. Increased levels of glucagon are also considered a factor in gastroparesis. It slows the rate at which food is delivered for digestion in the small intestine. All of these processes together lead to a decrease in fundic and antral motor activity, a reduction of interdigestive migration control, and an increase in digestive and gastric spasmodic problems.

The common symptoms associated with diabetic gastroparesis are early satiety, nausea, erratic glycemic control, weight loss, abdominal pain, and bloating.[23] In addition to gastrointestinal symptoms, diabetic gastroparesis can have a negative impact on the patient's quality of life and psychological health. When attempting treatment, it is important to exclude other known causes of altered gastric emptying, including, but not limited to, infection, gastric obstruction, or even some medications. Several therapies are available for the treatment of diabetic gastroparesis, although a combination of strict glycemic control, dietary changes, and medication therapy may result in the best outcome for the patient.[24]

METOCLOPRAMIDE

Metoclopramide is FDA approved for short-term use in the treatment of gastroparesis, but it should be reserved for severe refractory cases of the disease.[25] This medication acts on a diverse number of neurotransmitters: it is a serotonin-4 receptor ($5HT_4$) agonist, a weak serotonin-3 receptor ($5HT_3$) antagonist, a central and peripheral dopamine D_2 antagonist, and a cholinesterase inhibitor. Metoclopramide is prokinetic through $5HT_4$ receptor agonism and antagonism at the peripheral dopamine D_2 receptors, which decreases fundal relaxation and increases antral contractions, thereby improving gastric emptying. It also acts as an antiemetic through antagonism of $5HT_3$ receptors and the central dopamine D_2 receptors in the area postrema.

Metoclopramide is available in oral and parenteral forms. Onset of action is 30–60 min for oral, 10–15 min for intramuscular, and 1–3 min for intravenous administration. Metoclopramide is only 30% protein-bound and crosses the blood-brain barrier. The half-life for metoclopramide is 2.5–6 h, requiring multiple doses a day with meals.[25]

Despite its efficacy, use of metoclopramide is limited by the presence of unfavorable side effects, including neuroendocrine effects such as inappropriate lactation either in women without current maternal needs or in men, gynecomastia, impotence, and serious extrapyramidal symptoms such as tardive dyskinesia. Though increased gastric emptying is the goal, if achieved, it can also alter the absorption of coadministered medications. Plasma levels should be monitored initially for drugs with a narrow therapeutic index (e.g., lithium, digoxin) to ensure safety and efficacy. Metoclopramide is cleared renally, and the adjustment of metoclopramide dosing may be necessary in the renally impaired patient, as accumulation and toxicity may occur.[26] Metoclopramide has been shown to cross into breast milk, so caution is warranted when using metoclopramide in a breast-feeding patient.[24,25]

MACROLIDE ANTIBIOTICS: ERYTHROMYCIN

Erythromycin, a motilin agonist, induces high-amplitude gastric propulsive contractions and stimulates fundic contractility, mimicking the effect of the polypeptide motilin, which increases motility and improves gastric emptying of both liquids and solids.[26] In a systematic review of five clinical trials involving oral erythromycin for gastroparesis, 26 of 60 patients (43%) had an improvement in symptoms of gastroparesis, though the studies had a small sample size and a short duration.[27] Clinical responsiveness tends to wane after a few weeks, associated with tachyphylaxis, due to down regulation of the motilin receptor.[28] Common adverse effects of erythromycin include nausea/vomiting, diarrhea, abdominal pain, headache, rash, and possible cardiac QT interval prolongation. It is also a potent inhibitor and a substrate of the CYP3A4 enzyme, so care should be taken to avoid interactions with concurrent medications and food. Patients with a diagnosed heart rhythm disorder or a prolonged QT interval should receive erythromycin with caution, as this medication has been shown to cause ventricular arrhythmias of the torsade de pointes type. Erythromycin may be used with caution in pregnant patients and is considered safe for use in breast-feeding patients.[27]

Erythromycin is available in oral and intravenous form. It was found to be a more potent agent for treatment of diabetic gastroparesis when given intravenously; among oral formulations, suspension was found to be more effective than tablets. Finally, erythromycin efficacy is negatively affected by hyperglycemia, so adequate control of blood glucose must be established to maximize its effect. Newer motilin and synthetic ghrelin agonists are being researched to expand the options available for the treatment of gastroparesis.[29,30]

ERECTILE DYSFUNCTION

ED is the inability to achieve or maintain an erection sufficient for sexual intercourse. Causes for ED are multifactorial, and may relate to psychological, neurological, hormonal, vascular, mediation, or age factors, or a combination of these. Autonomic neurotransmission controls the corpora cavernosa and detrusor smooth muscle tone and function. Endothelial dysfunction is also a common cause of ED, as well as the common link between ED, diabetes, and subsequent vascular disease. Endothelial dysfunction in the pudendal penile arteries/arterioles leads to a loss of vascular patency and increased risk of atherosclerosis, thrombosis, plaque formation, and occlusive artery disease. The endothelium is responsible for release of nitric oxide into the smooth vascular cells, which ultimately increases release of cyclic guanosine monophosphate (cGMP), leading to increased relaxation of smooth vascular muscle cells. Endothelial dysfunction lowers nitric oxide formation and release, which was identified as a key contributor to ED.[3,24] Although therapy may be initiated to modify or treat ED, it is also recommended to educate the patient regarding other underlying conditions (e.g., diabetes mellitus, CVD), and make sure that control of these conditions is established to reduce any risk of further damage and worsening ED.[1]

PHOSPHODIESTERASE TYPE 5 INHIBITORS (PDE5-Is): SILDENAFIL, TADALAFIL, VARDENAFIL, AND AVANAFIL

Sildenafil was the first phosphodiesterase inhibitor studied for the treatment of ED, and has since been followed by vardenafil, tadalafil, and avanafil, which are more selective for phosphodiesterase type 5 (PDE5) (see Table 23.4). PDE5-Is, such as sildenafil, exert their action through blockade of cGMP-specific phosphodiesterase-5 degradation. Normally, the endothelium of the corpus cavernosum

Table 23.4—Phosphodiesterase Inhibitors[31]

Pde5-i	Dose/day	Onset of action	Duration	Comments
Sildenafil Available in tablets, suspension, and injectable	Initial p.r.n. dose: 50 mg Dose range: 25–100 mg >65 years: 25 mg	60 min	4 h	■ Possible color visual disturbances ■ Renal dosing: p.r.n. = CrCl 30–50 mL/min: max 5 mg OR 10 mg every 48 h. CrCl <30 mL/min: max 5 mg ■ Hepatic dosing: Child-Pugh Class A or B: max of 10 mg daily
Tadalafil Available in tablets	Initial p.r.n. dose: 10 mg Dose range (p.r.n.): 5–20 mg Initial daily dose: 2.5 mg Dose range (daily): 2.5–5 mg >65 years: 5 mg	30–45 min	Up to 36 h	■ Renal dosing: – p.r.n. = CrCl 30–50 mL/min: max 5 mg/day. CrCl <30 mL/min: max 5 mg/72 h – Daily = CrCl <30 mL/min: avoid use ■ Hepatic dosing: avoid use in Child-Pugh Class C
Vardenafil Available in tablets and ODT	Initial p.r.n. dose: 10 mg Dose range: 5–20 mg >65 years: 5 mg	60 min	5 h	■ Hepatic dosing: Child-Pugh Class B: start 5 mg x 1, max 10 mg per dose ■ Child-Pugh Class C: avoid use
Avanafil Available in tablets	Initial p.r.n. dosing: 100 mg Dose range: 50–200 mg	15–30 min	6 h	■ Renal dosing: CrCl <30 mL/min: avoid use ■ Hepatic dosing: avoid use in Child-Pugh Class C

ODT, orally dissolving tablet. *Source:* Huang.[31]

releases nitric oxide during sexual stimulation. The nitric oxide stimulates release of cGMP, which relaxes the smooth muscle of the corpus cavernosum and allows blood flow to occur. In ED, cGMP levels are decreased and smooth muscle relaxation may not occur, leading to the failure of erection. By inhibiting PDE5, sildenafil raises levels of cGMP and improves smooth muscle relaxation in the corpus cavernosum, improving erectile function. Repeated dosing is recommended, with continued exposure showing improved responses. Common adverse effects associated with PDE5-I use include headache, flushing, dizziness, and rash. Combined use of PDE5-Is with known CYP3A4 inhibitors (e.g., erythromycin, ketoconazole) may increase plasma concentrations of sildenafil through inhibition of metabolism, leading to a greater risk of side effects. Caution should also be exercised when using sildenafil in a patient with a previous history of cardiovascular events (e.g., MI, stroke). PDE5-Is should not be used concurrently with nitrate therapy, due to the additive effect of vasodilation and acute hypotension that could potentially lead to death.[24,31]

ALPROSTADIL

Alprostadil is a naturally occurring prostaglandin E found in the seminal vesicles and cavernous tissues of the penis. Alprostadil acts on the smooth muscles of the corpus cavernosum, thereby stimulating the activity of adenylate cyclase. As a result, an increase of intracellular cAMP and a decrease in intracellular calcium occur. A decrease in norepinephrine also occurs through this mechanism, leading to smooth muscle relaxation and increased blood flow. Additionally, alprostadil directly dilates cavernosal arteries, increasing arterial blood flow, and thereby enhancing erectile function.

Alprostadil is available as an intracavernosal injection and an intraurethrally applied tablet, allowing for administration of an ED medication in patients unable to take PDE5-Is (e.g., patients taking concurrent antianginal nitrates). Systemic absorption of alprostadil is minimal, with little to no adverse effects associated with this medication. No dosing adjustments are necessary for known disease states, such as hepatic or renal impairment. Side effects noted during use include hypotension and syncope. Alprostadil should be used cautiously in patients who have experienced priapism (erection ≥4 h). Although no dosing guidelines have been outlined for this medication, the manufacturer recommendations state initial dosing is to begin at 1.25 µg for injection and 125 µg per intraurethral tablet, with titration based on physiological response. Injections should be given no more than three times per week, with at least a 24 h period between doses following initial titration.[2,32]

MONOGRAPHS

Alprostadil injection: https://dailymed.nlm.nih.gov/dailymed/drugInfo.cfm?setid=4dec1dbd-c63b-4a1b-81cb-c8d29696cc40

Alprostadil suppository: https://dailymed.nlm.nih.gov/dailymed/drugInfo.cfm?setid=4c55f3f9-c4cf-11df-851a-0800200c9a66

Amitriptyline: https://dailymed.nlm.nih.gov/dailymed/drugInfo.cfm?setid=1e6d2c80-fbc8-444e-bdd3-6a91fe1b95bd

Avanafil: https://dailymed.nlm.nih.gov/dailymed/drugInfo.cfm?setid=a8726f90-9329-46ca-9379-2b50c78fe0e2

Capsaicin cream 0.075%: https://dailymed.nlm.nih.gov/dailymed/drugInfo.cfm?setid=5a9e970c-7e67-469d-b9ad-010c031ed35b

Carbamazepine: https://dailymed.nlm.nih.gov/dailymed/drugInfo.cfm?setid=8d409411-aa9f-4f3a-a52c-fbcb0c3ec053

Desipramine: https://dailymed.nlm.nih.gov/dailymed/drugInfo.cfm?setid=a3b4b25d-0ddb-4531-badb-f1ba3168ac07

Desvenlafaxine ER: https://dailymed.nlm.nih.gov/dailymed/drugInfo.cfm?setid =0f43610c-f290-46ea-d186-4f998ed99fce

Duloxetine: https://dailymed.nlm.nih.gov/dailymed/drugInfo.cfm?setid =2f7d4d67-10c1-4bf4-a7f2-c185fbad64ba

Erythromycin: https://dailymed.nlm.nih.gov/dailymed/drugInfo.cfm?setid= 86d6353c-2b58-4219-b31d-fb5b97789094

Gabapentin: https://dailymed.nlm.nih.gov/dailymed/drugInfo.cfm?setid =ee9ad9ed-6d9f-4ee1-9d7f-cfad438df388

Imipramine: https://dailymed.nlm.nih.gov/dailymed/drugInfo.cfm?setid =2f7d5e7f-79aa-4f3a-b9a6-758d9f3ce74d

Isosorbide dinitrate spray: https://health.gsk.sg/content/dam/global/Health/en_ SG/pdf/i/Isoket_Spray_PI_NCDS03SI_approved_2Oct14.pdf

Lidocaine patch 5%: https://dailymed.nlm.nih.gov/dailymed/drugInfo.cfm?setid =f1c40164-4626-4290-9012-c00e33420a33

Metoclopramide: https://dailymed.nlm.nih.gov/dailymed/drugInfo.cfm?setid =de55c133-eb08-4a35-91a2-5dc093027397

Nortriptyline: https://dailymed.nlm.nih.gov/dailymed/drugInfo.cfm?setid =e17dc299-f52d-414d-ab6e-e809bd6f8acb

Pregabalin: https://dailymed.nlm.nih.gov/dailymed/drugInfo.cfm?setid =60185c88-ecfd-46f9-adb9-b97c6b00a553

Sildenafil: https://dailymed.nlm.nih.gov/dailymed/drugInfo.cfm?setid=0b0be196- 0c62-461c-94f4-9a35339b4501

Tadalafil: https://dailymed.nlm.nih.gov/dailymed/drugInfo.cfm?setid=bcd8f8ab- 81a2-4891-83db-24a0b0e25895

Valproate: https://dailymed.nlm.nih.gov/dailymed/drugInfo.cfm?setid=6b4331f5- 4475-417a-6a9d-09c2f8334235

Vardenafil: https://dailymed.nlm.nih.gov/dailymed/drugInfo.cfm?setid =a01def95-c0ef-43b9-bd9e-5565b2385ad3

Venlafaxine ER: https://dailymed.nlm.nih.gov/dailymed/drugInfo.cfm?setid =53c3e7ac-1852-4d70-d2b6-4fca819acf26

REFERENCES

1. Vinik A. Diabetic sensory and motor neuropathy. *N Engl J Med* 2016;374:1455–1464

2. Sima AA, Kamiya H. Diabetic neuropathy differs in type 1 and type 2 diabetes. *Ann NY Acad Sci* 2006;1084:235–249

3. Vinik A, Nevoret M-L, Casellini C, Parson H. Diabetic neuropathy. In *Acute and Chronic Complications of Diabetes*. Poretsky L, Liao EP, Eds. Amsterdam, Elsevier, 2013, p. 747–787

4. Ziegler D, Papanas N, Vinik AI, Shaw JE. Epidemiology of polyneuropathy in diabetes and prediabetes. In *Diabetes and the Nervous System*. Zochodne DW, Malik RA, Eds. Vol. 126 of *Handbook of Clinical Neurology*. 3rd series. Amsterdam, Elsevier, 2014, p. 3–22

5. Rahman H, Jha MK, Suk K. Evolving insights into the pathophysiology of diabetic neuropathy: implications of malfunctioning glia and discovery of novel therapeutic targets. *Curr Pharm Des* 2016;22:738–757

6. Tomlinson DR, Gardiner NJ. Glucose neurotoxicity. *Nat Rev Neurosci* 2008;9:36–45

7. Hinder LM, Vivekanandan-Giri A, McLean LL, et al. Decreased glycolytic and tricarboxylic acid cycle intermediates coincide with peripheral nervous system oxidative stress in a murine model of type 2 diabetes. *J Endocrinol* 2013;216:1–11

8. Triplitt CL, Repas T, Alvarez C. Diabetes mellitus. In *Pharmacotherapy: A Physiological Approach*. 10th ed. Dipiro DT, Talbert RL, et al., Eds. New York, McGraw-Hill, 2017, p. 1174

9. Neurontin (gabapentin) Clinical Pharmacology. Pfizer Medical Information. Available from https://www.pfizermedicalinformation.com/en-us/neurontin/clinical-pharmacology. Accessed 5 May 2018

10. Bockbrader HN, Wesche D, Miller R, et al. A comparison of the pharmacokinetics and pharmacodynamics of pregabalin and gabapentin. *Clin Pharmacokinet* 2010;49(10):661–669

11. Wiffen PJ, Derry S, Bell RF, et al. Gabapentin for chronic neuropathic pain in adults. *Cochrane Database Syst Rev* 2017;6:CD007938

12. Arnold L, McCarberg B, Clair AG, et al. Dose-response of pregabalin for diabetic peripheral neuropathy, postherpetic neuralgia, and fibromyalgia. *Postgrad Med* 2017;129(8):921–933

13. Finnerup NB, Attal N, Haroutounian S, et al. Pharmacotherapy for neuropathic pain in adults: a systematic review and meta-analysis. *Lancet Neurol* 2015;14(2):162–173

14. Kristensen JH, Ilett KF, Hackett PL, Kohan R. Gabapentin and breastfeeding: a case report. *J Human Lactation* 2006;22(4):426–428

15. Saeed T, Nasrullah M, Ghafoor A, et al. Efficacy and tolerability of carbamazepine for the treatment of painful diabetic neuropathy in adults: a 12-week, open-label, multicenter study. *Int J Gen Med* 2014;7:339–343

16. Rakitin A. Does Valproic acid have potential in the treatment of diabetes mellitus? *Front Endocrinol* (Lausanne) 2017;8:147

17. Bril V, England J, Franklin GM, et al. Evidence-based guideline: treatment of painful diabetic neuropathy: report of the American Academy of Neurology, the American Association of Neuromuscular and Electrodiagnostic Medicine, and the American Academy of Physical Medicine and Rehabilitation. *Neurology* 2011;76(20):1758–1765

18. Sansone RA, Sansone LA. Pain, pain, go away: antidepressants and pain management. *Psychiatry* (Edgmont) 2008;5:16–19

19. Griebeler ML, Morey-Vargas OL, Brito JP, et al. Pharmacological interventions for painful diabetic neuropathy: an umbrella systematic review and comparative effectiveness network meta-analysis. *Ann Intern Med* 2014;161:639–649

20. Snyder MJ, Gibbs LM, Lindsay TJ. Treating painful diabetic peripheral neuropathy: an update. *Am Fam Physician* 2016;94(3):227–234

21. Lindsay TJ, Rodgers BC, Savath V, Hettinger K. Treating diabetic peripheral neuropathic pain. *Am Fam Physician* 2010;82(2):151–158

22. Wong MC, Chung JW, Wong TK. Effects of treatments for symptoms of painful diabetic neuropathy: systematic review. *BMJ* 2007;335(7610):87

23. Yuen K, Baker N, Rayman G. Treatment of chronic painful diabetic neuropathy with isosorbide dinitrate spray. *Diabetes Care* 2002;25(10):1699–1703

24. Pop-Busui R, Boulton AJ, Feldman EL, et al. Diabetic neuropathy: a position statement by the American Diabetes Association. *Diabetes Care* 2017;40(1):136–154

25. Kumar M, Chapman A, Javed S, et al. The investigation and treatment of diabetic gastroparesis. *Clin Ther* 2018;40(6):850–861

26. Youssef AS, Parkman HP, Nagar S. Drug-drug interactions in pharmacologic management of gastroparesis. *Neurogastroenterol Motil* 2015;27(11):1528–1541

27. Ali T, Hasan M, Hamadani M, Harty RF. Gastroparesis. *South Med J* 2007;100:281–286

28. Keshavarzian A, Isaac RM. Erythromycin accelerates gastric emptying of indigestible solids and transpyloric migration of the tip of an enteral feeding tube in fasting and fed states. *Am J Gastroenterol* 1993;88:193

29. Maganti K, Onyemere K, Jones MP. Oral erythromycin and symptomatic relief of gastroparesis: a systematic review. *Am J Gastroenterol* 2003;98:259

30. Camilleri M, Parkman HP, Shafi MA, et al.; American College of Gastroenterology. Clinical guideline: management of gastroparesis. *Am J Gastroenterol* 2013;108:18–37

31. Huang SA, Lie JD. Phosphodiesterase-5 (PDE5) inhibitors in the management of erectile dysfunction. *P T* 2013;38(7):407–419

32. Kamenov ZA. A comprehensive review of erectile dysfunction in men with diabetes. *Exp Clin Endocrinol Diabetes* 2015;123(3):141–158

Chapter 24
Medications for the Management of Nephropathy

Emmeline Tran, PharmD

INTRODUCTION

CKD resulting from diabetes is known as diabetic kidney disease (DKD) or diabetic nephropathy. DKD is typically characterized by the presence of albuminuria and/or reduced eGFR not attributable to other causes of renal injury.[1] This broad definition of DKD has made it difficult to compare and contrast relevant results from trials since renal endpoints in these trials have not always been consistent.

Approximately 20–40% of patients with diabetes have DKD.[1] Risk factors for DKD are both modifiable and nonmodifiable. Modifiable risk factors include poor glycemic control, hypertension, dyslipidemia, and obesity. Nonmodifiable risk factors include older age; male sex; early age of onset of diabetes; family history; African American, Native American, Hispanic, Asian, or Pacific Islander race or ethnicity; and genetics.[2,3] Progression of DKD to ESRD can occur. In fact, the major cause of ESRD in the U.S. is diabetes.[4] Moreover, patients with DKD have a substantial cost burden. This is principally driven by the strong association with CVD among this patient population and by the development of ESRD.[4-6]

The pathophysiology of DKD involves a multifactorial process driven by histological changes in the glomeruli. Mesangial expansion occurs initially followed by thickening of the glomerular basement membrane and, lastly, glomerular sclerosis.[7] Collectively, these changes result in glomerular hyperfiltration, glomerular hypertension, and renal hypertrophy, which are clinically manifested as albuminuria and hypertension.[7] The natural history of DKD aligns with the histological changes, moving from progressive albuminuria to declining GFR, and ultimately ESRD.[3] However, it must be noted that not all patients with DKD present in the conventional manner described. Some patients may present with GFR loss independent from albuminuria.[8]

GOALS OF TREATMENT

Considerable morbidity, mortality, and costs are associated with DKD.[4] Once DKD is established, it is only possible to slow progression. Additionally, DKD is strongly associated with CVD, and most patients with DKD die from CVD prior to needing dialysis.[3,9] Consequently, the goals of DKD treatment are to prevent DKD development and progression, to improve quality of life, and to reduce morbidity and mortality.

Despite limitations in these surrogate markers, it is generally accepted that GFR (estimating kidney function) and albuminuria (assessing kidney injury) are used to help identify and monitor DKD. In general, an eGFR of <60 mL/min/1.73 m^2, and a urinary albumin excretion (UAE) ≥30 mg/g creatinine are considered to be abnormal.[1] However, variations may be seen in the literature, especially in regard to studies examining the efficacy of treatment options in DKD. Of note, the terms "microalbuminuria" (30–300 mg/g creatinine) and "macroalbuminuria" (>300 mg/g creatinine) are no longer favored. Instead, reporting of urine albumin level as a continuous variable is preferred.[10] Although there is guidance correlating these laboratory parameters with initiation of pharmacological treatment, guidance on use of these parameters to monitor efficacy of the treatment implemented is less clear.[1,10] Furthermore, correlation of specific targets with improved patient-centered outcomes is inconclusive. A meta-analysis of two large clinical trials suggests that a 30% reduction in albuminuria may translate into a 30% reduction in risk of ESRD.[11]

MEDICATIONS

Development and progression of DKD is believed to be driven by glomerular hyperfiltration, and in turn, glomerular hypertension. Under diabetic conditions, afferent arterioles are dilated, and blood flow into the glomeruli is increased, causing elevated intraglomerular pressure. These changes induce inflammation and oxidative stress in the glomeruli, leading to the excessive production of extracellular matrix, which plays a key role in the development of glomerulosclerosis. Studies have shown that reducing intraglomerular pressure is associated with renal protection.[12,13] Medications targeting this pathogenesis mechanism are a central focus and therapeutic option in patients with DKD. Although inflammation, oxidative stress, and fibrosis also contribute to the pathogenesis of DKD, attempts to target these mechanisms have been less successful.

Although a targeted mechanistic approach on the kidneys is described, prevention and treatment of DKD lies heavily with glycemic control, hypertension, and cardiovascular risk reduction. Several landmark trials have proven the benefits of glycemic control on reducing progression of DKD in both patients with T1D[14,15] and patients with T2D.[16–20] The effect of antihypertensive therapy on DKD will be discussed below. Although statin therapy has not been found to inhibit the progression of kidney disease,[21] it has been shown to be beneficial in reducing CVD events and mortality in patients with non-dialysis-dependent CKD, with or without diabetes.[22] Conversely, benefits of statin therapy on CVD events or mortality have not been found in patients on dialysis.[23] Therefore, initiating statin therapy in patients on dialysis is not recommended. However, continuation of statin therapy in those who progress to dialysis may be considered.

RENIN-ANGIOTENSIN SYSTEM INHIBITORS

Renin-angiotensin system (RAS) inhibition, through the use of ACE inhibitors, ARBs, or direct renin inhibitors, is the most effective therapy for slowing the progression of DKD. ACE inhibitors, ARBs, and renin inhibitors favorably affect intraglomerular pressure by lowering systemic blood pressure and reducing efferent arteriolar vasoconstriction.[24]

Furthermore, the beneficial effects of ACE inhibitors and ARBs are found to be independent of their effects on systemic blood pressure.[25-29] Specifically, long-term renoprotective effects are believed to be related to an initial rise in serum creatinine of up to 30% and decreased intraglomerular pressure.[12,13] The level of evidence supporting the efficacy of these classes of medications on renal outcomes is driven by the studied patient population, specifically type of diabetes mellitus, presence of hypertension, and presence of albuminuria.

T1D with Hypertension and Albuminuria

The Captopril Study established the role of ACE inhibitors in the treatment of DKD in patients with T1D, mild to moderate hypertension (mean blood pressure of 139/86 mmHg), and established nephropathy (mean urinary protein excretion of 2,750 mg per 24 h).[25] Specifically, captopril statistically significantly reduced the risk of doubling of serum creatinine and the decline in creatinine clearance rate, and decreased the risk of the composite endpoint of death, dialysis, and transplantation compared with placebo over a median follow-up of 3 years. Moreover, remission of nephrotic syndrome in a subset of these patients with nephrotic-range proteinuria was established and sustained at approximately 8 years. Remission was defined as a decrease in proteinuria from >3,500 mg per 24 h to <1,000 mg per 24 h and sustained for at least 6 months at <1,500 mg per 24 h.[30,31]

T1D with Normotension and Albuminuria

Use of ACE inhibitors to prevent worsening renal function in patients with T1D who have albuminuria but no hypertension has been studied and was found to be efficacious. The combined results of two large clinical trials in patients with T1D, normotension (mean blood pressure of 122/77 mmHg), and albuminuria (geometric mean albumin excretion rate of 59 µg/min) showed that captopril statistically significantly decreased the risk of progression to overt clinical albuminuria, UAE rate, and decline in CrCl compared with placebo at 24 months.[32-34] Follow-up to one of the studies at 8 years found statistically significant benefits related to UAE rate, but not in rate of decline in GFR.[35]

A Cochrane review found that ACE inhibitors reduced the risk of new onset kidney disease by 29% and the risk of death by 16% in individuals with diabetes.[36] Clear renal benefits were observed among individuals without hypertension at baseline and in comparison to calcium channel blockers (CCBs). These effects were consistent regardless of type of diabetes, presence of hypertension, or comparator group (placebo-controlled studies or studies comparing ACE inhibitors to other blood pressure agents). In contrast, use of ARBs did not find the same benefits. Most ARB studies in this meta-analysis recruited mainly normotensive patients at lower renal and vascular risk. Consequently, study power was limited.[36]

T1D with Hypertension and Normoalbuminuria

Studies specifically examining DKD outcomes in patients with T1D, hypertension, and normoalbuminuria are lacking. This may be explained by the more common presence of microalbuminuria prior to the onset of hypertension in patients with T1D. The onset of hypertension appears to be an effect of DKD rather than a cause.[37]

T1D with Normotension and Normoalbuminuria

Literature supporting the use of RAS inhibitors in patients with normotension and normoalbuminuria is equivocal. Patients with T1D, normotension (median blood pressure of 122/80 mmHg), and mainly normoalbuminuria (84%) were studied to investigate the effects of lisinopril on prevention of diabetic nephropathy in the EUCLID study.[38] Although lisinopril was found to have a statistically significant effect on decreasing the progression of microalbuminuria in those with albuminuria at baseline, no difference was found in those with normoalbuminuria.

On the other hand, another study found benefits with the use of an ACE inhibitor on primary prevention of diabetic nephropathy. The Renal and Retinal Effects of Enalapril and Losartan in Type 1 Diabetes (RASS) study examined the renal preventative effects of enalapril and losartan in patients with T1D, normotension (mean blood pressure of 120/70 mmHg), and normoalbuminuria (median UAE rate of 5.1 µg/min).[39] When compared to placebo, enalapril statistically significantly prevented the increase of UAE rate and decreased the incidence of albuminuria at 5 years, but losartan did not. No effects on GFR were found with either medication.

The Diabetic Retinopathy Candesartan Trials Renal (DIRECT-Renal) study pooled three clinical trials to determine whether candesartan prevents the onset of albuminuria in patients with T1D or T2D.[40] Of the patients with diabetes, about 64% had T1D. All patients were normotensive and normoalbuminuric. Similarly, no difference was found on development of albuminuria (defined as a UAE rate of ≥20 µg/min) or on change in UAE rate compared with placebo.

T2D with Hypertension and Albuminuria

Although there has been much less information, similar findings with ACE inhibitors have been observed in patients with T2D. The MICRO-Heart Outcomes Prevention Evaluation (MICRO-HOPE) substudy of the HOPE trial assessed whether or not similar renal protective effects with ACE inhibitors seen in patients with T1D could be obtained in patients with T2D.[41] Approximately one-third of the patients were defined as having a urinary ACR of 17.7 mg/g creatinine or higher. Additionally, about 56% of patients had a history of hypertension, and the mean blood pressure at baseline was 142/80 mmHg. When compared with placebo, ramipril statistically significantly decreased the progression to overt nephropathy. In patients with normoalbuminuria, the risk of development of albuminuria was reduced, but not significantly. Of note, although the term is no longer in use, microalbuminuria, as defined by the study, is slightly different than what has been previously considered the cutoff (30–300 mg/g creatinine). Moreover, the benefit on mortality found in the trial can be attributable only to patients with T2D at an increased risk for CVD but without established diabetic nephropathy.

More data are available on the efficacy of ARBs in T2D than in T1D. As with the ACE inhibitors, efficacy findings correlate with level of albuminuria. The Irbesartan in Patients with Type 2 Diabetes and Microalbuminuria (IRMA-2) trial examined the effect of irbesartan on the development of diabetic nephropathy in patients with T2D, hypertension (mean blood pressure of 153/90 mmHg), and albuminuria between 20–200 µg/min (geometric mean UAE rate of 57 µg/min).[26] Irbesartan achieved statistical significance in decreasing the progression to overt nephropathy, reducing UAE rate, and restoring normoalbuminuria compared with placebo. No statistically significant difference was found in the rate of decline in CrCl. The MicroAlbuminuria Reduction With VALsartan (MARVAL) study examined a similar patient population (T2D, hypertension with mean blood pressure of 148/86 mmHg, and albuminuria between 20–200 µg/min with a mean of UAE rate of 57 µg/min), but compared an ARB (valsartan) to amlodipine instead of placebo.[27] Valsartan statistically significantly reduced the UAE rate compared with amlodipine regardless of baseline blood pressure.

Benefits of ARBs on patients with higher levels of albuminuria at baseline have also been established. The Irbesartan Diabetic Nephropathy Trial (IDNT)[28] and Reduction of Endpoints in NIDDM with the Angiotensin II Antagonist Losartan (RENAAL)[42] trials examined the effects of ARBs in patients with T2D, hypertension (mean blood pressures of 159/87 mmHg and 153/82 mmHg, respectively), and nephropathy (median UAE rate of 1,900 mg per 24 h and median urinary ACR of 1,249 mg/g creatinine, respectively). In the IDNT trial, irbesartan was associated with a statistically significant decrease in the risk of the composite endpoint (doubling of serum creatinine, onset of ESRD, or death) compared with amlodipine and placebo.[28] The composite outcome was driven mainly by statistically significant benefits achieved by irbesartan in decreasing the risk of doubling serum creatinine and ESRD. Losartan achieved similar results compared with placebo using the same composite endpoint in the RENAAL trial.[42]

Although most trials examining aliskiren were in combination with ACE inhibitors or ARBs, there are a few studies examining aliskiren monotherapy on progression of diabetic nephropathy. In a small exploratory study examining the effect of aliskiren in patients with T2D, hypertension (mean blood pressure of 146/76 mmHg), and albuminuria (median urinary ACR of 158 mg/g creatinine), aliskiren was found to reduce urinary ACR significantly, but not eGFR, at 28 days compared with baseline.[43] Another larger study compared the antiproteinuric effect of aliskiren to that of ramipril.[44] Patients had T2D, hypertension (mean blood pressure of 159/94 mmHg), and albuminuria defined as a UAE rate of >200 and <300 mg per day (mean UAE rate of 258 mg per day). Aliskiren was found to have a statistically significantly greater and more prolonged effect on decreasing UAE rate compared with ramipril. The authors attribute this finding to a higher degree of intrarenal renin-angiotensin-aldosterone system (RAAS) blockade.

T2D with Normotension and Albuminuria

A small trial compared the effects of enalapril to placebo on patients with T2D, normotension, and microalbuminuria defined as a UAE rate of 30–300 mg per 24 h.[45] Enalapril statistically significantly slowed progression to nephropathy compared with placebo. Benefits persisted through 7 years.

T2D with Hypertension and Normoalbuminuria

Use of an RAS inhibitor for primary prevention in patients with T2D is supported by a few trials. The Bergamo Nephrologic Diabetes Complication Trial (BENEDICT) trial examined the effects of trandolapril with verapamil, trandolapril monotherapy, verapamil monotherapy, or placebo on the development of albuminuria defined as an overnight UAE rate of ≥20 µg/min.[46] Patients had T2D, hypertension (mean blood pressure of 151/88 mmHg), and normoalbuminuria (median UAE rate of 5.3 µg/min). Development of albuminuria was significantly delayed in patients receiving trandolapril with verapamil or trandolapril monotherapy, but not verapamil monotherapy, compared with placebo.

Instead of an ACE inhibitor, the Randomized Olmesartan And Diabetes MicroAlbuminuria Prevention (ROADMAP) trial investigated the effects of an ARB (olmesartan) for primary prevention of albuminuria in patients with T2D and hypertension (mean blood pressure of 136/81 mmHg).[47] Albuminuria was defined as a urinary ACR of >35 mg/g creatinine in females and >25 mg/g creatinine in males. The geometric mean baseline urinary ACR was 6.1 mg/g creatinine. Olmesartan was associated with a statistically significantly longer time to the development of albuminuria compared with placebo.

T2D with Normotension and Normoalbuminuria

Again, in patients with normotension and normoalbuminuria, the literature is less clear. The Appropriate Blood Pressure Control in Diabetes (ABCD) study examining the effects of enalapril or nisoldipine on primary prevention of diabetic nephropathy found that a lower percentage of patients progressed from normoalbuminuria to microalbuminuria regardless of antihypertensive agent used, but observed no difference in CrCl.[48] Patients in this study had T2D and normotension (mean blood pressure of 136/84 mmHg). Approximately 66% of patients had normoalbuminuria. Similarly, another study in patients with T2D, normotension (mean systolic blood pressure of 97 mmHg), and normoalbuminuria (mean UAE rate of 11.2 mg per 24 h) found benefits of enalapril on decreasing the risk of new onset microalbuminuria and UAE, and preventing CrCl in declining substantially.[49]

Patients with T2D in the DIRECT-Renal study (36%) were generally normotensive or well controlled on antihypertensive medications.[40] All patients were normoalbuminuric. As previously mentioned, candesartan was not found to have a benefit in preventing the development of albuminuria or decreasing UAE rate when compared with placebo.

Of note, two randomized controlled trials examining the renoprotective effects of olmesartan in patients with T2D observed an increase in the number of cardiovascular-related deaths in the olmesartan group compared with the placebo group.[47,50] The FDA conducted a safety review and found no clear evidence of increased cardiovascular risk associated with the use of olmesartan in patients with diabetes. A recent meta-analysis also confirmed no difference in cardiovascular risk.[51]

ACE Inhibitors versus ARBs

Comparisons of ACE inhibitors to ARBs on their effects in diabetic nephropathy are relatively limited.[52] The majority of evidence from controlled clinical trials supports the use of ACE inhibitors in patients with T1D and ARBs in patients with T2D. A noninferiority study (Diabetics Exposed to Telmisartan And enaplaIL [DETAIL]) comparing the effect of telmisartan and enalapril on the change in GFR in patients with T2D, mild to moderate hypertension (mean blood pressure of 152/86 mmHg), and albuminuria with a UAE rate between

11–999 µg/min (median UAE rate 53 µg/min) found telmisartan to be not inferior to enalapril in change in GFR over 5 years.[53]

Limitations in comparative studies of ACE inhibitors and ARBs make it difficult to clearly define superiority of one class over another in the prevention and treatment of diabetic nephropathy. Mixed findings showing benefits of one class over another have been observed in reviews and meta-analyses.[52,54–57] Clinical determination of using one class over another may be driven by side-effect profile. ACE inhibitors have traditionally been associated with a dry cough whereas ARBs have not.[52]

In summary, studies investigating the use of RAS inhibitors on improving renal outcomes in patients with normotension and albuminuria are lacking. Furthermore, the data supporting use of RAS inhibitors in the setting of normoalbuminuria are inconsistent and suggest no clear benefit over other antihypertensive agents. In those patients with hypertension and albuminuria, it is generally accepted that the renal protective benefit is a class effect. However, studies examining specific dosing of each medication within each class are not available. Consequently, equivalent doses that may confer renoprotective effects are unknown when converting from one medication to another within a class.

SGLT2 INHIBITORS

SGLT2 inhibitors are believed to exert renoprotection through direct and indirect effects. The direct renal effects of SGLT2 inhibitors are thought to be related to activation of tubuloglomerular feedback through reduction in sodium reabsorption in the proximal tubules and consequently increased distal sodium delivery to the macula densa.[58] The increased sodium delivery is perceived as an increase in circulating volume causing constriction of the afferent renal arterioles and reduction in intraglomerular pressure. Indirect effects occur through suppression of renal glucose reabsorption for improved glycemic control.[58]

The potential efficacy of canagliflozin on progression of diabetic nephropathy was examined in the CANVAS-R[59] and CANagliflozin Treatment And Trial Analysis-Sulfonylurea (CANTATA-SU)[60] trials as secondary outcomes or analyses. All patients in the CANVAS-R trial had T2D (mean A1C of 8.2%) and high cardiovascular risk, 30% of patients had albuminuria, and 80% of patients were on a RAAS inhibitor at baseline.[59] Outcomes of *1*) progression to albuminuria and *2*) the composite endpoint of 40% reduction in GFR, need for renal replacement therapy, or death from renal causes occurred less frequently in patients receiving canagliflozin compared with placebo. Additionally, regression of albuminuria occurred more frequently among patients on canagliflozin compared with placebo. As with the CANVAS-R trial, all patients in the CANTATA-SU trials had T2D (mean A1C of 7.8%).[60] The median urinary ACR at baseline in the CANTATA-SU was 8.5 mg/g creatinine; approximately 16% of patients had a baseline urinary ACR ≥30 mg/g creatinine; and approximately 61% of patients received background RAAS inhibition. Canagliflozin at both the 100-mg and 300-mg dose was associated with a decreased rate of decline in GFR compared with glimepiride, and canagliflozin 300 mg was associated with a decreased urinary ACR compared with glimepiride. Changes in A1C were similar in both groups. Therefore, the renal benefits found are thought to be independent of the glycemic effects of canagliflozin.

A secondary analysis of prespecified renal outcomes was also conducted in the EMPA-REG OUTCOME trial to assess the renal effects of empagliflozin in patients with T2D (mean A1C of 8.1%) at high risk for cardiovascular events.[61] Approximately 30% of patients had a urinary ACR of 30–300 mg/g creatinine and ~13% had a urinary ACR of >300 mg/g creatinine. Most patients (82%) were on a RAAS inhibitor at baseline. Significant benefits were found in those receiving empagliflozin compared with placebo in incident or worsening nephropathy, progression to albuminuria of >300 mg/g creatinine, doubling of serum creatinine, and initiation of renal replacement therapy. However, no difference was found in regard to rate of incident albuminuria in patients with a normal albumin level at baseline. The CREDENCE trial was conducted to specifically examine the effects of empagliflozin on renal outcomes. Patients included had T2D (mean A1C of 8.3%) and were at high risk of kidney disease (median urinary ACR of 927 mg/g).[62] Although the specific findings of the trial have not yet been published, the trial was stopped early for positive efficacy findings.[63] The primary outcome was a composite endpoint of ESRD, doubling of serum creatinine, and renal or cardiovascular death.

Lastly, dapagliflozin was assessed for renal effects in patients with T2D (mean A1C of 8.4%) and moderate renal impairment, defined as eGFR values of 30–59 mL/min/1.73 m[2].[64] As with the other trials, renal outcomes were secondary objectives. The median urinary ACR was 73 mg/g creatinine, with about 71% of patients with diabetic nephropathy. RAAS inhibitor use was not reported. Individuals in the dapagliflozin group were more likely to regress to a lower UAE category than individuals in the placebo group.

Although not an FDA-approved indication, SGLT2 inhibitors have been studied in patients with T1D. In particular, the effects of empagliflozin were investigated in a small trial of patients with T1D, and were found to attenuate renal hypertension over a period of 8 weeks.[65]

Overall, although findings of these trials suggest benefits in the setting of diabetic nephropathy, the majority of patients examined did not have evidence of DKD at baseline. As such, it is difficult to ascertain whether or not SGLT2 inhibitors can be added to the pharmacologic armamentarium in treating diabetic nephropathy. Several clinical trials are being conducted to evaluate the effect of SGLT2 inhibitors in patients with DKD.

Common side effects related to this class include an increased risk of genital infections.[66] The FDA released a warning on the increased risk of a serious rare genital infection, Fournier's gangrene, with the use of SGLT2 inhibitors. Of note, renal function was not found to be a clinical risk factor in predicting genital fungal infections in patients taking SGLT2 inhibitors.[67] However, safety outcomes are still being explored. It is also important to take into account the FDA alerts regarding the risk of AKI in patients taking canagliflozin and dapagliflozin. A retrospective study published after the release of the FDA drug safety communication found no increased risk of AKI.[68] Further studies are needed to confirm these findings.

GLP-1 RAs AND DPP-4 INHIBITORS

In addition to their effects on glycemic control, GLP-1 RAs and DPP-4 inhibitors potentially have direct beneficial effects on renal function independent of their glucose-lowering effects. Most studies investigating the mechanisms of action of these medications on diabetic nephropathy have been in animal studies or models. Elucidated mechanisms of actions include inhibition of inflammatory markers, attenuation of angiotensin II–mediated effects, and modulation of sodium-water homeostasis.[69] Extrapolation of these findings to humans should be done cautiously, and data are insufficient to discriminate whether the effect of these medications on nephropathy is due to improvement of glycemic control or direct action on the kidneys.

In general, like the SGLT2 inhibitors, the renal effects of these medications are mainly derived from secondary analyses of trials with primary outcomes related to cardiovascular effects of these agents in patients with T2D.

The LEADER trial examined the effects of liraglutide on prespecified secondary renal outcomes in patients with T2D (mean A1C of 8.7%).[70] Microalbuminuria was present in 26.3% of patients and macroalbuminuria was present in 10.5% of patients at randomization. Approximately 84% of patients received RAAS inhibitors at baseline. The composite renal outcome of new-onset persistent macroalbuminuria, persistent doubling of serum creatinine and eGFR of 45 mL/min/1.73 m^2 or less, the need for renal replacement therapy, or death from renal disease occurred in fewer patients receiving liraglutide than in those receiving placebo. The statistical significance achieved in the composite outcome was driven primarily by differences found in new-onset persistent macroalbuminuria in those on liraglutide compared with placebo. Additionally, the urinary ACR increased less in patients receiving liraglutide compared with placebo. Although the decrease in eGFR was lower in the liraglutide group, this is likely not clinically significant (difference of 0.38 mL/min/1.73 m^2).

Semaglutide and its effects on renal function were investigated as a prespecified secondary outcome in the SUSTAIN-6 trial.[71] Patients had T2D (mean A1C of 8.7%), and a majority were on an ACE inhibitor or ARB (~84%). Albuminuria status at baseline was not reported. The same composite outcome used in the LEADER trial was examined and found to have similar results: patients in the semaglutide group experienced the composite outcome less frequently than those in the placebo group. Again, this was driven by benefits seen with semaglutide on the development of new-onset persistent macroalbuminuria.

Lixisenatide was found to decrease the percentage change in urinary ACR from baseline favorably compared with placebo in the ELIXA trial.[72] As with the previous trials, renal outcomes were considered to be an additional efficacy variable examined. Patients had T2D (mean A1C of 7.7%) and normoalbuminuria (median urinary ACR of 10.3 mg/g creatinine). About 85% of patients were taking an ACE inhibitor or ARB at baseline. The change in urinary ACR was found to be statistically significant in favor of lixisenatide. However, this may not be clinically significant (difference of 1.5 mg/g creatinine between groups).

Meta-analyses examining the effects of GLP-1 RAs on diabetic nephropathy have shown conflicting results.[73,74]

In regard to DPP-4 inhibitors, similar benefits on diabetic nephropathy have been seen, but, again, the data are limited and mainly derived from secondary analyses of controlled clinical trials.

A pooled analysis of all randomized, double-blind, and placebo-controlled trials of linagliptin was conducted to assess the renal effects of the medication.[75] Patients had T2D (mean A1C of 8.2%); 66% of patients had a urinary ACR of 30 mg/g creatinine or less. Approximately 45% of patients were on ACE inhibitors or ARBs at enrollment. The primary outcome examined was a composite of first occurrence of six individual and clinically relevant kidney disease endpoints. The six endpoints were new onset of moderate elevation of albuminuria, new onset of severe elevation of albuminuria, reduction in kidney function, halving of eGFR, incidence of acute renal failure, and death from any cause. This composite outcome occurred less frequently in patients receiving linagliptin compared with placebo, and was driven by differences seen with new onset of moderate elevation of albuminuria in favor of linagliptin. Changes in urinary ACR also favored linagliptin.

The SAVOR-TIMI 53[76, 77] (saxagliptin versus placebo), EXAMINE[78] (alogliptin versus placebo), and TECOS[79, 80] (sitagliptin versus placebo) trials reported renal outcomes as other efficacy or safety endpoints. Benefits in change in urinary ACR were seen with saxagliptin and sitagliptin compared with placebo in patients in which urinary ACR data were available. The difference in mean change in urinary ACR in patients receiving saxagliptin compared with placebo was mainly driven by differences in change in urinary ACR among patients with urinary ACRs >300 mg/g creatinine at baseline, but was statistically significant at any level of albuminuria.[77]

An observational cohort study was conducted to determine the renoprotective effects of DPP-4 inhibitors and found benefit with use of these agents, especially in patients with macroalbuminuria.[81] Patients with macroalbuminuria experienced significant reductions in albumin levels, but patients with normoalbuminuria or microalbuminuria did not. Similarly, reductions in eGFR were reversed in patients with macroalbuminuria or normoalbuminuria and slowed in patients with microalbuminuria.

Currently, not enough data are available to determine whether the effect of these two classes of medications on diabetic nephropathy is independent of its glycemic effects.

CCBs

The renoprotective role of CCBs is more equivocal than that of the RAS inhibitors. In part, this may be due to the fact that effects on nephropathy may be highly dependent on the individual CCB. In addition to blood pressure–lowering effects that impact the development and progression of diabetic nephropathy, certain CCBs have intrarenal effects. In general, nondihydropyridine calcium antagonists (NDCAs) reduce glomerular membrane permeability, especially to large molecules such as proteins.[82] On the other hand, dihydropyridine calcium antagonists (DCAs) preferentially vasodilate the afferent arteriole, increasing glomerular pressure and perhaps negating the beneficial effects of blood-pressure reduction.[83] However, there potentially are some exceptions.[84]

NDCAs versus DCAs

The difficulty in establishing the benefits of CCBs for renoprotection in patients with diabetes potentially stems from inconsistent findings in the literature when examining the medication class as a whole. However, when breaking down the class into subclasses, benefits are found beyond blood pressure–lowering effects with the NDCAs compared with the DCAs. A systematic review examining the differences in these subclasses and their effects on proteinuria in individuals with hypertension (mean blood pressure of 162/97 mmHg) found that although these two subclasses of calcium antagonists lower blood pressure to a similar degree, NDCAs provide greater reductions in proteinuria regardless of diabetes status or background ACE inhibitor or ARB therapy.[83] Of note, the number of studies examining patients with diabetes on concomitant calcium antagonists and RAS inhibitor therapy was limited, and of these, a majority examined ACE inhibitor and NDCA combinations.

CCBs versus RAS Inhibitors

In studies comparing calcium antagonists to ACE inhibitors or ARBs in patients with diabetes and albuminuria, renoprotection by calcium antagonists was often inferior. However, most of the head-to-head comparison trials included a DCA rather than an NDCA.

A small trial compared the effects of diltiazem to lisinopril on diabetic nephropathy.[85] Patients had T2D, hypertension (mean arterial blood pressure of 118 mmHg), and nephrotic-range proteinuria (mean urinary protein excretion of 4,100 mg per 24 h). Both medications reduced urinary protein excretion by relatively the same amount over 6 weeks.

The MARVAL trial was a larger study that also compared the renal effects of a CCB to an RAS inhibitor, but in patients with lower albuminuria levels.[27] Specifically, valsartan was compared with amlodipine to determine their effects on UAE rate in patients with T2D and albuminuria of 20–200 µg/min. Valsartan was more effective in lowering UAE rates compared with amlodipine. Similar findings were seen in the IDNT trial, but with irbesartan compared with amlodipine.[28]

MINERALOCORTICOID RECEPTOR ANTAGONISTS

Contribution of aldosterone to the development of renal fibrosis and sclerosis has mainly been shown in experimental models or animals.[86] Consequently, medications that reduce the concentration of aldosterone, and hence oxidative stress and inflammation leading to fibrosis and sclerosis, may play a renoprotective role in patients with DKD.

Studies examining mineralocorticoid receptor antagonist (MRA) monotherapy are limited. One study in patients with T1D and albuminuria, defined as a UAE rate of 30–300 mg per 24 h, observed a significant reduction in UAE rate in the spironolactone group compared with the placebo group.[87] Another study comparing the effect of spironolactone to concomitant spironolactone and losartan on diabetic nephropathy in patients with T2D and albuminuria defined as a urinary ACR of 20–200 mg/g creatinine (mean urinary ACR of 92 mg/g creatinine) found that patients on spironolactone monotherapy had a similar percentage achieve more than a 50% reduction in microalbuminuria as did patients on spironolactone and losartan combination.[88] Interestingly, no difference was found in mean serum potassium level after 3 months. The study was limited by sample size and duration.

COMBINATION THERAPY

DUAL RAS INHIBITORS

Several studies have investigated the combination of RAS inhibitors on further improving outcomes in patients with DKD. Combination ACE inhibitor and ARB treatment was studied in three large randomized controlled trials, two of which included only patients with T2D.

Benefits on albuminuria were seen with combination candesartan and lisinopril compared with either agent alone in patients with T2D, hypertension (mean blood pressure of 163/96 mmHg), and albuminuria defined as urinary ACR between 22 and 221 mg/g creatinine (geometric mean urinary ACR of 55 mg/g creatinine).[89] Specifically, combination therapy reduced urinary ACR to a greater extent than candesartan monotherapy, but not lisinopril monotherapy. No clinically significant difference was found in regard to potassium concentrations. On the other hand, the Veterans Affairs Nephropathy in Diabetes (VA-NEPHRON D) trial examining the effects of combination therapy with losartan and lisinopril was stopped early due to safety concerns related to hyperkalemia and AKI in the combination group compared with the monotherapy groups.[90]

The Ongoing Telmisartan Alone and in Combination with Ramipril Global Endpoint Trial (ONTARGET) study examined the effects of telmisartan, ramipril, or a combination of the two drugs on nephropathy as a secondary outcome.[91,92] Approximately 38% of patients had diabetes. In regard to the frequency of the composite renal outcome of dialysis, doubling of serum creatinine, and death, telmisartan and ramipril had similar effects. However, combination therapy resulted in an increased frequency of the composite endpoint. The composite endpoint was primarily driven by differences seen with acute dialysis. eGFR concentrations decreased at a greater rate in those in the telmisartan and combination groups compared with ramipril. Urinary ACRs increased to a lesser extent in those receiving telmisartan or combination therapy than in those receiving ramipril. Overall, although combination therapy reduced albuminuria to a greater extent, major renal outcomes were worse.

Combination therapy with aliskiren and an ACE inhibitor or ARB has also been examined and, like the above trials, found to have inconsistent results. The Aliskiren in the Evaluation of Proteinuria in Diabetes (AVOID) trial investigated aliskiren compared with placebo on top of losartan background therapy in patients with T2D, hypertension (mean blood pressure of 135/78 mmHg), and nephropathy defined as a urinary ACR of >300 mg/g creatinine (geometric mean urinary ACR of 533 mg/g creatinine).[93] Significantly greater reductions in urinary ACR were seen in the aliskiren group compared with the placebo group. Although there was a trend in increased serum potassium levels in those receiving aliskiren compared with those receiving placebo, it was not significant (percentage of patients with at least one value of serum potassium ≥6.0 mmol/L, 4.7% vs. 1.7%). Conversely, the Aliskiren Trial in Type 2 Diabetes Using Cardiovascular and Renal Disease Endpoints (ALTITUDE) trial examining the combination of aliskiren with an ACE inhibitor or ARB was stopped prematurely secondary to an increase in adverse effects.[94]

CCBs + RAS INHIBITORS

A greater reduction in intraglomerular pressure may be provided with the combined use of a calcium antagonist and RAS inhibitor due to effects of the calcium antagonist in reducing afferent arteriolar pressure and the RAS inhibitor in reducing efferent arteriolar pressure.

Direct comparison of the subclasses in an RAS inhibitor-calcium antagonist combination was examined in a study of patients with T2D, hypertension (mean blood pressure of 142/81 mmHg), and diabetic nephropathy (mean urinary ACR of 830 mg/g creatinine).[95] No difference was found on percentage change in urinary ACR from baseline to week 36 or final visit with trandolapril-verapamil SR compared with benazepril-amlodipine. This trial suggests that a dihydropyridine-RAS inhibitor combination may negate any negative effects DCAs may have on the kidneys. In fact, in the RENAAL trial examining the effects of losartan compared with placebo on the progression of nephropathy, a majority of patients were on a dihydropyridine at baseline and during study treatment.[42] Again, this suggests that DCAs, when used with an RAS inhibitor, do not counteract the benefits of the RAS inhibitor on nephropathy progression.

Another study observed significant reductions of proteinuria from baseline with a combination NDCA-ACE inhibitor (verapamil-trandolapril) over either agent alone.[96] This study examined patients with T2D, hypertension (mean blood pressure of 172/105 mmHg), and urinary protein excretion of >300 mg per day (mean UAE rate of 631 mg per day). However, the trial was relatively small, with 37 participants.

MRAs + RAS INHIBITORS

The concept of aldosterone breakthrough lends to the mechanistic understanding of combining an MRA and RAS inhibitor. Aldosterone breakthrough is typically defined as an elevated plasma aldosterone concentration after treatment compared with pretreatment concentrations.[97] In regard to diabetic nephropathy, aldosterone breakthrough can be thought of as sustained aldosterone synthesis during long-term RAS inhibitor therapy.

A systematic review of eight studies examined the effects of MRAs on albuminuria in patients with diabetes. Albuminuria was defined as at least 30 mg in 24-h urine collection or a urinary ACR of at least 30 mg/g creatinine.[98] Additionally, patients needed to have received an ACE inhibitor and/or ARB throughout the study. Albuminuria was reduced by 23–61% compared with standard treatment. However, this was at the expense of increased potassium levels, resulting in a drop-

Table 24.1—Medications and Dosing*

Class	Medication	Typical dose(s)	Renal dose adjustment(s)	Hepatic dose adjustment(s)
ACE Inhibitors	Captopril (Capoten)	Initial: 25 mg t.i.d.	Reduce initial dose and titrate slowly	None
	Enalapril (Vasotec)	Initial: 2.5 mg b.i.d. Max: 40 mg/day	CrCl ≤30 mL/min: initial 2.5 mg daily; titrate upward as needed HD: initial 2.5 mg after dialysis on dialysis days; adjust dose on non-dialysis days depending on blood pressure response	None or not specified
	Lisinopril (Prinivil, Zestril)	Initial: 2.5–5 mg daily Max: 80 mg/day	HD: initial 2.5 mg daily after dialysis	None or not specified
	Ramipril (Altace)	Initial: 1.25–2.5 mg daily Max: 20 mg/day	CrCl <40 mL/min: administer 25% of normal dose	None or not specified
ARBs	Candesartan (Atacand)	Initial: 4–8 mg daily Max: 32 mg/day	None or not specified	None or not specified
	Irbesartan (Avapro)	Initial: 150 mg daily Max: 300 mg/day	None or not specified	None or not specified
	Losartan (Cozaar)	Initial: 25–50 mg daily Max: 100 mg/day	None or not specified	Mild to moderate hepatic impairment: initial 25 mg once daily Severe hepatic impairment: not studied
	Olmesartan (Benicar)	Initial: 20 mg daily Max: 40 mg/day	None or not specified	None or not specified
	Telmisartan (Micardis)	Initial: 20–40 mg daily Max: 80 mg/day	None or not specified	Initiate therapy with low dose; titrate slowly and monitor closely
	Valsartan (Diovan)	Initial: 80 mg daily Max: 320 mg/day	None or not specified	None or not specified

(continued)

Table 24.1 (continued)

Class	Medication	Typical dose(s)	Renal dose adjustment(s)	Hepatic dose adjustment(s)
Direct Renin Inhibitor	Aliskiren (Tekturna)	Initial: 150 mg daily Max: 300 mg/day	None or not specified	None or not specified
SGLT2 Inhibitors	Canagliflozin (Invokana)	Initial: 100 mg daily Max: 300 mg/day	eGFR 45 to <60 mL/min/1.73 m^2: maximum dose 100 mg daily eGFR ≥30 to <45 mL/min/1.73 m^2: not recommended for initiation of therapy or when eGFR is persistently <45 mL/min/1.73 m^2 eGFR <30 mL/min/1.73 m^2, ESRD, or HD: contraindicated	None or not specified
	Dapagliflozin (Farxiga)	Initial: 5 mg daily Max: 10 mg/day	eGFR 30 to <60 mL/min/1.73 m^2: not recommended for initiation of therapy or when eGFR is persistently between 30 and <60 mL/min/1.73 m^2 eGFR <30 mL/min/1.73 m^2, ESRD, or HD: contraindicated	None or not specified
	Empagliflozin (Jardiance)	Initial: 10 mg daily Max: 25 mg/day	eGFR 30 to <45 mL/min/1.73 m^2: not recommended for initiation of therapy or when eGFR is persistently <45 mL/min/1.73 m^2 eGFR <30 mL/min/1.73 m^2, ESRD, or HD: contraindicated	None or not specified

(continued)

Table 24.1 (continued)

Class	Medication	Typical dose(s)	Renal dose adjustment(s)	Hepatic dose adjustment(s)
GLP-1 RAs	Liraglutide (Victoza)	Initial: 0.6 mg SQ daily for 1 week; then increase to 1.2 mg daily Max: 1.8 mg SQ daily	None or not specified	None or not specified
	Lixisenatide (Adlyxin)	Initial: 10 µg SQ daily for 14 days; on day 15 increase to 20 µg daily Maintenance dose: 20 µg SQ daily	eGFR <15 mL/min/1.73 m²: not recommended	None or not specified
	Semaglutide (Ozempic)	Initial: 0.25 mg SQ once weekly for 4 weeks then increase to 0.5 mg once weekly for at least 4 weeks Max: 1 mg SQ once weekly	None or not specified	None or not specified
DPP-4 Inhibitors	Alogliptin (Nesina)	25 mg daily	CrCl ≥30 to <60 mL/min: 12.5 mg daily CrCl ≥15 to <30 mL/min: 6.25 mg daily CrCl <15 mL/min or HD: 6.25 mg daily	None or not specified
	Linagliptin (Tradjenta)	5 mg daily	None or not specified	None or not specified
	Saxagliptin (Onglyza)	2.5–5 mg daily	eGFR <45 mL/min/1.73 m²: 2.5 mg daily HD: 2.5 mg daily; administer post dialysis	None or not specified
	Sitagliptin (Januvia)	100 mg daily	eGFR ≥30 to <45 mL/min/1.73 m²: 50 mg daily eGFR <30 mL/min/1.73 m²: 25 mg daily HD: 25 mg daily	None or not specified

(continued)

Table 24.1 (continued)

Class	Medication	Typical dose(s)	Renal dose adjustment(s)	Hepatic dose adjustment(s)
NDCAs	Diltiazem (Cardizem, Tiazac)	Initial: 120–180 mg daily Max: 480–540 mg/day	None or not specified	None or not specified
	Verapamil (Calan, Verelan)	Initial: 40–80 mg t.i.d. Max: 480 mg/day	None or not specified	Severe hepatic impairment: 30% of the normal dose
MRAs	Spironolactone (Aldactone)	Initial: 12.5–25 mg daily Max: 100–200 mg	Use with caution due to risk of hyperkalemia	None or not specified
	Eplerenone (Inspra)	Initial: 25 mg daily Max: 100 mg/day	Use with caution due to risk of hyperkalemia	None or not specified

ACE, angiotensin-converting enzyme; ARB, angiotensin receptor blocker; CrCl, creatinine clearance; DPP-4, dipeptidyl peptidase 4; eGFR, estimated glomerular filtration rate; ESRD, end-stage renal disease; GLP-1 RA, glucagon-like peptide-1 receptor agonist; HD, hemodialysis; MRA, mineralocorticoid receptor antagonist; NDCA, nondihydropyridine calcium antagonist; SGLT2, sodium-glucose cotransporter 2; SQ, subcutaneously. * Not inclusive of all medications within each class (focused on medications discussed in the chapter); § Oral route unless otherwise indicated; ∧ General doses, not necessarily specific to indication of diabetic nephropathy.

out rate of up to 17%. Unfortunately, findings may be clouded by the significant heterogeneity between the studies included. Similar results were confirmed with a Cochrane review evaluating the effects of MRAs in individuals with CKD with proteinuria, whereby the addition of MRAs to standard RAS inhibition reduces proteinuria, but is associated with hyperkalemia.[99] Not all studies included in the review were in patients with diabetes or DKD. Lastly, a meta-analysis of spirono-lactone as add-on therapy to standard antidiabetic-renoprotective antihypertensive treatment in patients with diabetic nephropathy confirmed the above findings.[100]

The combination of an MRA with an RAS inhibitor proved to be more effective in reducing urinary ACR than two RAS inhibitors.[101] This study in patients with primarily T2D (85%), hypertension (mean clinical blood pressure of 133/73 mmHg), and albuminuria defined as a urinary ACR ≥300 mg/g (geometric mean urinary ACR of 969 mg/g creatinine) on lisinopril 80 mg once daily found that patients receiving spironolactone had a greater decrease in urinary ACR than patients receiv-ing losartan when compared with placebo. Mean serum potassium concentrations were significantly higher in patients on losartan or spironolactone compared with placebo. Although potassium levels were higher in those in the spironolactone group compared with the losartan group, statistical significance was not met.

Due to concerns of adverse effects of traditional MRAs, newer MRAs with different properties are being developed and studied to overcome these limita-tions.[102] Specifically, finerenone has been found to have less incidence of hyperka-lemia, and higher potency and mineralocorticoid receptor selectivity than spironolactone or eplerenone.[102] Although not yet FDA approved, preliminary studies in patients with T2D and diabetic nephropathy on RAS inhibition therapy have shown promising results in reducing albuminuria without serious adverse effects.[103,104] Results on ongoing studies of finerenone in patients with DKD are pending.

SGLT2 INHIBITORS + RAS INHIBITORS

The different roles that SGLT2 inhibitors and RAS inhibitors play in the kidney may theoretically promote synergistic activity when used as combination therapy in DKD. Although this has mechanistically been seen in animal models, extrapolation to humans must be done with caution.[105] In general, in the random-ized controlled trials assessing cardiovascular outcomes with SGLT2 inhibitors, patients received background ACE inhibitor or ARB therapy (see previous "SGLT2 Inhibitors" section). One study specifically examined the effects of dapa-gliflozin on albuminuria in patients with T2D, hypertension (mean blood pressure of 152/91 mmHg), and albuminuria defined as a urinary ACR ≥30 mg/g creatinine (median urinary ACR of 77 mg/g creatinine).[106] This was a post hoc analysis of pooled randomized controlled phase 3 trials in patients on a stable dose of an ACE inhibitor or ARB. At 12 weeks, dapagliflozin resulted in greater reductions in albuminuria compared with placebo.

SGLT2 INHIBITORS + DPP-4 INHIBITORS

Analyses of secondary outcomes in trials of patients on combined SGLT2 inhibitors and DPP-4 inhibitors suggest potential benefit of this combination on renal outcomes. Specifically, one study found that combination empagliflozin-linagliptin had more patients regress in proteinuria compared with each medication at 52 weeks.[107]

COMBINATION PRODUCTS

CCBs + RAS INHIBITORS

- Amlodipine-benazepril (Lotrel)
- Verapamil-trandolapril (Tarka)

MONOGRAPHS

ACE INHIBITORS

Captopril (Capoten): https://dailymed.nlm.nih.gov/dailymed/drugInfo.cfm?setid=01cca91e-0374-4b89-a25a-be05e8b64346

Enalapril (Vasotec): https://dailymed.nlm.nih.gov/dailymed/drugInfo.cfm?setid=39631f1f-5d19-43c1-b504-bf56d991ed97

Lisinopril (Prinivil, Zestril): https://dailymed.nlm.nih.gov/dailymed/drugInfo.cfm?setid=27ccb2f4-abf8-4825-9b05-0bb367b4ac07

Ramipril (Altace): https://dailymed.nlm.nih.gov/dailymed/drugInfo.cfm?setid=0fc34cd8-86e6-4034-73bd-4263a68ba046

ARBs

Candesartan (Atacand): https://dailymed.nlm.nih.gov/dailymed/drugInfo.cfm?setid=a73e1339-9643-4eea-2cbe-e879c92fb50e

Irbesartan (Avapro): https://dailymed.nlm.nih.gov/dailymed/drugInfo.cfm?setid=7885b2a8-be4e-48ab-8113-4e6ab791eb98

Losartan (Cozaar): https://dailymed.nlm.nih.gov/dailymed/drugInfo.cfm?setid=5ac32c20-169d-475a-fc8a-934f758d6ab0

Olmesartan (Benicar): https://dailymed.nlm.nih.gov/dailymed/drugInfo.cfm?setid=33770d80-754f-11de-8dba-0002a5d5c51b

Telmisartan (Micardis): https://dailymed.nlm.nih.gov/dailymed/drugInfo.cfm?setid=cfb9309f-e0df-4a55-9542-0e869fce05fb

Valsartan (Diovan): https://dailymed.nlm.nih.gov/dailymed/drugInfo.cfm?setid=5ddba454-f3e6-43c2-a7a6-58365d2101213

DIRECT RENIN INHIBITORS

Aliskiren (Tekturna): https://dailymed.nlm.nih.gov/dailymed/drugInfo.
cfm?setid=3dd61fa5-1620-4ebf-bbdb-ede29b92fce2

SGLT2 INHIBITORS

Canagliflozin (Invokana): https://dailymed.nlm.nih.gov/dailymed/drugInfo.
cfm?setid=b9457d3b-b104-4f09-8a61-c61ef9d4a3f3

Dapagliflozin (Farxiga): https://dailymed.nlm.nih.gov/dailymed/drugInfo.
cfm?setid=72ad22ae-efe6-4cd6-a302-98aaee423d69

Empagliflozin (Jardiance): https://dailymed.nlm.nih.gov/dailymed/drugInfo.
cfm?setid=faf3dd6a-9cd0-39c2-0d2e-232cb3f67565

GLP-1 RAs

Liraglutide (Victoza): https://dailymed.nlm.nih.gov/dailymed/drugInfo.
cfm?setid=5a9ef4ea-c76a-4d34-a604-27c5b505f5a4

Lixisenatide (Adlyxin): https://dailymed.nlm.nih.gov/dailymed/drugInfo.
cfm?setid=1727cc16-4f86-4f13-b8b5-804d4984fa8c

Semaglutide (Ozempic): https://dailymed.nlm.nih.gov/dailymed/drugInfo.
cfm?setid=adec4fd2-6858-4c99-91d4-531f5f2a2d79

DPP-4 INHIBITORS

Alogliptin (Nesina): https://dailymed.nlm.nih.gov/dailymed/drugInfo.
cfm?setid=a3768c7e-aa4c-44d3-bc53-43bb7346c0b0

Linagliptin (Tradjenta): https://dailymed.nlm.nih.gov/dailymed/drugInfo.
cfm?setid=c797ea5c-cab7-494b-9044-27eba0cfe40f

Saxagliptin (Onglyza): https://dailymed.nlm.nih.gov/dailymed/drugInfo.
cfm?setid=c5116390-e0fe-4969-94cb-e9de5165fbab

Sitagliptin (Januvia): https://dailymed.nlm.nih.gov/dailymed/drugInfo.
cfm?setid=f85a48d0-0407-4c50-b0fa-7673a160bf01

NDCAs

Diltiazem (Cardizem, Tiazac): https://dailymed.nlm.nih.gov/dailymed/drugInfo.
cfm?setid=73b3607a-99d0-44d8-92ef-0074684c9d7d

Verapamil (Calan, Verelan): https://dailymed.nlm.nih.gov/dailymed/drugInfo.
cfm?setid=ed1e0c14-3571-43f9-88fc-5a4d2b598263

MRAs

Spironolactone (Aldactone): https://dailymed.nlm.nih.gov/dailymed/drugInfo.
cfm?setid=0fed2822-3a03-4b64-9857-c682fcd462bc

Eplerenone (Inspra): https://dailymed.nlm.nih.gov/dailymed/drugInfo.
cfm?setid=a55a39ff-1bd5-428b-a64f-c44262e2f3ed

REFERENCES

1. American Diabetes Association. 10. Microvascular Complications and Foot Care: *Standards of Medical Care in Diabetes—2018. Diabetes Care* 2018;41(Suppl. 1):S105–S118

2. Harjutsalo V, Groop PH. Epidemiology and risk factors for diabetic kidney disease. *Adv Chronic Kidney Dis* 2014;21(3):260–266

3. Alicic RZ, Rooney MT, Tuttle KR. Diabetic kidney disease: challenges, progress, and possibilities. *Clin J Am Soc Nephrol* 2017;12(12):2032–2045

4. Saran R, Robinson B, Abbott KC, et al. US renal data system 2017 annual data report: epidemiology of kidney disease in the United States. *Am J Kidney Dis* 2018;71(3S1):A7

5. Ozieh MN, Dismuke CE, Lynch CP, Egede LE. Medical care expenditures associated with chronic kidney disease in adults with diabetes: United States 2011. *Diabetes Res Clin Pract* 2015;109(1):185–190

6. United States Renal Data System. Chapter 6: healthcare expenditures for persons with CKD. Available from https://www.usrds.org/2017/view/v1_06.aspx. Accessed 30 April 2018

7. Toth-Manikowski S, Atta MG. Diabetic kidney disease: pathophysiology and therapeutic targets. *J Diabetes Res* 2015;2015:697010

8. Kramer HJ, Nguyen QD, Curhan G, Hsu CY. Renal insufficiency in the absence of albuminuria and retinopathy among adults with type 2 diabetes mellitus. *JAMA* 2003;289(24):3273–3277

9. Afkarian M, Sachs MC, Kestenbaum B, et al. Kidney disease and increased mortality risk in type 2 diabetes. *J Am Soc Nephrol* 2013;24(2):302–308

10. Tuttle KR, Bakris GL, Bilous RW, et al. Diabetic kidney disease: a report from an ADA Consensus Conference. *Diabetes Care* 2014;37(10):2864–2883

11. Heerspink HJ, Kropelin TF, Hoekman J, de Zeeuw D. Drug-induced reduction in albuminuria is associated with subsequent renoprotection: a meta-analysis. *J Am Soc Nephrol* 2015;26(8):2055–2064

12. Apperloo AJ, de Zeeuw D, de Jong PE. A short-term antihypertensive treatment-induced fall in glomerular filtration rate predicts long-term stability of renal function. *Kidney Int* 1997;51(3):793–797

13. Holtkamp FA, de Zeeuw D, Thomas MC, et al. An acute fall in estimated glomerular filtration rate during treatment with losartan predicts a slower decrease in long-term renal function. *Kidney Int* 2011;80(3):282–287

14. DCCT/EDIC Research Group. Effect of intensive diabetes treatment on albuminuria in type 1 diabetes: long-term follow-up of the Diabetes Control and Complications Trial and Epidemiology of Diabetes Interventions and Complications study. *Lancet Diabetes Endocrinol* 2014;2(10):793–800

15. de Boer IH, Sun W, Cleary PA, et al.; DCCT/EDIC Research Group. Intensive diabetes therapy and glomerular filtration rate in type 1 diabetes. *N Engl J Med* 2011;365(25):2366–2376

16. UK Prospective Diabetes Study (UKPDS) Group. Effect of intensive blood-glucose control with metformin on complications in overweight patients with type 2 diabetes (UKPDS 34). *Lancet* 1998;352(9131):854–865

17. Ismail-Beigi F, Craven T, Banerji MA, et al. Effect of intensive treatment of hyperglycaemia on microvascular outcomes in type 2 diabetes: an analysis of the ACCORD randomised trial. *Lancet* 2010;376(9739):419–430

18. Zoungas S, Arima H, Gerstein HC, et al. Effects of intensive glucose control on microvascular outcomes in patients with type 2 diabetes: a meta-analysis of individual participant data from randomised controlled trials. *Lancet Diabetes Endocrinol* 2017;5(6):431–437

19. Patel A, MacMahon S, Chalmers J, et al.; ADVANCE Collaborative Group. Intensive blood glucose control and vascular outcomes in patients with type 2 diabetes. *N Engl J Med* 2008;358(24):2560–2572

20. Zoungas S, Chalmers J, Neal B, et al. Follow-up of blood-pressure lowering and glucose control in type 2 diabetes. *N Engl J Med* 2014;371(15): 1392–1406

21. Haynes R, Lewis D, Emberson J, et al. Effects of lowering LDL cholesterol on progression of kidney disease. *J Am Soc Nephrol* 2014;25(8):1825–1833

22. Palmer SC, Craig JC, Navaneethan SD, et al Benefits and harms of statin therapy for persons with chronic kidney disease: a systematic review and meta-analysis. *Ann Intern Med* 2012;157(4):263–275

23. Palmer SC, Navaneethan SD, Craig JC, et al. HMG CoA reductase inhibitors (statins) for dialysis patients. *Cochrane Database Syst Rev* 2013(9):CD004289

24. Brown NJ, Vaughan DE. Angiotensin-converting enzyme inhibitors. *Circulation* 1998;97(14):1411–1420

25. Lewis EJ, Hunsicker LG, Bain RP, Rohde RD; for the Collaborative Study Group. The effect of angiotensin-converting-enzyme inhibition on diabetic nephropathy. *N Engl J Med* 1993;329(20):1456–1462

26. Parving HH, Lehnert H, Brochner-Mortensen J, et al. The effect of irbesartan on the development of diabetic nephropathy in patients with type 2 diabetes. *N Engl J Med* 2001;345(12):870–878

27. Viberti G, Wheeldon NM. Microalbuminuria reduction with valsartan in patients with type 2 diabetes mellitus: a blood pressure-independent effect. *Circulation* 2002;106(6):672–678

28. Lewis EJ, Hunsicker LG, Clarke WR, et al. Renoprotective effect of the angiotensin-receptor antagonist irbesartan in patients with nephropathy due to type 2 diabetes. *N Engl J Med* 2001;345(12):851–860

29. Kasiske BL, Kalil RS, Ma JZ, et al. Effect of antihypertensive therapy on the kidney in patients with diabetes: a meta-regression analysis. *Ann Intern Med* 1993;118(2):129–138

30. Hebert LA, Bain RP, Verme D, et al.; for the Collaborative Study Group. Remission of nephrotic range proteinuria in type I diabetes. *Kidney Int* 1994;46(6):1688–1693

31. Wilmer WA, Hebert LA, Lewis EJ, et al. Remission of nephrotic syndrome in type 1 diabetes: long-term follow-up of patients in the Captopril Study. *Am J Kidney Dis* 1999;34(2):308–314

32. Laffel LM, McGill JB, Gans DJ; on behalf of the North American Microalbuminuria Study Group. The beneficial effect of angiotensin-converting enzyme inhibition with captopril on diabetic nephropathy in normotensive IDDM patients with microalbuminuria. *Am J Med* 1995;99(5):497–504

33. Viberti G, Mogensen CE, Groop LC, Pauls JF, et al. Effect of captopril on progression to clinical proteinuria in patients with insulin-dependent diabetes mellitus and microalbuminuria. European Microalbuminuria Captopril Study Group. *JAMA* 1994;271(4):275–279

34. The Microalbuminuria Captopril Study Group. Captopril reduces the risk of nephropathy in IDDM patients with microalbuminuria. *Diabetologia* 1996;39(5):587–593

35. Parving HH, Hommel E, Jensen BR, Hansen HP. Long-term beneficial effect of ACE inhibition on diabetic nephropathy in normotensive type 1 diabetic patients. *Kidney Int* 2001;60(1):228–234

36. Lv J, Perkovic V, Foote CV, et al. Antihypertensive agents for preventing diabetic kidney disease. *Cochrane Database Syst Rev* 2012;12:CD004136

37. Van Buren PN, Toto R. Hypertension in diabetic nephropathy: epidemiology, mechanisms, and management. *Adv Chronic Kidney Dis* 2011;18(1): 28–41

38. The EUCLID Study Group. Randomised placebo-controlled trial of lisinopril in normotensive patients with insulin-dependent diabetes and normoalbuminuria or microalbuminuria. *Lancet* 1997;349(9068):1787–1792

39. Mauer M, Zinman B, Gardiner R, et al. Renal and retinal effects of enalapril and losartan in type 1 diabetes. *N Engl J Med* 2009;361(1):40–51

40. Bilous R, Chaturvedi N, Sjolie AK, et al. Effect of candesartan on microalbuminuria and albumin excretion rate in diabetes: three randomized trials. *Ann Intern Med* 2009;151(1):11–20, W13–14

41. Heart Outcomes Prevention Evaluation Study Investigators. Effects of ramipril on cardiovascular and microvascular outcomes in people with diabetes mellitus: results of the HOPE study and MICRO-HOPE substudy. *Lancet* 2000;355(9200):253–259

42. Brenner BM, Cooper ME, de Zeeuw D, et al. Effects of losartan on renal and cardiovascular outcomes in patients with type 2 diabetes and nephropathy. *N Engl J Med* 2001;345(12):861–869

43. Persson F, Rossing P, Schjoedt KJ, et al. Time course of the antiproteinuric and antihypertensive effects of direct renin inhibition in type 2 diabetes. *Kidney Int* 2008;73(12):1419–1425

44. Fogari R, Mugellini A, Zoppi A, et al. Time course of antiproteinuric effect of aliskiren in arterial hypertension associated with type 2 diabetes and microalbuminuria. *Expert Opin Pharmacother* 2013;14(4):371–384

45. Ravid M, Lang R, Rachmani R, Lishner M. Long-term renoprotective effect of angiotensin-converting enzyme inhibition in non-insulin-dependent diabetes mellitus. A 7-year follow-up study. *Arch Intern Med* 1996;156(3):286–289

46. Ruggenenti P, Fassi A, Ilieva AP, et al. Preventing microalbuminuria in type 2 diabetes. *N Engl J Med* 2004;351(19):1941–1951

47. Haller H, Ito S, Izzo JL Jr., et al. Olmesartan for the delay or prevention of microalbuminuria in type 2 diabetes. *N Engl J Med* 2011;364(10):907–917

48. Schrier RW, Estacio RO, Esler A, Mehler P. Effects of aggressive blood pressure control in normotensive type 2 diabetic patients on albuminuria, retinopathy and strokes. *Kidney Int* 2002;61(3):1086–1097

49. Ravid M, Brosh D, Levi Z, et al. Use of enalapril to attenuate decline in renal function in normotensive, normoalbuminuric patients with type 2 diabetes mellitus. A randomized, controlled trial. *Ann Intern Med* 1998;128(12 Pt 1):982–988

50. Imai E, Chan JC, Ito S, et al. Effects of olmesartan on renal and cardiovascular outcomes in type 2 diabetes with overt nephropathy: a multicentre, randomised, placebo-controlled study. *Diabetologia* 2011;54(12):2978–2986

51. Wang AC, Stellmacher U, Schumi J, et al. Assessment of the cardiovascular risk of olmesartan medoxomil-based treatment: meta-analysis of individual patient data. *Am J Cardiovasc Drugs* 2016;16(6):427–437

52. Strippoli GF, Craig M, Deeks JJ, et al. Effects of angiotensin converting enzyme inhibitors and angiotensin II receptor antagonists on mortality and renal outcomes in diabetic nephropathy: systematic review. *BMJ* 2004;329(7470):828

53. Barnett AH, Bain SC, Bouter P, et al. Angiotensin-receptor blockade versus converting-enzyme inhibition in type 2 diabetes and nephropathy. *N Engl J Med* 2004;351(19):1952–1961

54. Wu HY, Peng CL, Chen PC, et al. Comparative effectiveness of angiotensin-converting enzyme inhibitors versus angiotensin II receptor blockers for major renal outcomes in patients with diabetes: a 15-year cohort study. *PLoS One* 2017;12(5):e0177654

55. Casas JP, Chua W, Loukogeorgakis S, et al. Effect of inhibitors of the renin-angiotensin system and other antihypertensive drugs on renal outcomes: systematic review and meta-analysis. *Lancet* 2005;366(9502):2026–2033

56. Palmer SC, Mavridis D, Navarese E, et al. Comparative efficacy and safety of blood pressure-lowering agents in adults with diabetes and kidney disease: a network meta-analysis. *Lancet* 2015;385(9982):2047–2056

57. Wu HY, Huang JW, Lin HJ, et al. Comparative effectiveness of renin-angiotensin system blockers and other antihypertensive drugs in patients with diabetes: systematic review and bayesian network meta-analysis. *BMJ* 2013;347:f6008

58. Fioretto P, Zambon A, Rossato M, et al. SGLT2 inhibitors and the diabetic kidney. *Diabetes Care* 2016;39(Suppl. 2):S165–S171

59. Neal B, Perkovic V, Matthews DR. Canagliflozin and cardiovascular and renal events in type 2 diabetes. *N Engl J Med* 2017;377(21):2099

60. Heerspink HJ, Desai M, Jardine M, et al. Canagliflozin slows progression of renal function decline independently of glycemic effects. *J Am Soc Nephrol* 2017;28(1):368–375

61. Wanner C, Inzucchi SE, Lachin JM, et al. Empagliflozin and progression of kidney disease in type 2 diabetes. *N Engl J Med* 2016;375(4):323–334

62. Jardine MJ, Mahaffey KW, Neal B, et al. The Canagliflozin and Renal Endpoints in Diabetes with Established Nephropathy Clinical Evaluation (CREDENCE) study rationale, design, and baseline characteristics. *Am J Nephrol* 2017;46(6):462–472

63. Johnson & Johnson. Phase 3 CREDENCE renal outcomes trial of INVOKANA® (canagliflozin) is being stopped early for positive efficacy findings. Available from www.jnj.com/phase-3-credence-renal-outcomes-trial-of-invokana-canagliflozin-is-being-stopped-early-for-positive-efficacy-findings. Accessed 3 December 2018

64. Kohan DE, Fioretto P, Tang W, List JF. Long-term study of patients with type 2 diabetes and moderate renal impairment shows that dapagliflozin reduces weight and blood pressure but does not improve glycemic control. *Kidney Int* 2014;85(4):962–971

65. Cherney DZ, Perkins BA, Soleymanlou N, et al. Renal hemodynamic effect of sodium-glucose cotransporter 2 inhibition in patients with type 1 diabetes mellitus. *Circulation* 2014;129(5):587–597

66. Liu J, Li L, Li S, et al. Effects of SGLT2 inhibitors on UTIs and genital infections in type 2 diabetes mellitus: a systematic review and meta-analysis. *Sci Rep* 2017;7(1):2824

67. Thong KY, Yadagiri M, Barnes DJ, et al. Clinical risk factors predicting genital fungal infections with sodium-glucose cotransporter 2 inhibitor treatment: The ABCD nationwide dapagliflozin audit. *Prim Care Diabetes* 2018;12(1):45–50

68. Nadkarni GN, Ferrandino R, Chang A, et al. Acute kidney injury in patients on SGLT2 inhibitors: a propensity-matched analysis. *Diabetes Care* 2017;40(11):1479–1485

69. Filippatos TD, Elisaf MS. Effects of glucagon-like peptide-1 receptor agonists on renal function. *World J Diabetes* 2013;4(5):190–201

70. Mann JFE, Orsted DD, Brown-Frandsen K, et al. Liraglutide and renal outcomes in type 2 diabetes. *N Engl J Med* 2017;377(9):839–848

71. Marso SP, Bain SC, Consoli A, et al. Semaglutide and cardiovascular outcomes in patients with type 2 diabetes. *N Engl J Med* 2016;375(19):1834–1844

72. Pfeffer MA, Claggett B, Diaz R, et al. Lixisenatide in patients with type 2 diabetes and acute coronary syndrome. *N Engl J Med* 2015;373(23):2247–2257

73. Dicembrini I, Nreu B, Scatena A, et al. Microvascular effects of glucagon-like peptide-1 receptor agonists in type 2 diabetes: a meta-analysis of randomized controlled trials. *Acta Diabetol* 2017;54(10):933–941

74. Gargiulo P, Savarese G, D'Amore C, et al. Efficacy and safety of glucagon-like peptide-1 agonists on macrovascular and microvascular events in type 2 diabetes mellitus: a meta-analysis. *Nutr Metab Cardiovasc Dis* 2017;27(12):1081–1088

75. Cooper ME, Perkovic V, McGill JB, et al. Kidney disease end points in a pooled analysis of individual patient-level data from a large clinical trials program of the dipeptidyl peptidase 4 inhibitor linagliptin in type 2 diabetes. *Am J Kidney Dis* 2015;66(3):441–449

76. Scirica BM, Bhatt DL, Braunwald E, et al. Saxagliptin and cardiovascular outcomes in patients with type 2 diabetes mellitus. *N Engl J Med* 2013;369(14):1317–1326

77. Mosenzon O, Leibowitz G, Bhatt DL, et al. Effect of saxagliptin on renal outcomes in the SAVOR-TIMI 53 trial. *Diabetes Care* 2017;40(1):69–76

78. White WB, Cannon CP, Heller SR, et al. Alogliptin after acute coronary syndrome in patients with type 2 diabetes. *N Engl J Med* 2013;369(14):1327–1335

79. Green JB, Bethel MA, Armstrong PW, et al. Effect of sitagliptin on cardiovascular outcomes in type 2 diabetes. *N Engl J Med* 2015;373(3):232–242

80. Cornel JH, Bakris GL, Stevens SR, et al. Effect of sitagliptin on kidney function and respective cardiovascular outcomes in type 2 diabetes: outcomes from TECOS. *Diabetes Care* 2016;39(12):2304–2310

81. Kim YG, Byun J, Yoon D, et al. Renal protective effect of DPP-4 inhibitors in type 2 diabetes mellitus patients: a cohort study. *J Diabetes Res* 2016:1423191

82. Smith AC, Toto R, Bakris GL. Differential effects of calcium channel blockers on size selectivity of proteinuria in diabetic glomerulopathy. *Kidney Int* 1998;54(3):889–896

83. Bakris GL, Weir MR, Secic M, et al. Differential effects of calcium antagonist subclasses on markers of nephropathy progression. *Kidney Int* 2004;65(6):1991–2002

84. Murray KM. Calcium-channel blockers for treatment of diabetic nephropathy. *Clin Pharm* 1991;10(11):862–865

85. Bakris GL. Effects of diltiazem or lisinopril on massive proteinuria associated with diabetes mellitus. *Ann Intern Med* 1990;112(9):707–708

86. Bauersachs J, Jaisser F, Toto R. Mineralocorticoid receptor activation and mineralocorticoid receptor antagonist treatment in cardiac and renal diseases. *Hypertension* 2015;65(2):257–263

87. Nielsen SE, Persson F, Frandsen E, et al. Spironolactone diminishes urinary albumin excretion in patients with type 1 diabetes and microalbuminuria: a randomized placebo-controlled crossover study. *Diabet Med* 2012;29(8):e184–e190

88. Makhlough A, Kashi Z, Akha O, et al. Effect of spironolactone on diabetic nephropathy compared to the combination of spironolactone and losartan. *Nephrourol Mon* 2014;6(1):e12148

89. Mogensen CE, Neldam S, Tikkanen I, et al. Randomised controlled trial of dual blockade of renin-angiotensin system in patients with hypertension, microalbuminuria, and non-insulin dependent diabetes: the candesartan and lisinopril microalbuminuria (CALM) study. *BMJ* 2000;321(7274): 1440–1444

90. Fried LF, Emanuele N, Zhang JH, et al. Combined angiotensin inhibition for the treatment of diabetic nephropathy. *N Engl J Med* 2013;369(20): 1892–1903

91. Yusuf S, Teo KK, Pogue J, et al. Telmisartan, ramipril, or both in patients at high risk for vascular events. *N Engl J Med* 2008;358(15):1547–1559

92. Mann JF, Schmieder RE, McQueen M, et al. Renal outcomes with telmisartan, ramipril, or both, in people at high vascular risk (the ONTARGET study): a multicentre, randomised, double-blind, controlled trial. *Lancet* 2008;372(9638):547–553

93. Parving HH, Persson F, Lewis JB, et al. Aliskiren combined with losartan in type 2 diabetes and nephropathy. *N Engl J Med* 2008;358(23):2433–2446

94. Parving HH, Brenner BM, McMurray JJ, et al. Cardiorenal end points in a trial of aliskiren for type 2 diabetes. *N Engl J Med* 2012;367(23):2204–2213

95. Toto RD, Tian M, Fakouhi K, et al. Effects of calcium channel blockers on proteinuria in patients with diabetic nephropathy. *J Clin Hypertens* (Greenwich) 2008;10(10):761–769

96. Bakris GL, Weir MR, DeQuattro V, McMahon FG. Effects of an ACE inhibitor/calcium antagonist combination on proteinuria in diabetic nephropathy. *Kidney Int* 1998;54(4):1283–1289

97. Sato A, Saruta T. Aldosterone breakthrough during angiotensin-converting enzyme inhibitor therapy. *Am J Hypertens* 2003;16(9 Pt 1):781–788

98. Mavrakanas TA, Gariani K, Martin PY. Mineralocorticoid receptor blockade in addition to angiotensin converting enzyme inhibitor or angiotensin II receptor blocker treatment: an emerging paradigm in diabetic nephropathy: a systematic review. *Eur J Intern Med* 2014;25(2):173–176

99. Bolignano D, Palmer SC, Navaneethan SD, Strippoli GF. Aldosterone antagonists for preventing the progression of chronic kidney disease. *Cochrane Database Syst Rev* 2014;(4):CD007004

100. Hou J, Xiong W, Cao L, et al. Spironolactone add-on for preventing or slowing the progression of diabetic nephropathy: a meta-analysis. *Clin Ther* 2015;37(9):2086–2103.e10

101. Mehdi UF, Adams-Huet B, Raskin P, et al. Addition of angiotensin receptor blockade or mineralocorticoid antagonism to maximal angiotensin-converting enzyme inhibition in diabetic nephropathy. *J Am Soc Nephrol* 2009;20(12):2641–2650

102. Dojki FK, Bakris G. Nonsteroidal mineralocorticoid antagonists in diabetic kidney disease. *Curr Opin Nephrol Hypertens* 2017;26(5):368–374

103. Bakris GL, Agarwal R, Chan JC, et al. Effect of finerenone on albuminuria in patients with diabetic nephropathy: a randomized clinical trial. *JAMA* 2015;314(9):884–894

104. Katayama S, Yamada D, Nakayama M, et al. A randomized controlled study of finerenone versus placebo in Japanese patients with type 2 diabetes mellitus and diabetic nephropathy. *J Diabetes Complications* 2017;31(4):758–765

105. Zou H, Zhou B, Xu G. SGLT2 inhibitors: a novel choice for the combination therapy in diabetic kidney disease. *Cardiovasc Diabetol* 2017;16(1):65

106. Heerspink HJ, Johnsson E, Gause-Nilsson I, et al. Dapagliflozin reduces albuminuria in patients with diabetes and hypertension receiving renin-angiotensin blockers. *Diabetes Obes Metab* 2016;18(6):590–597

107. DeFronzo RA, Lewin A, Patel S, et al. Combination of empagliflozin and linagliptin as second-line therapy in subjects with type 2 diabetes inadequately controlled on metformin. *Diabetes Care* 2015;38(3):384–393

Chapter 25
Medications for the Management of Retinopathy

Emmeline Tran, PharmD

INTRODUCTION

Diabetic retinopathy is a microvascular complication of diabetes resulting from changes in the blood vessels of the retina.[1] It is the leading cause of vision loss in individuals aged 20–74 years old. Vision loss secondary to diabetic retinopathy occurs as a result of increased vascular permeability and or capillary nonperfusion, distortion of the retina from the development of new blood vessels and fibrous tissue, hemorrhaging of new blood vessels, and damage to retinal neurons.[1]

Global prevalence of diabetic retinopathy is estimated to be about 35%, with a prevalence of 7% for PDR and 7% for diabetic macular edema (DME).[2] Major risk factors for diabetic retinopathy include poor glycemic control, hypertension, dyslipidemia, duration of diabetes, and nephropathy.[3-7] The lifetime risk of diabetic retinopathy is up to approximately 98% in individuals with T1D and up to approximately 80% in individuals with T2D.[8,9]

Diabetic retinopathy occurs in several stages at a slow, nonlinear progression.[1] Initially, patients may present with mild nonproliferative diabetic retinopathy (NPDR) characterized by microaneurysms. Without treatment, patients may progress to moderate or severe NPDR whereby the blood vessels in the retina begin to change shape and become deprived of blood supply. Lack of blood supply causes the body to secrete factors that promote new blood vessel growth leading to the next stage, PDR. The fragile state of the new blood vessels makes them susceptible to leakage and bleeding. Scar tissue can then form and may cause retinal detachment and subsequently permanent vision loss. At any stage, patients can develop macular edema. Macular edema is the swelling of the macula, an area in the center of the retina. Increased vascular permeability due to the breakdown of the blood-retina barrier causes fluid from blood vessels to leak into the retina, resulting in the swelling and thickening of the macula.[1,10] Clinically, patients report blurred vision. In the short term, reductions in visual acuity may be reversible. However, persistent edema may result in irreversible damage and permanent vision loss.[11]

GOALS OF TREATMENT

Unfortunately, treatment of diabetic retinopathy usually does not restore lost vision. Additionally, baseline retinopathy greatly shapes the development of this complication. Patients with more severe baseline retinopathy are more likely to progress to vision-threatening retinopathy.[12] Consequently, first and foremost, the goal is to prevent progression of diabetic retinopathy with appropriate management of blood glucose, blood pressure, and lipids. In fact, decreases in the incidence and risk of progression of diabetic retinopathy over the past few decades are a result of improved management in glycemia, blood pressure, and lipid concentration.[13-15]

Tight control of blood glucose in both T1D[16] and T2D[17,18] cannot be overstated in decreasing the risk of development or progression of diabetic retinopathy. The risk of diabetic retinopathy is lowered by approximately 30–50% with each percent reduction in A1C[16,17,19] and effects are long lasting despite loss of glycemic control later on.[20,21] Despite agreement that glycemic control is important in prevention and treatment of diabetic retinopathy, the degree of glucose control is less clear. The ADVANCE trial showed no difference in the development of retinopathy between patients receiving conventional therapy (achieved mean A1C of 7.3%) or intensive therapy (achieved mean A1C of 6.5%) for glucose control.[22] Balancing the risks of hypoglycemia with potential benefit on diabetic retinopathy should be taken into consideration. Additionally, it is important to note that glycemic control may not be the only factor in impacting the incidence and progression of diabetic retinopathy. A1C accounted for only 11% of the risk of retinopathy in the DCCT trial.[23]

Similar to intensive glycemic control, tight blood pressure control has benefits in reducing the risks of diabetic retinopathy progression. The UKPDS study found that the risk for vision loss was decreased by 47%, and need for laser treatment by 34% in patients with T2D.[24] Again, the degree of blood pressure control has been difficult to characterize. The UKPDS study found benefits in lowering systolic blood pressure from a mean of 160 mmHg to a mean of 144 mmHg compared with a mean of 154 mmHg.[24] On the other hand, the ACCORD study did not find a benefit in lowering systolic blood pressure from a median of 137 mmHg to a median of 117 mmHg compared with a median of 133 mmHg.[18] In contrast to glycemic control, benefits seen are only maintained with ongoing blood pressure control.[21]

The impact of lipid control has been more difficult to assess. Although dyslipidemia is a known risk factor for diabetic retinopathy, treatments targeted at lowering lipids have yielded inconsistent results.[25,26] Statin therapy has been evaluated, but studies have mostly been small with conflicting results. Larger studies examining statins were not designed to specifically address diabetic retinopathy outcomes.[25,26] Favorable data regarding lipid-lowering agents have mainly been centered on fenofibrate.

Once diabetic retinopathy develops, the goal is to prevent or arrest progression to avoid vision loss and improve quality of life. The impact of diabetic retinopathy on functions of daily living is significant. Among those with severe NPDR or PDR, approximately half have difficulties with at least one visual function task.[27] Studies examining the effects of certain interventions on diabetic retinopathy have used visual acuity as a marker for improvement in vision. Clinically significant improvement in visual acuity in these studies has generally been defined as a gain of ≥5–15 letters or 1–3 three lines from baseline on the ETDRS chart.[28,29]

Clinically significant macular edema is defined as retinal thickening of the macula or within 500 μm of it, presence of hard exudates at or within 500 μm of the center of the retina with thickening of the adjacent retina, or presence of a zone of retinal thickening one disk area or larger in size, any part of which is within one disk diameter of the center of the retina.[30] This definition generally refers to the threshold at which laser photocoagulation is indicated. Macular edema as defined by central subfield thickness has been described as ≥275 μm on time-domain optical coherence tomography (TD-OCT) with a corresponding Snellen visual acuity decrease of 20/40 to 20/320.[31] This has become a more common measure of clinically significant macular edema in studies examining pharmacologic agents in the treatment of diabetic retinopathy.

MEDICATIONS

In general, outside of medications targeted at metabolic control, pharmacological therapies for diabetic retinopathy are limited, and even then are often costly and require a vitreoretinal ophthalmologist specialist for administration. Pharmacologic treatment options mainly include anti-vascular endothelial growth factor (anti-VEGF) agents and intravitreal corticosteroids. Prior to the advent of anti-VEGF agents, nonpharmacological therapies such as focal laser photocoagulation and panretinal laser photocoagulation (PRP) were standards of care.[30,32,33] Laser photocoagulation improves oxygen availability, thus reducing the secretion of VEGFs and regressing neovascularization.[34] In general, a shift away from these nonpharmacological options has transpired, especially in the setting of DME.

Initiation of treatment is guided by the presence of DME and stage of diabetic retinopathy. The threshold for initiation of treatment in DME is the presence of central-involved DME (CIDME). CIDME is defined as edema affecting the diameter of 1 mm in the retinal central subfield.[1] In regard to stage of diabetic retinopathy, treatment may be considered with the development of severe NPDR and recommended with PDR. Table 25.1 summarizes treatment recommendations for initiation of intraocular interventions. These treatment options do not reverse vision loss, but instead work to minimize development and progression of vision loss by primarily targeting the angiogenesis and inflammatory pathways.

ANTI-VEGF AGENTS

Angiogenesis is a key component in the pathogenesis of diabetic retinopathy, especially in the later stages. Overexpression of VEGFs induces proliferation of blood vessel development and vascular leakage.[35] Currently, there are two FDA-approved anti-VEGF agents, ranibizumab and aflibercept. Additionally, bevacizumab and pegaptanib have been used off-label for diabetic retinopathy. Bevacizumab is repackaged in aliquots containing approximately 1/500th of the systemic dose used in cancer therapy.[36] These compounds differ in structure, VEGF-binding affinity, and VEGF isoform specificity.[37,38] The effect of these differences in terms of clinical efficacy is not fully known.

Table 25.1—Recommended Intraocular Treatment Based on Stage of Diabetic Retinopathy and Presence of DME[1]

Presence of DME	Intraocular treatment
No	None
Yes, non-CIDME	None
Yes, CIDME	Anti-VEGF therapy ± macular laser Alternative: intravitreous steroids
Stage	Intraocular treatment
No diabetic retinopathy	None
Mild NPDR	None
Moderate NPDR	None
Severe NPDR	Consider early PRP for patients with T2D
PDR	PRP or anti-VEGF therapy

CIDME, central-involved diabetic macular edema; DME, diabetic macular edema; NPDR, nonproliferative diabetic retinopathy; PDR, proliferative diabetic retinopathy; PRP, panretinal laser photocoagulation; VEGF, vascular endothelial growth factor. *Source:* Solomon.[1]

DME

Data supporting the use of anti-VEGF agents are mainly in the treatment of DME. Several randomized controlled trials have established the efficacy of ranibizumab,[39,40] aflibercept,[41] and bevacizumab[42] in visual acuity gain and central retinal thickness reduction when compared with laser therapy. Moreover, a Cochrane review found that use of ranibizumab, aflibercept, and bevacizumab were all more effective than laser photocoagulation for improving vision by three or more lines at 1 year.[43] Data supporting use of pegaptanib in the treatment of DME have been limited to comparison with sham treatment.[44]

Few data are available to guide selection of which VEGF inhibitor should be initiated compared with the others. A large randomized controlled trial compared three agents—aflibercept, bevacizumab, and ranibizumab—and found that all improved vision, but the effect was dependent on baseline visual acuity. In patients who presented with worse baseline levels of visual acuity (20/50 or worse), improvement in vision was greatest with aflibercept.[36] A subsequent post hoc analysis of the trial found a preferential sustained benefit of aflibercept in visual acuity improvement over 2 years compared with bevacizumab, but not ranibizumab among patients with 20/50 or worse vision.[45] Superiority of aflibercept may also be seen in patients with PDR at baseline.[46]

Findings suggesting benefits of aflibercept and ranibizumab over bevacizumab were observed in persistent DME. Persistent DME occurs when, despite anti-VEGF therapy, complete resolution of DME is lacking. A post hoc analysis found that persistent DME at 24 weeks was more common in patients receiving bevacizumab compared with aflibercept or ranibizumab.[47] For patients with persistent DME through 24 weeks, the probability of chronic persistent DME was lower with aflibercept compared with bevacizumab, but not with ranibizumab. However, no difference was found among the anti-VEGF agents in patients with persistent DME with regard to gain of at least 10 letters from baseline through 2 years for patients with chronic persistent DME compared with those without chronic persistent DME. Consequently, these results suggest that meaningful benefits in vision can be gained regardless of anti-VEGF agent given or persistence of DME through 2 years with little risk of vision loss.[47]

Despite the strong evidence supporting the use of anti-VEGF agents for the treatment of DME, real-world considerations present certain challenges. Administration of these agents is intravitreal and requires multiple injections. Most clinical trials investigating these drugs used at least monthly injections. However, in the real world, patients appear to receive anti-VEGF injections less frequently, resulting in less efficacy than that seen in original trials.[48] Studies have been conducted to determine the potential for tapering the number of injections over a period of time, and suggest no difference in outcomes.[49,50]

Additional considerations center on cost. Anti-VEGF agents have established cost-effectiveness compared with other interventions in the treatment of DME.[51] The substantial difference in cost with bevacizumab compared with ranibizumab or aflibercept (approximately 20- to 40-fold less) make it an attractive option.[52] A cost-effectiveness study of the three agents emphasized this cost discrepancy, finding that aflibercept and ranibizumab are not cost-effective compared with bevacizumab for the treatment of DME.[53] Conversely, bevacizumab must be compounded to use intravitreally. Issues surrounding compounding such as sterility or requirements for patient-specific prescriptions may limit access to compounded bevacizumab.[52,54]

PDR

Limited data are available on the use of anti-VEGF agents in the treatment of PDR. Standard of care has traditionally been PRP. A noninferiority study (Protocol S) compared PRP with ranibizumab.[55] The mean treatment group difference in visual acuity letter score improvement between groups was greater than the prespecified noninferiority limit of −5.0 letters. As such, ranibizumab was found to be noninferior to PRP. Another noninferiority study (CLARITY) examined the use of aflibercept compared with PRP and found aflibercept to be noninferior and superior in visual acuity improvement.[56]

Reviews of the literature also emphasize the lack of efficacy and safety outcomes available with the use of anti-VEGF agents in the treatment of PDR over standard therapy options. In particular, a Cochrane review, including studies primarily investigating bevacizumab, found potential benefits with the use of anti-VEGF agents, but results were heterogeneous and supported by very low-quality evidence. Limitations of the studies included indirect assessment of visual acuity, lacking of blinding, attrition bias, selective reporting, and lack of prespecified sample size. The review also suggested that a reduction in risk of intraocular bleeding in individuals with PDR is associated with anti-VEGFs.[57] Considerations for use of anti-VEGF agents over PRP may include scenarios in which there is difficulty in performing PRP such as dense cataracts or vitreous hemorrhage, when PRP has failed in preventing PDR progression, and in patients with DME with PDR.[58]

As with DME, a potential drawback in the use of anti-VEGF therapy in the management of PDR is the increased number of visits and treatment compared with PRP.[58,59] Consequently, lack of adherence is a major concern. Of those allocated to the anti-VEGF group, approximately 6% of participants in the Protocol S trial and 9% of participants in the CLARITY trial were loss to follow-up.[55,56] A retrospective cohort study found that 22.1% of patients receiving anti-VEGF therapy were loss to follow-up over a period of about 4 years, but statistically significantly more patients who received PRP were loss to follow-up (28.0%).[60]

Cost evaluations comparing PRP to anti-VEGF therapy have been conducted. One cost study used a Markov-style analysis and found PRP to be less expensive than intravitreal ranibizumab for PDR, taking into account both facility and non-facility settings.[61] In patients with PDR with concomitant vision-impairing DME, ranibizumab monotherapy may be a more cost-effective option than PRP. However, this cost benefit is lost in patients with PDR without baseline vision-impairing DME.[62]

Safety

In general, most clinical trials have reported a favorable safety profile for these agents. However, it must be noted that these studies often do not have adequate power to detect safety events, especially if rare. A systematic review and meta-analysis found an association between aflibercept or ranibizumab and potential increased risk for death, cerebrovascular accidents, and vascular death.[63] An increased risk for MI and thrombotic events was not seen. Other reviews or meta-analyses have not observed similar signals for cardiovascular events or death.[43,64] Further data are needed to clarify the safety profile of these agents in patients with diabetes who already have increased cardiovascular risk.

Other adverse events to be aware of include endophthalmitis (incidence reported up to 1.6%), intraocular inflammation, intraocular pressure elevation (often transient and self-limiting), retinal detachment, and ocular hemorrhage.[65,66]

CORTICOSTEROIDS

Inflammatory pathway activation is a proposed mechanism in DME. Therefore, medications such as corticosteroids that suppress pathways of inflammation are potential treatment options. Additionally, corticosteroids have been found to inhibit the expression of VEGFs in vascular smooth muscle cells and thus reduce blood vessel formation.[67]

DME

Data supporting the use of intravitreal corticosteroids is less promising than anti-VEGF agents. Superior efficacy and safety outcomes of intravitreal triamcinolone over focal or grid photocoagulation in patients with primarily DME (61%) and mild to moderately severe NPDR (61%) were not observed.[68] Although there were benefits in visual acuity at 4 months in individuals receiving triamcinolone, those benefits were no longer present by 1 year. Additionally, by 2 years, patients receiving laser therapy showed improved visual acuity compared with patients receiving triamcinolone. Results regarding effects on retinal thickening paralleled the visual acuity results. In terms of safety, there was an increased percentage of patients with ocular hypertension and/or glaucoma and cataract surgery in the triamcinolone group compared with the laser therapy group. A follow-up study at 3 years showed similar results.[69]

Another study also found no benefit to the use of a corticosteroid compared with laser therapy. Study eyes with DME received prompt laser monotherapy, ranibizumab with prompt laser therapy, ranibizumab with deferred laser therapy, or triamcinolone with prompt laser therapy.[70,71] No difference was found in patients receiving the triamcinolone-laser therapy combination compared with laser monotherapy. Reduction in mean central subfield thickness was seen in all three medication-laser therapy combination groups compared with laser monotherapy at 1 year. However, benefits were lost in those patients receiving triamcinolone-laser therapy at 2 years with an increase in mean central subfield thickness from the 1- to 2-year visit. As with previous studies, intraocular pressure and cataract surgery were more frequent in patients receiving triamcinolone.

Intravitreal steroid injections require repeated administrations. Consequently, to reduce the need for repeated intravitreal injections, intravitreal corticosteroid implants have been developed and studied. Two steroids in three different implant products are available in the U.S.: dexamethasone (Ozurdex) and fluocinolone (Iluvien and Retisert). However, although studied in patients with DME, Retisert is not FDA approved for this indication.

Pooled results from an analysis of the dexamethasone intravitreal implant (Macular Edema: Assessment of Implantable Dexamethasone in Diabetes [MEAD] trial) found that a greater number of patients in the implant group had at least a ≥15-letter improvement in visual acuity and reduction in central retinal thickness than patients in the sham group.[72] Cataract-related adverse events in patients with phakic eyes were greater in those receiving the implant than in those receiving the sham.

A direct comparison of a corticosteroid implant with an anti-VEGF agent was examined in the Intravitreal Bevacizumab Versus Intravitreal Dexamethasone for Persistent Diabetic Macular Oedema (BEVORDEX) study.[73] This study compared dexamethasone implant with bevacizumab in patients with CIDME. Similar percentages of eyes achieved vision improvement by 10 or more letters with each group. Conversely, those eyes that received the dexamethasone implant achieved a greater reduction in mean central macular thickness. However, a greater number of eyes were associated with vision loss in the dexamethasone group secondary to cataract development. A greater number of injections were seen with the bevacizumab group. Of note, the benefits seen with reduction in mean central macular thickness with dexamethasone were lost at 24 months.[74]

Fluocinolone implants have been investigated in two studies. One study examined intravitreal implants releasing 0.2 μg/day or 0.5 μg/day of fluocinolone compared with sham injections in patients with persistent DME.[75] The two doses of fluocinolone each achieved greater percentages of patients who gained at least a ≥15–letter score compared with the sham group at 36 months (28.7% low dose, 27.8% high dose vs. 18.9% sham). A similar percentage was observed between the different doses. The incidence of cataracts and intraocular-related adverse events were higher in those patients receiving the steroid implant than the sham. Another study examined the Retisert implant delivering fluocinolone 0.59 mg.[76] Compared with standard of care, patients with persistent or recurrent DME randomized to receive the implant saw a greater improvement of visual acuity of at least three lines at 6 months and 2 years. This significance was lost at 3 years. Findings regarding retinal thickening at the center of the macula generally paralleled the above findings. Intraocular pressure and cataracts were greater in the implanted eyes.

With the introduction of anti-VEGF agents and concerns with safety, corticosteroids are rarely used first line, and when used, have been confined to select patient populations.[35] Frequent administrations and high cost of anti-VEGF agents may make sustained-release corticosteroid products attractive in comparison. However, the risk of adverse effects of corticosteroids often outweighs these benefits. Steroid therapy may be considered in patients who have conditions, such as recent cardiovascular events, in which the systemic adverse effects of anti-VEGF agents—although associations are limited—should be avoided; who have not responded to anti-VEGF therapy, especially in those with pseudophakic eyes; and post-vitrectomy patients with CIDME.[77]

RAS INHIBITORS

Good blood pressure control is central to preventing and arresting progression of diabetic retinopathy. However, data thus far supporting preferential selection of an antihypertensive agent have been inconclusive.

T1D

Three major controlled trials examined the effects of ACE inhibitors or ARBs in patients with T1D. The EUCLID trial examined the effects of lisinopril compared with placebo on retinopathy as a secondary endpoint. Patients had T1D (mean A1C of 7.1%), normotension (mean blood pressure of 123/81 mmHg), and primarily normoalbuminuria (85% of patients; median UAE rate of 7 μg/min).[78] Approximately 80% of patients had minimal NPDR or no retinopathy at baseline. Patients who received lisinopril had less progression of retinopathy by at least 1 level, by two or more grades, and to proliferative retinopathy compared with placebo. However, the study had limitations in terms of differences in baseline glycemia between the two groups and short follow-up (24 months).

Another trial (RASS) found similar benefits with an ACE inhibitor and an ARB.[79] When compared with placebo, both agents (enalapril and losartan) statistically significantly reduced the progression of retinopathy by two or more steps independent of changes in blood pressure. Patients had T1D (mean A1C of 8.5%), normotension (mean blood pressure of 120/70 mmHg), and normoalbuminuria (median UAE rate of 5.1 μg/min). At baseline, 74% of patients had minimal NPDR or no retinopathy. The retinopathy outcome was added a priori shortly after the study began.

Lastly, the DIRECT-Prevent 1 and DIRECT-Protect 1 studies examined the incidence and progression of retinopathy in patients with T1D, normotension, and normoalbuminuria on candesartan compared with placebo.[80] At baseline, those in the DIRECT-Prevent 1 trial had a mean A1C of 8.1%, mean blood pressure of 116/72 mmHg, and no retinopathy. Comparatively, those in the DIRECT-Protect 1 trial had a mean A1C of 8.5%, mean blood pressure of 117/74 mmHg, and a majority of patients had retinopathy at a level of 20 or 35 in the worst eye using the ETDRS scale (91%). With adjustment for blood pressure, candesartan statistically significantly reduced the incidence of retinopathy, defined as at least a three-step increase on the ETDRS scale. No significant difference was found in progression of diabetic retinopathy with the use of candesartan compared with placebo.

T2D

As with patients with T1D, the role of ACE inhibitors or ARBs in patients with T2D in preventing progression of diabetic retinopathy is conflicting. The BENEDICT trial was explored to determine the effects of trandolapril on diabetic retinopathy.[81] This was a prespecified secondary endpoint. Patients had T2D, normoalbuminuria, and hypertension or were on antihypertensive agents. A majority of patients did not have diabetic retinopathy (83.6%). They were randomized to trandolapril, verapamil, or combination therapy. In those individuals receiving trandolapril monotherapy or combination therapy, regression occurred more frequently compared with those receiving verapamil.

A similar study to the DIRECT-Protect 1 trial was conducted in patients with T2D (DIRECT-Protect 2).[82] In this study, patients with T2D (mean A1C of 8.2%), normotension or treated with antihypertensive agents (mean blood pressure of 123/76 mmHg in normotensive group, and 139/80 mmHg in the treated hypertensive group), and normoalbuminuria (mean UAE rate of 5.5 μg/min) were allocated to candesartan or placebo. Most patients had a retinopathy level of 20 or 35 in the worst eye based on the ETDRS scale (83%). No significant difference was found in progression of retinopathy. However, there was a statistically significant increase in risk of regression over the 4-year trial duration. It is unknown what a 5% difference between the two groups may mean clinically.

A retrospective cohort study using an insurance database in patients with T2D was conducted to investigate the risk of sight-threatening diabetic retinopathy (STDR) in patients receiving antihypertensive agents.[83] Interestingly, ACE inhibitors or ARBs and CCBs were associated with a significantly greater risk of developing STDR compared with β-blockers.

A systematic review and meta-analysis found beneficial effects of RAS inhibitors on reducing the risk of diabetic retinopathy and increasing the potential for regression of diabetic retinopathy, specifically in patients with normotension and T1D or T2D.[84] In patients with hypertension, RAS inhibitors were not associated with a difference in either outcome. When broken down by class, ACE inhibitors were found to decrease the risk of progression and increase the chance of regression, while ARBs were found to only increase the chance of regression.

Based on the literature above, it is difficult to ascertain the role of a specific class of antihypertensive agent in the treatment of diabetic retinopathy. Most evidence examining the effects of ACE inhibitors or ARBs is in patients with T1D or T2D with normotension and normoalbuminuria. Patients with retinopathy often have concomitant nephropathy, in which RAS inhibitors have been shown to have a strong benefit in preventing progression.[6,59]

PPAR-α

The mechanism of action of a PPAR-α in the management of diabetic retinopathy is not fully elucidated. In addition to its lipid effects, fenofibrate has antiinflammatory, antiangiogenic, antiapoptotic, and antioxidant effects that theoretically may be protective in diabetic retinopathy.[85]

The Fenofibrate Intervention and Event Lowering in Diabetes (FIELD) study was conducted in patients with T2D (mean A1C of 6.9%) to investigate coronary events.[86] However, retinopathy outcomes were examined as other endpoints. The mean blood pressure was 141/82 mmHg and mean LDL cholesterol was 119 mg/dL. Approximately 8% of patients had retinopathy at baseline. The fenofibrate group needed fewer laser treatments for retinopathy than the placebo group. A substudy of the FIELD trial examined patients without retinopathy at baseline.[87] Similarly, patients who received fenofibrate had a statistically significantly lower rate in needing laser treatment for diabetic retinopathy when compared with placebo. In patients with preexisting retinopathy, fewer experienced progression. No difference was seen in deterioration of visual acuity.

Diabetic retinopathy outcomes were examined in a substudy of the ACCORD trial.[18] In contrast with the FIELD study, patients in the ACCORD trial had a higher prevalence of preexisting diabetic retinopathy at baseline and a longer duration of diabetes. Regardless, the results of the study were consistent with those observed in the FIELD study. Patients in the fenofibrate group had a lower rate of retinopathy progression over the 4-year study period compared with the simvastatin group. No difference was seen in deterioration of visual acuity.

Due to limitations of its effects on cardiovascular outcomes, fenofibrate is often avoided as first-line therapy for the treatment of dyslipidemia. However, based on the above studies, considerations may be made for the use of fenofibrate in diabetic retinopathy progression.

ASPIRIN

Aspirin has been found to prevent leukocyte vascular occlusion and decrease production of inflammatory markers in diabetic retinopathy.[88] These mechanisms of action make it an attractive treatment option. However, clinical outcomes to support this hypothesis have not been well supported. In particular, the ETDRS study found that aspirin 650 mg daily had no effect on the progression of diabetic retinopathy or risk of vision loss.[89] Of note, aspirin also did not have an effect on the risk of vitreous hemorrhage among patients with PDR.[90] Therefore, although strong supporting evidence for the role of aspirin in the treatment of diabetic retinopathy is lacking, aspirin is safe to use in patients with diabetic retinopathy for its cardioprotective benefits.[59]

GLP-1 RAs

GLP-1 RAs are believed to exert neuroprotective effects that may be beneficial in the treatment of diabetic retinopathy beyond their effects on glycemic control.[91] Moreover, studies have shown the presence of GLP-1 receptors in human retinas, which helps support the idea that GLP-1 RAs may be useful in preventing or arresting retinal neurodegeneration.[91]

Currently, there is a lack of literature supporting the role of GLP-1 RAs in the treatment of diabetic retinopathy. When examined as secondary outcomes in major controlled trials examining primarily cardiovascular outcomes, effects of GLP-1 RAs were found to be neutral or even harmful. Specifically, the SUSTAIN-6 trial observed that patients who received semaglutide had an increase in the progression of retinopathy compared with placebo.[92] Again, it must be emphasized that retinopathy was examined as a secondary outcome. Therefore, this finding must be taken into context and with caution. Analyses of other studies examining semaglutide did not have similar outcomes.[93,94] It is proposed that the worsening of retinopathy is associated with the speed and magnitude of improvement in glycemic control and not related to the medication itself.[93] A meta-analysis supported the idea that this is not a class effect; outside of semaglutide, GLP-1 RAs appear to have no specific effect to beneficial effects on retinopathy.[95] More data are needed to define the role of this class of medication in the treatment of diabetic retinopathy.

COMBINATION THERAPY

Combination therapy may be a promising avenue for the treatment of diabetic retinopathy, particularly in cases not responding to initial therapy or with more severity. Currently, further studies are needed to solidify initial findings.

ANTI-VEGF + LASER THERAPY

The Ranibizumab Monotherapy or Combined with Laser Versus Laser Monotherapy for Diabetic Macular Edema (RESTORE) study found that ranibizumab combination therapy, in addition to ranibizumab monotherapy, was superior to laser treatment alone for DME. However, no differences in efficacy were found between the ranibizumab monotherapy or combination groups.[39] Similarly, patients receiving combination treatment with bevacizumab and macular photocoagulation did not experience better outcomes in terms of visual acuity or reduction in macular thickness than patients receiving monotherapy with bevacizumab.[96]

A potential role for combination therapy was alluded to in the Ranibizumab for Edema of the mAcula in Diabetes (READ-2) trial.[97] The study found that combined ranibizumab with macular laser photocoagulation may be beneficial in reducing the number of injections. Another role for combination therapy may be in PDR. A systematic review and meta-analysis found that anti-VEGF agents in patients with PDR may be used as an adjunct to PRP or pars plana vitrectomy.[64] Potential benefits of adjunctive use include improved visual activity and central retinal thickness, less intraoperative bleeding, decreased duration of surgery, and fewer retinal breaks.

CORTICOSTEROID + LASER THERAPY

Combination therapy with laser photocoagulation after 1 month was examined in the Primary Laser with Adjunctive Implantable Dexamethasone in DME (PLACID) trial.[98] Patients were allocated to dexamethasone implant or sham implant. Both groups received laser therapy at 1 month. Although no difference in

Table 25.2—Medications and Dosing

Medication	Typical dose(s)	Renal dose adjustment(s)	Hepatic dose adjustment(s)
Aflibercept (Eylea)*	2 mg once every 4 weeks for the first 5 injections, followed by 2 mg (0.05 mL) once every 8 weeks**	None	None
Bevacizumab (Avastin)	1.25 mg, may repeat every 4 weeks depending on response	None	None
Dexamethasone (Ozurdex)*	0.7-mg implant	None	None
Fluocinolone (Iluvien)*	0.19-mg implant	None	None
Fluocinolone (Retisert)	0.59-mg implant	None	None
Pegaptanib (Macugen)	0.3 mg once every 6 weeks	None	None
Ranibizumab (Lucentis)*	0.3 mg once a month	None	None
Triamcinolone (Triesence)	4 mg once	None	None

*FDA approved for diabetic macular edema **Some patients may require dosing every 4 weeks after the first 20 weeks. *Source*: refs. 36,68,76,103–108.

percentage of patients who gained ≥10 letters in visual acuity at 12 months was found, the group who received the implant had significantly greater improvement at 1 month and 9 months. Cataract-related adverse events were more common in phakic study eyes that received the dexamethasone implant than the sham implant.

A few small studies have been conducted examining the combination of laser photocoagulation with intravitreal corticosteroids on diabetic retinopathy in patients primarily with PDR. These studies found improvement in visual acuity and central macular thickness with combination therapy compared with laser photocoagulation alone.[99,100]

ANTI-VEGF + CORTICOSTEROIDS

A phase 2 randomized clinical trial suggests that in patients with persistent DME, addition of a steroid may be harmful.[101] At 24 weeks, patients receiving ranibizumab and dexamethasone combination had a greater reduction in central subfield thickness compared with the ranibizumab monotherapy group. Of note, although no difference was found in mean visual acuity improvement, the study was not sufficiently powered to identify a difference. A higher proportion of patients developed a statistically significant increase in intraocular pressure in the combination group compared with the monotherapy group.

The efficacy of combination therapy with an anti-VEGF agent and steroid for the treatment of DME was analyzed in a meta-analysis.[102] The meta-analysis found that bevacizumab with intravitreal triamcinolone improved visual acuity at 3 months, but no difference was found at 6 months. Similarly, benefits of combination therapy were seen in central macular thickness at 3 months, but not at 6 months. Ocular hypertension ranged from 0 to 8.3% in the combination group, and there were no cases among the bevacizumab group. Results of the meta-analysis were limited by the short duration of the studies included.

MONOGRAPHS

Aflibercept (Eylea): https://dailymed.nlm.nih.gov/dailymed/drugInfo.cfm?setid=f96cfd69-da34-41ee-90a9-610a4655cd1c

Bevacizumab (Avastin): https://dailymed.nlm.nih.gov/dailymed/drugInfo.cfm?setid=939b5d1f-9fb2-4499-80ef-0607aa6b114e

Dexamethasone (Ozurdex): https://dailymed.nlm.nih.gov/dailymed/drugInfo.cfm?setid=4b204f44-6e8a-4d17-803c-268f0b04679f

Fluocinolone (Iluvien): https://dailymed.nlm.nih.gov/dailymed/drugInfo.cfm?setid=4400e471-7402-11df-93f2-0800200c9a66

Fluocinolone (Retisert): https://dailymed.nlm.nih.gov/dailymed/drugInfo.cfm?setid=1ab0f849-2a0d-47ce-ad05-768094da8cc9

Pegaptanib (Macugen): https://dailymed.nlm.nih.gov/dailymed/drugInfo.cfm?setid=45d03177-5d52-492c-b2e0-01afc7c8d2e0

Ranibizumab (Lucentis): https://dailymed.nlm.nih.gov/dailymed/drugInfo.cfm?setid=de4e66cc-ca05-4dc9-8262-e00e9b41c36d

Triamcinolone (Triesence): https://dailymed.nlm.nih.gov/dailymed/drugInfo.cfm?setid=3f045347-3e5e-4bbd-90f8-6c3100985ca5

REFERENCES

1. Solomon SD, Chew E, Duh EJ, et al. Diabetic retinopathy: a position statement by the American Diabetes Association. *Diabetes Care* 2017;40(3): 412–418

2. Yau JW, Rogers SL, Kawasaki R, et al. Global prevalence and major risk factors of diabetic retinopathy. *Diabetes Care* 2012;35(3):556–564

3. Xu J, Xu L, Wang YX, et al. Ten-year cumulative incidence of diabetic retinopathy. The Beijing Eye Study 2001/2011. *PLoS One* 2014;9(10):e111320

4. Jin P, Peng J, Zou H, et al. The 5-year onset and regression of diabetic retinopathy in Chinese type 2 diabetes patients. *PLoS One* 2014;9(11):e113359

5. Hammer SS, Busik JV. The role of dyslipidemia in diabetic retinopathy. *Vision Res* 2017;139:228–236

6. Lee MK, Han KD, Lee JH, et al. Normal-to-mildly increased albuminuria predicts the risk for diabetic retinopathy in patients with type 2 diabetes. *Sci Rep* 2017;7(1):11757

7. Klein R, Knudtson MD, Lee KE, et al. The Wisconsin Epidemiologic Study of Diabetic Retinopathy: XXII the twenty-five-year progression of retinopathy in persons with type 1 diabetes. *Ophthalmology* 2008;115(11):1859–1868

8. Klein R, Klein BE, Moss SE, et al. The Wisconsin epidemiologic study of diabetic retinopathy. II. Prevalence and risk of diabetic retinopathy when age at diagnosis is less than 30 years. *Arch Ophthalmol* 1984;102(4):520–526

9. Klein R, Klein BE, Moss SE, et al. The Wisconsin epidemiologic study of diabetic retinopathy. III. Prevalence and risk of diabetic retinopathy when age at diagnosis is 30 or more years. *Arch Ophthalmol* 1984;102(4):527–532

10. Wong TY, Cheung CM, Larsen M, et al. Diabetic retinopathy. *Nat Rev Dis Primers* 2016;2:16012

11. Romero-Aroca P, Baget-Bernaldiz M, Pareja-Rios A, et al. Diabetic macular edema pathophysiology: vasogenic versus inflammatory. *J Diabetes Res* 2016:2156273

12. Klein R, Klein BE, Moss SE, Cruickshanks KJ. The Wisconsin epidemiologic study of diabetic retinopathy. XIV. Ten-year incidence and progression of diabetic retinopathy. *Arch Ophthalmol* 1994;112(9):1217–1228

13. Klein R, Lee KE, Gangnon RE, Klein BE. The 25-year incidence of visual impairment in type 1 diabetes mellitus the Wisconsin epidemiologic study of diabetic retinopathy. *Ophthalmology* 2010;117(1):63–70

14. Klein R, Klein BE. Are individuals with diabetes seeing better? a long-term epidemiological perspective. *Diabetes* 2010;59(8):1853–1860

15. Nathan DM, Zinman B, Cleary PA, et al. Modern-day clinical course of type 1 diabetes mellitus after 30 years' duration: the diabetes control and complications trial/epidemiology of diabetes interventions and complications and Pittsburgh epidemiology of diabetes complications experience (1983–2005). *Arch Intern Med* 2009;169(14):1307–1316

16. Nathan DM, Genuth S, Lachin J, et al. The effect of intensive treatment of diabetes on the development and progression of long-term complications in insulin-dependent diabetes mellitus. *N Engl J Med* 1993;329(14):977–986

17. UK Prospective Diabetes Study (UKPDS) Group. Intensive blood-glucose control with sulphonylureas or insulin compared with conventional treatment and risk of complications in patients with type 2 diabetes (UKPDS 33). *Lancet* 1998;352(9131):837–853

18. Chew EY, Ambrosius WT, Davis MD, et al. Effects of medical therapies on retinopathy progression in type 2 diabetes. *N Engl J Med* 2010;363(3): 233–244

19. The Diabetes Control and Complications Trial Research Group. The relationship of glycemic exposure (HbA1c) to the risk of development and progression of retinopathy in the diabetes control and complications trial. *Diabetes* 1995;44(8):968–983

20. Lachin JM, Genuth S, Cleary P, et al. Retinopathy and nephropathy in patients with type 1 diabetes four years after a trial of intensive therapy. *N Engl J Med* 2000;342(6):381–389

21. Holman RR, Paul SK, Bethel MA, Matthews DR, Neil HA. 10-year follow-up of intensive glucose control in type 2 diabetes. *N Engl J Med* 2008;359(15):1577–1589

22. Patel A, MacMahon S, Chalmers J, et al. Intensive blood glucose control and vascular outcomes in patients with type 2 diabetes. *N Engl J Med* 2008;358(24):2560–2572

23. Hirsch IB, Brownlee M. Beyond hemoglobin A1c—need for additional markers of risk for diabetic microvascular complications. *JAMA* 2010;303(22):2291–2292

24. UK Prospective Diabetes Study Group. Tight blood pressure control and risk of macrovascular and microvascular complications in type 2 diabetes: UKPDS 38. *BMJ* 1998;317(7160):703–713

25. Ioannidou E, Tseriotis VS, Tziomalos K. Role of lipid-lowering agents in the management of diabetic retinopathy. *World J Diabetes* 2017;8(1):1–6

26. Modjtahedi BS, Bose N, Papakostas TD, et al. Lipids and diabetic retinopathy. *Semin Ophthalmol* 2016;31(1-2):10–18

27. Willis JR, Doan QV, Gleeson M, et al. Vision-related functional burden of diabetic retinopathy across severity levels in the United States. *JAMA Ophthalmol* 2017;135(9):926–932

28. Beck RW, Maguire MG, Bressler NM, et al. Visual acuity as an outcome measure in clinical trials of retinal diseases. *Ophthalmology* 2007;114(10): 1804–1809

29. Fortin P, Mintzes B, Innes M. A systematic review of intravitreal bevacizumab for the treatment of diabetic macular edema [Internet], 2012. Ottawa, Canadian Agency for Drugs and Technologies in Health. Available from https://www.ncbi.nlm.nih.gov/books/NBK169468/

30. Early Treatment Diabetic Retinopathy Study research group. Photocoagulation for diabetic macular edema. Early Treatment Diabetic Retinopathy Study report number 1. *Arch Ophthalmol* 1985;103(12):1796–1806

31. Nguyen QD, Brown DM, Marcus DM, et al. Ranibizumab for diabetic macular edema: results from 2 phase III randomized trials: RISE and RIDE. *Ophthalmology* 2012;119(4):789–801

32. The Diabetic Retinopathy Study Research Group. Preliminary report on effects of photocoagulation therapy. *Am J Ophthalmol* 1976;81(4):383–396

33. Evans JR, Michelessi M, Virgili G. Laser photocoagulation for proliferative diabetic retinopathy. *Cochrane Database Syst Rev* 2014(11):CD011234

34. Stefansson E. The therapeutic effects of retinal laser treatment and vitrectomy: a theory based on oxygen and vascular physiology. *Acta Ophthalmol Scand* 2001;79(5):435–440

35. Antonetti DA, Klein R, Gardner TW. Diabetic retinopathy. *N Engl J Med* 2012;366(13):1227–1239

36. Wells JA, Glassman AR, Ayala AR, et al. Aflibercept, bevacizumab, or ranibizumab for diabetic macular edema. *N Engl J Med* 2015;372(13):1193–1203

37. Simo R, Hernandez C. Intravitreous anti-VEGF for diabetic retinopathy: hopes and fears for a new therapeutic strategy. *Diabetologia* 2008;51(9):1574–1580

38. MacDonald DA, Martin J, Muthusamy KK, et al. Aflibercept exhibits VEGF binding stoichiometry distinct from bevacizumab and does not support formation of immune-like complexes. *Angiogenesis* 2016;19(3):389–406

39. Mitchell P, Bandello F, Schmidt-Erfurth U, et al. The RESTORE study: ranibizumab monotherapy or combined with laser versus laser monotherapy for diabetic macular edema. *Ophthalmology* 2011;118(4):615–625

40. Ishibashi T, Li X, Koh A, et al. The REVEAL Study: Ranibizumab monotherapy or combined with laser versus laser monotherapy in Asian patients with diabetic macular edema. *Ophthalmology* 2015;122(7):1402–1415

41. Korobelnik JF, Do DV, Schmidt-Erfurth U, et al. Intravitreal aflibercept for diabetic macular edema. *Ophthalmology* 2014;121(11):2247–2254

42. Michaelides M, Kaines A, Hamilton RD, et al. A prospective randomized trial of intravitreal bevacizumab or laser therapy in the management of diabetic macular edema (BOLT study) 12-month data: report 2. *Ophthalmology* 2010;117(6):1078–1086.e2

43. Virgili G, Parravano M, Evans JR, et al. Anti-vascular endothelial growth factor for diabetic macular oedema: a network meta-analysis. *Cochrane Database Syst Rev* 2017;6:CD007419

44. Sultan MB, Zhou D, Loftus J, et al. A phase 2/3, multicenter, randomized, double-masked, 2-year trial of pegaptanib sodium for the treatment of diabetic macular edema. *Ophthalmology* 2011;118(6):1107–1118

45. Jampol LM, Glassman AR, Bressler NM, et al. Anti-vascular endothelial growth factor comparative effectiveness trial for diabetic macular edema: additional efficacy post hoc analyses of a randomized clinical trial. *JAMA Ophthalmol* 2016;134(12)

46. Bressler SB, Liu D, Glassman AR, et al. Change in diabetic retinopathy through 2 years: secondary analysis of a randomized clinical trial comparing aflibercept, bevacizumab, and ranibizumab. *JAMA Ophthalmol* 2017;135(6):558–568

47. Bressler NM, Beaulieu WT, Glassman AR, et al. Persistent macular thickening following intravitreous aflibercept, bevacizumab, or ranibizumab for central-involved diabetic macular edema with vision impairment: a secondary analysis of a randomized clinical trial. *JAMA Ophthalmol* 2018;136(3): 257–269

48. Blinder KJ, Dugel PU, Chen S, et al. Anti-VEGF treatment of diabetic macular edema in clinical practice: effectiveness and patterns of use (ECHO Study Report 1). *Clin Ophthalmol* 2017;11:393–401

49. Elman MJ, Ayala A, Bressler NM, et al. Intravitreal ranibizumab for diabetic macular edema with prompt versus deferred laser treatment: 5-year randomized trial results. *Ophthalmology* 2015;122(2):375–381

50. Schmidt-Erfurth U, Lang GE, Holz FG, et al. Three-year outcomes of individualized ranibizumab treatment in patients with diabetic macular edema: the RESTORE extension study. *Ophthalmology* 2014;121(5): 1045–1053

51. Pershing S, Enns EA, Matesic B, et al. Cost-effectiveness of treatment of diabetic macular edema. *Ann Intern Med* 2014;160(1):18–29

52. Martin DF, Maguire MG. Treatment choice for diabetic macular edema. *N Engl J Med* 2015;372(13):1260–1261

53. Ross EL, Hutton DW, Stein JD, et al. Cost-effectiveness of aflibercept, bevacizumab, and ranibizumab for diabetic macular edema treatment: analysis from the diabetic retinopathy clinical research network comparative effectiveness trial. *JAMA Ophthalmol* 2016;134(8):888–896

54. Yannuzzi NA, Klufas MA, Quach L, et al. Evaluation of compounded bevacizumab prepared for intravitreal injection. *JAMA Ophthalmol* 2015;133(1):32–39

55. Gross JG, Glassman AR, Jampol LM, et al. Panretinal photocoagulation vs intravitreous ranibizumab for proliferative diabetic retinopathy: a randomized clinical trial. *JAMA* 2015;314(20):2137–2146

56. Sivaprasad S, Prevost AT, Vasconcelos JC, et al. Clinical efficacy of intravitreal aflibercept versus panretinal photocoagulation for best corrected visual acuity in patients with proliferative diabetic retinopathy at 52 weeks (CLARITY): a multicentre, single-blinded, randomised, controlled, phase 2b, non-inferiority trial. *Lancet* 2017;389(10085):2193–2203

57. Martinez-Zapata MJ, Marti-Carvajal AJ, Sola I, et al. Anti-vascular endothelial growth factor for proliferative diabetic retinopathy. *Cochrane Database Syst Rev* 2014;(11):CD008721

58. Osaadon P, Fagan XJ, Lifshitz T, Levy J. A review of anti-VEGF agents for proliferative diabetic retinopathy. *Eye* (Lond) 2014;28(5):510–520

59. American Diabetes Association. 10. Microvascular complications and foot care: *Standards of Medical Care in Diabetes—2018*. *Diabetes Care* 2018; 41(Suppl. 1):S105–S118

60. Obeid A, Gao X, Ali FS, et al. Loss to follow-up in patients with proliferative diabetic retinopathy after panretinal photocoagulation or intravitreal anti-VEGF injections. *Ophthalmology* 2018;125(9):1386–1392

61. Lin J, Chang JS, Smiddy WE. Cost evaluation of panretinal photocoagulation versus intravitreal ranibizumab for proliferative diabetic retinopathy. *Ophthalmology* 2016;123(9):1912–1918

62. Hutton DW, Stein JD, Bressler NM, et al. Cost-effectiveness of intravitreous ranibizumab compared with panretinal photocoagulation for proliferative diabetic retinopathy: secondary analysis from a diabetic retinopathy clinical research network randomized clinical trial. *JAMA Ophthalmol* 2017;135(6):576–584

63. Avery RL, Gordon GM. Systemic safety of prolonged monthly anti-vascular endothelial growth factor therapy for diabetic macular edema: a systematic review and meta-analysis. *JAMA Ophthalmol* 2016;134(1):21–29

64. Simunovic MP, Maberley DA. Anti-vascular endothelial growth factor therapy for proflierative diabetic retinopathy: a systematic review and meta-analysis. *Retina* 2015;35(10):1931–1942

65. Gupta A, Sun JK, Silva PS. Complications of intravitreous injections in patients with diabetes. *Semin Ophthalmol* 2018;33(1):42–50

66. Falavarjani KG, Nguyen QD. Adverse events and complications associated with intravitreal injection of anti-VEGF agents: a review of literature. *Eye* (Lond) 2013;27(7):787–794

67. Nauck M, Karakiulakis G, Perruchoud AP, et al. Corticosteroids inhibit the expression of the vascular endothelial growth factor gene in human vascular smooth muscle cells. *Eur J Pharmacol* 1998;341(2–3):309–315

68. Diabetic Retinopathy Clinical Research Network. A randomized trial comparing intravitreal triamcinolone acetonide and focal/grid photocoagulation for diabetic macular edema. *Ophthalmology* 2008;115(9):1447–1449, 1449.e1–10

69. Beck RW, Edwards AR, Aiello LP, et al. Three-year follow-up of a randomized trial comparing focal/grid photocoagulation and intravitreal triamcinolone for diabetic macular edema. *Arch Ophthalmol* 2009;127(3):245–251

70. Elman MJ, Aiello LP, Beck RW, et al. Randomized trial evaluating ranibizumab plus prompt or deferred laser or triamcinolone plus prompt laser for diabetic macular edema. *Ophthalmology* 2010;117(6):1064–1077.e1035

71. Elman MJ, Bressler NM, Qin H, et al. Expanded 2-year follow-up of ranibizumab plus prompt or deferred laser or triamcinolone plus prompt laser for diabetic macular edema. *Ophthalmology* 2011;118(4):609–614

72. Boyer DS, Yoon YH, Belfort R Jr., et al. Three-year, randomized, sham-controlled trial of dexamethasone intravitreal implant in patients with diabetic macular edema. *Ophthalmology* 2014;121(10):1904–1914

73. Gillies MC, Lim LL, Campain A, et al. A randomized clinical trial of intravitreal bevacizumab versus intravitreal dexamethasone for diabetic macular edema: the BEVORDEX study. *Ophthalmology* 2014;121(12):2473–2481

74. Fraser-Bell S, Lim LL, Campain A, et al. Bevacizumab or dexamethasone implants for DME: 2-year results (the BEVORDEX study). *Ophthalmology* 2016;123(6):1399–1401

75. Campochiaro PA, Brown DM, Pearson A, et al. Sustained delivery fluocinolone acetonide vitreous inserts provide benefit for at least 3 years in patients with diabetic macular edema. *Ophthalmology* 2012;119(10):2125–2132

76. Pearson PA, Comstock TL, Ip M, et al. Fluocinolone acetonide intravitreal implant for diabetic macular edema: a 3-year multicenter, randomized, controlled clinical trial. *Ophthalmology* 2011;118(8):1580–1587

77. Regillo CD, Callanan DG, Do DV, et al. Use of corticosteroids in the treatment of patients with diabetic macular edema who have a suboptimal response to anti-VEGF: recommendations of an expert panel. *Ophthalmic Surg Lasers Imaging Retina* 2017;48(4):291–301

78. Chaturvedi N, Sjolie AK, Stephenson JM, et al. Effect of lisinopril on progression of retinopathy in normotensive people with type 1 diabetes. The EUCLID Study Group. EURODIAB Controlled Trial of Lisinopril in Insulin-Dependent Diabetes Mellitus. *Lancet* 1998;351(9095):28–31

79. Mauer M, Zinman B, Gardiner R, et al. Renal and retinal effects of enalapril and losartan in type 1 diabetes. *N Engl J Med* 2009;361(1):40–51

80. Chaturvedi N, Porta M, Klein R, et al. Effect of candesartan on prevention (DIRECT-Prevent 1) and progression (DIRECT-Protect 1) of retinopathy in type 1 diabetes: randomised, placebo-controlled trials. *Lancet* 2008;372(9647):1394–1402

81. Ruggenenti P, Iliev I, Filipponi M, et al. Effect of trandolapril on regression of retinopathy in hypertensive patients with type 2 diabetes: a prespecified analysis of the benedict trial. *J Ophthalmol* 2010:106384

82. Sjolie AK, Klein R, Porta M, et al. Effect of candesartan on progression and regression of retinopathy in type 2 diabetes (DIRECT-Protect 2): a randomised placebo-controlled trial. *Lancet* 2008;372(9647):1385–1393

83. Lin JC, Lai MS. Antihypertensive drugs and diabetic retinopathy in patients with type 2 diabetes. *Ophthalmologica* 2016;235(2):87–96

84. Wang B, Wang F, Zhang Y, et al. Effects of RAS inhibitors on diabetic retinopathy: a systematic review and meta-analysis. *Lancet Diabetes Endocrinol* 2015;3(4):263–274

85. Noonan JE, Jenkins AJ, Ma JX, et al. An update on the molecular actions of fenofibrate and its clinical effects on diabetic retinopathy and other microvascular end points in patients with diabetes. *Diabetes* 2013;62(12):3968–3975

86. Keech A, Simes RJ, Barter P, et al. Effects of long-term fenofibrate therapy on cardiovascular events in 9795 people with type 2 diabetes mellitus (the FIELD study): randomised controlled trial. *Lancet* 2005;366(9500): 1849–1861

87. Keech AC, Mitchell P, Summanen PA, et al. Effect of fenofibrate on the need for laser treatment for diabetic retinopathy (FIELD study): a randomised controlled trial. *Lancet* 2007;370(9600):1687–1697

88. Kohner EM. Aspirin for diabetic retinopathy. *BMJ* 2003;327(7423): 1060–1061

89. Early Treatment Diabetic Retinopathy Study Research Group. Effects of aspirin treatment on diabetic retinopathy. ETDRS report number 8. *Ophthalmology* 1991;98(5 Suppl.):757–765

90. Chew EY, Klein ML, Murphy RP, et al. Effects of aspirin on vitreous/preretinal hemorrhage in patients with diabetes mellitus. Early Treatment Diabetic Retinopathy Study report no. 20. *Arch Ophthalmol* 1995;113(1):52–55

91. Hernandez C, Bogdanov P, Corraliza L, et al. Topical administration of GLP-1 receptor agonists prevents retinal neurodegeneration in experimental diabetes. *Diabetes* 2016;65(1):172–187

92. Marso SP, Bain SC, Consoli A, et al. Semaglutide and cardiovascular outcomes in patients with type 2 diabetes. *N Engl J Med* 2016;375(19): 1834–1844

93. Vilsboll T, Bain SC, Leiter LA, et al. Semaglutide, reduction in glycated haemoglobin and the risk of diabetic retinopathy. *Diabetes Obes Metab* 2018;20(4):889–897

94. Pratley RE, Aroda VR, Lingvay I, et al. Semaglutide versus dulaglutide once weekly in patients with type 2 diabetes (SUSTAIN 7): a randomised, open-label, phase 3b trial. *Lancet Diabetes Endocrinol* 2018;6(4):275–286

95. Dicembrini I, Nreu B, Scatena A, et al. Microvascular effects of glucagon-like peptide-1 receptor agonists in type 2 diabetes: a meta-analysis of randomized controlled trials. *Acta Diabetol* 2017;54(10):933–941

96. Lee SJ, Kim ET, Moon YS. Intravitreal bevacizumab alone versus combined with macular photocoagulation in diabetic macular edema. *Korean J Ophthalmol* 2011;25(5):299–304

97. Nguyen QD, Shah SM, Khwaja AA, et al. Two-year outcomes of the ranibizumab for edema of the mAcula in diabetes (READ-2) study. *Ophthalmology* 2010;117(11):2146–2151

98. Callanan DG, Gupta S, Boyer DS, et al. Dexamethasone intravitreal implant in combination with laser photocoagulation for the treatment of diffuse diabetic macular edema. *Ophthalmology* 2013;120(9):1843–1851

99. Kang SW, Sa HS, Cho HY, Kim JI. Macular grid photocoagulation after intravitreal triamcinolone acetonide for diffuse diabetic macular edema. *Arch Ophthalmol* 2006;124(5):653–658

100. Maia OO Jr., Takahashi BS, Costa RA, et al. Combined laser and intravitreal triamcinolone for proliferative diabetic retinopathy and macular edema: one-year results of a randomized clinical trial. *Am J Ophthalmol* 2009;147(2):291–297.e292

101. Maturi RK, Glassman AR, Liu D, et al. Effect of adding dexamethasone to continued ranibizumab treatment in patients with persistent diabetic macular edema: a DRCR network phase 2 randomized clinical trial. *JAMA Ophthalmol* 2018;136(1):29–38

102. Jin E, Luo L, Bai Y, Zhao M. Comparative effectiveness of intravitreal bevacizumab with or without triamcinolone acetonide for treatment of diabetic macular edema. *Ann Pharmacother* 2015;49(4):387–397

103. Aflibercept (Eylea) injection, for intravitreal use [product information]. Tarrytown, NY, Regeneron Pharmaceuticals, May 2017

104. Rajendram R, Fraser-Bell S, Kaines A, et al. A 2-year prospective randomized controlled trial of intravitreal bevacizumab or laser therapy (BOLT) in the management of diabetic macular edema: 24-month data: report 3. *Arch Ophthalmol* 2012;130(8):972–979

105. Dexamethasone (Ozurdex) implant, for intravitreal use [product information]. Madison, NJ, Allergan, May 2018

106. Fluocinolone (Iluvien) implant, for intravitreal use [product information]. Alpharetta, GA, Alimera Sciences, November 2016

107. Rinaldi M, Chiosi F, dell'Omo R, et al. Intravitreal pegaptanib sodium (Macugen) for treatment of diabetic macular oedema: a morphologic and functional study. *Br J Clin Pharmacol* 2012;74(6):940–946

108. Ranibuzumab (Lucentis) injection, for intravitreal use [product information]. South San Francisco, CA, Genentech USA, Inc., March 2018

Chapter 26

Medications for the Management of Depression

Megan Willson, PharmD, BCPS

INTRODUCTION

Depression is one of the most common mental health disorders. The DSM-V defines MDD as having five or more of the following symptoms during a 2-week period. These symptoms must include a depressed mood or loss of interest or pleasure. Other symptoms are changes in weight, changes in sleep, agitation or slowing, lack of energy, worthlessness or guilt, decreased ability to concentrate, or recurrent thoughts of death.[1] Depression symptoms can range from mild to severe and are truly different from just being sad. According to the Substance Abuse and Mental Health Services Administration (SAMHSA), 16.2 million adults, or almost 7% of the U.S. adult population, had one episode of depression in 2016. The prevalence of depression increased with female sex and is highest in patients aged 18–25 years and reporting two or more racial/ethnic backgrounds.[2] Risk factors for depression are both medical and social. Some medical-related risk factors are biochemical, genetic, sleep disorders, and serious medical illness including diabetes. Social-related risk factors can include abuse, gender, social support systems, and life events. Other factors to consider include substance use and abuse and certain medications.[3]

Serious chronic illnesses such as diabetes are known risk factors for MDD, but MDD is also a risk factor for diabetes. Evidence also demonstrates additive effects of comorbid MDD and diabetes to both morbidity and mortality. The bidirectional association has been observed in effect of treatment outcomes of both disease states.[4] Patients with diabetes have a 1.6 times greater risk of depression than those without diabetes.[5] Another study showed that patients with newly diagnosed diabetes were 30% more likely to have had an episode of depression in the past 3 years than individuals without diabetes. A meta-analysis also demonstrated that suicidal ideation and suicide attempts were increased in patients with depression and diabetes.[6] Patients with T2D had a 24% increased risk of developing MDD.[4] Mezuk and colleagues proposed the strongest correlation exists for MDD leading to diabetes.[7]

The causal relationship between diabetes and depression is multifactorial. General factors for depression impacting diabetes are antidepressant use, weight gain, obesity, and lack of physical activity.[4,8] Further exploration of antidepressant use has led to associations beyond the impact on weight gain or direct impact on glycemic control. Higher doses of antidepressants used for longer periods of time have led to increases in rates of diabetes. The factors associated with diabetes that led to depression include emotional stress, metabolic syndrome, genetics, and obesity.[4,8,9]

Depression has a significant impact on both morbidity and mortality associated with diabetes as well, including worse glycemic control and insulin resistance, more micro- and macrovascular complications, as well as increased rates of mortality.[4,10,11] Research has demonstrated a relationship between diabetes outcomes and emotional stress and health-related quality of life.[12,13] Depression has been linked to poor self-care, diet, and medication adherence, which lead to decreased glycemic control. Patients with comorbid depression and diabetes treated with antidepressant medications are more likely to achieve good glycemic control than those not treated,[14] which indicates the strong need to recognize and treat depression in this population. The identification and treatment of the associated emotional distress is also important to address when treating the depression. Hyperglycemia and poor glycemic control are well-recognized contributing factors to macrovascular complications necessitating the management of co-morbid depression.

Due to the significant impact that treatment of depression can have on diabetes morbidity and mortality, this chapter will discuss the following major classes of antidepressants commonly used today: SSRIs; SNRIs; TCAs, atypical antidepressants, and serotonin modulators. A limited number of trials are focused on patients with diabetes, so most evidence is derived for treatment of depression in population-based studies.

Depression treatment follows some general rules or principles for treatment. Depression treatment begins with the acute phase, followed by the continuation phase, and concluded with the maintenance phase. The acute phase consists of initiation of pharmacotherapy, psychotherapy, or a combination of pharmacotherapy and psychotherapy or electroconvulsive therapy. Pharmacotherapy should be initiated at a low dose and titrated up to achieve symptom resolution while still maintaining a tolerable side-effect profile. If side effects occur, a reduction of dose can sometimes alleviate the symptoms. The acute phase should be continued for at least 6–12 weeks. Symptom relief can occur as early as 1–2 weeks but may take 4–6 weeks to show improvement with pharmacotherapy. A trial of 4–8 weeks at the maximal tolerated dose is adequate to determine if therapy is not effective. Full benefit with pharmacotherapy occurs at around 12 weeks. The continuation phase should continue for 4–9 months with the same therapy that induced remission of depression. The continuation phase should be used to prevent relapse. The maintenance phase should be used in patients with chronic depression, patients with three or more episodes of MDD, and those at high risk of relapse.[15]

Table 26.1—Goals of Therapy

- Remission of depression
- Preventing relapse of depression
- Avoiding adverse effects of pharmacotherapy
- Improving daily functioning

SSRIs

SSRIs are considered a first-line therapy, with or without combination psychotherapy, for the treatment of mild to moderate depression. This class is considered first line because of efficacy in clinical trials and overall tolerability. SSRIs used in combination with psychotherapy are also recommended as first line for severe forms of MDD. SSRIs can also be useful for the treatment of anxiety disorders.[12]

Class effects as well as individual medication characteristics must be considered when selecting an agent in the SSRI medication class. No medication in this class is considered superior to another. Also, no specific medication classes have been found to be superior to another class based on efficacy.[15] Each medication should be selected based on differences in side-effect profile and/or tolerability for the patient, dosing, or other drug characteristics. Most medications have a long elimination half-life allowing for once-daily dosing, except fluvoxamine, which should be taken twice daily.[16]

Although SSRIs are considered better tolerated than tricyclics or monoamine oxidase inhibitors, patients can still commonly experience side effects. Citalopram and escitalopram can cause a dose-related corrected QT (QTc) interval prolongation.[17,18] Paroxetine is more likely to cause sedation and upset stomach or nausea.[19] Sertraline is activating and has a high rate of diarrhea.[20] Fluoxetine is also considered to be activating.[21] Note also that paroxetine, fluvoxamine, and fluoxetine are metabolized by cytochrome enzymes, leading to drug interactions.[18,21] In a survey of approximately 400 patients, more than 50% complained of side effects during initial treatment with SSRIs. The three most commonly reported side effects were sexual dysfunction (17%), drowsiness (17%), and weight gain (12%).[22]

The side effect of weight gain is particularly troubling for patients with comorbid diabetes. Weight gain generally occurs over time with longer courses of therapy, which may be necessary with the treatment of depression. Differences are seen between individual medications in the class. In a trial comparing weight changes for fluoxetine, paroxetine, and sertraline, fluoxetine demonstrated a nonsignificant weight decrease, sertraline a nonsignificant weight increase, and paroxetine a significant weight gain.[23] One case-control study demonstrated that use of SSRIs not only increased weight but also increased the incidence of diabetes. High to moderate doses of SSRIs when used for longer than 2 years were associated with doubling of the risk of diabetes (incidence rate ratio 2.06, 95% CI 1.20–3.52). In reviewing individual medications, fluvoxamine and paroxetine had significantly positive incidence rate ratios influencing the overall weight gain associated with the SSRI medication class.[24]

SNRIs

SNRIs, like SSRIs, are considered first line for treatment of depression due to efficacy of treatment and tolerability of the medications. This class of medication may also be a good choice because of the benefit in chronic pain conditions like DPN. SNRIs are also approved to treat anxiety disorders.[15] The FDA has approved desvenlafaxine, duloxetine, milnacipran, levomilnacipran, and venlafaxine for the treatment of depression. Efficacy for treatment of depression is similar among the medications in this class.[15] Selection of a specific medication is dependent on side-effect profile, patient-specific symptoms, drug interactions, and other patient-specific factors.

The SNRI medications share some general characteristics but have unique profiles as well. SNRIs treat depression by blocking the reuptake of serotonin and norepinephrine. The effect on receptors is dose dependent. Venlafaxine blocks mostly serotonin at lower doses, but at doses of 225 mg and higher norepinephrine is affected.[25] Dosing in patients with severe renal and hepatic insufficiency may need to be reduced or avoided; however, medication doses should be titrated to the individualized patient effect. The most common side effects experienced were nausea and dizziness.[26–28] Elevations of blood pressure are seen with all medications except duloxetine.[26] Duloxetine demonstrated an initial decrease in weight of 0.4 kg compared to baseline in the first 12 weeks. At the end of the 34-week trial, however, patients receiving duloxetine had a weight increase of approximately 1 kg from baseline.[29] Levomilnacipran is weight neutral.[28] Abrupt discontinuation of medications in this class leads to decontamination syndrome, so these medications should be tapered to avoid withdrawal symptoms.[15] Sexual dysfunction can be problematic with this class of medications.[15]

TRICYCLIC ANTIDEPRESSANTS

Tricyclic and tetracyclic antidepressants are effective treatment for depression. These medications have also been shown to have similar efficacy to SSRIs and SNRIs; however, they are no longer used as a first-line treatment for depression. Medications in this class are considered equally efficacious. Due to significant side effects, this class of medication is used as second line or for resistant forms of depression. The tricyclics are also effective for the treatment of anxiety disorders, panic disorders, and neuropathy.[15]

Common medications used in this class are amitriptyline, imipramine, desipramine, and nortriptyline. The medications block reuptake of both serotonin and norepinephrine. Use-limiting side effects include cardiovascular effects such as arrhythmias and hypotension; anticholinergic effects such as constipation, dry eyes and mouth, sedation, and weight gain; and falls.[15] These medications also have varying degrees of affinity for histamine and muscarinic receptors, leading to the unwanted side-effect profile of weight gain, sedation, and other anticholinergic effects. Nortriptyline appears to have the least effect on histamine and muscarinic receptors and may be better tolerated. Most of these medications have therapeutic drug levels that may be monitored for efficacy or response and adherence to the medication. Some other adverse effects beyond the anticholinergic and antihistaminic effects are cardiac and lowering of the seizure threshold. Cardiac effects can include arrhythmias, heart block, sudden death, and orthostatic hypotension. These medications can also be fatal in cases of overdose.[15]

ATYPICAL ANTIDEPRESSANTS

The atypical antidepressants include bupropion and mirtazapine. These medications are different from other antidepressant medication classes due to different mechanisms of action. The mechanism of action of bupropion is not completely clear. It is classified as a dopamine and norepinephrine reuptake inhibitor with a majority of the effect on norepinephrine. It is generally used to treat MDD and seasonal affective disorder. The medication is also approved to assist in smoking cessation.[30] However, unlike other antidepressants, bupropion is not indicated in the treatment of anxiety. The clinical efficacy of bupropion for MDD is considered less than that of an SSRI for treatment of depression and anxiety.[15] Bupropion is not used for first-line treatment of depression for this reason. This medication may be considered when patients also need assistance in smoking cessation or have side effects with other antidepressants. The side-effect profile includes the potential for weight loss, anxiety, dry mouth, nausea, insomnia, and seizures. Sexual dysfunction is less acute with bupropion than with other antidepressants, so it may be considered a good alternative in patients who experience sexual dysfunction with other antidepressant classes.[30]

Mirtazapine is a tetracyclic compound with an unknown mechanism for its antidepressant properties. The antidepressant effects are thought to be through antagonism of central α-2 receptors, leading to increased central noradrenergic and serotonergic activity. It also has some antagonism to histamine receptors, peripheral α-1 adrenergic receptors, and muscarinic receptors.[31] Mirtazapine is similar in efficacy to SSRIs.[15] The adverse effects of mirtazapine include dry mouth, drowsiness, sedation, increased appetite, and weight gain.[31] Sedation is more prominent at lower doses and tends to go away at doses ≥30 mg per day.[32]

SEROTONIN MODULATORS

Serotonin modulators include trazodone, vilazodone, and vortioxetine. The serotonin modulators' effects are not completely understood but are thought to affect depression through inhibition of serotonin reuptake. The serotonin modulators have proven benefit in the treatment of depression compared to placebo.[33–35] Generally, trazodone is used more for its sedation effect than as a first-line therapy in the treatment of depression.[15] Common side effects for trazodone are sedation, dizziness, dry mouth, and nausea.[33] For vortioxetine, nausea and sexual dysfunction are the only adverse effects occurring in >10% of patients.[34] Patients taking vilazodone commonly experienced diarrhea, nausea, and headache.[35]

COMMON PRECAUTIONS

All medications can cause adverse reactions for patients. Some adverse events of concern for antidepressant agents are withdrawal syndrome with discontinuation of pharmacotherapy, an increased risk of suicidal thoughts or actions, and serotonin syndrome. Discontinuation syndrome can occur with most antidepressants,

Table 26.2—Dose and Dosage Adjustment for Commonly Used Medications

Drug	Initial dose (mg/day)	Usual dose (mg/day)	Dose adjustments
SSRIs			
Citalopram	20	20–40	Maximum dose of 20 mg daily in patients over age 60, hepatic impairment, and poor metabolizers of CYP2C19 or taking CYP2C19 inhibitors.
Escitalopram	10	10–20	Maximum dose of 10 mg daily in elderly and those with hepatic impairment. Use with caution in severe renal impairment.
Fluoxetine	20	20–80	No renal adjustments. May require a reduced dose or frequency in hepatic dysfunction, elderly, or in patients with multiple comorbidities.
Paroxetine	20	20–50	Doses should not exceed 40 mg in elderly, debilitated, or severe renal or hepatic failure. Initial dose in this population should be 10 mg daily.
Sertraline	50	50–200	For mild hepatic impairment, the starting dose is 25 mg daily and the maximum dose is 100 mg daily. Avoid in moderate or severe hepatic impairment.
SNRIs			
Venlafaxine, immediate release	75	75–375	Reduce dose by 50% in patients with mild to moderate hepatic impairment. Reduce dose by 25% in mild to moderate renal impairment and 50% for patients on hemodialysis.
Venlafaxine, extended release	37.5–75	75–225	Reduce dose by 50% in patients with moderate hepatic impairment. Reduce dose by 25–50% in mild to moderate renal impairment and 50% for patients on hemodialysis.
Desvenlafaxine	50	50	Reduce dose for CrCl <30 mL/min to 25 mg per day or 50 mg every other day.
Duloxetine	40	40–120	Not recommended for patients with CrCl <30 mL/min or patients with hepatic impairment.
Tricyclic Antidepressants			
Amitriptyline	25–50	100–300	No renal or hepatic adjustments.
Nortriptyline	25	50–200	No renal or hepatic adjustments.
Atypical Antidepressants			
Bupropion, immediate release	200	300–450	Moderate to severe hepatic impairment, 75 mg daily. Mild hepatic impairment or renal impairment, a dose and/or frequency reduction should be considered.
Bupropion, sustained release	150	300–400	Moderate to severe hepatic impairment, 100 mg daily or 150 mg every other day. Mild hepatic impairment or renal impairment, a dose and/or frequency reduction should be considered.
Bupropion, extended release	150	300	Moderate to severe hepatic impairment, 150 mg every other day. Mild hepatic impairment or renal impairment, a dose and/or frequency reduction should be considered.
Mirtazapine	15	15–45	No renal or hepatic adjustments.

(continued)

Table 26.2 (continued)

Drug	Initial dose (mg/day)	Usual dose (mg/day)	Dose adjustments
Serotonin Modulators			
Trazodone	150	150–600	No renal or hepatic adjustments.
Vilazodone	10	20–40	No renal or hepatic adjustments.
Vortioxetine	10	20	No renal or hepatic adjustments. Maximum recommended dose for poor metabolizers of CYP2D6 is 10 mg daily.

Source: refs. 17–21,26–28,30,31,33–35,37–42.

but is more common in agents with shorter half-lives. Some symptoms of discontinuation syndrome are similar to the flu, such as nausea, aches, chills, and some neurologic symptoms. Relapse of depression can occur with abrupt discontinuation. Serotonin syndrome is a rare condition that may occur as a result of too much serotonin in the body. This is more likely when using multiple medications that increase serotonin. Suicide and suicidal ideation are severe complications of depression. This is thought to be sometimes increased with the initiation of antidepressants, specifically in adolescents and young adults. Providers should assess patients for thoughts of suicide prior to initiation of therapy and monitor patients closely while on therapy.[15]

COMBINATION THERAPY

Achieving resolution of depressive symptoms is important to a patient's quality of life. Sometimes treatment with combination therapy is warranted to achieve remission. Combinations can often include addition of psychotherapy or the use of additional medications. Combination pharmacotherapy with psychotherapy should be considered as initial therapy for patients with severe depression or in hospitalized patients, and as augmentation to pharmacotherapy for patients not reaching remission on pharmacotherapy alone. Psychotherapy can come in many forms, such as family/marital, psychodynamic, group, problem-solving, interpersonal, and cognitive and behavioral therapies. Psychotherapies and pharmacotherapy have a synergistic benefit compared to either therapy alone. Pharmacotherapeutic combinations can also be used in individuals with incomplete response to single-agent therapy. Medications can be combined with another medication with a different mechanism of action.[15]

PHARMACOTHERAPY COMBINATIONS

When attempting combination or therapy augmentations, one should consider patient risk for side effects, comorbid conditions, and tolerability. Bupropion has shown synergistic effects when added to SSRI therapy, although caution should be used with the potential for drug-drug interactions. Also, mirtazapine has demonstrated beneficial effects when added to an SSRI or venlafaxine. Augmentation with second-generation antipsychotics can be used in patients who have depression with psychotic features but has also demonstrated benefit in patients who have incomplete response. The additional efficacy is not without risk. Increased weight gain, lipid alterations, as well as development of diabetes are significantly increased.[15] Symbyax is a combination of olanzapine and fluoxetine approved for bipolar 1 with depression.[36] Stimulant medications such as methylphenidate or modafinil have been used as add-on therapy to help with somnolence and fatigue.[15]

MONOGRAPHS

SSRI MEDICATIONS

Citalopram (Celexa): https://dailymed.nlm.nih.gov/dailymed/drugInfo.cfm?setid=6c96373f-6744-49d4-aec5-3720bc993fab

Escitalopram (Lexapro): https://dailymed.nlm.nih.gov/dailymed/drugInfo.cfm?setid=d5fbc8ce-bd41-4bd0-b413-0dea97e596c3

Fluoxetine (Prozac): https://dailymed.nlm.nih.gov/dailymed/drugInfo.cfm?setid=45454555-7402-41cb-a452-e6a76e04f387

Fluvoxamine (Luvox): https://dailymed.nlm.nih.gov/dailymed/drugInfo.cfm?setid=85b61f83-ab47-470d-8673-02fea29247be

Paroxetine (Paxil): https://dailymed.nlm.nih.gov/dailymed/drugInfo.cfm?setid=89dd7e24-85fc-4152-89ea-47ec2b48a1ed

SNRI MEDICATIONS

Duloxetine (Cymbalta): https://dailymed.nlm.nih.gov/dailymed/drugInfo.cfm?setid=7436185e-c738-48ee-a9b4-49656e21f303

Levomilnacipran (Fetzima): https://dailymed.nlm.nih.gov/dailymed/drugInfo.cfm?setid=f371258d-91b3-4b6a-ac99-434a1964c3af

Venlafaxine (Effexor): https://dailymed.nlm.nih.gov/dailymed/drugInfo.cfm?setid=3423487c-80e3-6bff-e054-00144ff88e88

TRICYCLIC ANTIDEPRESSANTS

Amitriptyline (Elavil): https://dailymed.nlm.nih.gov/dailymed/drugInfo.cfm?setid=1e6d2c80-fbc8-444e-bdd3-6a91fe1b95bd

Nortriptyline (Pamelor): https://dailymed.nlm.nih.gov/dailymed/drugInfo.cfm?setid=765d726b-fd4b-4ef7-afd7-9e7e9bf8cae6

ATYPICAL ANTIDEPRESSANTS

Bupropion (Wellbutrin XL): https://dailymed.nlm.nih.gov/dailymed/drugInfo.
cfm?setid=1a2a5385-ec04-448f-8bdb-d1cc3eb5f1c0

Mirtazapine (Remeron): https://dailymed.nlm.nih.gov/dailymed/drugInfo.
cfm?setid=0039f505-7cd0-4d79-b5dd-bf2d172571a0

SEROTONIN MODULATORS

Trazodone (Desyrel): https://dailymed.nlm.nih.gov/dailymed/drugInfo.cfm?setid
=71961ab1-951d-1493-f76c-2ff25cca2a85

Vilazodone (Viibryd): https://dailymed.nlm.nih.gov/dailymed/drugInfo.cfm?setid
=4c55ccfb-c4cf-11df-851a-0800200c9a66

Vortioxetine (Trintellix): https://dailymed.nlm.nih.gov/dailymed/drugInfo.
cfm?setid=1a5b68e2-14d0-419d-9ec6-1ca97145e838

REFERENCES

1. American Psychiatric Association. *Diagnostic and Statistical Manual of Mental Disorders*. 5th ed., 2013

2. National Institute of Mental Health Information Resource Center. Available from https://www.nimh.nih.gov/health/statistics/major-depression. shtml#part_155028. Last updated November 2017. Accessed 25 April 2018

3. Healthline Editorial Team. Risk factors for depression [Internet]. Medically reviewed by Timothy J. Legg, 27 October 2016. Available from https:// www.healthline.com/health/depression/risk-factors#1. Accessed 25 April 2018

4. Semenkovich K, Brown ME, Svrakic DM, Lustman PJ. Depression in type 2 diabetes mellitus: prevalence, impact and treatment. *Drugs* 2015;75: 577–587

5. Ali S, Stone MA, Peters JL, et al. The prevalence of co-morbid depression in adults with type 2 diabetes: a systematic review and meta-analysis. *Diabet Med* 2006;23(11):1165–1173

6. Elamoshy R, Bird Y, Thorpe L, Moraros J. Risk of depression and suicidality among diabetic patients: systematic review and meta-analysis. *J Clin Med* 2018;7:445

7. Mezuk B, Eaton WW, Albrecht S, Golden SH. Depression and type 2 diabetes over the lifespan. *Diabetes Care* 2008;31(12):2383–2390

8. Atasoy S, Johar H, Fang X, et al. Cumulative effect of depressed mood and obesity on type 2 diabetes incidence: findings from the MONICA/KORA cohort study. *J Psychosom Res* 2018;115:66–70

9. Xuan L, Zhao Z, Jia X, et al. Type 2 diabetes is causally associated with depression: a Mendelian randomization analysis. *Front Med* 2018;12(6):678–687. DOI:10.1007/s11684-018-0671-7. [Epub ahead of print]

10. Lustman PJ, Anderson RJ, Freedland KE, et al. Depression and poor glycemic control: a meta-analytic review of the literature. *Diabetes Care* 2000; 23(7):934–942

11. de Groot M, Anderson R, Freedland KE, et al. Association of depression and diabetes complications: a meta-analysis. *Psychosom Med* 2001;63(4):619–630

12. Burns RJ, Deschênes SS, Schmitz N. Cyclical relationship between depressive symptoms and diabetes distress in people with Type 2 diabetes mellitus: results from the Montreal Evaluation of Diabetes Treatment Cohort Study. *Diabetic Med* 2015;32:1272–1278

13. van Bastlaar KM, Pouwer F, Geelhoed-Duijvestijn PH, et al. Diabetes-specific emotional distress mediates the association between depressive symptoms and glycaemic control in Type 1 and Type 2 diabetes. *Diabet Med* 2010;27:798–803

14. Brieler JA, Lustman PJ, Scherrer JF, et al. Antidepressant medication use and glycaemic control in comorbid type 2 diabetes and depression. *Family Practice* 2016;33(1):30–36

15. American Psychiatric Association. *The Practice Guideline for the Treatment of Patients with Major Depressive Disorder.* 3rd ed, 2010. Available from https://www.psychiatry.org/psychiatrists/practice/clinical-practice-guidelines

16. Fluvoxamine maleate [package insert]. Research Triangle Park, NC, Synthon Pharmaceuticals, Inc., 2007

17. Celexa (citalopram) [package insert]. St. Louis, MO, Forest Pharmaceuticals, Inc., 2017

18. Lexapro (escitalopram oxalate) [package insert]. St. Louis, MO, Forest Pharmaceuticals, Inc., 2017

19. Paxil (paroxetine) [package insert]. Research Triangle Park, NC, GlaxoSmithKline, 2016

20. Zoloft (sertraline) [package insert]. New York, Roerig, 2018

21. Prozac (fluoxetine) [package insert]. Indianapolis, IN, Eli Lilly and Company, 2017

22. Hu XH, Bull SA, Hunkeler EM, et al. Incidence and duration of side effects and those rated as bothersome with selective serotonin reuptake inhibitor treatment for depression: patient report versus physician estimates. *J Clin Psychiatry* 2004;65:959–965

23. Fava M, Judge R, Hoog SL, et al. Fluoxetine versus sertraline and paroxetine in major depressive disorder: changes in weight with long-term treatment. *J Clin Psychiatry* 2000;61(11):863–867

24. Andersohn F, Schade R, Suissa S, Garbe E. Long-term use of antidepressants for depressive disorders and the risk of diabetes mellitus. *Am J Psychiatry* 2009;166:591–598

25. Debonnel G, Saint-André E, Hébert C, et al. Differential physiological effects of a low dose and high doses of venlafaxine in major depression. *Int J Neuropsychopharmacol* 2007;10(1):51–61

26. Cymbalta (duloxetine hydrochloride) [package insert]. Indianapolis, IN, Eli Lilly and Company, 2017

27. Effexor XR (venlafaxine hydrochloride) [package insert]. Philadelphia, PA, Wyeth Pharmaceuticals Inc., 2018

28. Fetizma (levomilnacipran) [package insert]. Irvine, CA, Allergan USA, Inc., 2017

29. Hudson JI, Wohlreich MM, Kajdasz DK, et al. Safety and tolerability of duloxetine in the treatment of major depressive disorder: analysis of pooled data from eight placebo-controlled clinical trials. *Hum Psychopharmacol* 2005;20:327–341

30. Wellbutrin XL (bupropion hydrochloride) [package insert]. Bridgewater, NJ, Valeant Pharmaceuticals North America LLC, 2017

31. Remeron (mirtazapine) [package insert]. Roseland, NJ, Organon USA Inc., 2018

32. Grasmäder K, Verwohlt PL, Kühn KU, et al. Relationship between mirtazapine dose, plasma concentration, response, and side effects in clinical practice. *Pharmacopsychiatry* 2005;38(3):113–117

33. Trazodone hydrochloride [package insert]. Weston, FL, Apotex Corp, 2017

34. Trintellix (vortioxetine hydrobromide) [package insert]. Deerfield, IL, Takeda Pharmaceuticals America, Inc., 2018

35. Viibryd (vilazodone hydrochloride) [package insert]. Madison, NJ, Allergan USA, Inc., 2018

36. Symbyax (olanzapine and fluoxetine hydrochloride) [package insert]. Indianapolis, IN, Eli Lilly and Company, 2018

37. Effexor (venlafaxine hydrochloride) [package insert]. Cranbury, NJ, Sun Pharmaceutical Industries, Inc., 2016

38. Pristiq (desvenlafaxine) [package insert]. Philadelphia, PA, Wyeth Pharmaceuticals Inc., 2018

39. Amitriptyline hydrochloride [package insert]. Chestnut Ridge, NY, Par Pharmaceuticals, 2017

40. Nortriptyline hydrochloride [package insert]. Greenville, NC, Mayne Pharma, 2016

41. Bupropion hydrochloride [package insert]. Weston, FL, Apotex Corp, 2017

42. Wellbutrin SR (bupropion hydrochloride) [package insert]. Research Triangle Park, NC, GlaxoSmithKline, 2017

Chapter 27

Medications for the Management of Hypoglycemia

Megan Giruzzi, PharmD, BCPS

INTRODUCTION

Hypoglycemia is a common complication of both T1D and T2D treatment that affects anywhere from 6 to 45% of the population.[1] Hypoglycemia is considered the major limiting factor for glycemic control in many patients with T1D or T2D.[2] Hypoglycemia has been defined in several different ways, and the definition has evolved over time. Despite the changes in the definition of hypoglycemia, the treatment recommendations and medication options for hypoglycemia have been consistent over the past decade.

Since the early 1930s, hypoglycemia has been defined as the presence of the Whipple triad. The Whipple triad consists of signs and symptoms of low blood glucose, low blood glucose levels, and the reversal of these signs and symptoms with administration or ingestion of glucose. In recent years there has been a growing concern regarding the incidence of hypoglycemic unawareness. Recent studies have observed hypoglycemia unawareness in 8–10% of patients with T1D and T2D.[3,4] With prolonged hypoglycemia, secondary to hypoglycemia unawareness, neurological complications such as behavioral changes, cognitive impairment, seizures, coma, and mortality are increased sixfold, affecting an estimated 4.9–9% of individuals.[5,6] This led the American Diabetes Association to redefine hypoglycemia and to create five classifications of it in 2013.[7] Most recently, the International Hypoglycemia Study Group redefined the classifications for hypoglycemia into three levels.[8] The first level is classified as the hypoglycemia alert value, where an SMBG or laboratory measurement of ≤70 mg/dL (3.9 mmol/L) is observed. Patients meeting this criterion can typically be treated with any form of fast-acting carbohydrate and should have their glycemic control regimen adjusted to prevent a future event. The second level is classified as clinically significant hypoglycemia, due to the risk for serious, potentially fatal consequences, where an SMBG or laboratory measurement is found to be <54 mg/dL (3.0 mmol/L). The third level is classified as severe hypoglycemia. For this classification, there is no specified glucose threshold; however, these patients will have hypoglycemia associated with severe cognitive impairment requiring assistance from another individual for recovery.[8] The second and third levels may require treatment with a parenteral formulation of dextrose or glucagon to reverse hypoglycemia and prevent complications. These three classifications were adapted by the American Diabetes Association in 2017 and are currently used to define and classify hypoglycemia within the *Standards of Medical Care in Diabetes*.[2]

When an individual's blood glucose level begins to fall, multiple systems in the body are triggered to help resolve the hypoglycemic episode. The initial response of the body occurs when the blood glucose falls between 80 and 90 mg/dL. At this time, the pancreas begins to decrease the production of insulin and will begin to counterregulate by increasing glucagon production. The liver will quickly detect the increase in glucagon and respond by increasing both glycogenolysis and gluconeogenesis. In some patients, the glucagon production will be sufficient to resolve the hypoglycemic episode. In other patients, especially those whose glucose drops below 70 mg/dL, the adrenaline hormones will begin to play a key role to ensure the brain has a constant supply of glucose by limiting the use of glucose by nonessential tissues.[9–11]

The counterregulatory response is further carried out by the adrenal glands, which begin producing and releasing epinephrine. The epinephrine acts on certain body tissues, such as muscle, to decrease glucose use, as well as on the kidneys to decrease glucose clearance. Another counterregulatory response involves the peripheral nervous system, mediating an increase in acetylcholine. Acetylcholine and epinephrine then begin to trigger an autonomic response to alert the patient that their blood glucose is low. Lastly, cortisol and growth hormone are released and play a minor role in slowing the consumption of glucose by nonessential tissues to aid in the increase of blood glucose levels.[9–11]

During episodes of hypoglycemia, patients can experience a variety of symptoms that can be classified as either autonomic or neuroglycopenic. As previously mentioned, epinephrine and acetylcholine trigger the body's autonomic response. Typical symptoms of this response include tremors, diaphoresis, hunger, palpitations, anxiety, and sometimes pallor. It is important to note that medications such as β-blockers can mask the autonomic response, resulting in patients being unable to notice a hypoglycemic episode until the event progresses to the neuroglycopenic symptoms. Neuroglycopenic symptoms are caused by a lack of glucose in the CNS and are typically more distressing and severe. These symptoms include cognitive impairment, confusion, behavioral changes, anger, irritability, blurred vision, headaches, seizures, and loss of consciousness, leading to coma and even death.[11,12]

Acute hypoglycemia has been linked to a number of different consequences. In some cases, its effect can go beyond just the patient to affect others, especially if the episode is associated with a fall, motor vehicle accident, or other injury.[2] Hypoglycemia is associated with an increased risk for cardiovascular events, such as MI, stroke, and cardiovascular death. It has also been shown to cause QT prolongation and life-threatening ventricular arrhythmias.[13,14] Studies have found that patients with hypoglycemia are at an increased risk of developing dementia, both vascular and Alzheimer's disease. In adults, the degree of cognitive impairment has been associated with the frequency of severe hypoglycemia.[2,15] Patients with cognitive dysfunction may have difficulty identifying and treating low blood glucose levels; therefore, the risk of developing severe hypoglycemia may be greater. Lastly, numerous studies have documented the effect of hypoglycemia on quality of life. Patients with episodes of hypoglycemia report decreased overall health, mental health issues, and increased anxiety.

There are a number of factors that can contribute to hypoglycemia. The most common cause of hypoglycemia is antidiabetic medications. Antidiabetic oral medications with the highest risk of hypoglycemia include sulfonylureas and meglitinides. When used as monotherapy, they have been associated with an increased relative risk of 2–8; when used as part of a combination therapy, they are associated with a four- to eightfold increase in the frequency of hypoglycemic events.[16] Other oral medications that may be associated with a risk of hypoglycemia include aspirin, warfarin, allopurinol, and probenecid when used in combination with antidiabetic medications. When analyzing patients who are treated with insulin, the rates of hypoglycemia are greater than 15 times those of patients treated with oral medications. With several formulations of insulin on the market, there are profound variabilities in their pharmacokinetic and pharmacodynamic properties. Compared to longer-acting basal analogs such as insulin glargine and insulin detemir, NPH has been found to have a greater variability in its absorption profile and duration of action.[17] Furthermore, due to a lower variability profile, the basal analogs insulin detemir and insulin glargine are associated with a 31% risk reduction of nocturnal hypoglycemia and a 27% risk reduction of severe hypoglycemia in T1D and a 54% reduction in nocturnal hypoglycemia and 31% reduction in symptomatic hypoglycemia in T2D.[18,19] Other factors that contribute to hypoglycemia include alcohol ingestion, hot weather, stress, acute illness, exercise, weight loss, CKD, and hepatic disease. Elderly patients are at an increased risk of hypoglycemic events due to polypharmacy, cognitive impairment, and deteriorating renal function.

As mentioned previously, hypoglycemia unawareness is a growing concern. Hypoglycemia unawareness is defined as the asymptomatic onset of hypoglycemia. Patients will typically not recognize the autonomic warning symptoms and therefore are at an increased risk for morbidity and mortality. Studies have found that the increased risk of all-cause mortality remains for 4 years following a severe hypoglycemic event.[20] The major risk factors for hypoglycemia unawareness include duration of the disease, number of prior hypoglycemic events, frequent nocturnal hypoglycemia, aging, and more stringent glycemic control.[3] Major consequences of hypoglycemia unawareness include major macrovascular events, major microvascular events, venous thromboembolisms, severe arrhythmias, and cognitive dysfunction. Unfortunately, hypoglycemic unawareness can also lead to an increased risk of depression, missed days of work, and financial burdens.

HYPOGLYCEMIC PREVENTION

The prevention of hypoglycemic episodes is a critical component of diabetes management. The importance of SMBG should be stressed to patients at their initial diagnosis and reinforced longitudinally throughout management of their diabetes. In some patients, SMBG is not enough, and they will need CGM to detect hypoglycemia. Patients must be educated to understand situations that increase their risk of hypoglycemia, including fasting for blood tests or procedures, delaying meals, during or after exercise, and while asleep. Education regarding these situations may not prevent all hypoglycemic episodes, but may increase a patient's self-awareness of their body's glucose demands in specific situations. All hypoglycemic events should be discussed and evaluated at every visit. The evaluation should include frequency of events, timing of events, current treatment regimen, and severity. Treatment regimens should be reevaluated if the patient is experiencing frequent or severe hypoglycemia. In certain situations of recurrent hypoglycemia, relaxing blood glucose targets for a couple of weeks may prevent unnecessary hypoglycemic episodes and reverse hypoglycemia unawareness.

TREATMENT OPTIONS

The backbone to hypoglycemic management is the consumption of pure glucose or fast-acting carbohydrates when a patient's glucose level falls below 70 mg/dL (3.9 mmol/L). Studies have found that either glucose or carbohydrates are effective; however, some data suggest that a hypoglycemic event will resolve faster with pure glucose. There are a number of fast-acting, oral glucose products that are readily available and easy to administer. Available glucose products include chewable tablets, oral gels, and liquids, which can be found at the local pharmacy (see Table 27.1). Although these products are readily available, they are not the only option. A patient can consume any type of fast-acting carbohydrate that is readily available, as long as the patient is conscious and demonstrates no difficulty in breathing or swallowing.

Patients being treated with medications that can cause hypoglycemia must be counseled on the appropriate amount of glucose to consume in order to raise their blood glucose quickly. In conscious individuals with a blood glucose <70 mg/dL (3.9 mmol/L), administration of 15–20 g of glucose is advised. Fifteen minutes after treatment, patients should recheck their blood glucose, and if they show continued hypoglycemia, the treatment should be repeated. This administration of 15 g of carbohydrates, followed by rechecking blood glucose levels in 15 min is often referred to as the "Rule of 15." Once a patient's SMBG returns to normal, they should consume a meal or snack to prevent the recurrence of hypoglycemia. This meal or snack should include a blend of carbohydrates, fats, and protein. Examples of snacks that a patient can consume include, but are not limited to, a peanut butter and jelly sandwich, cheese and crackers, or a granola bar. Patients should be advised to not overeat after these situations, as this may lead to a hyperglycemic state.

Education regarding hypoglycemia and management is important and should be revisited regularly with patients. All patients with diabetes should be counseled to carry a source of fast-acting glucose with them at all times. The "Rule of 15" further applies to the quantity of fast-acting candy sources such as M&Ms and Skittles. It is recommended that a patient self-treat with 15 M&Ms or 15 Skittles during a hypoglycemic event.[20] Other options for fast-acting glucose sources that patients may use other than oral glucose products include 4 ounces of regular fruit juice or regular soda (not diet); 2 tablespoons of raisins; 1 tablespoon of corn syrup, table sugar, or honey; 8 ounces of nonfat or 1% milk; hard candy or jellybeans (see package for number to consume); or a spoonful of commercial cake frosting. All of these sources will rapidly raise blood glucose levels. Patients experiencing hypoglycemia should initially avoid ingesting high-fat or protein-based foods or drinks. Both protein and fats will impact and slow the

Table 27.1—Fast–Acting Glucose Products

Product (manufacturer)*	Carbohydrate amount	Dose
Liquids		
Dex4 (Perrigo)	15 g per bottle	1 bottle
TRUEplus Glucose Shot (Trividia Health)		
Gels		
Dex4 (Perrigo)	15 g per pouch	1 pouch
Glutose 15 (Perrigo)	15 g per tube	1 tube
Glutose 45 (Perrigo)	45 g per tube	1/3 of tube
Insta-Glucose (Valeant Pharmaceuticals)	24 g per tube	1 tube
Transcend (Transcend Foods)	15 g per pouch	1 pouch
TRUEplus Glucose Gel (Trividia Health)	15 g per pouch	1 pouch
Powder		
Elovate 15 (Diasan Corp)	15 g per packet	1 packet
Tablets		
Dex4 (Perrigo)	4 g per tablet	4 tablets, for 16 g carbohydrates
Glucolift (Jungell)		
Optimum (Magno-Humphries Labs)		
TRUEplus Glucose Tablets (Trividia Health)		
TRUEplus Soft Tabs (Trividia Health)		

*Store-brand glucose products contain the same amount of fast-acting glucose as the name-brand version and may serve as a cost-effective alternative.

absorption of glucose into the system, prolonging the acute hypoglycemic episode.

All patients that experience a hypoglycemic episode should continue to regularly monitor their glucose throughout the remainder of the day, while resuming a regular eating schedule. A patient should also contact their physician and discuss the hypoglycemic episode and determine whether adjustment with their treatment regimen is needed. If a patient is unable to self-administer oral glucose products due to swallowing difficulties or unconsciousness, another option that may be used is parenteral glucagon.

GLUCAGON

Glucagon is produced by the α-cells in the pancreas and is released when the concentration of glucose in the blood falls between 80 and 90 mg/dL. When released, it works to raise blood glucose levels and prevent or reverse hypoglycemia. When the body is not able to produce enough glucagon, other systems in the body respond to alert patients to the hypoglycemic event. Unfortunately, some patients will lose consciousness before being able to adequately treat the event. In these situations, exogenous glucagon is available as a hypoglycemic antidote and may be administered for the management of hypoglycemia. Therefore, glucagon should be prescribed for all individuals at increased risk of clinically significant hypoglycemia. This includes, but is not limited to, all T1D patients, children with diabetes, and any patient who has experienced a hypoglycemic event of <54 mg/dL (3.0 mmol/L).

When released and/or administered, glucagon triggers adenylate cyclase in the liver to stimulate the conversion of AMP to cAMP. The increase in cAMP leads to a degradation of stored glycogen to rapid-acting glucose. This process is known as glycogenolysis, resulting in return to a euglycemic state rapidly, reversing hypoglycemia. In order for this mechanism to be effective at increasing blood glucose levels, there must be a preexisting hepatic glycogen store for breakdown. Patients at risk of having depleted glycogen stores include geriatric patients, patients with low body weight, and chronic alcoholics. These patients have been found to have a reduced response or no response to glucagon. In situations where glycogen stores are depleted, other methods of raising blood glucose must be employed, including the administration of intravenous dextrose.

Glucagon, when used for the emergent treatment of hypoglycemia, is administered parenterally via an intravenous, intramuscular, or subcutaneous injection. For adults and pediatrics weighing more than 44 lbs (20 kg), administration of a 1 mg dose is appropriate. In patients weighing less than 44 lbs (20 kg), a 0.5 mg dose or a dose equivalent to 20–30 µg/kg, not exceeding 1 mg, would be appropriate (see Table 27.2). Prior to administration, glucagon kits will need to be reconstituted. Patients and family members should be counseled on how to reconstitute the solution and to not inject the solution unless the solution is clear and a water-like consistency. The glucagon injection should be administered in the patient's buttock, arm, or thigh. The patient should then be turned on their side, due to the risk of vomiting. Following administration of glucagon, immediately call 911. A clinical response and return to consciousness should occur within 15 min of administration. If there is a delayed response, administration of an additional dose of glucagon is appropriate. Replacement with intravenous 50% dextrose solution may be preferred in these situations to ensure that an adequate glucose response is achieved. After consciousness is obtained, patients should ingest carbohydrates to prevent hypoglycemic recurrence and assist in the replenishment of glucose to replace glycogen stores in the liver. Patients should consume a fast-acting carbohydrate, followed by a long-acting carbohydrate that can be combined with some protein and small amounts of fat as mentioned previously.

Recently, intranasal glucagon has made its way back into clinical trials as a potential alternative for injectable glucagon. It was first studied more than 20 years ago; however, none of those studies led to the FDA approval of a nonparenteral

Table 27.2—Glucagon Prescribing Information for Treatment of Hypoglycemia

Medication	Available formulations	Dosage
Glucagon	Kit and solution for reconstitution	IM, IV, Subcutaneous: Dose may be repeated in 15 min as needed
		Adults & Pediatrics >44 lbs (20 kg): 1 mg by injection
		Pediatrics <44 lbs (20 kg): 0.5 mg or dose equivalent to 20–30 µg/kg
		If a patient fails to respond to glucagon injection, IV dextrose must be given

IM, intramuscular; IV, intravenous.

glucagon preparation.[21] Many challenges have been reported with the reconstitution of injectable glucagon, such as opening the package, removing the needle sheath, mixing the ingredients, bending the needle, and time to reconstitution (ranging from 2.5–3 min on average).[22,23] Intranasal glucagon has the ability to overcome most of these obstacles since there is no need for reconstitution because of its dry powder formulation. When evaluating intranasal glucagon's efficacy, it has been found to be noninferior to injectable glucagon; however, in studies, the time to resolution of a hypoglycemic event when blood glucose is <50 mg/dL was 16 min with intranasal glucagon versus 13 min with injectable glucagon.[21,24] Although statistically there was a 3 min difference, when taking into account the time to reconstitute the injectable glucagon, both formulations work in about the same amount of time; therefore, there is no clinical difference. At this time, intranasal glucagon has not yet been FDA approved. However, a phase 3 trial studying intranasal glucagon has concluded, and another trial comparing nasal versus intramuscular glucagon is in process. With the favorable outcomes that have currently been reported, there is promise that intranasal glucagon may be approved in the coming years.

Glucagon is a well-tolerated medication, with nausea and vomiting being the most common side effect associated with its injectable formulation. This effect may be compounded by the body's natural hypoglycemic response. In clinical trials, the common adverse effects associated with intranasal glucagon include nasal irritation, ocular irritation, head or facial discomfort, and some nausea and vomiting. Glucagon has positive inotropic and chronotropic effects; therefore, patients with underlying cardiovascular conditions such as arrhythmias and hypertension should be monitored closely following administration. Monitoring parameters should include blood pressure, blood glucose, ECG, heart rate, and mentation. Glucagon carries contraindications for administration in patients with known hypersensitivity, pheochromocytoma, insulinoma, and glucagonoma.

In terms of special populations, glucagon is a pregnancy risk category B, as adverse events have not been observed in animal studies. However, there are not any adequate well-controlled studies in pregnant women. It is unknown whether this medication is excreted in human milk; therefore, caution should be exercised in nursing women. There are no dosing adjustments required for patients with renal or hepatic impairment.

There is not an extensive list of drug interactions for concern; however, the use of glucagon in combination with vitamin K antagonists such as warfarin may enhance the bleeding risk. This interaction is noted with much larger doses of glucagon than are used in hypoglycemic management. Nonetheless, patients at a high risk for bleeding should be monitored for fluctuations in INR and signs/symptoms of bleeding.

SUMMARY

Hypoglycemia is a commonly encountered complication of glycemic control. It affects a patient's quality of life and can be an economic burden. It is important to properly educate patients to be able to recognize the early signs and symptoms of hypoglycemia and appropriately manage their hypoglycemic event with fast-acting carbohydrates or injectable glucagon. Furthermore, patients should be counseled to follow up with their provider after a hypoglycemic event to have their glycemic regimen adjusted as necessary to prevent future events.

MONOGRAPH

Glucagon: https://dailymed.nlm.nih.gov/dailymed/drugInfo.cfm?setid=e4be1c0e-0fe6-45a0-9229-5cde98434b84&audience=consumer

REFERENCES

1. Edridge CL, Dunkley AJ, Bodicoar DH, et al. Prevalence and incidence of hypoglycaemia in 532,542 people with type 2 diabetes on oral therapies and insulin: a systematic review and meta-analysis of population based studies. *PLoS One* 2015;10(6):e0126427

2. American Diabetes Association. 6. Glycemic targets: *Standards of Medical Care in Diabetes—2018. Diabetes Care* 2018;41(Suppl. 1):S55–S64

3. Czyzewska K, Czerniawska E, Szadkowska A. Prevalence of hypoglycemia unawareness in patients with type 1 diabetes. *Pediatr Diabet* 2012;13 (Suppl. 17):77

4. Schopman JE, Geddes J, Frier BM. Prevalence of impaired awareness of hypoglycaemia and frequency of hypoglycaemia in insulin-treated type 2 diabetes. *Diabetes Res Clin Pract* 2010;87:64–68

5. Marrett E, Radican L, Davies MJ, Zhang Q. Assessment of severity and frequency of self-reported hypoglycemia on quality of life in patients with

type 2 diabetes treated with oral antihyperglycemic agents: a survey study. *BMC Res Notes* 2011;4:251

6. Martin-Timon I, Canizon-Gomez FJ. Mechanisms of hypoglycemia unawareness and implications in diabetic patients. *World J Diabetes* 2015;6(7):912–926

7. Seaquist ER, Anderson J, Childs B, et al. Hypoglycemia and diabetes: a report of a work group of the American Diabetes Association and the Endocrine Society. *Diabetes Care* 2013;36:1384–1395

8. International Hypoglycaemia Study Group. Glucose concentrations of less than 3.0 mmol/L (54 mg/dL) should be reported in clinical trials: a joint position statement of the American Diabetes Association and the European Association for the Study of Diabetes. *Diabetes Care* 2017;40:155–157

9. Briscoe VJ, Davis SN. Hypoglycemia in type 1 and type 2 diabetes: physiology, pathophysiology, and management. *Clin Diabetes* 2006;24:115–121

10. Cryer PE, Davis SN, Shamoon H. Hypoglycemia in diabetes. *Diabetes Care* 2003;26:1902–1912

11. Kenny C. When hypoglycemia is not obvious: diagnosing and treating under-recognized and undisclosed hypoglycemia. *Prim Care Diabetes* 2014;8:3–11

12. White JR. The contribution of medications to hypoglycemia unawareness. *Diabetes Spectrum* 2007;20(2):77–80

13. Frier BM. Hypoglycemia in diabetes mellitus: epidemiology and clinical implications. *Nat Rev Endocrinol* 2014;10:711–722

14. Zoungas S, Patel A, Chalmers J, et al. Severe hypoglycemia and risks of vascular events and death. *N Engl J Med* 2010;363:1410–1418

15. Punthakee Z, Miller ME, Launer LI, et al. ACCORD Group of Investigators: ACCORD-MIND Investigators. Poor cognitive function and risk of severe hypoglycemia in type 2 diabetes: post hoc epidemiologic analysis of the ACCORD trial. *Diabetes Care* 2012;35:787–793

16. Phung OJ, Scholle JM, Talwar M, Coleman CI. Effect of noninsulin antidiabetic drugs added to metformin therapy on glycemic control, weight gain, and hypoglycemia in type 2 diabetes. *JAMA* 2010;303:1410–1418

17. Vora J, Heise T. Variability of glucose-lowering effect as a limiting factor in optimizing basal insulin therapy: a review. *Diabetes Obes Metab* 2013;15:701–712

18. Monami M, Marchionni N, Mannucci E. Long-acting insulin analogues verses NPH human insulin in type 1 diabetes. A meta-analysis. *Diabetes Obes Metab* 2009;11;372–378

19. Monami M, Marchionni N, Mannucci E. Long-acting insulin analogues verses NPH human insulin in type 2 diabetes: a meta-analysis. *Diabetes Res Clin Pract* 2008;81:184–189

20. Morales J, Schneider D. Hypoglycemia. *Am J Med* 2014;127(10 Suppl.):S17–S24

21. Rickels MR, Ruedy KJ, Foster CN, et al. Intranasal glucagon for treatment of insulin-induced hypoglycemia in adults with type 1 diabetes: a randomized crossover noninferiority study. *Diabetes Care* 2016;39(2):264–270

22. Pontiroli AE. Intranasal glucagon: a promising approach for treatment of severe hypoglycemia. *J Diabetes Sci Technol* 2015;9(1):38–43

23. Yale JF, Dulede H, Egeth M, et al. Faster use and fewer failures with needle-free nasal glucagon versus injectable glucagon in severe hypoglycemia rescue: a simulation study. *Diabetes Technol Ther* 2017;19(7):423–432

24. Boido A, Ceriani V, Pontiroli AE. Glucagon for hypoglycemic episodes in insulin-treated diabetic patients: a systematic review and meta-analysis with a comparison of glucagon with dextrose and of different glucagon formulations. *Acta Diabetol* 2015;52(2):405–412

Chapter 28
Medications for the Management of Obesity

Nicholas R. Giruzzi, PharmD, BCPS

INTRODUCTION

O besity is a chronic medical condition that is the result of a long-term mismatch in energy balance, in which daily energy intake exceeds daily energy use.[1] The daily energy balance is affected by multiple factors including metabolic rate, appetite, diet, and physical activity.[1] Obesity is associated with many health risks, including hypertension, hyperlipidemia, T2D, CHD, stroke, gallbladder disease, osteoarthritis, sleep apnea, respiratory problems, and some cancers.[2] Obesity has also been associated with an increased risk of all-cause and cardiovascular mortality. The 1998 overweight and obesity clinical guidelines[3] defined overweight as a BMI of 25–29.9 kg/m² and obesity as a BMI of ≥30 kg/m². According to reports from the CDC, more than one-third (36.5%) of U.S. adults have obesity.[4] In 2008, the estimated medical cost of obesity in the U.S. was $147 billion.[4] The average medical costs were $1,429 more in those who were obese than those with a normal weight.[4]

As confirmed by multiple studies, there is strong evidence showing that weight management can delay or even prevent the progression from prediabetes to T2D and may be beneficial in the treatment.[5] Evidence-based research strongly suggests that medical nutrition therapy provided by a registered dietitian who is experienced in the management of diabetes is clinically effective.[6] Outcomes from randomized controlled nutrition therapy studies have documented decreases in A1C of approximately 1% in patients with newly diagnosed T1D, 2% in patients with newly diagnosed T2D, and 1% in patients with a long-standing history of T2D (average duration of 4 years).[6]

Weight loss can be attained with lifestyle modifications and programs that help the patient achieve a daily energy deficit,[5] and maintaining this over the long term is done by maintaining a neutral energy deficit. There are many benefits associated with weight loss, including decreased A1C, lipid levels, and blood pressure, that may be seen with as little as 5% weight loss.[7] However, a sustained weight loss over the long term of ≥7% is the optimal scenario. Many different diets have been studied, such as those restricting certain foods (high fat or high carbohydrate), which creates the necessary energy deficit that leads to weight loss.[5] Healthcare professionals play an important role not only in educating patients about dietary changes but also in providing ongoing support and encouragement for these patients.

Although diet and exercise are the backbone of therapy for weight management, those interventions alone may not be sufficient to achieve weight loss goals.

This circumstance is when pharmacological therapies should be considered. The FDA defines the indication for obesity pharmacotherapy as a BMI >30 kg/m² or a BMI >27 kg/m² with at least one obesity-associated comorbid condition.[8] This means a very large percentage of the U.S. adult population meets the criteria for pharmacological weight management therapy. The goals of weight management therapy include the prevention of further weight gain, reduction of body weight, and maintaining weight loss over the long term.[9,10]

PHARMACOLOGICAL MANAGEMENT OF OBESITY

PHENTERMINE

Phentermine (Lomaira; Adipex-P) is classified as a CNS stimulant and anorexiant. Phentermine has FDA approval as a short-term weight management agent in appropriate patients, but it is often prescribed off-label for long-term use.[11] Phentermine is a federally controlled (C-IV) medication. A meta-analysis[7] of six randomized, controlled trials of phentermine lasting 2–24 weeks reported patients on phentermine 15–30 mg/day lost an average of 3.6 kg more than patients receiving placebo, with a mean total weight loss of 6.3 kg.

Pharmacology

Mechanism of Action
Phentermine is a sympathomimetic amine.[12,13] Its mechanism in reducing appetite is secondary to its CNS effects: phentermine stimulates the hypothalamus to release norepinephrine, which leads to a reduction in hunger and signals fat cells to break down stored fat, resulting in weight loss.[12,13]

Pharmacokinetics
Phentermine is available as both capsules and tablets, with the onset of action varying depending on the timing of administration and meals.[12,13] Phentermine is well absorbed, with maximal plasma concentrations reached within 3–4 h. Less than 20% of the dose is protein-bound, and phentermine is minimally metabolized by the liver.[12,13] Between 62 and 85% of the drug is excreted unchanged in the urine, with an elimination half-life of approximately 20 h.[12,13]

Treatment Advantages and Disadvantages

Clinical use of phentermine should be limited to short-term weight management in appropriate patients.[9,12,13] Phentermine is an effective adjunct to diet, exercise, and behavioral modification for producing weight loss compared to placebo. A clinical downside of phentermine use is that it should only be used for short-term management (<12 weeks), and typically patients will experience some weight regain after discontinuation, which can be discouraging.[12,13]

Therapeutic Considerations

Warnings and Precautions
Phentermine use is contraindicated in patients with a history of CVD, within 14 days of MAOI use, and in those with hyperthyroidism.[12,13] Phentermine can

also cause CNS depression, and use is associated with primary pulmonary hypertension (PPH), for which patients usually present initially with dyspnea.[12,13] Treatment should be discontinued in patients who develop new and unexplained symptoms of dyspnea.[12,13] Phentermine has also been associated with direct cardio-toxic effects, including HF and valvular heart disease; its use should be cautioned in patients with a history of these diseases.[12,13] Patients with a history of substance abuse, agitation, hyperthyroidism, glaucoma, or recent (within 14 days) use of MAOI therapy should also avoid the use of phentermine.[12,13]

Special Populations

Phentermine is an FDA pregnancy category X medication.[12,13] The use of phentermine is contraindicated during pregnancy due to lack of potential benefit and possible fetal harm. It is unknown whether phentermine is excreted in human milk; however, other amphetamines are present in human milk, and the risk/benefit of using phentermine should be considered prior to use. Safety and efficacy in children under the age of 18 years have not been evaluated, so use in this population should be avoided. Caution is warranted in patients with kidney disease. A dose reduction is recommended in patients with severe kidney disease (eGFR 15–29 mL/min/1.73 m²), limiting the dose to 15 mg daily. Use in patients with an eGFR <15 mL/min/1.73 m², including hemodialysis, has not been studied and should be avoided.[12,13]

Adverse Effects and Monitoring

All patients using phentermine should be monitored for PPH, valvular heart disease, CNS side effects, and withdrawal effects including weight gain. Common adverse effects associated with phentermine use include dry mouth, dizziness, headache, insomnia, and restlessness.[9,12,13]

Drug Interactions

Concomitant use with MAOIs is contraindicated, and should only be initiated after a minimum of 14 days following discontinuation of MAOI use. All patients under consideration for phentermine therapy should be checked for potential drug interactions. See Table 28.1 for more drug interaction information.[12,13]

Dosage and Administration

Dosage and administration of phentermine varies depending on the product formulation. Lomaira comes as a tablet and should be dosed at 8 mg by mouth three times daily approximately 30 min prior to a meal. Adipex-P comes as a tablet or capsule and should be dosed at 15–37.5 mg/day in one dose or two divided doses. It should be dosed before a meal or 1–2 h after a meal. Dosing for both formulations should be maintained at the lowest effective doses. Administration of either formulation should be avoided in the late evening to prevent insomnia, due to its amphetamine-like characteristics. See Table 28.2 or refer to the full prescribing information for more dosing guidance.[12,13]

LORCASERIN

Lorcaserin is a selective serotonin-2c (5-HT$_{2C}$) receptor agonist and is classified as an anorexiant agent.[14] This agent was approved by the FDA in 2012 under the brand name Belviq for chronic weight management as an adjunct to lifestyle modifications in adults with either an initial BMI of ≥30 kg/m² or an initial BMI of ≥27 kg/m² and at least one weight-related comorbid condition.[14] Lorcaserin is

Table 28.1—Drug Interactions for Weight Loss–Management Agents

Substance	Interaction
Phentermine (Lomaira; Adipex-P)	
Acebrophylline	May enhance stimulatory effect of CNS stimulants; Risk X: Avoid combination
Alcohol (Ethyl)	May enhance the adverse/toxic effect of phentermine; Risk C: Monitor
Alkalinizing Agents	May decrease the excretion of amphetamines; Risk D: Consider modification
Ammonium Chloride	May decrease the serum concentration of amphetamines, likely due to enhanced excretion of amphetamines in urine; Risk C: Monitor
Antacids	May decrease the excretion of amphetamines; Risk C: Monitor
Antihistamines	May diminish the sedative effect of antihistamines; Risk C: Monitor
Antihypertensive Agents	May diminish the antihypertensive effects; Risk C: Monitor
Antipsychotic Agents	May diminish stimulatory effect of amphetamines; Risk C: Monitor
Ascorbic Acid	May decrease serum concentration of amphetamines; Risk C: Monitor
Atomoxetine	May enhance hypertensive and tachycardic effect of sympathomimetic; Risk C: Monitor
Bupropion	May enhance neuroexcitatory and/or seizure potentiating effects; Risk C: Monitor
Cannabinoid-Containing Products	May enhance tachycardic effect of sympathomimetic; Risk C: Monitor
Carbonic Anhydrase Inhibitors	May decrease excretion of amphetamines; Risk C: Monitor
Cocaine (Topical)	May enhance hypertensive effects; Risk D: Consider Modification
CYP2D6 Inhibitors	May increase serum concentration of amphetamines; Risk C: Monitor
Ethosuximide	Amphetamines may diminish the therapeutic effect of ethosuximide; Risk C: Monitor
Linezolid	May enhance the hypertensive effect of sympathomimetics; Risk D: Consider Modification
Lithium	May diminish stimulatory effect of amphetamines; Risk C: Monitor
Methenamine	May decrease the serum concentration of amphetamines; Risk C: Monitor
MAOIs	May enhance hypertensive effect; at least 14 days should elapse between discontinuation of an MAOI and initiation of treatment with bupropion; Risk X: Avoid Combination
Multivitamins	May decrease the serum concentration of amphetamines; Risk C: Monitor
Opioid Analgesics	Amphetamines may enhance the analgesic effect of opioid analgesics; Risk C: Monitor
Phenobarbital	Amphetamines may decrease the serum concentration of phenobarbital; Risk C: Monitor

(continued)

Table 28.1 (continued)

Substance	Interaction
Phenytoin	Amphetamines may decrease the serum concentration of phenytoin; Risk C: Monitor
Seizure Threshold–lowering Drugs	Extreme caution with concomitant use; Risk C: Monitor
Tricyclic Antidepressants	May enhance stimulatory effect of amphetamines and may also potentiate the cardiovascular effects of amphetamines; Risk C: Monitor
Urinary Acidifying Agents	May decrease serum concentration of amphetamines; Risk C: Monitor
Lorcaserin (Belviq) and Lorcaserin XR (Belviq XR)	
CYP2D6 Substrates or Inhibitors	Caution with concomitant use
Phosphodiesterase 5 Inhibitors	Lorcaserin may enhance the adverse/toxic effect of PDE5 inhibitors; specifically, the risk of developing a priapism may be increased
Serotonergic Agents	Caution with concomitant use; serotonin syndrome or NMS may be precipitated with use of multiple serotonergic agents
Orlistat (Xenical, Alli)	
Amiodarone	A reduction in serum concentration of amiodarone with coadministration; Risk C: Monitor
Anticonvulsants	Convulsions have been reported in patients taking orlistat with antiepileptic drugs; Exceptions: fosphenytoin, pentobarbital, thiopental; Risk C: Monitor
Antiretroviral Drugs	Loss of virological control has been reported in HIV-infected patients. Patients should be monitored frequently for changes in HIV RNA levels; Drugs include: atazanavir, ritonavir, tenofovir disoproxil fumarate, emtricitabine and combinations; Risk C: Monitor
Cyclosporine	Reductions in cyclosporine plasma levels were observed. Administer orlistat at least 3 h before or after cyclosporine and monitor for decreased serum concentrations even with dose separation; Risk D: Consider Modification
Fat-Soluble Multivitamins	Coadministration may decrease efficacy and absorption of vitamins; therefore, separation of orlistat by 2–4 h is advised; Risk D: Consider Modification
Levothyroxine	Concomitant use may result in decreased levothyroxine levels
Paricalcitol	Decreased serum concentration with coadministration; when combination must be used, consider administering paricalcitol at least 1 h before or 4–6 h after the administration of orlistat; Risk D: Consider Modification
Propafenone	Coadministration may decrease serum concentrations; Risk C: Monitor
Vitamin D Analogs	Coadministration may decrease serum concentration of vitamin D analogs by inhibiting absorption; Risk D: Consider Modification
Warfarin	Concomitant use may result in an enhanced anticoagulant effect; Risk C: Monitor
Liraglutide (Saxenda)	
α-Lipoic Acid	May enhance hypoglycemic effect of antidiabetic agents; Risk C: Monitor

(continued)

Table 28.1 (continued)

Substance	Interaction
Androgens	May enhance the hypoglycemic effect of blood glucose–lowering agents; Risk C: Monitor
Guanethidine	May enhance the hypoglycemic effects of antidiabetic agents; Risk C: Monitor
Hypoglycemia-Associated Agents	Antidiabetic agents used in combination (oral and noninsulin injectables) may enhance the hypoglycemic effect; Risk C: Monitor
Insulins	May enhance hypoglycemic effects of insulins; Risk D: Consider Modification
MAOIs	May enhance the hypoglycemic effects; Risk C: Monitor
Pegvisomant	May enhance the hypoglycemic effects of blood glucose–lowering agents; Risk C: Monitor
Prothionamide	May enhance the hypoglycemic effects of blood glucose–lowering agents; Risk C: Monitor
Quinolones	Quinolones may diminish the therapeutic effect of blood glucose–lowering agents; Risk C: Monitor
Salicylates	May enhance the hypoglycemic effect of blood glucose–lowering agents; Risk C: Monitor
Selective Serotonin Reuptake Inhibitors	May enhance the hypoglycemic effect of blood glucose–lowering agents; Risk C: Monitor
Sulfonylureas	May enhance the hypoglycemic effects of sulfonylureas; Risk D: Consider Modification
Thiazide and Thiazide-like Diuretics	May diminish the therapeutic effect of antidiabetic agents; Risk C: Monitor
Phentermine/Topiramate (Qsymia)	
Please see Phentermine section for specific interactions related to that component	
Antiepileptic Medications	Concomitant administration of phenytoin or carbamazepine with topiramate in patients with epilepsy decreased plasma concentrations of topiramate by 48% and 40%, respectively Concomitant administration of valproic acid and topiramate has been associated with hyperammonemia with and without encephalopathy. The combination has also been associated with hypothermia
Carbonic Anhydrase Inhibitors	Concomitant use may increase the severity of metabolic acidosis and may also increase the risk of kidney stone formation
CNS Depressants including Alcohol	Concomitant use with alcohol or CNS depressants may potentiate CNS depression such as dizziness or cognitive adverse reactions or other centrally mediated effects of these agents
MAOIs	Phentermine use within 14 days of MAOIs is contraindicated due to risk of hypertensive crisis
Non-Potassium Sparing Diuretics	Concomitant use may potentiate potassium-wasting action of the diuretics, monitor for hypokalemia

(continued)

Table 28.1 (continued)

Substance	Interaction
Oral Contraceptives	Qsymia decreased the exposure of ethinyl estradiol by 16% and increased exposure to norethindrone by 22%. Increased risk of pregnancy is not anticipated; however, irregular bleeding (spotting) may occur more frequently due to both the increased exposure to progestin and lower exposure to estrogen
Naltrexone/Bupropion Extended Release (Contrave)	
CYP2B6 Inducers	May reduce the efficacy by reducing bupropion exposure
CYP2B6 Inhibitors	Drugs such as ticlopidine or clopidogrel can increase concentrations of bupropion exposure, leading to increased adverse reactions
CYP2D6 Substrates	Bupropion inhibits CYP2D6 and can increase concentrations of drugs metabolized by CYP2D6, leading to increased adverse reactions
Dopaminergic Drugs	CNS toxicity can occur when used concomitantly with Contrave
Drug-Laboratory Test Interactions	Contrave can cause false-positive urine test results for amphetamines
MAOI	Increased risk of hypertensive reactions can occur when used concomitantly
Seizure Threshold–lowering Drugs	Extreme caution with concomitant use

NMS, Neuroleptic Malignant Syndrome.

federally classified as a schedule IV substance.[14] Lorcaserin comes as both an immediate release and extended-release tablet.[14] A clinical trial demonstrated that more patients completing 1 year of treatment with lorcaserin lost ≥5% of their body weight than with the placebo (47.5% vs. 20.3%).[15–17] Patients with T2D treated with lorcaserin lost approximately 5% of their body weight and achieved a 0.9% improvement in A1C compared to 1.5% weight loss and 0.4% A1C improvement in the placebo group.[14]

Pharmacology

Mechanism of Action

Lorcaserin is believed to activate the serotonin 5-HT_{2C} receptors, which stimulate proopiomelanocortin (POMC) neurons in the arcuate nucleus of the hypothalamus, leading to increased release of α-melanocortin stimulating hormone at melanocortin-4 receptors, resulting in satiety and decreased food intake.[14]

Pharmacokinetics

Following oral administration, lorcaserin is absorbed in the gastrointestinal tract with peak plasma concentrations occurring 1.5–2 h after dosing.[14] Steady-state concentrations are typically reached in 3 days after twice-daily dosing; lorcaserin may be administered without regard to food.[14] Lorcaserin is moderately bound to human plasma proteins, and can be distributed in the CNS and cerebrospinal fluid.[14] Metabolism is extensively in the liver by multiple enzymatic pathways and 92% is excreted in the urine as metabolites.[14] The elimination half-life of lorcaserin/lorcaserin XR is approximately 11–12 h.[14]

Table 28.2 — Prescribing Information for Weight Loss–Management Agents

Generic (brand)	Ingredient/strength	Dosage*
Phentermine (Lomaira)	Tablet, 8 mg	Adults ■ 8 mg by mouth three times daily. Individualize to achieve adequate response with lowest effective dose.
Phentermine (Adipex-P)	Tablet, 37.5 mg Capsule: ■ 15 mg ■ 30 mg ■ 37.5 mg	Adults ■ 15–37.5 mg/day in one dose or two divided doses. Individualize to achieve adequate response with lowest effective dose
Lorcaserin HCl (Belviq) Locaserin HCl XR (Belviq XR)	Tablets: ■ IR: 10 mg ■ XR: 20 mg	Adults ■ IR: 10 mg by mouth twice daily ■ XR: 20 mg by mouth once daily ■ Max daily dosing 20 mg/day Severe Hepatic (Child-Pugh Class C) & Renal (CrCl <30 mL/min) impairment ■ Use not recommended
Orlistat (Xenical) Orlistat (Alli)	Capsule, 120 mg Capsule, 60 mg	Adults: ■ Rx: Recommended dosing is 120 mg by mouth three times per day with each meal containing fat ■ OTC: 60 mg by mouth three times daily with each main meal containing fat (maximum: 180 mg/day)
Liraglutide (Saxenda)	Subcutaneous Pen, 6 mg/mL, 3 mL	Adults: Daily Dose ■ Week 1: 0.6 mg ■ Week 2: 1.2 mg ■ Week 3: 1.8 mg ■ Week 4: 2.4 mg ■ Week 5: 3 mg (target dose)
Phentermine/Topiramate (Qsymia)	Extended-release Capsules: ■ 3.75/23 mg ■ 7.5/46 mg ■ 11.25/69 mg ■ 15/92 mg	Adults: ■ Take once daily in morning to prevent insomnia ■ Recommended: 3.75/23 mg daily for 14 days; increase to 7.5/46 mg daily ■ Discontinue or dose escalation if 3% weight loss not achieved after 12 weeks ■ Discontinue is 5% weight loss not achieved on maximum dose of 15/92 mg daily

(continued)

Table 28.2 (continued)

Generic (brand)	Ingredient/strength	Dosage*
Naltrexone/Bupropion Extended Release (Contrave)	Tablet, 8/90 mg	Adults: Morning/Evening Dose • Week 1: 1 tablet (8/90 mg)/None • Week 2: 1 tablet (8/90 mg)/1 tablet (8/90 mg) • Week 3: 2 tablets (16/180 mg)/1 tablet (8/90 mg) • Week 4: 2 tablets (16/180 mg)/2 tablets (16/180 mg) Moderate to Severe Renal Impairment • 1 tablet twice daily Hepatic Impairment • Maximum dose of 1 tablet daily

*All therapies are adjunct to a reduced-calorie diet and increased physical activity.

Therapeutic Considerations

Warnings and Precautions

Lorcaserin is contraindicated in pregnancy.[14] Lorcaserin is a serotonergic agent, so its use with other serotonergic agents should be limited and carefully monitored to reduce the risk of serotonin syndrome or neuroleptic malignant syndrome (NMS).[14] Caution is advised in patients with valvular heart disease, psychiatric disorders, PPH, and hematological effects.[14]

Special Populations

Lorcaserin is listed as an FDA pregnancy category X medication, because weight loss during pregnancy offers no clinical benefit and increases potential risks to the fetus and its growth.[14] Lorcaserin may alter maternal serum prolactin concentrations, affecting the body's ability to make breast milk.[14] Although it has not been studied in breast-feeding, due to the potential for serious adverse reactions, use is not recommended.[14] The safety and efficacy of lorcaserin in children <18 years of age has not been studied and should be avoided.[14] There are no dosing adjustments in patients with moderate renal impairment; however, its use is not recommended in patients with severe renal impairment (CrCl <30 mL/min).[14] There are no dosing adjustments provided for those with severe hepatic impairment (Child-Pugh Class C) as it has not been studied; however, caution should be used due to extensive hepatic metabolism.[14]

Adverse Effects and Monitoring

The most common adverse effects (>10% incidence) associated with the use of lorcaserin include headache, dizziness, hypoglycemia, abnormal lymphocytes, back pain, upper respiratory tract infection, and nasopharyngitis.[14,15] Patients should be advised to self-monitor their weight and waist circumference if they are able.[14] The patient's healthcare provider should monitor complete blood count, blood glucose (patients with diabetes), prolactin levels, depression, and signs and symptoms of serotonin syndrome, NMS, or valvular heart disease, along with weight and waist circumference.[14]

Drug Interactions

Use of lorcaserin with other medications that affect the serotonin pathways should be done with caution, and patients should be closely monitored and counseled on signs and symptoms of serotonin syndrome. Lorcaserin is also a moderate CYP2D6 inhibitor; therefore, it can increase exposure to CYP2D6 substrates. See Table 28.1 for more drug interaction information.[14]

Dosage and Administration

Patients should be initiated on either lorcaserin 10 mg by mouth twice daily or lorcaserin XR 20 mg by mouth once daily, with a maximum dose of either form of 20 mg per day. Response should be evaluated by week 12.[14] If a patient loses ≥5% of their weight from baseline, they will likely continue losing weight, with a 1-year weight loss exceeding 10%. In patients who do not lose ≥5% of baseline body weight, therapy should be discontinued.[14] There are no dosing adjustments in patients with moderate renal impairment; however, its use is not recommended in patients with severe renal impairment (CrCl <30 mL/min). There are no dosing adjustments provided for those with severe hepatic impairment (Child-Pugh Class C) as it has not been studied; however, caution should be used due to extensive hepatic metabolism.[14] See Table 28.2 or refer to the full prescribing information for further guidelines.[14]

ORLISTAT

Orlistat is the only noncentrally acting medication with FDA approval for obesity management. Orlistat should be used in conjunction with a reduced-calorie diet in adults with either an initial BMI of ≥30 kg/m² or an initial BMI of ≥27 kg/m² and at least one weight-related comorbid condition.[18] Orlistat is a gastric and pancreatic lipase inhibitor, available as both a prescription (Xenical) and over the counter (Alli) at half the strength.[18] The Xenical in the Prevention of Diabetes in Obese Subjects (XENDOS) trial was conducted to assess the efficacy of orlistat in preventing T2D in obese patients.[19] The study demonstrated that orlistat plus behavioral counseling led to meaningful weight loss through 4 years of therapy, with twice as much weight loss compared to the placebo.[19] Those in the orlistat group lost 10.6 kg at 1 year and maintained a loss of 5.8 kg at 4 years, compared to 6.2 kg and 3.0 kg, respectively, in the placebo group.[19] In patients with T2D, those treated with orlistat experienced a reduction in body weight more than the placebo.[20]

Pharmacology

Mechanism of Action

Orlistat is a reversible inhibitor of gastrointestinal and pancreatic lipases.[18] It works by exerting its therapeutic activity in the lumen of the stomach and small intestine by forming a covalent bond with the active serine residue site of gastric and pancreatic lipase.[18] The inactivated enzymes are thus unavailable to hydrolyze dietary fat, in the form of triglycerides, into absorbable free fatty acids and monoglycerides.[18] The undigested triglycerides are not absorbed, and the resulting caloric deficit leads to weight loss.[18]

Pharmacokinetics

Systemic exposure to orlistat is minimal and >99% bound to lipoproteins and albumin.[18] The onset of action is between 24 and 48 h, with a duration of action between 48 and 72 h.[18] Orlistat has an elimination half-life of 1–2 h. Approximately 97% of the drug is excreted in the feces, 83% unchanged.[18]

Therapeutic Considerations

Warnings and Precautions

Orlistat is contraindicated in pregnancy, chronic malabsorption syndrome, cholestasis, and known hypersensitivity.[18] There have been postmarketing reports indicating severe liver injury, so patients should be closely monitored.[18] There have also been reports of increased urinary oxalate, resulting in acute renal disease.[18] As such, renal function should be monitored. Substantial weight loss has been associated with an increase in the risk of cholelithiasis.[18]

Special Populations

Orlistat is contraindicated in pregnancy and is listed as an FDA pregnancy category X medication.[18] Caution should be exercised in nursing mothers since secretion in human milk is unknown.[18] Safety for use in patients below the age of 12 years and patients over the age of 65 years has not been established.[18]

Adverse Effects and Monitoring

Orlistat is associated with a variety of side effects mainly resulting from its mechanism of action in the gastrointestinal tract. Common adverse effects (≥5% incidence and at least twice that of placebo) associated with the use of orlistat include oily spotting, flatus with discharge, fecal urgency, fatty/oily stool, oily evacuation, increased defecation, and fecal incontinence.[18] Patients should have their BMI, diet (calorie and fat intake), thyroid function, liver function, and renal function monitored throughout their duration of medication therapy.[18]

Drug Interactions

The use of orlistat is associated with interactions with cyclosporine, fat-soluble vitamin supplements, levothyroxine, anticoagulants, amiodarone, antiepileptic, and antiretroviral therapy.[18] Orlistat can decrease the absorption of these medications, altering their efficacy.[18] See Table 28.1 for more drug interaction information.

Dosage and Administration

The recommended dosage depends on the formulation. Dosing for prescription orlistat (Xenical) is 120 mg by mouth three times daily with each main meal containing fat. The dose may be given during or up to 1 h after the meal and may be omitted if the meal is occasionally missed or contains no fat.[18] Dosing for the OTC formulation of orlistat (Alli) is 60 mg by mouth three times daily with each main meal containing fat, up to a maximum of 180 mg per day.[18] Patients on orlistat should be maintained on a nutritionally balanced, reduced-calorie diet that contains approximately 30% of calories from fat.[18] The manufacturer does not have any dosing recommendations for hepatic or renal impairment.[18] See Table 28.2 or refer to the full prescribing information for further guidelines.

LIRAGLUTIDE

Liraglutide (Saxenda), a GLP-1 RA, was approved by the FDA in 2016 for chronic weight management.[21] Liraglutide is also marketed under the brand name Victoza, which is FDA approved for the management of T2D, but at a lower dosage (max of 1.8 mg/day).[21] Liraglutide, while not the only diabetes medication that aids in weight loss, is the only diabetes medication with FDA approval for weight management.[21] As part of the Satiety and Clinical Adiposity—Liraglutide Evidence in Nondiabetic and Diabetic Individuals (SCALE) program, there were three trials with a primary outcome of weight loss.[22] The SCALE Maintenance trial treated nondiabetic patients with liraglutide or placebo following a 12-week, low-calorie-diet run-in period in which they achieved ≥5% weight loss.[22] After 1 year, liraglutide-treated patients achieved significantly greater weight loss than those treated with the placebo (6.2% vs. 0.2%, $P < 0.0001$).[22] Significantly more patients in the SCALE Maintenance trial lost ≥5% of body weight in the treatment group after randomization than in the placebo group.[22]

The SCALE Obesity and Prediabetes trial was a 2-year extension of the SCALE Maintenance trial.[23] The goal of the 2-year extension was to evaluate the proportion of overweight and obese individuals with prediabetes who progressed to a diagnosis of T2D.[23] At 160 weeks, 26 (2%) participants treated with liraglutide versus 46 (6%) participants in the placebo group were diagnosed with T2D.[23] These results indicate that liraglutide may reduce the risk of developing diabetes in obese patients with prediabetes.[23]

The SCALE Diabetes trial was designed to investigate efficacy and safety of liraglutide (3.0 mg and 1.8 mg) versus placebo for weight management in overweight or obese adults with T2D.[24] A ≥5% weight loss occurred in 54.3% and 40.4% of patients treated with liraglutide 3.0 mg and 1.8 mg, respectively, compared with 21.4% of patients treated with placebo. A ≥10% weight loss occurred in 25.2% and 15.9% of patients treated with liraglutide 3.0 mg and 1.8 mg, respectively, compared with 6.7% of patients treated with placebo.[24] These results indicate that liraglutide, in conjunction with lifestyle changes, is more effective than placebo at reducing weight.[24]

Pharmacology

Mechanism of Action

Liraglutide is a long-acting analog of human GLP-1, an incretin hormone.[25] Like other GLP-1 RAs, liraglutide has multiple mechanisms of action, including increasing glucose-dependent insulin secretion, decreasing inappropriate glucagon secretion, increasing β-cell growth and replication, and slowing gastric emptying.[25] GLP-1 RAs also act centrally on neurons in the hypothalamus, leading to a satiety-inducing effect that is believed to be the most relevant to its role in weight loss.[25]

Pharmacokinetics

Following the subcutaneous administration of liraglutide, maximum concentrations are achieved between 8 and 12 h after dosing.[25] Exposure to the drug increased proportionally in the dose range of 0.6–3 mg.[25] Liraglutide is extensively bound to plasma proteins (>98%). The elimination half-life of liraglutide is approximately 13 h, making it suitable for once-daily administration.[25]

Therapeutic Considerations

Warnings and Precautions

Liraglutide is contraindicated in patients who are pregnant and those with a personal or family history of medullary thyroid carcinoma or multiple endocrine neoplasia type 2.[25] Use of liraglutide has also been associated with thyroid C-cell tumors, acute pancreatitis, gallbladder disease, serious hypoglycemia with the use of additional secretagogue agents, heart rate increase, and renal impairment.[25] Caution should be used in patients with a history of any of these conditions.[25]

Special Populations

Liraglutide (Saxenda) is contraindicated in pregnancy.[25] There is no available data on the presence of liraglutide in human milk, the effects on a breast-fed infant, or on milk production.[25] There is limited experience with liraglutide in patients with renal impairment; however, there have been postmarketing reports of acute renal failure and worsening of chronic renal failure with liraglutide use.[25] Caution should be used in those with hepatic impairment, although data are limited.[25] Liraglutide slows gastric emptying, so use should be cautioned in patients with a history of gastroparesis.[25]

Adverse Effects and Monitoring

Common adverse effects associated with the use of liraglutide include nausea (39%), hypoglycemia (monotherapy 16%), diarrhea (21%), constipation (19%), vomiting (16%), headache (14%), decreased appetite (10%), dyspepsia (10%), fatigue (8%), dizziness (7%), abdominal pain (5%), and increased lipases (5%).[25] Monitoring while using liraglutide includes blood glucose, renal function, signs or symptoms of pancreatitis and gallbladder disease, triglycerides, and body weight at 16 weeks.[25]

Drug Interactions

As stated previously, liraglutide causes delays in gastric emptying; thus, use may impact the absorption of all concomitantly administered oral medications.[25] In clinical trials, liraglutide did not affect the absorption of orally administered medications to a clinically relevant degree.[25] Due to the effect liraglutide has on lowering blood glucose levels, the administration with additional diabetes medications dramatically increases the risk of hypoglycemia compared with monotherapy (in T2D, combination therapy with sulfonylurea: 44%; monotherapy: 16%; nondiabetic: 2–3%).[25] See Table 28.1 for more drug interaction information.

Dosage and Administration

Liraglutide (Saxenda) is a subcutaneously administered medication. The recommended target dose for chronic weight management is 3 mg daily.[25] This recommended target dose should be attained by a titration schedule. Patients should start with 0.6 mg/day at baseline and increase daily dose by 0.6 mg every week as tolerated.[25] Patients should adhere to the dosing escalation recommendations until achieving the 3-mg dosage.[25] If patients do not tolerate an increased dose during dose escalation, consider delaying the escalation by an additional week and rechallenge.[25] The slow titration helps to minimize side effects, especially those related to the gastrointestinal tract. Clinical judgment should be used when determining whether to continue the medication in patients unable to tolerate the 3-mg per day dose. If patients are experiencing a benefit from a lower dose, it may be reasonable to maintain the maximum tolerated dose; however, liraglutide doses of <3 mg have not been FDA approved for weight management.[25] The FDA recommends evaluation of weight loss after 16 weeks of therapy. Clinical trials assessing weight loss have shown that patients who lose ≥4% of baseline weight during this 16-week time frame will likely continue to lose weight,[25] while those who lose <4% of baseline weight are unlikely to lose significantly more weight with therapy continued beyond 16 weeks. There are no dosing adjustments necessary in patients with renal or hepatic impairment, although caution is advised.[25] See Table 28.2 or refer to the full prescribing information for further guidelines.

COMBINATION PRODUCTS

PHENTERMINE-TOPIRAMATE EXTENDED RELEASE (ER)

Phentermine/topiramate ER is a combination product that was approved by the FDA in 2012 for weight management under the brand name Qsymia.[26] This medication is classified as a schedule IV controlled substance.[26] The EQUIP trial provided an evaluation of the safety and efficacy of phentermine-topiramate ER (3.75/23 mg and 15/92 mg) versus placebo on weight loss and metabolic improvements when added to a reduced-calorie diet.[27] Patients lost an average 5.1% (3.75/23 mg dose), 10.9% (15/92 mg dose), and 1.6% (placebo) of their baseline body weight.[27] The percentage of patients achieving weight loss of ≥5% was significantly more in the treatment groups versus the placebo.[27]

The CONQUER clinical trial was a 56-week phase 3 trial designed to assess the efficacy and safety of two doses of phentermine plus topiramate ER as an adjunct to diet and lifestyle modification for weight loss and metabolic risk reduction in individuals who were overweight and obese, with two or more risk factors.[28] Patients were assigned to placebo, once-daily phentermine 7.5/46 mg, or once-daily phentermine 15/92 mg.[28] At 56 weeks, weight losses of 1.4 kg, 8.1 kg, and 10.2 kg were recorded in the placebo, 7.5/46-mg, and 15/92-mg groups, respectively.[28] Patients achieving at least 5% weight loss were 21%, 62%, and 70% in the placebo, 7.5/46-mg, and 15/92-mg groups, respectively.[28] This study concluded that the combination of phentermine and topiramate may be a valuable treatment for obesity in comparison to the placebo.[28]

The SEQUEL randomized clinical trial was a 52-week extension study in eligible patients that completed the CONQUER study and complied with treatment.[29] The objective of this study was to evaluate the long-term efficacy and safety of phentermine/topiramate ER combination in overweight and obese subjects.[29] After the 52-week extension (week 108), the phentermine/topiramate ER combination was associated with significant, sustained weight loss, indicating that this is a potentially effective option for the sustained treatment of obesity.[29]

Pharmacology

Mechanism of Action

Phentermine, as discussed previously, is a sympathomimetic amine with a mechanism of reducing appetite secondary to the CNS effects, which include the stimulation of the hypothalamus to release norepinephrine leading to a reduction in hunger and signaling fat cells to break down stored fat, resulting in weight loss.[26]

The mechanism of topiramate on chronic weight management is not fully understood, although it may be due to its effects on both appetite suppression and satiety enhancement, induced by a combination of pharmacologic effects.[26]

Pharmacokinetics

High-fat meals do not affect the pharmacokinetic profiles of either medication in combination.[26] Phentermine is approximately 17.5% bound to plasma proteins, while topiramate is 15–41% protein-bound.[26] Phentermine is primarily metabolized by CYP3A4 with a mean terminal half-life of approximately 20 h.[26] Topiramate does not show extensive hepatic or renal metabolism, with about 70% of the dose existing as unchanged metabolites.[26] Minor amounts are metabolized in the liver via hydroxylation, hydrolysis, and glucuronidation. Topiramate has a mean terminal half-life of approximately 65 h.[26]

Therapeutic Considerations

Warnings and Precautions

The use of phentermine/topiramate ER is contraindicated during pregnancy due to an increased risk of oral clefts (cleft lip and/or palate). Its use is also associated with an increased heart rate, suicidal behavior and ideation, acute myopia and secondary angle closure glaucoma, mood and sleeping disorders, cognitive impairment, and elevations in creatinine and metabolic acidosis.[26] Patients should be advised against abrupt discontinuation of phentermine/topiramate as it can precipitate seizure activity due to the topiramate component.[26]

Special Populations

Phentermine/topiramate ER is contraindicated in pregnancy and is listed as an FDA category X medication.[26] Because topiramate is a known teratogen (cleft lip and/or palate), pregnancy should be ruled out prior to initiating phentermine/topiramate ER, and women of childbearing age should be advised to use contraception and to have monthly pregnancy testing during use.[26] Topiramate and amphetamine derivatives such as phentermine are excreted into human milk; therefore, its use should be avoided in breast-feeding. In patients with renal impairment (CrCl <50 mL/min) and those with moderate hepatic impairment, dosing should not exceed 7.5/46 mg once daily.[26]

Adverse Effects and Monitoring

Common adverse effects (≥5% incidence and at least 1.5 times placebo) that are associated with the use of phentermine/topiramate ER include paresthesia, dizziness, dysgeusia, insomnia, constipation, and dry mouth.[26] Patients on phentermine/topiramate ER should have their blood chemistries—including bicarbonate, creatinine, potassium, and glucose—monitored at baseline and periodically throughout treatment.[26] Monthly pregnancy testing is recommended for female patients while using this medication.[26] Patients should also monitor their weight. If after 12 weeks on the recommended 7.5/46-mg daily dosing a 3% weight loss has not been achieved, the medication should be discontinued or escalated to the next dose of 11.25/69 mg daily.[26]

Drug Interactions

Phentermine/topiramate ER has many potential drug interactions, including with MAOIs, oral contraceptives, CNS depressants such as alcohol, non-potassium sparing diuretics, antiepileptics, and carbonic anhydrase inhibitors.[26] See Table 28.1 for more detailed drug interaction information.

Dosage and Administration

Patients should be advised to take phentermine/topiramate ER by mouth, once daily in the morning with or without food. Treatment should be initiated with the 3.75/23-mg tablet for 14 days and then should be increased to the 7.5/46-mg tablet, the recommended target dose.[26] If a 3% weight loss is not achieved in 12 weeks, the dose may be escalated to 11.25/69 mg daily for 14 days followed by 15/92 mg once daily.[26] If at this time a 5% weight loss is not achieved after an additional 12 weeks on the 15/92-mg dose, the medication should be discontinued.[26] In patients with a CrCl <50 mL/min or moderate hepatic impairment, dosing should not exceed 7.5/46-mg once daily.[26] In patients who have been stabilized, the dose should gradually be decreased if discontinuation is desired.[26] Patients should be advised to take the dose every other day for at least 1 week prior to discontinuation to avoid precipitating a seizure. See Table 28.2 or refer to the full prescribing information for further guidelines.[26]

NALTREXONE-BUPROPION SR

Naltrexone-bupropion SR is another combination product marketed for weight management under the brand name Contrave.[30] This medication is an anorexiant agent approved for weight management.[30] Naltrexone-bupropion SR is not approved for use in the treatment of major depressive disorder or other psychiatric disorders.[30] Several randomized trials have shown weight loss and improvements in obesity-related comorbid conditions, including a trial of naltrexone-bupropion SR in patients with obesity and T2D.[31] Those treated with the medication for 1 year lost 5.9% of initial body weight and had an A1C reduction of 0.6% compared to 2.2% weight loss and 0.1% A1C reduction with the placebo.[31]

Pharmacology

Mechanism of Action

Naltrexone-bupropion SR has two components: naltrexone, an opioid receptor antagonist, and bupropion, a relatively weak inhibitor of the neuronal reuptake of dopamine and norepinephrine.[30] The exact neurochemical effects of naltrexone-bupropion leading to weight loss are not fully understood.[30] Studies suggest that naltrexone and bupropion have effects on two separate areas of the brain involved in the regulation of food intake.[30] Those areas are located in the hypothalamus, which is the appetite regulatory center, and the mesolimbic dopamine circuit, which is also known as the reward center.[30] Besides decreasing appetite, the combination also decreases cravings for high-calorie, pleasurable foods.[30]

Pharmacokinetics

Following oral administration, the time to peak concentration is 2 h for naltrexone and 3 h for bupropion.[30] When taken with a high-fat meal, the food effect increased the AUC and C_{max} for naltrexone and bupropion.[30] Thus, naltrexone-bupropion SR should not be taken with a high-fat meal, as it may increase the systemic exposure of the active ingredients.[30] Naltrexone is not metabolized by cytochrome P450 enzymes, while bupropion inhibits CYP2D6 and is metabolized by CYP2B6.[30] Bupropion is metabolized into three active metabolites (erythrohydrobupropion, threohydrobupropion, and hydroxybupropion), which have longer elimination half-lives.[30] Following oral administration of naltrexone-bupropion

SR, the mean elimination half-life was approximately 5 h for naltrexone and 21 h for bupropion.[30]

Therapeutic Considerations

Warnings and Precautions

This medication contains bupropion, thus patients with major depressive disorder may experience worsening of their depression and/or suicidal ideation.[30] However, in clinical trials with naltrexone-bupropion SR, no suicides or attempts were reported. Patients should be appropriately counseled about this risk.[30] Bupropion may cause seizures, so use is cautioned in patients with a history of seizures.[30] Due to the naltrexone component, patients using opioid medications are at risk for an opioid overdose and/or opioid withdrawal, and use of this medication is contraindicated.[30] Naltrexone-bupropion SR may increase blood pressure, and therefore is contraindicated in patients with uncontrolled hypertension.[30]

Special Populations

Naltrexone-bupropion SR is contraindicated in pregnancy and carries an FDA category X label, because weight loss therapy is not recommended in pregnant women, and there have been inconsistent reports of adverse fetal events such as cardiovascular malformations following maternal use of bupropion.[30] The constituents and metabolites of this combination are known to be secreted in human milk; therefore, use in nursing mothers is not recommended.[30] A pooled analysis of naltrexone-bupropion SR suggests no clinically meaningful differences in patients based on sex and race.[30] Although this medication has not been specifically studied in patients with hepatic failure, the individual components have. Patients with hepatic impairment should have the dose reduced to a maximum dose of 8/90 mg twice daily (50% reduction).[30] Similarly, in patients with renal impairment, the dose should be reduced, and its use is not recommended in those with ESRD.[30] Naltrexone-bupropion should be used with caution in elderly patients due to a greater risk of drug accumulation when used chronically, precipitating adverse drug reactions.[30]

Adverse Effects and Monitoring

Common adverse effects (≥10% incidence) that are associated with the use of naltrexone-bupropion include nausea, constipation, headache, vomiting, insomnia, dry mouth, and diarrhea.[30] Patients, especially those with a psychiatric disorder, should also be monitored for changes in mood. Patients should be monitored for weight loss.[30]

Drug Interactions

The use of naltrexone-bupropion should be cautioned with medications that can lower the seizure threshold, as well as other dopaminergic drugs (e.g., levodopa and amantadine), as this can lead to CNS toxicity.[30] Bupropion is a CYP2D6 inhibitor; therefore, this medication can increase exposure to CYP2D6 substrates. See Table 28.1 for more drug interaction information.[30]

Dosage and Administration

When initiating this medication, patients should be started on a low dose and then titrate the dose every week until a maximum dosage of two tablets in the morning and two tablets in the evening is established.[30] This phased titration greatly improves the tolerability of this medication.[30] Although the weekly dose escalation was forced in clinical trials regardless of tolerability, patients who continue to experience side effects may benefit from a slower dose titration over several months.[30] If a patient has not lost at least 5% of their baseline body weight after 12 weeks at the target dose of two tablets (16/180 mg) twice daily, therapy should be discontinued. In clinical trials, naltrexone-bupropion SR was administered with meals, but high-fat meals should be avoided.[30] Similar to liraglutide, early weight loss of ≥5% at 16 weeks predicted better long-term weight loss with naltrexone-bupropion at 1 year compared to those with <5% weight loss.[32] In patients with moderate or severe renal impairment, the maximum recommended dose is one tablet (8/90 mg) twice daily, and its use is not recommended for those with ESRD.[30] In patients with hepatic impairment, the maximum dosage is one tablet (8/90 mg) daily. Caution should be exercised in elderly patients due to a greater risk of accumulation leading to adverse drug reactions.[30] See Table 28.2 or refer to full prescribing information for further guidelines.

SUMMARY

Obesity is a chronic medical condition that results from a long-term mismatch in energy balance and affects almost 40% of U.S. adults. There are many health risks that are associated with obesity, including T2D, cardiovascular effects, osteoarthritis, respiratory problems, and even some cancers. These risks can be decreased by implementing an appropriate, personalized weight loss regimen. The regimen should include lifestyle modifications to diet and exercise and may include the use of pharmacotherapy. Decreasing the health risks associated with obesity will have long-term benefits that may also include a decreased financial burden. Goals of therapy are preventing further weight gain, an eventual weight loss, and maintaining this lower weight over the long term. There are many agents that can be used as adjunct therapy to diet and exercise. Selection ultimately comes down to patient-specific factors, and the cost and benefit seen with these medications.

MONOGRAPHS

Liraglutide (Saxenda): https://dailymed.nlm.nih.gov/dailymed/drugInfo.cfm?setid=3946d389-0926-4f77-a708-0acb8153b143

Lorcaserin HCl (Belviq; Belviq XR): https://dailymed.nlm.nih.gov/dailymed/drugInfo.cfm?setid=7cbbb12f-760d-487d-b789-ae2d52a3e01f

Naltrexone/Bupropion ER (Contrave): https://dailymed.nlm.nih.gov/dailymed/drugInfo.cfm?setid=ed2da3a6-0614-4bea-8e82-962cbaae6428

Orlistat (Xenical; Alli): https://dailymed.nlm.nih.gov/dailymed/drugInfo.cfm?setid=5bbdc95b-82a1-4ba5-8185-6504ff68cc06

Phentermine (Lomaira; Adipex-P): https://dailymed.nlm.nih.gov/dailymed/drugInfo.cfm?setid=737eef3b-9a6b-4ab3-a25c-49d84d2a0197

Phentermine/Topiramate (Qsymia): https://dailymed.nlm.nih.gov/dailymed/drugInfo.cfm?setid=40dd5602-53da-45ac-bb4b-15789aba40f9

REFERENCES

1. Delaet D, Schauer D. Obesity in adults. *Clin Evid Handbook* 2010;216–217

2. American College of Cardiology/American Heart Association Task Force on Practice Guidelines, Obesity Expert Panel, 2013. Expert Panel Report: Guidelines (2013) for the management of overweight and obesity in adults. *Obes* (Silver Spring) 2014;22(Suppl. 2):S41–S410. DOI:10.1002/oby.20660

3. National Institutes of Health. Clinical guidelines on the identification, evaluation, and treatment of overweight and obesity in adults—the evidence report. *Obes Res* 1998(6 Suppl. 2):51S–209S

4. Centers for Disease Control and Prevention. Adult Obesity Facts [Internet], 29 August 2017. Available from https://www.cdc.gov/obesity/data/adult.html. Accessed 29 January 2018

5. American Diabetes Association. 7. Obesity management for the treatment of type 2 diabetes: *Standards of Medical Care in Diabetes—2018. Diabetes Care* 2018;41(Suppl. 1):S65–S72

6. Pastors JC, Warshaw H, Daly A, et al. The evidence for the effectiveness of medical nutrition therapy in diabetes management. *Diabetes Care* 2002;25(3):608–613

7. Franz MJ, Boucher JL, Rutten-Ramos S, VanWormer JJ. Lifestyle weight-loss intervention outcomes in overweight and obese adults with type 2 diabetes: a systematic review and meta-analysis of randomized clinical trials. *J Acad Nutr Diet* 2015;115:1447–1463

8. Kahan S, Fujioka K. Obesity pharmacotherapy in patients with type 2 diabetes. *Diabetes Spectrum* 2017;30(4):250–257

9. World Health Organization (WHO). Fact sheet: obesity and overweight. [article online], 2017. Available from http://www.who.int/en/news-room/fact-sheets/detail/obesity-and-overweight. Accessed 25 April 2018

10. Jensen MD, Ryan DH, Apovian CM, et al. 2013 AHA/ACC/TOS guideline for the management of overweight and obesity in adults: a report of the American College of Cardiology/American Heart Association Task Force on Practice Guidelines and the Obesity Society. *J Am Coll Cardiol* 2014;63:2985–3023

11. Patel D. Pharmacotherapy for the management of obesity. *Metabolism* 2015;64:1376–1385

12. Adipex-P (phentermine) [package insert]. Horsham, PA, Teva Select Brands, March 2017. Available from https://dailymed.nlm.nih.gov/dailymed/drugInfo.cfm?setid=f5b2f9d8-2226-476e-9caf-9d41e6891c46

13. Lomaira (phentermine) [package insert]. Newtown, PA, KVK-Tech, September 2016. Available from https://dailymed.nlm.nih.gov/dailymed/drugInfo.cfm?setid=cde9fb09-e5af-434d-8874-e4f9f974d893

14. Belviq IR & XR (lorcaserin & XR) [package insert]. Woodcliff Lake, NJ, Eisai Inc., May 2017. Available from https://dailymed.nlm.nih.gov/dailymed/drugInfo.cfm?setid=7cbbb12f-760d-487d-b789-ae2d52a3e01f

15. Smith SR, Weissman NJ, Anderson CM, et al.; Behavioral Modification and Lorcaserin for Overweight and Obesity Management (BLOOM) Study Group. Multicenter, placebo-controlled trial of lorcaserin for weight management. *N Engl J Med* 2010;363:245–256

16. Smith SR, O'Neil PM, Astrup A, et al. Early weight loss while on lorcaserin, diet and exercise as a predictor of week 52 weight loss outcomes. *Obes* (Silver Spring) 2014;22:2137–2146

17. Yanovski SZ, Yanovski JA. Long-term drug treatment for obesity: a systematic and clinical review. *JAMA* 2014;311:74–86

18. Xenical (orlistat) [package insert]. South San Francisco, CA, Genentech USA Inc., December 2017. Available from https://dailymed.nlm.nih.gov/dailymed/drugInfo.cfm?setid=5bbdc95b-82a1-4ba5-8185-6504ff68cc06

19. Torgerson JS, Hauptman J, Boldrin MN, Sjostrom L. XENical in the prevention of diabetes in obese subjects (XENDOS) study: a randomized study of orlistat as an adjunct to lifestyle changes for the prevention of type 2 diabetes in obese patients. *Diabetes Care* 2004;27:155–161

20. Rucker D, Padwal R, Li SK, et al. Long term pharmacotherapy for obesity and overweight: updated meta-analysis. *BMJ* 2007;335:1194–1199

21. Fujioka K, O'Neil PM, Davies M, et al. Early weight loss with liraglutide 3.0 mg predicts 1-year weight loss and is associated with improvements in clinical markers. *Obes* 2016;24:2278–2288

22. Wadden TA, Hollander P, Klein S, et al. Weight maintenance and additional weight loss with liraglutide after low-calorie-diet-induced weight loss: the SCALE maintenance randomized study. *Int J Obes* 2013;37:1443–1451

23. Le Roux CW, Astrup A, Fujioka K, et al. 3 years of liraglutide versus placebo for type 2 diabetes risk reduction and weight management in individuals with prediabetes: a randomized, double-blind trial. *Lancet* 2017;380:1399–1409

24. Davies MJ, Bergenstal R, Bode B, et al. Efficacy of liraglutide for weight loss among patients with type 2 diabetes: the SCALE diabetes randomized clinical trial. *JAMA* 2015;314(7):687–699

25. Saxenda (liraglutide) [package insert]. Plainsboro, NJ, Novo Nordisk Inc., May 2017. Available from https://dailymed.nlm.nih.gov/dailymed/drugInfo.cfm?setid=3946d389-0926-4f77-a708-0acb8153b143

26. Qsymia (phentermine/topiramate) [package insert]. Campbell, CA, Vivus Inc., June 2017. Available from https://dailymed.nlm.nih.gov/dailymed/drugInfo.cfm?setid=40dd5602-53da-45ac-bb4b-15789aba40f9

27. Allison DB, Gadde KM, Garvey WT, et al. Controlled-release phentermine/topiramate in severely obese adults: a randomized controlled trial (EQUIP). *Obes* 2012;20:330–342

28. Gaddle KM, Allison DB, Ryan DH, et al. Effects of low-dose, controlled-release, phentermine plus topiramate combination on weight and associated comorbidities in overweight and obese adults (CONQUER): a randomized, placebo-controlled, phase 3 trial. *Lancet* 2011;377(9774):1341–1352

29. Garvey WT, Ryan DH, Look M, et al. Two-year sustained weight loss and metabolic benefits with controlled-release phentermine/topiramate in obese and overweight adults (SEQUEL): a randomized, placebo-controlled, phase 3 extension study. *Am J Clin Nutr* 2012;95:297–308

30. Contrave (naltrexone/bupropion) [package insert]. Deerfield, IL, Takeda Pharmaceuticals America, Inc., September 2014. Available from https://dailymed.nlm.nih.gov/dailymed/drugInfo.cfm?setid=ed2da3a6-0614-4bea-8e82-962cbaae6428

31. Hollander P, Gupta AK, Plodkowski RA, et al. Effects of naltrexone sustained-release/bupropion sustained-release combination therapy on body weight and glycemic parameters in overweight and obese patients with type 2 diabetes. *Diabetes Care* 2013;36:4022–4029

32. Fukioka K, Plodkowski R, O'Neil PM, et al. The relationship between early weight loss and weight loss at one year with naltrexone ER/bupropion ER combination therapy. *Int J Obes* 2016;40:1369–1375

Chapter 29

Immunizations and Diabetes

Kimberly C. McKeirnan, PharmD, BCACP
Nicole M. Perea, PharmD

INTRODUCTION

Complications from vaccine-preventable diseases lead to hospitalization and sometimes death. The CDC considers T1D and T2D to be high-risk health conditions that can result in serious and long-term health consequences due to illness from vaccine-preventable diseases.[1] Patients with T1D or T2D are at higher risk for serious complications from contracting these diseases, even when diabetes is well managed. Patients with diabetes are at an increased risk of glycemic fluctuations, increased risk of hepatitis B infection, and even an increased risk of death by vaccine-preventable diseases.[1] This chapter will provide an overview of available vaccines, recommendations specifically for people with diabetes, and information about available vaccine resources.

VACCINATION SCHEDULES

Vaccination schedules are available from the CDC as a guide for which vaccines are needed and recommended timing of administration. Vaccination schedules developed for healthcare providers are available categorized by patient age (birth to 18 years, 19 years and older) and also by medical condition.[2] Patient-friendly schedules are also available categorized by age for infants and children, preteens and teens, and adults.[2] Catch-up schedules are available for patients who need immunizations that were recommended at younger ages.

The Advisory Committee on Immunization Practices (ACIP) also has useful vaccination resources for specific medical conditions. Figure 29.1 displays an informational table called Vaccinations for Adults with Diabetes.[3] This resource lists common adult vaccinations along with recommendations on the need for vaccines indicated specifically for patients with diabetes. The CDC also has helpful condition-specific patient infographics explaining the importance of being vaccinated and which vaccines are recommended. The diabetes infographic is shown in Figure 29.2.[4]

VACCINES

The CDC vaccination schedules provide a foundation for the vaccines that everyone should receive. However, additional recommendations are provided for peo-

Vaccinations for Adults with Diabetes

The table below shows which vaccinations you should have to protect your health if you have diabetes. Make sure you and your healthcare provider keep your vaccinations up to date.

Vaccine	Do you need it?
Hepatitis A (HepA)	**Maybe.** You need this vaccine if you have a specific risk factor for hepatitis A* or simply want to be protected from this disease. The vaccine is usually given in 2 doses, 6–12 months apart.
Hepatitis B (HepB)	**Yes!** All adults with diabetes who are younger than 60 and have never received or completed a series of HepB vaccine, should get vaccinated now. If you are 60 or older and diabetic, discuss your need for HepB vaccine with your healthcare provider.
Hib *(Haemophilus influenzae* type b)	**Maybe.** Some adults with certain high-risk conditions, for example, lack of a functioning spleen, need vaccination with Hib. Talk to your healthcare provider to find out if you need this vaccine.
Human papillomavirus (HPV)	**Yes!** You need this vaccine if you are a woman age 26 or younger or a man age 21 or younger. Men age 22 through 26 with a risk condition* also need vaccination. All other men age 22 through 26 who want to be protected from HPV may receive it too. The vaccine is usually given in 3 doses over a 6-month period.
Influenza	**Yes!** You need a dose every fall (or winter) for your protection and for the protection of others around you.
Measles, mumps, rubella (MMR)	**Maybe.** You need at least 1 dose of MMR vaccine if you were born in 1957 or later. You may also need a second dose.*
Meningococcal ACWY (MenACWY)	**Maybe.** You may need MenACWY vaccine if you have one of several health conditions,* for example, if you do not have a functioning spleen. You need MenACWY if you are age 21 or younger and a first-year college student living in a residence hall and you either have never been vaccinated or were vaccinated before age 16.
Meningococcal B (MenB)	**Maybe.** You should consider MenB vaccine if you are age 23 or younger (even if you don't have a high-risk medical condition). You may need MenB vaccine if you have one of several health conditions,* for example, if you do not have a functioning spleen.
Pneumococcal (Pneumovax 23, PPSV23; Prevnar 13, PCV13)	**Yes!** If you're younger than 65 and have diabetes, you need to get vaccinated with Pneumovax. If you haven't been vaccinated, you should get 1 dose now. You may also need a 1-time dose of Prevnar, depending on whether you have a certain high-risk condition,* such as immunosuppression, or you lack a functioning spleen. At age 65 (or older), you will need a dose of Prevnar (if you haven't received it previously) and a second dose of Pneumovax, provided at least 5 years have passed since your first dose. Prevnar and Pneumovax are usually spaced 1 year apart.
Tetanus, diphtheria, whooping cough (pertussis) (Tdap, Td)	**Yes!** If you have not received a dose of Tdap during your lifetime, you need to get a Tdap shot now (the adult whooping cough vaccine). And all women need to get a dose during each pregnancy. After that, you need a Td booster dose every 10 years. Consult your healthcare provider if you haven't had at least 3 tetanus and diphtheria toxoid-containing shots sometime in your life or if you have a deep or dirty wound.
Varicella (Chickenpox)	**Maybe.** If you've never had chickenpox, never were vaccinated, or were vaccinated but received only 1 dose, talk to your healthcare provider to find out if you need this vaccine.*
Zoster (shingles)	**Yes!** If you are age 50 or older, you should get the 2-dose series of the Shingrix brand of shingles vaccine, even if you already were vaccinated with Zostavax.

* Consult your healthcare provider to determine your level of risk for infection and your need for this vaccine.

Are you planning to travel outside the United States? Visit the Centers for Disease Control and Prevention's (CDC) website at wwwnc.cdc.gov/travel/destinations/list for travel information, or consult a travel clinic.

immunization
action coalition

immunize.org

Saint Paul, Minnesota • 651-647-9009 • www.immunize.org • www.vaccineinformation.org

Technical content reviewed by the Centers for Disease Control and Prevention

www.immunize.org/catg.d/p4043.pdf • Item #P4043 (6/18)

Figure 29.1—ACIP Table Vaccinations for Adults with Diabetes.[3]

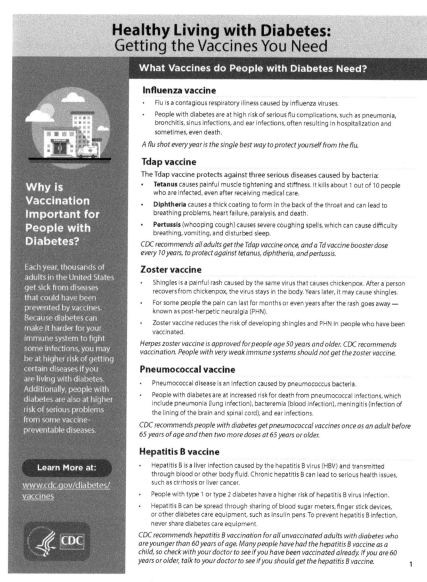

Figure 29.2—CDC Infographic.[4]

ple with specific medical conditions. For patients with diabetes, the CDC specifically recommends vaccination against influenza, hepatitis B, pneumococcal diseases, herpes zoster (shingles), and the combination vaccine for tetanus, diphtheria, and pertussis.

INFLUENZA

Influenza is a respiratory illness affecting the nose, throat, and lungs caused by infection with the influenza virus. Complications from influenza can lead to pneumonia, bronchitis, sinus infections, and ear infections in all people, but it can also cause blood glucose fluctuations in those with diabetes. Acute illness may cause hyperglycemia, but dietary inconsistency due to the general malaise and feeling not well during the course of illness can also lead to hypoglycemia in patients taking antihyperglycemic agents. Many flu medications contain high levels of sugar. It is good practice to recommend increasing the frequency of blood glucose testing during this time. Annual influenza vaccinations are recommended by the CDC and are FDA approved for people with diabetes.[5] The influenza vaccine comprises three (trivalent) or four (quadrivalent) influenza viruses that researchers believe will be most common in the upcoming flu season. The vaccine is generally administered intramuscularly in one dose.[5] Other routes of administration include intradermal and intranasal. For patients over the age of 65 years, the high-dose influenza vaccine is recommended for increased protection.[5] The flu vaccine has been shown to reduce the risk of getting sick with the flu, as well as to reduce the risk of having a serious flu outcome if infected, such as a stay in the hospital.[5]

HEPATITIS B

Hepatitis B is a vaccine-preventable liver infection caused by the hepatitis B virus (HBV), which is transmitted by bodily fluid. People with diabetes have higher rates of hepatitis B, because outbreaks associated with blood glucose monitoring procedures have occurred.[6] There is approximately a 60% increase in prevalence in patients with diabetes for contracting HBV and up to a twofold increase in acquiring the virus.[7] In most people, hepatitis B is an acute illness, but in patients with reduced immune function, hepatitis B can become a chronic infection leading to cirrhosis, cancer, liver failure, or death.[6] The hepatitis B vaccine is available as a two- or three-dose series of intramuscular injections, although one hepatitis B vaccine has an FDA-approved four-dose accelerated schedule.

PNEUMOCOCCAL DISEASE

Infection with pneumococcal bacteria can lead to meningitis, pneumonia, and bacteremia. Two different pneumococcal vaccines, pneumococcal conjugate vaccine (PCV13) and pneumococcal polysaccharide vaccine (PPSV23), are available to prevent illness from pneumococcal bacteria.[8] Since these two vaccines protect in part against different types of pneumococcal bacteria, both are recommended for all people aged 65 years and over. PPSV23 is also recommended for people with an increased risk for infection, including patients with diabetes, even when under the age of 65 years. PCV13 may not be needed prior to age 65 even in those with diabetes unless the patient has an additional immunocompromising condition.[2] Both pneumococcal vaccines are administered individually as a one-dose intramuscular or subcutaneous injection. People with diabetes potentially will receive three adult pneumococcal vaccines: PPSV23 prior to age 65, PPSV23 at or after age 65 years, and PCV13 at or after age 65 years.[8] These vaccines are generally separated by 1 year and are not given at the same time.[8] Once the patient reaches age 65 years, PPSV23 should be administered if the patient has not received the vaccine prior. After receiving this dose of PPSV23, they should receive PCV13 at least 1 year later. If the patient has previously been vaccinated with PPSV23 before the age of 65 years, they should receive the PCV13 vaccine at age 65 years, at least 1 year after their last pneumococcal vaccine. The patient should then receive an additional dose of PPSV23 at least 5 years after receiving the PCV13 dose.[8]

HERPES ZOSTER

Herpes zoster, also known as shingles, is caused by the chickenpox virus in the form of reactivating the varicella zoster virus, which remains dormant in the nervous system after infection. Shingles presents as a painful rash that develops on one side of the body. The rash usually resolves in 2–4 weeks, but some patients have complications, such as postherpetic neuralgia, which can cause pain lasting for years. Two vaccines, zoster vaccine live and recombinant zoster vaccine, are available to protect against shingles. The CDC recommends all people over the age of 50 years receive a zoster vaccine. The newer recombinant zoster vaccine is a two-dose series and was FDA approved in 2017. This is compared to the single dose of the zoster vaccine live that was previously recommended. Even people who were previously vaccinated with zoster vaccine live should receive the full schedule of the new recombinant vaccine in order to more adequately prevent shingles and the complications caused by the disease.[9]

TETANUS, DIPHTHERIA, PERTUSSIS

Tetanus is a vaccine-preventable infection that is caused by Clostridium tetani bacteria. Tetanus primarily presents as painful muscle contractions in the jaw, also known as "lockjaw." Tetanus itself is not spread among humans. The Clostridium tetani bacteria spreads through mediums such as soil, dust, or manure. Pertussis is also known as whooping cough. This is a respiratory disease that is caused by the Bordetella pertussis bacteria. It is known for the violent, uncontrollable coughing associated with the disease that often makes it hard to breathe.[10] Protection against these infections is offered in a variety of combination products. For patients who are younger than 7 years of age, diphtheria and tetanus (DT) and diphtheria, tetanus, and pertussis (DTaP) combinations are offered. For patients who are 7 years of age or older, the same combinations of diphtheria and tetanus (Td) and diphtheria, tetanus, and pertussis (Tdap) exist with differing doses of the diphtheria component. According to the CDC, this is to be used as a booster that should be updated every 10 years in diabetic patients.[11]

CONCLUSION

T1D and T2D increase risk for complications from vaccine-preventable diseases even when the diabetes is well managed. The CDC recommends that patients with diabetes be up to date with the flu vaccine and the tetanus, diphtheria, pertussis vaccine, and for these patients to maintain an altered schedule when receiving the pneumococcal series, the hepatitis B series, and protection against herpes zoster.[1,2] Following these recommended schedules and reducing complications from vaccine-preventable diseases will lead to lower hospitalization rates and fewer deaths for patients with diabetes.

REFERENCES

1. Centers for Disease Control and Prevention (CDC). Diabetes type 1 and type 2 and adult vaccination [Internet], 2 May 2016. Updated 1 November 2016. Available from https://www.cdc.gov/vaccines/adults/rec-vac/health-conditions/diabetes.html. Accessed 3 August 2018

2. CDC. Information for adult patients: 2018 recommended immunizations for adults: by age [Internet]. Available from https://www.cdc.gov/vaccines/schedules/downloads/adult/adult-schedule-easy-read.pdf. Accessed 3 August 2018

3. Immunization Action Coalition. Vaccinations for adults with diabetes [Internet], June 2018. Available from http://www.immunize.org/catg.d/p4043.pdf. Accessed 3 August 2018

4. CDC. Healthy living with diabetes: getting the vaccines you need [Internet], May 2018. Available from https://www.cdc.gov/vaccines/adults/rec-vac/health-conditions/diabetes/infographic/images/global/footer/diabates_en.pdf. Accessed 3 August 2018

5. CDC. Flu and people with diabetes [Internet], 25 August 2016. Updated 2 February 2017. Available from https://www.cdc.gov/flu/diabetes/index.htm. Accessed 3 August 2018

6. CDC. Viral hepatitis [Internet], 31 May 2015. Available from https://www.cdc.gov/hepatitis/hbv/index.htm. Accessed 3 August 2018

7. Hepbtalk. Hepatitis B precautions for people living with diabetes [Internet], 20 March 2018. Hepatitis B Foundation and Baruch S. Blumberg Institute. Available from www.hepb.org/blog/hepatitis-b-precautions-people-living-diabetes/

8. CDC. Pneumococcal vaccination [Internet], 6 September 2017. Available from https://www.cdc.gov/pneumococcal/vaccination.html. Accessed 3 August 2018

9. CDC. Shingles (herpes zoster) [Internet], 25 January 2018. Updated 3 August 2018. Available from https://www.cdc.gov/shingles/vaccination.html. Accessed 3 August 2018

10. CDC. Epidemiology and prevention of vaccine-preventable diseases. The Pink Book [Internet]. Available from https://www.cdc.gov/vaccines/pubs/pinkbook/downloads/pert.pdf

11. CDC. Tetanus [Internet], 10 January 2017. Available from https://www.cdc.gov/tetanus/about/index.html. Accessed 3 August 2018

Index

Note: Page numbers followed by *f* refer to figures. Page numbers followed by *t* refer to tables. Page numbers in **bold** indicate an in-depth discussion of the topic.

A

A1C
α-glucosidase inhibitor, 72, 168, 170–171
biguanide, 67–68
bile acid sequestrant, 223–225, 347
cardiovascular outcome trial, 266*t*–267*t*
chronic kidney disease, 292
diabetic retinopathy, 440
dipeptidyl peptidase-4 (DPP-4) inhibitor, 73, 178, 184
dopamine-2 receptor agonist, 234
duloxetine, 303
gastroparesis, 402
glinide, 71, 140–141, 146
glucagon-like peptide 1 (GLP-1) receptor agonist, 75, 194–195, 202–203
glycemic recommendation, 10
insulin therapy, 2–4, 32, 34, 35*f*, 42, 76
medical nutrition therapy, 482
naltrexone/bupropion SR, 497
niacin, 345*t*
pramlintide, 211–213, 215
renin-angiotensin system (RAS) inhibitor, 446–447
sodium–glucose cotransporter 2 (SGLT2) inhibitor, 73, 158, 417
sulfonylurea, 70, 126
thiazolidinedione, 72, 105–108, 117

type 2 diabetes, 48–51
α₂ adrenergic receptor agonist, 383
α4β2 neuronal nicotinic acetylcholine receptor (nAchR), 376
AACE/ACE guidelines, 224–225, 234
α-adrenergic receptor blockade, 401
ABCD study, 416
abdominal pain, 171, 218, 228, 345*t*, 403–404, 494
abemaciclib, 90
abuse, 460. *See also* substance use/abuse
acarbose, 56*t*, 71–72, 168–174
acebrophylline, 485*t*
ACE inhibitor. *See* angiotensin-converting-enzyme (ACE) inhibitor
α-cell, 125, 477
acetylcholine, 473
acid-reducing medication, 359
acromegaly, 233
Action for Health in Diabetes (Look AHEAD) trial, 263
Action in Diabetes and Vascular Disease: Preterax and Diamicron Modified Release Controlled Evaluation (ADVANCE) trial, 127, 440
Action in Diabetes and Vascular Disease: Preterax and Diamicron MR Controlled Evaluation–Blood Pressure (ADVANCE BP) trial, 244, 245*t*

Action to Control Cardiovascular Risk in Diabetes (ACCORD) trial, 292, 346, 440, 448
Action to Control Cardiovascular Risk in Diabetes blood pressure (ACCORD BP) trial, 244, 245*t*, 246, 257
activation adhesion molecule, 356
Actos Now for the Prevention of Diabetes (ACT NOW) study, 106
acute coronary syndrome (ACS), 254, 258, 261, 342, 359–360, 362–363, 364*t*–365*t*
acute kidney injury (AKI), 156, 161, 198, 250, 290, 418, 422
ADA Professional Practice Committee, 241, 286
adenosine diphosphate (ADP) receptor, 358
adenosine monophosphate (AMP), 477
adenylate cyclase, 406, 477
A Diabetes Outcome Progression Trial (ADOPT), 110–111, 126
adipex-P, 484
adipocyte, 104
adipose tissue, 110
adlyxin, 206
Admelog, 13, 29
adolescent
    ADA treatment target recommendation, 10
    bupropion SR, 381
    diabetic retinopathy, 297
    dipyridamole/aspirin, 361
    glycemic goal, 11*t*
    metformin, 21
    nicotine replacement therapy, 373
    nortriptyline, 386
    severe hypoglycemia, 2
    smoking cessation, 371*t*
    suicidal ideation, 466
    type 1 diabetes, 8
adrenal gland, 473
adrenaline hormone, 473
adrenal insufficiency, 142
Advicor, 347
Advisory Committee on Immunization Practices (ACIP), 503

aflibercept, 299, 441–444, 450*t*, 451
African-American population, 171, 411
Agency for Healthcare Research and Quality (AHRQ), 68
aging-related condition, 84–85
agitation, 484
α-glucosidase enzyme, 71, 168
α-glucosidase inhibitor (AGIs), 56*t*, 71–72, 88, **168–175**
agranulocytosis, 129, 361
alanine transaminase (ALT), 109, 113, 229
albiglutide, 74, 190, 265
albumin, 14, 30–31, 288, 290, 418, 420
albumin-creatinine ratio (ACR). *See* urinary albumin-to-creatinine ratio
albuminuria
    antihypertensive treatment, 246
    cardiovascular risk factor, 242, 249*t*, 250–251, 255*t*, 260
    chronic kidney disease, 287–295
    diabetic kidney disease, 411–412, 417–420
    hypertension, 323, 328
    lipid, 342*t*
    mineralocorticoid receptor antagonist, 423
    nephropathy, 421–422, 428
    sodium–glucose cotransporter 2 (SGLT2) inhibitor, 155
    thiazolidinedione, 106
    type 1 diabetes, 413–414
albuterol, 39
alcohol
    aspirin therapy, 357
    bupropion SR, 381
    clonidine, 384
    hypertension, 322
    hypertriglyceridemia, 256
    insulin, 39
    metformin, 86
    nortriptyline, 387
    phentermine/topiramate, 487*t*, 496–497
    triglyceride, 340
    varenicline, 379
    vitamin B$_{12}$ supplementation, 88

alcohol (ethyl), 485*t*
alcoholic, 477
aldosterone, 421, 423
aldosterone antagonist, 163, 325*t*, 331*t*
alirocumab, 255, 343, 344*t*, 349*t*, 351
aliskiren, 415, 422, 425*t*, 429
alkaline phosphatase, 229
alkalinizing agent, 485*t*
alkyldiguanide synthalin A, 80
all-cause mortality, 106–107, 111, 141,
 154, 196, 253, 265, 268*t*, 340, 482
allergic reaction, 36, 119*t*, 129, 180,
 358, 361
allopurinol, 474
alogliptin
 adverse effects and monitoring, 182
 antihyperglycemic medication with
  metformin, 93*t*
 cardiovascular outcome trial, 179–
  180, 266*t*–268*t*, 269
 cost, 56*t*
 dipeptidyl peptidase-4 (DPP-4)
  inhibitor, 177
 dosage and administration, 183,
  184, 426*t*
 drug interaction, 182
 metformin and, 185*t*
 monograph, 185, 430
 pioglitazone and, 118*t*, 185*t*
 special population, 181
 type 2 diabetes, 73
alpha 1 β blocker, 326*t*
alpha-2 adrenergic agonist, 327*t*
alpha-lipoic acid, 89, 115, 487*t*
alpha-melanocortin stimulating
 hormone, 488
alprostadil, 406
ALTITUDE trial, 422
Alzheimer's disease, 473
American Association for the Study of
 Liver Disease (AASLD), 111
American Association of Clinical
 Endocrinologists (AACE), 194
American College of Cardiology,
 "Pathway for Tobacco Cessation
 Treatment", 371
American College of Cardiology/
 American Heart Association, 246

American College of Cardiology/
 American Heart Association ASCVD
 risk calculator (Risk Estimator Plus),
 242
American College of Cardiology
 Foundation, 260
American College of Obstetricians and
 Gynecologists (ACOG), 247
American Diabetes Association (ADA)
 aspirin recommendation, 260
 atherosclerotic cardiovascular
  disease recommendation, 340
 children and adolescents with T1D,
  10
 "Diabetes and Hypertension", 242
 Diabetes Forecast, 17, 41
 "Diabetic Neuropathy", 301
 foot examination recommendation,
  305
 glucagon recommendation, 16
 hyperglycemia in T2D, 66–67
 hypoglycemia classification, 472
 insulin therapy recommendation, 9
 pharmacologic treatment approach,
  138
 recommendation, 10
 (SGLT2) inhibitor
  recommendation, 154–155
 smoking cessation, 370, 371*t*
 Standards of Medical Care in Diabetes,
  3, 16, 33, 36–37, 82, 194, 224, 234,
  241, 269, 286, 472
 sulfonylurea, 124
 treatment algorithm, 131
 "Type 1 Diabetes Through the Life
  Span", 2, 20
American Diabetes Association
 and the European Association for
 the Study of Diabetes (EASD)
 Consensus Report, 194
American Diabetes Association/
 European Association for the Study
 of Diabetes, "Management of
 Hyperglycemia in Type 2 Diabetes,
 2018", 49, 66–67
*American Diabetes Association/JDRF
 Type 1 Diabetes Sourcebook*, 1

American Heart Association (AHA), 260, 355
AMIGO trial, 195t
amiloride, 90, 327t
amino acid, 31
amino acid sequence, 11
amiodarone, 145, 229t, 486t, 492
amitriptyline, 398t, 400–401, 406, 463, 465t, 467
amlodipine, 324t, 331t, 332–333, 415, 421
amlodipine/benazepril, 423, 429
ammonium chloride, 485t
amphetamine, 484, 485t–486t, 488t, 496
AMP kinase, 67
amputation, 106, 155–156, 161, 304–305, 307
amylin, 3, 20, 211
amylin mimetic, 57t
amylinomimetic agent, 20
amyloid fibril, 211
amyotrophic, 396t
anaphylaxis, 180, 182, 237
androgen, 89, 115, 487t
anemia, 48, 69, 113, 129, 172, 291t, 362
anesthetic administration, 397
angina, 106, 256, 263, 265, 268t, 327t, 328, 339
angina pectoris, 357
angioedema, 180, 182, 325t, 379
angiogenesis, 441
angioplasty, 304
angiotensin-converting-enzyme (ACE) inhibitor
  calcium channel blocker, 332
  cardiovascular disease, 261, 263
  chronic kidney disease, 287, 290, 295
  combination therapy, 329–330, 422–423
  diabetic retinopathy, 299
  dipyridamole/aspirin, 361
  diuretic and, 332
  hypertension, 248, 249t, 250–251, 323, 325t, 328, 332
  insulin therapy, 38–39

  metformin, 90
  nephropathy, 412–417, 419–423, 424t, 429
  pregnancy, 247
  renin-angiotensin system (RAS) inhibitor, 412–413, 446–447
  sodium–glucose cotransporter 2 (SGLT2) inhibitor, 163, 428
  thiazolidinedione, 114–115
  type 1 diabetes, 446
  type 2 diabetes, 447
angiotensin receptor blockers (ARBs)
  cardiovascular disease, 261, 263
  chronic kidney disease, 287, 290, 295
  combination therapy, 329–330, 422–423
  diabetic retinopathy, 299
  diuretic and, 332
  dosing, 424t
  hypertension, 248, 249t, 250–251, 323, 325t, 328, 332–333
  insulin and, 38–39
  monograph, 429
  nephropathy, 412–423, 429
  pregnancy, 247
  renin-angiotensin system (RAS) inhibitor, 412–413, 446–447
  sodium–glucose cotransporter 2 (SGLT2) inhibitor, 163, 428
  type 1 diabetes, 446
  type 2 diabetes, 447
angle-closure glaucoma, 382, 386, 496
anhidrosis, 396t
ankle-brachial index, 305–306
anorexia, 218, 237, 381
anorexiant agent, 488, 497
antacid, 172, 485t
antiadrenergic medication, 39
antibiotic, 229t, 307
anticholinergic agent, 304, 384, 387
anticholinergic effect, 463
anticoagulant, 358, 361–362, 401, 492
anticonvulsant, 361, 397–400, 486t
antidepressant medication, 380, 382, 386, 398t, 400–401, 460–461
antidiabetic agent, 70f, 77t, 473–474, 487t

antidiabetic-renoprotective antihypertensive treatment, 423
antidiuretic hormone, 129
anti-drug antibody, 203
antiepileptic medication, 381, 486*t*–487*t*, 492, 497
antifungal, 115
antihistamine, 485*t*
antihistaminic effect, 463
antihyperglycemic activity, 104
antihyperglycemic medication
  cardiovascular outcome trial, 266*t*–268*t*
  combination products, 91
  cost, 50–51, 55*t*–57*t*
  drug interaction, 88
  drug-specific and patient factors, 52*t*–53*t*
  hypoglycemia, 39
  insulin, 11–15
  metformin, containing, 99
  pharmacokinetic, 11
  renal effect, 292
  T2D weight gain, 38
  type 2 diabetes, 67
antihypertensive medication
  acute kidney injury, 290
  bromocriptine, 235
  cardiovascular event, 294
  chronic kidney disease, 289
  clonidine, 384
  diabetic kidney disease, 412
  diabetic retinopathy, 447
  nephropathy, 416–417
  overview and rationale, 323, 328–329, 330*t*–331*t*
  phentermine, 485*t*
  pregnancy, 246–248
  resistant hypertension, 250
  treatment strategies, 248
antihypertensive therapy, 243–244, 246–247, 294–295, 322–323, 328
antioxidant, 356, 396
antiplatelet, **355–369**
  aspirin, 357, 360–361
  cilostazol, 361
  clopidogrel, 358–359
  combination therapy, 362–365

coronary heart disease, 362–363
dipyridamole, 360–361
dual therapy, duration of, 364*t*
goals of therapy, 356*t*
medication, doses and dose adjustment, 365*t*
monograph, 365–366
myocardial infarction, 362–363
peripheral arterial disease, 364
prasugrel, 358
stroke, 363
therapy, 258, 356*t*, 357–362
ticagrelor, 359–360
vorapaxar, 362
antipsychotic medication, 39, 145, 382, 384, 467, 485*t*
antiretroviral therapy, 486*t*, 492
Antithrombotic Trialists' Collaboration, 259
anti–vascular endothelial growth factor (anti-VEGF) agent, 296–297, 299, 441–446, 449, 451
anti-VEGF/corticosteroid, 450–451
anti-VEGF/laser therapy, 449
antral motor activity, 403
anuria, 330*t*
anxiety disorder, 379, 382, 462–464
appetite, 464, 482, 494
arachidonic acid metabolism, 356
area under the curve (AUC), 88–89, 163, 497
arginine, 14, 30, 193
arrhythmia, 386, 463, 474, 478
ARRIVE (Aspirin to Reduce Risk of Initial Vascular Events), 259
arteriolar pressure, 423
arteriosclerosis, 339
arthralgia, 341, 344*t*
ASCEND (A Study of Cardiovascular Events iN Diabetes) trial, 259, 261
ascorbic acid, 485*t*
Asian population, 84, 171, 348*t*, 411
asinitial pharmacologic treatment, 300
asparagine, 14, 30
aspartate transaminase (AST), 229
aspirin, 357–363, 365, 448, 474
aspirin/dipyridamole, 365*t*

aspirin/extended-release dipyridamole, 365
aspirin resistance, 261
aspirin therapy, 258–261, 263, 297, 345*t*
ASPREE (Aspirin in Reducing Events in the Elderly), 259
asthenia, 237, 327*t*
asthma, 38, 60
atazanavir, 145
atenolol, 326*t*
atherosclerosis, 21, 339, 355–356, 404
atherosclerotic cardiovascular disease (ASCVD)
   antiplatelet agent, 258–260
   cardiovascular disease, 262–263, 269
   glucagon-like peptide 1 (GLP-1) receptor agonist, 194
   glucose-lowering medication, 293–294
   hypertension/blood pressure control, 242–244, 246, 250–251
   lipid management, 251–258, 339–343, 346–347
   primary prevention, 340
   risk management, 241–242
   secondary prevention, 340
   symptoms, 356*t*
   type 2 diabetes, 48–51, 67–68
Atherothrombosis Intervention in Metabolic Syndrome with Low HDL/High Triglycerides: Impact on Global Health Outcomes (AIM-HIGH) trial, 257, 346
atomoxetine, 485*t*
atorvastatin, 256*t*, 343*t*–344*t*, 348*t*, 350
ATP-dependent potassium ion channel, 124–125, 139
ATP-sensitive potassium channel, 71
atrial fibrillation, 328
atypical antidepressant, 461, 464, 465*t*, 468
autoimmunity, 8
autonomic nervous system, 191
autonomic neuropathy. *See* diabetic autonomic neuropathy
autonomic response, 473–474

avanafil, 404–406
average wholesale prices (AWP), 51, 54, 58
AVOID trial, 422
AWARD trial, 195*t*
axonal change, 395–396

B
back pain, 344*t*
bacteremia, 506
balance loss, 395, 399
barbiturate, 145, 381, 384
bare metal stent (BMS), 364*t*
barium study of the stomach, 302
Basaglar, 14, 30
basement membrane thickening, 395
β-blocker. *See* beta blocker
β-cell
   amylin, 20, 211
   dipeptidyl peptidase-4 (DPP-4) inhibitor, 176
   glinide, 71, 139, 141
   glucagon-like peptide 1 (GLP-1) receptor agonist, 74, 194
   incretin-based therapy, 21
   insulin, 26
   pramlintide, 3, 20
   sulfonylurea, 69, 124–127
   type 1 diabetes, 1, 3, 8–9
Beers Criteria, 130, 144
behavioral change, 472. *See also* lifestyle intervention
belching, 344*t*
benazepril, 330*t*, 332
benazepril/amlodipine, 423, 429
BENEDICT trial, 415, 447
benzodiazepine, 374, 381
Berhanu, Paulos, 70*f*
β-1-selective adrenergic blocker, 326*t*
β-adrenergic blocker, 90, 326*t*
beta blocker
   biguanide, 90
   blood glucose level, 39
   bupropion SR, 382
   cardiovascular disease, 261, 263
   diabetic retinopathy, 447
   dipyridamole/aspirin, 361

glinide, 142
hypertension, 250, 326*t*, 328, 331*t*, 333
hypoglycemia, 128, 142, 145, 473
nicotine replacement therapy, 374
repaglinide, 145
sulfonylurea, 130
bevacizumab, 299, 441–443, 445, 449, 450*t*, 451
BEVORDEX study, 445
bictegravir, 90
BIDS: bedtime insulin daytime
sulfonylurea, 132
biguanide, **80–102**
combination products, 91, 99
cost, 55*t*
dosage and administration, 91
mechanism of action, 80–81
monograph, 99
pharmacology, 80–81
therapeutic consideration, 85–90
treatment advantages/
disadvantages, 81–85
type 2 diabetes, 67–69
bile acid, 223–224
bile acid sequestrant, **223–232**
adverse effects and monitoring, 228–229
cost, 57*t*
dosage and administration, 230
drug interaction, 229
fat-soluble vitamin, 226
hypertension, 345*t*
mechanism of action, 223–224
monograph, 230, 351
pharmacogenomics, 228
pharmacokinetic/
pharmacodynamics, 224
pharmacology, 223
serum triglyceride, 226
special population, 227–228
statins and, 347
therapeutic consideration, 226–230
treatment advantages/
disadvantages, 224–225
warnings/precautions, 226–227
biliary cirrhosis, 349*t*
bipolar disorder, 382, 386, 467

birth defect, 199. *See also* pregnancy
bisoprolol, 326*t*, 331*t*
black patient, 328
bladder cancer, 107, 109–111, 113, 162
bladder dysfunction, 302
bladder infection, 396*t*
bladder tone, 396*t*
bleeding, 226, 258–260, 344*t*, 347, 356*t*, 357–363, 488*t*
blindness, 198, 297
bloating, 228, 345*t*, 403
blood glucose
diabetic retinopathy, 440
fasting, 10*t*
insulin dosage, 1–2
monitoring, 19. *see also* continuous glucose monitor
postprandial, 2, 10, 12–13, 141, 168, 203
preprandial, 10
testing, 114
blood glucose level. *See also*
hyperglycemia; hypoglycemia
bile acid sequestrant, 224
bromocriptine, 234
cardiovascular risk factor, 355–356
correction dose, 19
gastroparesis, 402
inhaled human insulin, 58
insulin dosing, 33
lorcaserin, 491
recommendation, 10
T2D insulin therapy, 48
type 1 diabetes, 9
blood glucose–lowering agent, 487*t*
blood pressure. *See also* hypertension
bupropion SR, 381
calcium channel blocker, 420–421
chronic kidney disease, 287, 291, 291*t*, 294–295
clonidine, 383–384
control, 242–244, 246–251
diabetic retinopathy, 296, 299, 440
dopamine-2 receptor agonist, 237
glucagon-like peptide 1 (GLP-1)
receptor agonist, 203
hypertension, 322
NDCA *vs* DCA, 420–421

nephropathy, 413–414, 420–421
nicotine replacement therapy, 374
pharmacologic intervention, 248
pregnancy, 246–248
randomized controlled trial, 244, 245*t*
renin-angiotensin system (RAS) inhibitor, 413–414, 446–447
resistant hypertension, 250–251
screening and diagnosis, 243
self-monitoring, 322–323
serotonin-norepinephrine reuptake inhibitor, 463
sodium–glucose cotransporter 2 (SGLT2) inhibitor, 156
statin and combination treatment recommendation, 255*t*
thiazolidinedione, 108
treatment goals, 243–244
treatment recommendation, 249*f*
treatment strategies, 247–248
type 1 diabetes, 446–447
type 2 diabetes, 447
blood-thinning medication, 357
blood vessel, 395, 439, 444
blurred vision, 386, 399
body mass index (BMI), 82, 482–483, 488, 491–492
bone deformity, 306
bone density, 72
bone fracture, 159, 162
bone health, 111
Bordetella pertussis bacteria, 507
bowel obstruction, 226, 228
bradyarrhythmia, 324*t*, 326*t*
brain, 190
breast-feeding
  α-glucosidase inhibitor, 171
  bile acid sequestrant, 227
  dipeptidyl peptidase-4 (DPP-4) inhibitor, 181
  erythromycin, 404
  GABA analog, 399
  glinide, 143
  glucagon, 479
  glucagon-like peptide 1 (GLP-1) receptor agonist, 199
  lorcaserin, 490

metoclopramide, 403
naltrexone/bupropion SR, 498
orlistat, 492
phentermine, 484
phentermine/topiramate ER, 496
pramlintide, 216
sulfonylurea, 128
thiazolidinedione, 110
tricyclic antidepressant, 401
venlafaxine, 400
vorapaxar, 362
Briggs, *Drugs in Pregnancy and Lactation*, 227, 236
bromocriptine, 57*t*, 233–238
bromocriptine QR, 233–235, 237
buccal mucosa, 375–376
buformin, 80
bulimia, 381
bumetanide, 326*t*
bupropion, 90, 464, 465*t*, 466, 468, 485*t*, 488*t*, 497–498
bupropion SR, 372, 378, 380–382, 388*t*, 389, 465*t*
buspirone, 386
bydureon BCise, 206
byetta, 206
Bypass Angioplasty Revascularization Investigation in Type 2 Diabetes (BARI 2D) trial, 302

C

cabergoline, 233
calcium, 71, 125, 356, 406
calcium antagonist, 421, 423
calcium channel α2-δ subunit ligand, 303
calcium channel blocker (CCB), 172, 249*t*, 324*t*, 333, 413, 420–421, 423, 429, 447
calcium channel blocker/ACE inhibitor, 332
calcium scoring, 263
callus, 305
caloric intake, 263
canagliflozin
  adverse effects and monitoring, 161–163

cardiovascular outcome trial, 51,
154–155, 264–265, 266*t*–268*t*,
270, 293–294
cost, 56*t*, 156
diabetic nephropathy, 417–418, 430
dosage and administration, 164*t*,
425*t*
lower limb amputation, 156
metformin and, 94*t*–95*t*, 165
monograph, 165
nephropathy, 425*t*
renal outcome trial, 417–418
sodium–glucose cotransporter 2
(SGLT2) inhibitor, 153
special population, 158
type 2 diabetes, 67, 73–74
urogenital infection, 157
Canagliflozin and Renal Endpoints
in Diabetes with Established
Nephropathy Clinical Evaluation
(CREDENCE), 155, 293, 418
Canagliflozin Cardiovascular
Assessment Study (CANVAS), 264
cancer, 83–84, 482, 506
candesartan, 325*t*, 414, 416, 422, 424*t*,
429, 446–447
cannabinoid-containing product, 485*t*
CANTATA-SU trial, 417
CANVAS (Canagliflozin
Cardiovascular Assessment Study),
155–156, 266*t*–268*t*, 270, 293–294
CANVAS-Renal (CANVAS-R) trial,
156, 264, 266*t*–268*t*, 417
Cao, X, 84
capsaicin, 303, 398*t*, 402, 406
captopril, 413, 424*t*, 429
Captopril Study, 413
carbamazepine, 145, 303, 382, 399–
400, 407, 487*t*
carbohydrate
α-glucosidase inhibitor, 71, 168,
170–171, 173
bile acid sequestrant, 224
glycemic management in people
with T1D, 9, 13, 18
hypoglycemia, 16, 37, 472, 475,
476*t*, 477

insulin therapy in people with T1D,
33
metabolism, 80
pramlintide, 212, 219–220
"rule of 15", 16, 37
carbohydrate counting, 2, 18
carbonic anhydrase inhibitor, 90, 485*t*,
487*t*, 497
cardiac autonomic neuropathy (CAN),
300–302
cardiac effect, 463
cardiac myocyte, 125
cardiac QT interval prolongation, 404
cardiac tissue, 190
cardiovascular
collapse, 85
complication, 397
effect, 74, 195
morbidity, 144, 259, 370
outcome, 169, 179, 205, 218, 244,
328, 370–371
system, 396
toxicity, 386
cardiovascular disease (CVD), **241–
285**
antihyperglycemic medication
outcome trial, 266*t*–268*t*
antihyperglycemic therapies and
cardiovascular outcomes, 263–265,
269–270
antihypertensive therapy, 295
antiplatelet therapy, 258–261, 355
asymptomatic patient, 262–263
cardiac testing, 262
cardiovascular outcome trial, 267*t*
chronic kidney disease, 289, 294–
295
cost, 355
diabetic kidney disease, 411
dopamine-2 receptor agonist, 234
glinide, 144
hypertension/blood pressure
control, 242–251
lifestyle intervention, 247–248, 263
lipid management, 251–258
nicotine replacement therapy, 373
pharmacologic intervention, 263
phentermine, 484

recommendation, 261–262
risk calculator, 242
smoking, 370, 374*f*
sodium–glucose cotransporter 2
  (SGLT2) inhibitor, 156
sulfonylurea, 129
thiazolidinedione, 107
type 2 diabetes, 53*t*, 67, 68*f*
varenicline, 378
cardiovascular event
  antiplatelet therapy, 355–356
  bromocriptine, 235
  chronic kidney disease, 287
  cigarette smoking, 370
  fenofibrate/simvastatin, 257, 346
  hypoglycemia, 473
  nicotine replacement therapy, 373
  sildenafil, 406
  statin/ezetimibe, 342
  steroid therapy, 446
  varenicline, 379
cardiovascular mortality
  albuminuria, 289
  angiotensin converting enzymes
    inhibitor, 290
  angiotensin receptor blocker, 290
  antihyperglycemic medication and
    metformin, 269
  aspirin, 259, 261
  blood pressure, 294
  cardiovascular outcome trial, 263–
    265, 267*t*, 269
  chronic kidney disease, 291
  cigarette smoking, 370
  dipeptidyl peptidase-4 (DPP-4)
    inhibitor, 179
  evolocumab, 256
  glinide, 141–142, 144
  glucagon-like peptide 1 (GLP-1)
    receptor agonist, 195–196
  metformin, 49
  obesity, 482
  rosiglitazone, 106–107
  sodium–glucose cotransporter 2
    (SGLT2) inhibitor, 154–155
  sulfonylurea, 127, 129
  thiazolidinedione, 72
  ticagrelor, 359

cardiovascular outcome trials (CVOT),
  73, 179–180, 197, 263–265, 267*t*,
  269, 293
cardiovascular risk
  American Diabetes Association
    recommendation, 355
  antiplatelet therapy, 356*t*
  biguanide, 82
  bile acid sequestrant, 223, 225
  chronic kidney disease, 287–288,
    290–291
  diabetic nephropathy, 412, 417
  glinide, 144
  hypertension, 322–323, 329
  management, 241
  sulfonylurea, 70–71, 127, 129
carotid bruits, 261
carvedilol, 326*t*, 331*t*, 333
catabolism, 34, 35*f*, 48
cataract, 297, 443, 445–446, 450
cationic drug, 89–90
Caucasian population, 171
Centers for Disease Control and
  Prevention (CDC), 8, 482, 503,
  505–507
Centers for Medicare & Medicaid
  Services, 307
central alpha 2 receptor, 464
central autonomic neuropathy, 402
central dopamine D_2 antagonist, 403
central involved diabetic macular
  edema (CIDME), 297, 299, 441,
  442*t*, 445–446
central nervous system (CNS), 191,
  234, 373, 376, 383–384, 473, 483–
  484, 485*t*
central nervous system depressant,
  487*t*, 496
central nervous system depression, 399
central nervous system toxicity, 488*t*,
  498
cephalexin, 90, 229*t*
cerebrovascular accident, 444
cerebrovascular disease, 241, 355
C-fiber afferent neuron, 402
cGMP-specific phosphodiesterase- 5
  degradation, 405
CHANCE trial, 363

Charcot foot, 304, 306, 396*t*
Charcot neuroarthropathy, 306–307
Chen, CB, 84
chickenpox, 504*f*, 507
children. *See also* pediatric patient
  ADA treatment target
    recommendation, 10
  bile acid sequestrant, 227
  bupropion SR, 381
  diabetic retinopathy, 297
  dipyridamole/aspirin, 361
  glycemic goal, 11*t*
  hypoglycemia, 477
  lorcaserin, 490
  nortriptyline, 386
  phentermine, 484
  severe hypoglycemia, 2
  smoking, 371*t*
  type 1 diabetes, 8
chloramphenicol, 145
chlorpropamide, 124–125, 128–130,
  132*t*–133*t*, 134
chlorthalidone, 249*t*, 330*t*, 333
chlorthalidone hydrochlorothiazide,
  324*t*
cholecystitis, 228
cholelithiasis, 203, 228, 492
cholestasis, 492
cholesterol, 21, 252, 339–340. *See also*
  HDL cholesterol; LDL cholesterol
cholesterol absorption inhibitor, 344*t*,
  349*t*, 351
cholesterol-lowering drug, 340
Cholesterol Treatment Trialists'
  Collaboration, 254, 341
cholestyramine, 223–225, 227, 230,
  345*t*, 349*t*, 351
cholinesterase inhibitor, 403
chronic depression, 461
chronic heart failure (CHF), 107, 109,
  113. *See also* heart failure
chronic inflammatory demyelinating
  neuropathy, 301
chronic kidney disease (CKD), **286–
  295**. *See also* diabetic kidney disease;
  kidney
    acute kidney injury, 290
    albuminuria, 288

antihypertensive medication, 246
ASCVD risk factor, 342*t*
cardiovascular disease and blood
  pressure, 294–295
cardiovascular risk factor, 355
complication, 291*t*
diagnosis, 288
epidemiology of diabetes and, 287
estimated glomerular filtration rate,
  288
glucagon-like peptide 1 (GLP-1)
  receptor agonist, 75
glucose-lowering medication,
  292–294
glycemic target, 292
insulin, 37
intervention, 291–295
mineralocorticoid receptor
  antagonist, 423
nephrologist referral, 295
nephropathy medication, 411
nutrition intervention, 291
recommendation, 286–295
staging of, 289–290
statin therapy, 255*t*
surveillance, 290–291
type 2 diabetes, 48–51, 67, 68*f*
ulcer and amputation risk, 305
Chronic Kidney Disease
  Epidemiology Collaboration (CKD-
  EPI) equation, 288
chronic lung disease, 60
chronic malabsorption syndrome, 492
chronic obstructive pulmonary disease
  (COPD), 38, 60, 378, 381
cigarette, 370, 374*f*. *See also* smoking;
  tobacco
ciglitazone, 103
cilostazol, 361, 365*t*, 366
cimetidine, 89, 379, 382
circadian rhythm, 233
cirrhosis, 110, 170, 506
citalopram, 462, 465*t*, 467
clarithromycin, 145, 360
CLARITY study, 443–444
claudication, 261, 305–306, 361, 365*t*
clomiphene, 90

clonidine, 39, 327*t*, 372, 383–384, 388*t*, 389
clopidogrel, 115, 145, 258, 261, 358–359, 362–363, 365*t*, 366, 488*t*
Clostridium tetani bacteria, 507
C_{max}, 88–89, 104, 112, 116, 153–154, 163, 497
coagulation, 355
cocaine (topical), 485*t*
Cochrane review, 140–141, 247, 413, 423, 442–443
cognitive dysfunction, 473–474
cognitive function, 258
cognitive impairment, 472–473, 496
colesevelam, 57*t*, 223–225, 227, 230, 345*t*, 347, 349*t*, 351
colestimide, 223
colestipol, 223–225, 227, 230, 345*t*, 350*t*
colonic ulceration, 72, 170
colorectal cancer (CRC), 83–84
coma, 386, 472
Combination of Prescription Omega-3 With Simvastatin (COMBOS) study, 347
comorbidity, 246
computed tomography angiography, 262–263
computed tomography calcium scoring, 262–263
confusion, 399
congenital abnormality, 128, 216
congestive heart failure (CHF), 53*t*, 68, 72, 85, 106–107, 262, 288. *See also* heart failure
CONQUER clinical trial, 495
constipation
    bile acid sequestrant, 226, 228, 230, 345*t*
    bromocriptine, 237
    clonidine, 384
    diabetic autonomic neuropathy, 301
    HMG-CoA reductase inhibitor, 344*t*
    liraglutide, 494
    nondihydropyridine calcium channel blocker, 324*t*
    nortriptyline, 386

tricyclic antidepressant, 463
continuous glucose monitor (CGM), 2, 17–19, 474
continuous subcutaneous insulin infusion (CSII), 2, 9, 16–17, 33, 41
contraception, 108, 116
contrave, 488*t*
convulsion, 486*t*
corn, 305
coronary arteriosclerosis, 339
coronary artery bypass graft (CABG), 357*t*, 362, 364*t*
coronary artery calcium, 262
coronary artery disease, 226, 261–262
coronary computed tomography angiography, 260
coronary death, 258
coronary heart disease (CHD), 126, 241, 253, 259, 261, 355, 362–363, 370, 482
coronary revascularization, 339
coronary syndrome, 179, 339
corpus cavernosum, 405–406
corticosteroid, 39, 88, 172, 357, 444–446, 450–451
corticosteroid/laser therapy, 449–450
cortisol, 473
cough, 325*t*, 328
creatinine acidosis, 496
creatinine clearance rate (CrCl), 413, 415–416, 424*t*, 426*t*, 465*t*
creatinine kinase, 344*t*
CREDO trial, 362–363
CURE trial, 362
cyanocobalamin level, 68–69
cyclic-3'5'-adenosine monophosphate (cAMP), 360–361
cyclic adenosine monophosphate (cAMP), 224, 406, 477
cyclic guanosine monophosphate (cGMP), 404–405
cyclooxygenase, 360
cyclosporine, 145, 229*t*, 486*t*, 492
CYP1A2 enzyme, 400
CYP2B6 enzyme, 358, 382, 497
CYP2B6 inducer, 488*t*
CYP2B6 inhibitor, 488*t*

CYP2C8 inhibitor, 114–117, 139, 145, 183, 348*t*
CYP2C8 substrate, 348*t*
CYP2C9 enzyme, 358
CYP2C9 inhibitor, 114, 128, 140, 145, 348*t*
CYP2C9 substrate, 348*t*
CYP2C19 enzyme, 358–359, 361
CYP2C19 inhibitor, 361, 365*t*, 465*t*
CYP2D6 enzyme, 382, 385, 387, 400, 466*t*
CYP2D6 inhibitor, 177, 382, 485*t*–486*t*, 491, 497–498
CYP2D6 substrate, 486*t*, 488*t*, 491
CYP3A4/5 inhibitor, 177–178, 182–183
CYP3A4 enzyme, 358, 360–362, 404, 496
CYP3A4 inducer, 237
CYP3A4 inhibitor, 114, 139–140, 145, 153, 177, 234, 237, 348*t*–349*t*, 365*t*, 405
CYP3A4 substrate, 349*t*
CYP3A inhibitor, 362
CYP450 3A4/5 inhibitor, 181
CYP450 3A4 enzyme, 178
CYP450 3A4 inducer, 182–183
CYP450 enzyme, 182
CYP450 inhibitor, 145
CYP450-mediated interaction, 163
CYP P450 2C19 enzyme, 359
cytisine, 376
Cytisus labarnum (false tobacco), 376
cytochrome enzyme, 462
cytochrome P450 enzyme, 114, 358
cytokine-induced apoptosis, 191

D

dabrafenib, 115
Dagogo-Jack, Sam, 70*f*
daily energy balance, 482, 497–499
dairy, 322
dalfampridine, 90
DAPA-CKD trial, 155
dapagliflozin
  antihyperglycemic medication and metformin, 95*t*
  bladder cancer, 162
  chronic kidney disease, 294
  cost, 56*t*, 156
  diabetic nephropathy, 418, 428
  dosage and administration, 164*t*, 425*t*
  metformin hydrochloride and, 165
  monograph, 165, 430
  nephropathy, 425*t*
  saxagliptin and, 165
  sodium–glucose cotransporter 2 (SGLT2) inhibitor, 151, 153, 163
  special population, 158–159
  type 2 diabetes, 73
  urogenital infection, 157
  weight loss, 155
Davidson, MB, 110–111
death. *See* all-cause mortality; cardiovascular mortality; mortality
DECLARE trial, 155
decontamination syndrome, 463
deferasirox, 229*t*
dehydration, 85, 199, 329
dementia, 473
depression
  atypical antidepressant, 464, 468
  bupropion, 498
  bupropion SR, 382
  clonidine, 384
  combination therapy, 466–467
  diabetes and, 460–461
  lorcaserin, 491
  medication adverse effect, 326*t*
  medication dosage, 465*t*–466*t*
  medication for the management of, **460–471**
  monograph, 467
  nortriptyline, 384–386
  pharmacotherapy, 461
  pharmacotherapy combination, 466–467
  precaution, 464, 466
  psychotherapy, 461
  risk factor, 460
  selective serotonin-norepinephrine reuptake inhibitor, 462–463, 467
  selective serotonin reuptake inhibitor, 461–462, 467

serotonin modulator, 464, 468
symptoms, 460
treatment, 461
tricyclic antidepressant, 463, 467
varenicline, 379
vorapaxar, 362
weight gain, 462
dermatological rash, 172
dermatological reaction, 88
desipramine, 407, 463
desvenlafaxine, 400, 462, 465*t*
desvenlafaxine ER, 407
DETAIL study, 416
Dex4, 476*t*
dexamethasone, 445
dexamethasone implant, 449–451
dexamethasone intravitreal implant
(MEAD trial), 445
dexterity issues, 17, 39, 41–42
diabetes. *See under specific type*
Diabetes Control and Complications
Trial (DCCT), 2, 9, 76, 440
Diabetes Control and Complications
Trial (DCCT)/Epidemiology
of Diabetes Interventions and
Complications (EDIC) study, 292
Diabetes Epidemiology: Collaborative
analysis of Diagnostic criteria in Asia
(DECODA), 141
Diabetes Epidemiology: Collaborative
analysis of Diagnostic criteria in
Europe (DECODE), 141
Diabetes Forecast (ADA), 17, 41
diabetes morbidity, 461
Diabetes Prevention Program, 82
Diabetes Prevention Program
Outcomes Study (DPPOS), 49
Diabetes Reduction Assessment
with Ramipril and Rosiglitazone
Medication (DREAM) study, 106
diabetic autonomic neuropathy
(DAN), 243, 300–302, 329, 395–397
diabetic gastroparesis. *See*
gastroparesis
diabetic glomerulopathy, 295
diabetic-induced neuropathic pain,
398

diabetic ketoacidosis (DKA). *See also*
ketoacidosis
α-glucosidase inhibitor, 170
bile acid sequestrant, 225
bromocriptine, 234
dipeptidyl peptidase-4 (DPP-4)
inhibitor, 178, 180
glinide, 142
glucagon-like peptide 1 (GLP-1)
receptor agonist, 198
metformin, 85, 92*t*
sodium–glucose cotransporter 2
(SGLT2) inhibitor, 52*t*, 157
sulfonylurea, 127
thiazolidinedione, 108
type 1 diabetes, 8
diabetic kidney disease (DKD), 53*t*,
263, 287–288, **411–438**. *See also*
chronic kidney disease
diabetic macular edema (DME), 439,
441–446, 449–451
diabetic nephropathy. *See* chronic
kidney disease; diabetic kidney
disease; nephropathy
"Diabetic Neuropathy" (ADA), 301
diabetic peripheral neuropathy (DPN),
48, 69, 300–302, 304–305, 462
diabetic polyneuropathy (DPN), 395,
397*t*
diabetic retinopathy (DR)
antihypertensive treatment, 246
combination products, 451
combination therapy, 447, 449–451
diabetic kidney disease, 288
goals of treatment, 439–441
intraocular treatment
recommendation, 442*t*
medication, 441–449, 450*t*
medication for the management of,
439–459
monograph, 451
pregnancy, 298
recommendation, 296–297
screening, 297–299
semaglutide, 198
type 1 diabetes, 298
type 2 diabetes, 298

Diabetic Retinopathy Clinical Research Network, 299
Diabetic Retinopathy Study (DRS), 298
Diagnostic and Statistical Manual of Mental Disorders (DSM-5), 460
dialysis, 94*t*–96*t*, 160, 183, 192, 287, 412–413, 422
diarrhea
  α-glucosidase inhibitor, 171
  β-adrenergic blocker, 326*t*
  cilostazol, 361
  diabetic autonomic neuropathy, 301
  dopamine-2 receptor agonist, 237
  erythromycin, 404
  glucagon-like peptide 1 (GLP-1) receptor agonist, 202
  HMG-CoA reductase inhibitor, 344*t*
  liraglutide, 494
  metformin, 88
  niacin, 345*t*
  sertraline, 462
  vilazodone, 464
diet, 248, 251, 256, 287, 291, 403, 461, 482–483
Dietary Approaches to Stop Hypertension (DASH), 247, 251
digoxin, 90, 115, 163, 172, 183, 229*t*, 382
dihexamer, 15, 32
dihydropyridine calcium antagonists (DCAs), 420–421, 423
dihydropyridine calcium channel blocker, 248, 249*t*, 250–251, 295, 323, 324*t*, 328, 331*t*
dihydropyridine- RAS inhibitor, 423
diltiazem, 229*t*, 331*t*, 333, 421, 427*t*, 430
diltiazem SR, 324*t*
dipeptidyl peptidase-4 (DPP-4) inhibitor, **176–189**
  adverse effects and monitoring, 182
  antidiabetic medication attributes, 77*t*
  cardiovascular outcomes trial, 263, 266*t*–268*t*
  combination products, 185*t*

  combination therapy, 50, 184
  cost, 56*t*, 179
  dosage and administration, 183, 184*t*, 426*t*
  drug interaction, 182–183
  gastroparesis, 304
  glucagon-like peptide 1 (GLP-1) receptor agonist, 190, 196–197
  heart failure, 269
  hypoglycemia, 178
  incretin-based therapy in T1D, 21
  mechanism of action, 176–177
  monograph, 185, 430
  nephropathy, 418–420, 426*t*, 428, 430
  pharmacokinetic, 177–178
  pharmacology, 176–179
  sodium–glucose cotransporter 2 (SGLT2) inhibitor and, 428
  special population, 181
  sulfonylurea, 127, 131
  therapeutic consideration, 179–185
  treatment advantages/ disadvantages, 178–179
  type 2 diabetes, 53*t*, 61, 67, 68*f*, 73
  warnings/precautions, 179–180
diphtheria, 504*f*, 505, 507
diplopia, 362
dipyridamole, 360–361
dipyridamole/aspirin, 360
DIRECT-Prevent 1 study, 446
DIRECT-Protect 1 study, 446–447
DIRECT-Protect 2 trial, 447
DIRECT-Renal study, 414, 416
direct vasodilator, 327*t*
disaccharide, 168
discontinuation syndrome, 464, 466
disopyramide, 39
distal sensorimotor polyneuropathy, 301
distal symmetric polyneuropathy, 300, 302
distal symmetric sensorimotor polyneuropathy (DSPN), 395–396, 399–401
diuretic, 39, 72, 161–163, 247–248, 249*t*, 287, 290, 329, 332–333, 361
diuretics—potassium sparing, 327*t*

dizziness, 237, 324*t*–327*t*, 384, 386, 399–400, 405, 464, 494
DNA technology, 11, 26
docosahexaenoic acid (DHA), 347
dofetilide, 90
dolutegravir, 90
domperidone, 304
dopamine, 233, 376, 377*f*, 380, 401, 464, 497
dopamine-2 receptor agonist, 57*t*, **233–240**
dopamine level, 234
dopaminergic drug, 488*t*, 498
drowsiness, 237, 462, 464
droxidopa, 304
drug eluting stent (DES), 364*t*
drug-laboratory test interaction, 488*t*
Drugs in Pregnancy and Lactation (Briggs), 227, 236
dry eye, 463
dry mouth, 381, 384, 386, 463–464
Du, L, 83
dual antiplatelet therapy (DAPT), 363, 364*t*
dual combination therapy, 48–49
dual RAS inhibitor, 422
dulaglutide, 57*t*, 68*f*, 74, 190, 192*t*, 193, 195–197, 201*t*, 202, 205
duloxetine, 300, 302–303, 398*t*, 400, 407, 462–463, 465*t*, 467
duloxetine/pregabalin, 402
DURATION study, 195*t*
Dutch DAMOCLES (Does Applying More Oxygen Cure Lower Extremity Sores?) trial, 307
dysesthesia, 301
dysgeusia, 88
dyslipidemia
    cardiovascular risk factor, 355
    coronary arteriosclerosis, 339
    diabetic kidney disease, 411
    diabetic retinopathy, 297, 299, 440
    dopamine-2 receptor agonist, 233–234
    fenofibrate, 448
    HDL cholesterol, 256
    pioglitazone, 104, 108
dyspepsia, 228, 237, 494
dysphagia, 225, 227
dyspnea, 326*t*, 360, 484

E
Early Treatment Diabetic Retinopathy Study (ETDRS), 298–299, 440, 447-448
eating disorder, 381
eating pattern, 131, 142
eating plan, 304. *See also* diet
echocardiography, 262
Edelman, S, 213, 214*t*
edema, 72, 107, 109, 112–113, 115–116, 327*t*, 399, 441
education, 41, 54, 204–205, 305–306, 474
efavirenz, 382
eicosapentanoic acid (EPA), 347
1800 Rule, 19
elderly patient. *See also* geriatric patient
    α-glucosidase inhibitor, 170–171
    blood pressure, 246
    diabetic retinopathy, 465*t*
    duloxetine, 400
    glinide, 142
    hypoglycemia, 142–143, 474
    naltrexone/bupropion XR, 498–499
    pramlintide, 217
    sodium–glucose cotransporter 2 (SGLT2) inhibitor, 156, 161
    statin therapy, 253
    sulfonylurea, 128, 130
    thiazolidinedione, 107, 112
electrocardiogram (ECG), 261–262
electroconvulsive therapy, 461
electrolyte abnormalities, 291*t*
electronic cigarettes (e-cigarettes), 370
electronic nicotine delivery systems (ENDS), 372
electrophysiological testing, 301
Elovate 15, 476*t*
embryo-fetal mortality, 199

emotional stress, 461
empagliflozin
   antihyperglycemic medication with
     metformin, 96*t*
   cardiovascular outcome trial, 51,
     263–265, 266*t*–268*t*, 269, 293–
     294, 417–418
   cost, 56*t*, 156
   dosage and administration, 164*t*,
     425*t*
   drug interaction, 163
   hypersensitivity, 162
   linagliptin and, 165
   metformin hydrochloride and, 165
   nephropathy, 425*t*, 430
   sodium–glucose cotransporter 2
     (SGLT2) inhibitor, 151, 153–154
   special population, 159–160
   type 2 diabetes, 67, 73–74
   urogenital infection, 157
empagliflozin/linagliptin, 428
EMPA-REG OUTCOME [BI 10773
   (Empagliflozin) Cardiovascular
   Outcome Event Trial in Type 2
   Diabetes Mellitus Patients], 154–155,
   263, 266*t*–268*t*, 269, 293–294, 417
enalapril, 325*t*, 330*t*, 332, 414–416,
   424*t*, 429, 446
encephalopathy, 487*t*
endometrial cancer, 83
endophthalmitis, 444
endothelial dysfunction, 104, 108, 404
endovascular arterial revascularization,
   364
end-stage liver disease, 110
end-stage renal disease (ESRD)
   alogliptin, 181
   antihyperglycemic medication with
     metformin, 94*t*–96*t*
   cardiovascular outcome trial,
     293–295
   chronic kidney disease, 287
   dapagliflozin, 164*t*
   diabetic kidney disease, 411–412
   empagliflozin, 160, 418
   exenatide, 192

exenatide XR, 193
   glucagon-like peptide 1 (GLP-1)
     receptor agonist, 199
   hepatitis B vaccination, 291
   irbesartan, 415
   naltrexone/bupropion XR, 498–499
   prasugrel, 358
   sitagliptin, 183
epilepsy, 487*t*
epinephrine, 39, 473
eplerenone, 325*t*, 331*t*, 427*t*, 428, 430
EQUIP trial, 495
erectile dysfunction, 301–302, 304,
   325*t*–326*t*, 396*t*, 404–406
ergot derivative, 237
ertugliflozin, 56*t*, 73, 151, 154, 157,
   160–161, 163, 164
erythromycin, 145, 304, 403–404, 407
escitalopram, 462, 465*t*, 467
esophageal difficulties, 397
esophageal dysmotility, 301
esophagogastroduodenoscopy, 302
estimated glomerular filtration rates
   (eGFR)
   acute kidney injury, 290
   α-glucosidase inhibitor, 72
   antihyperglycemic medications
     containing metformin, 92*t*,
     94*t*–97*t*
   antihypertensive medication,
     330*t*–331*t*
   canagliflozin, 158
   chronic kidney disease, 286–295
   dapagliflozin, 158–159, 418
   diabetic kidney disease, 411–412
   dipeptidyl peptidase-4 (DPP-4)
     inhibitor, 178, 183, 184*t*, 419–420,
     426*t*
   dual RAS inhibitor, 422
   empagliflozin, 159–160
   glucagon-like peptide 1 (GLP-
     1) receptor agonist, 200*t*–201*t*,
     419–420, 426*t*
   nephropathy, 411–412, 415, 422,
     426*t*
   phentermine, 484

saxagliptin, 178, 426t
sitagliptin, 178, 426t
sodium–glucose cotransporter 2
(SGLT2) inhibitor, 158–160, 164t,
425t
type 2 diabetes, 49, 68f, 69
estrogen, 39, 146, 172
ethanol, 86, 116, 129
ethinyl estradiol, 116, 488t
ethnicity, 84, 87, 112, 171, 217, 411,
460
ethosuximide, 485t
EUCLID trial, 414, 446
euglycemic diabetic ketoacidosis
(eDKA), 21
European Association for the Study of
Diabetes (EASD), 66–67
European Associations for the Study
of the Liver, Diabetes, and Obesity
(EASL, EASD, EASO), 111
European Medicines Agency, 302, 304
Evaluation of Lixisenatide in Acute
Coronary Syndrome (ELIXA) trial,
265, 266t–268t, 419
evolocumab, 255–256, 343, 344t, 349t,
351
Examination of Cardiovascular
Outcomes with Alogliptin versus
Standard of Care (EXAMINE), 179,
266t–268t, 269, 420
exenatide
adverse effects and monitoring,
202–205
availability, dosing, and
administration requirements, 200t
cardiovascular outcome trial, 195t,
196–197, 265, 266t–268t, 269
cost, 57t
glucagon-like peptide 1 (GLP-1)
receptor agonist, 190–192
glucose-lowering medication in
T2D, 68f
hepatic impairment, 199
injection, 177
insulin and, 4
renal impairment, 199
type 2 diabetes, 68f, 74

Exenatide Study of Cardiovascular
Event Lowering (EXSCEL) trial,
265, 266t–268t
exenatide XR, 190, 192t, 193, 195–197,
199, 201t, 202–203, 205
exendin-4, 74, 190–193, 203
exercise, 288, 303, 396t
exfoliative skin condition, 180
extrapancreatic mechanism, 70, 125
eye examination, 296–298
ezetimibe, 252, 254, 258, 341–343,
344t, 347, 349t, 351

F

fall risk, 384, 395, 463
farnesoid X receptors (FXR), 224
fasting plasma glucose (FPG)
α-glucosidase inhibitor, 71, 168
bile acid sequestrant, 223, 225
dipeptidyl peptidase-4 (DPP-4)
inhibitor, 184
glinide, 141
glucagon-like peptide 1 (GLP-1)
receptor agonist, 191–193, 203
injectable therapy for T2D, 35f
insulin, 32, 34, 42, 54, 60
sulfonylurea, 126
thiazolidinedione, 108
fat, 2, 304, 322, 475–476, 497
fatigue, 237, 324t, 326t–327t, 344t,
400, 467, 494
fat mass, 112
fat-soluble multivitamin, 486t
fatty acid oxidation, 345t
fecal impaction, 228
fecal incontinence, 301
fecal stool, abnormal, 361
felodipine, 324t, 331t
fenofibrate, 257, 299, 345t, 346, 349t,
351, 440, 448
fertility, 81, 90
fetal neuro-teratogenicity, 373
Fiasp, 13, 28t, 29
fiber, 304
fibrate, 39, 257, 346
fibrate/statin combination, 346

fibric acid derivative, 345*t*, 349*t*–350*t*, 351
fibrosis, 106, 110
fibrotic complication, 237
FIELD study, 448
finerenone, 428
fishy taste, 344*t*
"5 A's" model, 371, 372*t*, 374*f*
5-hydroxytryptamine (5-HT) agonist, 237
500 Rule, 18–19
fixed-dose combination (FDC) insulin, 43*t*
fixed-ratio combination (FRC) insulin pen, 42
flatulence, 171, 228, 345*t*
fluconazole, 145
fluocinolone, 445–446, 450*t*, 451
fluoxetine, 39, 462, 465*t*, 467
flushing, 324*t*, 345*t*, 405
fluvastatin, 343*t*–344*t*, 348*t*–349*t*, 350
fluvastatin XL, 256*t*
fluvastatin XR, 348*t*
fluvoxamine, 462, 467
focal laser photocoagulation, 441
focal neuropathy, 395, 396*t*
food insecurity, 128–129, 144
foot, 300, 395
foot care, 304–307
foot deformity, 305
foot infection, 307
foot ulceration, 301, 304–305, 307, 395
footwear, 305–306
forced expiratory volume in one second (FEV₁), 38
fortamet, 92*t*
fosinopril, 330*t*
Fournier's gangrene, 418
fracture, 107, 110–111, 113
frailty, 246
Framingham Risk Score, 262
free fatty acid, 104, 234
free radical, 396
French lilac, 80
fruit, 322
fundic motor activity, 403
fundus photograph, 298

furosemide, 89, 326*t*, 331*t*, 333
Further Cardiovascular Outcomes Research with PCSK9 Inhibition in Subjects with Elevated Risk (FOURIER) trial, 255, 343

G
GABA analog, 397–399
gabapentin, 300, 303, 397–399, 407
gabapentin/morphine, 402
gabapentin/nortriptyline, 402
galega officinalis, 80
gallbladder disease, 482, 494
gallstone, 345*t*
gamma-aminobutyric acid (GABA), 397
gamma-L-glutamyl, 31
gastric cancer, 84
gastric electrical stimulation, 304
gastric emptying
  erythromycin, 403–404
  gastrointestinal neuropathy, 302
  gastroparesis, 402–404
  glucagon-like peptide 1 (GLP-1) receptor agonist, 191, 196, 199, 204
  liraglutide, 494
  metoclopramide, 403
  pramlintide, 211–212, 216, 218
  type 1 diabetes, 20
gastric lipase inhibitor, 491
gastric motility, 216, 218
gastric outlet obstruction, 302
gastrointestinal
  bleeding, 259–260
  disease, 199
  disorder, 226
  motility, 304
  motor control, 402
  neuropathy, 397
  reaction, 87–88, 91
  side effect, 68, 71, 75, 170–171, 196, 202, 218, 225, 235, 237, 373
  surgery, 228
  symptom, 302
  system, 258, 347, 396

gastrointestinal (GI) tract, 73, 152–153, 190, 224, 228, 492
gastrointestinal neuropathy, 301–302
gastroparesis, 13, 29, 199, 216, 226, 301–302, 304, 397, 402–404, 494
gemfibrozil, 115, 145, 257, 345t, 346, 348t–349t, 351
gender, 87, 112, 217, 236, 460
genetic risk factor, 411, 461
genital infection, 157, 418
genital mycotic infection, 162
genitourinary disturbance, 301–302
genitourinary neuropathy, 397
genitourinary system, 396
geriatric patient. *See also* elderly patient
  α-glucosidase inhibitor, 170–171
  β-blocker, 331t
  biguanide, 87
  bile acid sequestrant, 227–228
  canagliflozin, 158
  cilostazol, 361
  clopidogrel, 359
  dapagliflozin, 159
  dopamine-2 receptor agonist, 236
  empagliflozin, 159
  ertugliflozin, 160
  glucagon-like peptide 1 (GLP-1) receptor agonist, 199
  hepatic glycogen, 477
  lovastatin XR, 348t
  prasugrel, 363
  thiazide, 330t
  vorapaxar, 362
gestational diabetes, 36, 82, 298
gestational hypertension, 247
GETGOAL trial, 195t
Gila monster, 74, 190
glaucoma, 297, 445, 484
glibenclamide, 125
glimepiride, 55t, 119t, 124, 126–129, 131, 132t–133t, 134, 417
glinide, **138–150**
  adverse effects and monitoring, 144–146
  combination pills, 146
  dosage and administration, 146, 147t

drug interaction, 145–146
  hyperglycemia, 145
  hypoglycemia, 141–142, 144–145
  mechanism of action, 138–139
  monograph, 146
  pharmacokinetic, 139–140
  pharmacology, 138–140
  special population, 142
  sulfonylurea and, 141
  therapeutic consideration, 142
  treatment advantages/disadvantages, 140–141
  type 2 diabetes, 71
  warnings/precautions, 142
glipizide, 55t, 97t, 124–126, 128–129, 131, 132t–133t, 134
glomerular filtration, 151–152
glomerular filtration rate (GFR), 36–37, 155–156, 192, 250, 290–291, 411–413, 416–417
glomerular hyperfiltration, 411–412
glomerular hypertension, 411–412
glomerular membrane permeability, 420
glomeruli, 411–412
glomerulosclerosis, 412
GLP-1 receptor agonists (GLP-1 RAs). *See* glucagon-like peptide 1 (GLP-1) receptor agonist
glucagon, 16, 20–21, 75, 125, 130, 170, 176, 402, 473, 477–479
glucagon injection, 477
glucagon-like peptide (GLP-1 7–37), 74
glucagon-like peptide 1 (GLP-1), 176–177, 224
glucagon-like peptide 1 (GLP-1) receptor agonist, **190–210**
  A1C, 75, 194–195, 202–203
  adverse effects and monitoring, 202–203
  antidiabetic medication attributes, 77t
  availability, dosing, and administration requirements, 200t–201t
  basal insulin products and, 205t
  cardiovascular disease, 262

cardiovascular outcome trial, 264–
265, 266*t*–268*t*, 269, 294
C-cell tumor, 75
chronic kidney disease, 286–287,
293
cost, 51, 57*t*, 197
diabetic nephropathy, 419
diabetic retinopathy, 448–449
dipeptidyl peptidase-4 (DPP-4)
inhibitor and, 73, 177, 196–197
dosage and administration, 204–
206, 426*t*
drug interaction, 204
efficacy and safety, 195*t*
gastrointestinal adverse effect, 75,
202
gastroparesis, 304
hypoglycemia, 75, 195, 198, 202–
204
iDegLira, 196
iGlarLixi, 196
incretin-based therapy, 21
insulin and, 42, 43*t*, 60, 196, 198,
202–204
liraglutide, 493
lixisenatide, 265
mechanism of action, 191
meglitinide, 202
metformin, 202
monograph, 206, 430
nephropathy, 418–420, 426*t*
pancreatitis, 75
pharmacokinetic, 191
pharmacology, 191–194
renal effect, 292–293
special population, 198–199
sulfonylurea, 127, 131, 202
therapeutic consideration, 197–206
thiazolidinedione, 110
treatment advantages/
disadvantages, 194–197
type 1 diabetes, 4, 198
type 2 diabetes, 34, 35*f*, 48, 50,
52*t*–53*t*, 67, 68*f*, 74–75
warnings/precautions, 197–198
weight loss, 38, 75
glucagonoma, 478
glucagon secretion, 198, 211–212

glucocorticoid, 145
Glucolift, 476*t*
gluconeogenesis, 473
glucophage XR, 92*t*
glucose. *See also* blood glucose
control, 300, 397
excretion, 73
glucagon-like peptide 1 (GLP-1)
receptor agonist, 191
homeostasis, 151, 177, 211–212
hypoglycemia, 472, 475–476
intolerance, 234
metabolism, 26, 70, 104
niacin, 345*t*
reabsorption, 151–152
toxicity, 126
transport, 26, 151–152
uptake, 76, 81
glucose-dependent insulinotropic
polypeptide (GIP) hormone, 73,
176–177, 190
glucose intolerance, 234
glucose-lowering medication, 68*f*, 289,
292
glucose transporter (GLUT1), 72, 104
glucose transporter (GLUT2), 72
glucose transporter (GLUT4), 104
glucosuria, 157
glucuronide metabolite, 154
glumetza, 92*t*
glutamate/ N-methyl-D-aspartate
(NMDA) receptor-mediated
neuronal excitation, 399
Glutose, 476*t*
GLUTs (glucose transporter protein),
152
glyburide, 55*t*, 88, 97*t*, 124–126, 128,
130–131, 132*t*–133*t*, 134, 141, 172
glycated hemoglobin A1c (A1C). *See*
A1C
Glycemia Reduction Approaches
in Diabetes: a Comparative
Effectiveness Study (GRADE), 127
glycemic control
chronic kidney disease, 292
depression, 461
diabetic gastroparesis, 403

diabetic kidney disease, 411–412, 417
diabetic retinopathy, 296–297
foot care, 305
gastrointestinal neuropathy, 302
glucagon-like peptide 1 (GLP-1) receptor agonist, 195
hypertension, 340
insulin, 30, 32
lipid management, 251
metformin, 21
neuropathy, 300, 302
pramlintide, 20
sulfonylurea, 125
glycemic management
adjunctive drug therapies in T1D, 20–21
antihyperglycemic drug therapy in T1D, 10–17
injection site reaction, 16
insulin dosing in T1D, 17–20
patient-centered approach, 69*f*
recommendation, 10*t*
treatment goals, 10
type 1 diabetes, 8–21
glycine, 14, 30
glycogenolysis, 473, 477
glycoprotein, 381
glycopyrrolate, 90
goat's rue, 80
gram-positive cocci, 307
Grave's disease, 227
growth alteration, 199
growth hormone, 473
guanethidine, 39, 89, 115, 487*t*
guanidine, 80
gustatory sweating, 396*t*
gynecomastia, 325*t*, 403

H

H$_1$-histaminergic receptor blockade, 401
hallucination, 237
Harmony Outcomes trial, 265
HDL cholesterol, 106, 251–252, 256–257, 339–340, 346
headache, 182, 237, 324*t*–325*t*, 327*t*, 360–361, 404–405, 464, 494
Health Canada, 302
healthcare provider, 371, 374*f*
heartbeat, 397
heart block, 463
heart failure (HF)
antihyperglycemic drug therapy, 269–270
antihyperglycemic medication with metformin, 97*t*–98*t*
antihypertensive medication, 328
cardiovascular disease, 241–242, 250
cilostazol, 361
dipeptidyl peptidase-4 (DPP-4) inhibitor, 73, 179–180
hypertension, 322, 324*t*
metformin, 82
phentermine, 484
pregabalin, 116
sodium–glucose cotransporter 2 (SGLT2) inhibitor, 154
thiazolidinedione, 107, 109, 111, 113, 118*t*–119*t*
type 2 diabetes, 48–51, 67, 68*f*
heart failure with preserved ejection fraction (HFpEF), 241–242
heart failure with reduced ejection fraction (HFrEF), 242, 263
Heart Protection Study, 254
Heart Protection Study 2—Treatment of HDL to Reduce the Incidence of Vascular Events (HPS2-THRIVE) trial, 257, 346
heart rate, 203, 373–374, 384, 494, 496
heat-not-burn (HNB) product, 370
hematocrit, 113
hematological effect, 88, 490
hematology, 108
hemodialysis (HD), 106, 424*t*, 426*t*, 465*t*, 484
hemoglobin, 113
hemolytic anemia, 129
hemorrhage, 227, 259–260
hemorrhagic stroke, 363
hemorrhoid, 226
hepatic

disease, 181
dysfunction, 112, 128, 143, 362
enzyme, 71, 361
failure, 109, 143, 180, 361, 465*t*
function, 86, 344*t*
gluconeogenesis, 234
glucose production, 54, 67, 76,
  80–81, 212
glycogen, 477
insufficiency, 86, 128, 142, 217
hepatic glucokinase expression, 104
hepatic impairment
  antihypertensive medication,
    330*t*–331*t*
  antiplatelet, 360
  atypical antidepressant, 465*t*
  bile acid sequestrant, 228
  bupropion SR, 380
  canagliflozin, 158
  cilostazol, 361
  clopidogrel, 359
  dapagliflozin, 159
  dopamine-2 receptor agonist, 236
  empagliflozin, 160
  ertugliflozin, 160
  glinide, 143
  glucagon-like peptide 1 (GLP-1)
    receptor agonist, 199
  insulin, 37
  liraglutide, 494
  lorcaserin, 490–491
  losartan, 424*t*
  naltrexone/bupropion SR, 498–499
  nephropathy, 427*t*
  nondihydropyridine calcium
    antagonist, 427*t*
  phentermine/topiramate ER, 496
  prasugrel, 358
  retinopathy, 465*t*
  rosiglitazone, 105
  selective serotonin-norepinephrine
    reuptake inhibitors, 400, 465*t*
  selective serotonin reuptake
    inhibitors, 465*t*
  sodium–glucose cotransporter
    2 (SGLT2) inhibitor, 158–160,
    164*t*–165*t*
  statin therapy, 349*t*–350*t*
  sulfonylurea, 131
  ticagrelor, 360
  type 1 diabetes, 199
  verapamil, 427*t*
hepatitis A (HepA), 504*f*
hepatitis B (HepB), 291, 504*f*, 505–506
hepatocellular carcinoma, 110
hepatotoxicity, 109, 115
herpes zoster, 507
heterozygous familial
  hypercholesterolemia, 227
hexadecanoic acid, 31
Hib (*Haemophilus influenzae* type b),
  504*f*
high blood pressure. *See* blood
  pressure; hypertension
high-density lipoprotein cholesterol
  (HDL-C), 81
high-density lipoproteins (HDL). *See*
  HDL cholesterol
high-intensity statin therapy, 341
Hinshaw, L, 213
Hispanic population, 411
histamine receptor, 463–464
histone deacetylase (HDAC) enzyme,
  399
HIV (human immunodeficiency
  viruses), 486*t*
HIV protease inhibitor, 146
HMG-CoA reductase inhibitor, 344*t*,
  348*t*, 350
homelessness, 128–129, 144
homeostasis, 355
hormonal contraceptive, 146
hospitalization, 268*t*
human papil loma virus (HPV), 504*f*
hybrid closed-loop pump system, 2, 17
hydralazine, 247, 327*t*
hydrochlorothiazide (HCTZ), 330*t*,
  332–333
hydrocortisone cream, 375
hydrophilic polymer, 224
hyperalgesia, 402
hyperammonemia, 487*t*
hyperbaric oxygen therapy (HBOT),
  307
hypercalcemia, 324*t*, 327*t*
hypercholesterolemia, 223, 255, 343

hyperglycemia, **8–25**
  adjunctive drug therapies in T1D, 20–21
  α-glucosidase inhibitor, 71
  antihyperglycemic drug therapy in T1D insulin therapy, 10–17
  antihypertensive medication, 326*t*
  chronic kidney disease, 37
  correction dose, 19
  depression, 461
  diabetic retinopathy, 297
  distal symmetric sensorimotor polyneuropathy, 395
  drug interaction, 134
  dual combination therapy, 49–50
  erythromycin, 404
  gestational diabetes, 36
  glinide, 141, 145
  glucagon-like peptide 1 (GLP-1) receptor agonist, 191
  glycemic goal for children and adolescent with T1D, 11*t*
  glycemic management in T1D, 9–21
  glycemic recommendation, 10*t*
  glycemic treatment goals in T1D, 10
  hypoglycemia, 16
  influenza, 506
  insulin, 18
  insulin dosing in T1D, 17–20
  kidney damage, 288
  monograph, 21–22
  nortriptyline, 386
  pathophysiology, 8
  pharmacokinetic, 11
  prednisone, 88
  quinolone, 89, 116
  regular human insulin, 28
  symptom, 8
  T2D insulin therapy, 48
  thiazolidinedione, 105, 114
  type 1 diabetes, 1, **8–25**
  type 2 diabetes, 34, 66, 105
hyperkalemia, 158, 161, 250–251, 290, 295, 325*t*, 329–330, 422–423, 427*t*, 428
hyperlipidemia, 223, 225, 482

hyperprolactinemia, 233
hyperprothrombinemia, 226
hypersensitivity
  α-glucosidase inhibitor, 170
  antihyperglycemic medication with metformin, 92*t*–98*t*
  bile acid sequestrant, 228
  bromocriptine, 236
  clopidogrel, 359
  dipeptidyl peptidase-4 (DPP-4) inhibitor, 180, 182
  glinide, 142
  glucagon, 478
  glucagon-like peptide 1 (GLP-1) receptor agonist, 198
  metformin hydrochloride, 85
  orlistat, 492
  pramlintide, 216
  sodium–glucose cotransporter 2 (SGLT2) inhibitor, 162
  sulfonylurea, 127
  thiazolidinedione, 118*t*–119*t*
  ticagrelor, 360
  varenicline, 379
hypertension, **322–338**. *See also* antihypertensive medication; blood pressure
  antihypertensive medication dosage, 330*t*–331*t*
  atomoxetine, 485*t*
  blood pressure control, 242–248, 250–251
  bupropion SR, 381
  calcium channel blocker/RAS inhibitor, 423
  cardiovascular risk factor, 355
  chronic kidney disease, 286–288, 294–295
  clonidine, 384
  combination products, 332
  combination therapy, 329–330, 428, 430
  diabetic kidney disease, 411–412
  glucagon, 478
  goals of treatment, 323
  lifestyle and pharmacologic interventions, 263
  MAOI, 488*t*

medication, overview of and
rationale for, 323, 324t–327t,
328–329
mineralocorticoid receptor
antagonist/RAS inhibitor
combination, 428
monograph, 332–333
nephropathy, 411–412, 421
obesity, 482
pregnancy, 243, 246–248
randomized controlled trial, 244,
245t
resistant hypertension, 250–251
retinopathy, 297
statin and combination treatment
recommendation, 342t
trandolapril, 447
treatment recommendation, 249f
type 1 diabetes, 413–414
Hypertension Optimal Treatment
(HOT) trial, 244, 245t
hyperthyroidism, 227–228, 484
hypertriglyceridemia, 1, 226, 256, 340,
347
hyperuricemia, 324t, 326t–327t
hypochloremia, 326t
hypoglycemia
ACE inhibitor, 114
α-glucosidase inhibitor, 170, 172
alert level, 472
alpha-lipoic acid, 115
androgen, 115
angiotensin converting enzymes
(ACE) inhibitor, 90
antiadrenergic medication, 39
aspirin therapy, 361
autonomic response, 473–474
basal insulin, 54
β-blocker, 90
carbohydrate, 472, 475–476
chronic kidney disease, 37
clinically significant, 472
clopidogrel, 115
diabetic retinopathy, 440
dipeptidyl peptidase-4 (DPP-4)
inhibitor, 178
drug interaction, 39
glinide, 71, 141–142, 144–145

glucagon, 477–479
glucagon-like peptide 1 (GLP-1)
receptor agonist, 75, 195, 198,
202–204
glucagon prescribing information,
478t
glucose, fast-acting, 476t
glucose-lowering medication T2D,
68
glycemic goal, 10
guanethidine, 115
hyperglycemia, 16
influenza, 506
insulin, 2, 11, 13–15, 30–32, 34, 35f,
36t, 37
insulin/insulin secretagogue, 162
intramuscular (IM) insulin delivery,
3
liraglutide, 487t, 494
medication for the management of,
472–481
metformin, 86
monograph, 479
neuroglycopenic symptom, 473
nocturnal, 2, 14–15, 30–32, 54, 474
nortriptyline, 386
pharmacologic therapy, 49–50
pramlintide, 215–218
prevention, 474–475
quinolone, 89, 116
"rule of 15", 16
sodium–glucose cotransporter 2
(SGLT2) inhibitor, 74, 155, 163
sulfonylurea, 70, 115, 126–131
symptoms, 15t, 16, 36t
T2D insulin therapy, 76
thiazolidinedione, 106, 108, 114
thiazolidinedione/insulin, 108
thiazolidinedione/sulfonylurea, 108
treatment options, 475–476
type 1 diabetes, 1, 9, 472, 474, 477
type 2 diabetes, 34
weight gain, 16
hypoglycemia-associated agent, 487t
hypoglycemia unawareness, 10, 16, 34,
37, 216, 301, 472, 474–475
hypogonadism, 304

hypokalemia, 34, 36, 116, 290, 324*t*, 326*t*, 487*t*
hypomagnesemia, 324*t*, 326*t*
hyponatremia, 129, 324*t*
hypoperfusion, 329
hypophosphatemia, 324*t*
hypoprolactinemia, 237
hypotension
    alprostadil, 406
    autonomic neuropathy, 397
    dipyridamole/aspirin, 361
    dopamine-2 receptor agonist, 235, 237
    hypertension, 327*t*, 328, 330
    orthostatic, 303–304, 384
    phosphodiesterase type 5 inhibitor, 406
    sodium–glucose cotransporter 2 (SGLT2) inhibitor, 156, 161
    tricyclic antidepressant, 463
hypothalamus, 233–234, 483, 488, 493, 495, 497
hypothermia, 487*t*
hypothyroidism, 227–228, 301
hypovolemia, 329
hypoxia, 85, 395

I
icosapent ethyl, 344*t*, 350
iDegLira, 196, 205*t*
IDNT trial, 415, 421
iGlarLixi, 196, 205*t*
illness, 1
imipramine, 407, 463
immune-mediated diabetes. *See* type 1 diabetes
immunization, **503–508**
immunogenicity, 196, 203
immunosuppressive therapy, 146
impaired glucose tolerance (IGT), 211, 395
impaired hepatic function, 86
impaired hepatic function (Child-Pugh grade B/C), 112
impaired myocardial contractility, 386
impaired nitric oxide (NO) synthesis, 402

impotence, 403. *See also* erectile dysfunction
IMProved Reduction of Outcomes: Vytorin Efficacy International Trial (IMPROVE-IT), 254, 342
incontinence, 396*t*
incretin-based therapy, 21
incretin hormone, 73, 176, 190
indapamide, 249*t*
indigestion, 344*t*–345*t*
infection, 17, 258, 301, 307, 347, 361
inflammatory bowel disease, 72, 170
inflammatory cytokines, 108
inflammatory marker, 448
inflammatory pathway, 441, 444
influenza, 344*t*, 504*f*, 505–506
injectable combination therapy, 67
injectable glucose-lowering drug, 3
injectable therapy, 50–51, 74–76
injection. *See also* multiple daily injection (MDI)
    pen device, 204–205, 216, 220
    site, 11, 27, 220
    site reaction, 16, 32, 38, 202–203, 218
    site rejection, 16
    syringe, 3, 32
    technique, 3
insomnia, 373, 377, 381, 464, 484
Insta-Glucose, 476*t*
insulin, **26–47**. *See also* continuous subcutaneous insulin infusion (CSII); injection
    absorption, 3, 27
    action, 26, 72, 125
    adjustment in T1D, 19–20
    administration, 38–39, 41–42
    adverse effect, 15–17, 37–38
    α-glucosidase inhibitor and, 172
    allergic reaction, 36
    analog, 11, 26–27
    antihyperglycemic drug therapy in T1D, 10–17
    aspart, 12–13, 21, 28*t*, 29, 40*t*, 43, 59*t*–60*t*
    attributes, 77*t*
    basal, 1, 9, 13–14, 18, 30, 33–34, 35*f*, 50, 54, 58, 59*t*, 60, 68*f*, 202

basal/bolus, 196
basal/prandial regimen, 60
BIDS: bedtime insulin daytime sulfonylurea, 132
bromocriptine and, 234
chronic kidney disease, 37, 292
colesevelam, 225
combination therapy, 42, 43*t*, 50
concentrated, 58, 59*t*
correction dose, 19
cost, 12–13, 29–30, 54, 58, 59*t*–60*t*, 61
degludec, 2, 12*t*, 15, 22, 28*t*, 31–32, 41*t*, 42, 43*t*, 44, 58, 59*t*–60*t*, 68*f*, 196
degludec/liraglutide, 60
delivery mode, 16–17
detemir, 12*t*, 13–14, 22, 28*t*, 30–31, 40*t*, 42, 44, 54, 59*t*, 474
diabetic ketoacidosis, 127
dosage, 1, 17–20, 31, 33–34, 38–39, 40*t*–41*t*, 42, 58
drug interaction, 38–39
dual combination therapy, 49–50
duration of action, 12–15, 28–32
fixed-dose combination, 43*t*
fixed dose/glucagon-like peptide 1 (GLP-1) receptor agonist, 43*t*
glargine, 2, 12*t*, 13–15, 22, 28*t*, 30–31, 41*t*, 42, 43*t*, 44, 54, 58, 59*t*–60*t*, 68*f*, 127, 196, 474
glargine/lixisenatide, 60
glinide, 71
glucagon-like peptide 1 (GLP-1) receptor agonist, 196, 198
glulisine, 12, 22, 28*t*, 29, 40*t*, 44, 59*t*
hepatic impairment, 37
human, 11–12, 27*f*, 28–29
hyperglycemia, 50, 67
hypersensitivity, 36
hypoglycemia, 34, 36*t*, 37, 108, 473–474
hypokalemia, 34, 36
Iletin, 26
inhalation, 2, 17, 22, 41–42
inhaled human, 12*t*, 13, 22, 28*t*, 29, 38–39, 40*t*, 44, 58, 59*t*, 60
initiation, 18, 33

intermediate-acting, 2, 13, 29–30, 59*t*
isophane, 13, 40*t*
linagliptin and, 183
liraglutide, 43*t*, 60*t*, 487*t*
lispro, 12–13, 22, 28*t*, 29, 40*t*, 43*t*, 44, 58, 59*t*–60*t*
lixisenatide, 43*t*, 60*t*
long-acting, 2, 13–15, 17, 30–32
mechanism of action, 26–30
microprecipitate, 30
mixing, 42
monitoring, 37–38
monograph, 43–44
nicotine replacement therapy, 374
NPH, 12*t*, 13, 22, 28*t*, 29–30, 40*t*, 42, 43*t*, 44, 54, 58, 59*t*–60*t*, 142, 474
NPH/regular, 61
overdose, 32
patch technology, 17
pen, 17, 32, 39, 41, 58
pharmacokinetic properties, 11, 27, 28*t*
pharmacology, 26–32
pramlintide, 213, 215–216, 218–219
prandial, 1–2, 9, 11, 17–18, 28, 33–34, 35*f*, 58, 60, 177
pregnancy, 36
premixed, 42, 58, 60*t*
preprandial, 10, 146
products, 12*t*, 21–22, 40*t*–41*t*, 43–44
pulmonary adverse event, 38
rapid-acting, 2, 9, 12–13, 17–19, 29, 33, 41–42, 58, 59*t*
regular, 22, 28*t*, 32, 40*t*, 42, 43*t*, 54, 58, 60*t*
regular human insulin, 11–12, 28–29, 42, 44, 59*t*
renal impairment, 36–37
resistance, 106–108, 110–111
secretagogue, 37
secretion, 73–74, 124, 176, 190–192, 202
sensitivity, 81, 90, 104, 106

short-acting, 2, 11–12, 17–18, 28–29, 59*t*. *see also* regular human insulin
special population, 36–37
storage, 40*t*–41*t*
sulfonylurea and, 131
syringe, 17
temperature variation, 11
therapeutic consideration, 34, 35*f*, 36–39, 40*t*, 41–42
titration, 14–15, 18, 31–33, 35*f*, 54, 58
treatment advantages/ disadvantages, 32–34
type 1 diabetes, 1–3, 8–9, 33
type 2 diabetes, 33–34, 75–76
ultra-long-acting, 17, 31
vial, 17, 39, 58
warnings/precautions, 34, 36
weight gain, 16, 38
insulinoma, 478
insulin pump therapy, 1–2, 17, 41, 213, 215
insulin receptor activation, 26
insulin resistance, 11, 32, 233, 340, 461
Insulin Resistance Intervention After Stroke (IRIS) trial, 107, 111
insulin-stimulated glucose transport, 80–81
insulin-to-carbohydrate ratio (I:C ratio), 18–19
intensive blood pressure control, 323
intensive diabetes management, 2, 297
intensive glycemic control, 292, 298
inter-digestive migration control, 403
International Hypoglycemia Study Group, 472
international normalized ratio (INR), 204, 401, 479
International Working Group on the Diabetic Foot, 307
intestinal disease, 170
intestinal obstruction, 170
intestine, 168–169
intracavernosal injection, 406
intracellular cholesterol biosynthesis, 339
intracorporeal prostaglandin, 304

intracranial hemorrhage, 360, 362
intraglomerular pressure, 412–413, 417, 423
intramuscular (IM) insulin delivery, 3
intranasal glucagon, 477–478
intraocular bleeding, 443
intraocular inflammation, 444
intraocular pressure, 445–446, 450
intraocular treatment, 441
intrarenal hemodynamic, 290
intraurethrally applied tablet, 406
intraurethral prostaglandin, 304
intravascular depletion, 330*t*
intravascular volume, 290
intravascular volume contraction, 156
intravascular volume–related adverse event, 158–160
intravitreal agent, 198
intravitreal corticosteroid, 441
intravitreal corticosteroid implant, 445, 450
intravitreal injection, 299
intravitreal steroid injection, 445
intravitreous injection, 296–297
intravitreous steroid, 442*t*
iodinated contrast imaging, 292–293
iodinated contrast media, 85
irbesartan, 330*t*, 414–415, 421, 424*t*, 429
IRMA-2 trial, 414
iron deficiency anemia, 172
isavuconazonium, 90
ischemic stroke, 111, 125, 257, 346, 357, 360, 363
isoniazid, 39, 146
isosorbide dinitrate spray, 398*t*, 402, 407
itraconazole, 115, 145

J

Jian-Yu, E, 83
juvenile diabetes. *See* type 1 diabetes

K

ketoacidosis, 1, 4, 157, 161. *See also* diabetic ketoacidosis

ketoconazole, 115, 145, 178, 182, 358, 360
ketosis, 157
kidney. *See also* chronic kidney disease; diabetic kidney disease; diabetic nephropathy
  damage, 290
  disease, 250, 288, 328, 484
  edema, 113
  epinephrine, 473
  failure, 341
  function, 420
  glucagon-like peptide 1 (GLP-1) receptor agonist, 75
  impairment, 161
  injury, 156, 161, 198, 250, 290
  insulin, 36
  sodium–glucose cotransporter 2 (SGLT2) inhibitor, 73–75, 151–153, 155
  stone, 487*t*
  sulfonylurea, 125–126
  thiazolidinedione, 106
  transplantation, 287
  weight gain, 109
Kidney Disease: Improving Global Outcomes (KDIGO), 289

L

labetalol, 247, 326*t*, 331*t*
lactation, 158–160, 199, 216, 227, 236, 403
lactic acidosis, 49, 69, 80, 85–87, 90, 92*t*, 119*t*
lamotrigine, 90
Lantus, 14, 30
laropiprant, 257–258, 346
laser photocoagulation surgery, 297, 299, 441–442, 450
laser therapy, 440, 444–445, 448–450
Latino population, 171
L cell, 190
LDL cholesterol, 21, 68, 72, 106, 162, 223–225, 252–258, 263, 339–343, 346–347
LEADER (Liraglutide Effect and Action in Diabetes: Evaluation of Cardiovascular Outcome Results), 195, 266*t*–268*t*, 293–294, 418
Lee, M, 107
lethargy, 327*t*
leukocyte vascular occlusion, 448
leukotriene receptor antagonist, 116
levomilnacipran, 462–463, 467
levothyroxine, 229*t*, 486*t*, 492
Li, X, 83
lidocaine, 398*t*, 401–402, 407
lifestyle intervention, 38, 49, 67, 82, 155, 251–252, 322–323, 340, 482
linagliptin, 56*t*, 73, 93*t*, 177–183, 184, 185, 419–420, 426*t*, 430
linezolid, 485*t*
lipases, 494
lipid, **339–354**
  antipsychotic medication, 467
  bile acid sequestrant, 226, 228
  combination products, 347
  combination therapy, 341–343
  diabetic retinopathy, 440
  goals of treatment, 340
  level, 3–4, 226, 251, 340, 482
  management, 251–258, 296
  medication, doses and dose adjustment, 348*t*–350*t*
  medication, overview of and rationale for, 340–341, 344*t*–345*t*
  metabolism, 80
  monograph, 350–351
  panel, 344*t*
  profile, 72, 104, 106, 108, 252
  statin and combination treatment recommendation, 342*t*
  statin/omega-3 fatty acid, 347
  weight loss, 482
lipid-lowering therapy, 242, 253, 258, 341, 342*t*
lipoatrophy, 3, 16, 38
lipohypertrophy, 3, 16, 38
lipoprotein, 339
liraglutide
  cardiovascular outcome trial, 51, 264–265, 266*t*–268*t*, 269, 293–294
  cost, 57*t*

glucagon-like peptide 1 (GLP-1) receptor agonist, 190, 192*t*, 193, 195–197, 200*t*, 202, 205
  hypoglycemia, 487*t*, 494
  monograph, 499
  nephropathy, 418, 426*t*, 430
  noninsulin treatment for T1D, 4
  sulfonylurea, 127
  type 2 diabetes, 68*f*, 74–75
  weight loss, 489*t*
Liraglutide Effect and Action in Diabetes: Evaluation of Cardiovascular Outcome Results (LEADER) trial, 264
lisinopril, 325*t*, 330*t*, 332, 414, 421–422, 424*t*, 428–429, 446
lithium, 485*t*
lithium salt, 39
liver
  cirrhosis, 170
  disease, 37, 112, 348*t*–350*t*
  failure, 180, 506
  function, 109, 113, 143, 172, 180, 229, 344*t*, 492
  function test, 345*t*
  Hepatitis B, 506
  hypoglycemia, 473
  orlistat, 492
  pramlintide, 212
  sulfonylurea, 125–126, 131
  thiazolidinedione, 106
lixisenatide, 74, 190, 192, 195–197, 200*t*, 202–204, 266*t*–268*t*, 419, 426*t*, 430
lixisenatide/glargine, 68*f*
lockjaw, 507
lomaira, 484
loop diuretic, 156, 326*t*, 331*t*
lopinavir, 382
lorcaserin, 486*t*, 488, 489*t*, 490–491, 499
lorcaserin XR, 486*t*, 489*t*
losartan, 325*t*, 330*t*, 332–333, 414–415, 421–423, 424*t*, 428–429, 446
loss of balance, 395
loss of protective sensation (LOPS), 301, 305–306

lovastatin, 256*t*, 343*t*–344*t*, 347, 348*t*, 350, 360
lovastatin XR, 348*t*
low-density lipoprotein cholesterol (LDL-C), 81
low-density lipoproteins (LDL). *See* LDL cholesterol
lower-extremity complication, 305
lower limb amputation, 264. *See also* amputation
lumen membrane, 152
lung cancer, 84
luteinizing hormone, 82
lysine, 14, 30–31

M

macroalbuminuria, 293, 412, 418–420
macrolide antibiotic, 403–404
macrovascular complication, 8, 461, 474
macula, 439, 441
macular edema, 114, 296–299. *See also* diabetic macular edema
macular laser, 442*t*
macular laser photocoagulation, 449
magnesium, 356
major cardiovascular event (MACE), 51
major depressive disorder (MDD), 378, 460–462, 464
malignancies, 301
"Management of Hyperglycemia in Type 2 Diabetes, 2018" (American Diabetes Association/European Association for the Study of Diabetes), 49
Mannucci, E, 107
Mantel-Haenszel odds ratio, 129
MAOI, 382, 386, 484, 485*t*, 487*t*–488*t*, 496
Markov-style analysis, 444
MARVAL trial, 415, 421
masked hypertension, 243, 322
maternal hypoglycemia, 128
maternal weight loss, 199
maturity-onset diabetes of the young (MODY), 124, 138

MEAD trial, 445
measles, mumps, rubella (MMR), 504*f*
medical nutrition therapy (MNT), 251, 482
Mediterranean diet, 251
medullary thyroid cancer, 75
medullary thyroid carcinoma (MTC), 197, 265, 494
mefenamic acid, 163
meglitinide, 56*t*, 86, 130–131, 202, 474. *See also* glinide
melanocortin-4 receptor, 488
meningitis, 506
meningococcal ACWY (MenACWY), 504*f*
meningococcal B (MenB), 504*f*
menses, 81–82, 325*t*
menstruation, 288
mental illness, 379, 382
mesolimbic dopamine circuit, 497
metabolic acidosis, 85, 291*t*, 487*t*, 496
metabolic bone disease, 291*t*
metabolic rate, 482
metabolic syndrome, 106, 461
metabolite, 125, 131, 139–140, 153, 169
metformin
  acarbose and, 170, 172
  ACE inhibitor, 90
  adverse effects and monitoring, 87–88
  agents that decrease the effect of, 90
  agents that enhance effects of, 89
  alcohol, 86, 88
  alogliptan and, 93*t*
  antihyperglycemic agent, 88
  antihyperglycemic medication containing, 92*t*–98*t*
  antihyperglycemic treatment in T2D, 52*t*
  β-blocker, 90
  bromocriptine and, 234
  canagliflozin and, 94*t*–95*t*
  cancer, 83–84
  cardiovascular outcome trial, 266*t*, 269
  cardiovascular risk, 82

cationic drug, 89–90
chronic kidney disease, 292–293
clomiphene, 90
colesevelam, 225
combination products, 91
congestive heart failure, 262
cost, 55*t*
dapagliflozin, 95*t*
dermatological reaction, 88
dipeptidyl peptidase-4 (DPP-4) inhibitor, 184, 185*t*
dosage and administration, 91
drug interaction, 88–90
dysgeusia, 88
empagliflozin, 96*t*
ethnicity, 87
extended release, 88
furosemide interaction, 89
gastrointestinal reaction, 87–88
gender, 87
geriatric patient, 87
glipizide, 97*t*
glucagon-like peptide 1 (GLP-1) receptor agonist, 194, 202
glyburide, 97*t*
hematological reaction, 88
hepatic insufficiency, 86
historical use, 80
hyperglycemia in T1D, 21
hypoglycemia, 86
hypoxic state, 85
impaired hepatic function, 86
lactic acidosis, 87, 90
linagliptin and, 93*t*
miglitol and, 172
monograph, 99
monotherapy failure, 126
nonalcoholic fatty liver disease, 110
noninsulin treatment for T1D, 3–4
pediatric patient, 87
pioglitazone and, 97*t*–98*t*, 119*t*
polycystic ovary syndrome, 81–82
pregnancy, 82
quinolone, 89
radiological studies, 85
renal function, 85
renal tubular transport system, 89
repaglinide and, 94*t*

rosiglitazone and, 106–107, 112
saxagliptin and, 93t
sitagliptin and, 93t–94t
special population, 86–87
sulfonylurea and, 134
surgical procedure, 86
T2D prevention, 82
thiazolidinedione, 97t
trospium, 89
type 2 diabetes, 48–51, 61, 67–69,
  77t
vitamin B12 deficiency, 86
warnings/precautions, 85–86
methenamine, 485t
methotrexate, 361
methyldopa, 247
methylphenidate, 467
metoclopramide, 304, 403, 407
metoprolol, 326t
metronidazole, 229t
Mezuk, B, 460
microalbuminuria, 412, 414, 416,
  419–421
MICRO-HOPE sub-study of the
  HOPE trial, 414
microsphere, 13, 29
microvascular complication, **286–321**
  chronic kidney disease, 48–51, 67,
    68f, 75, 246, 286–295
  depression, 461
  diabetic retinopathy, 198, 246,
    296–299
  foot care, 304–307
  glycemic control in T1D, 8
  histone deacetylase (HDAC)
    enzyme, 400
  hypertension, 322–323
  hypertension/blood pressure
    control, 242, 244
  hypoglycemia unawareness, 474
  neuropathy, 49, 300–304, 395
midodrine, 304
miglitol, 56t, 71, 168–174
M-III (keto derivatives), 105
Mills, EP, 110
milnacipran, 462

mineralocorticoid receptor antagonist
  (MRAs), 249t, 250–251, 295, 328–
  329, 421, 423, 427t, 428, 430
mineralocorticoid receptor antagonist/
  RAS inhibitor combination, 423, 428
mirtazapine, 464, 465t, 466–468
M-IV (hydroxy derivatives), 105
modafinil, 467
monoamine oxidase inhibitor (MAOI),
  39, 89, 130, 145, 381, 462
monofilament testing, 300–301, 304,
  306
mood disorder, 496
μ-opioid receptor agonism, 303
morphine, 90
mortality. *See also* all-cause mortality;
  cardiovascular mortality
    depression, 461
    diabetic autonomic neuropathy, 397
    empagliflozin, 155
    hepatitis B, 506
    hypoglycemia, 472, 474
    nephropathy, 413, 417–420, 422
    nonalcoholic fatty liver disease, 110
    peripheral diabetic retinopathy, 444
motilin agonist, 403–404
motor nerve function, 396t
multihexameric chain, 15, 32
multiple daily injection (MDI), 1–2, 9,
  16–17, 33
multiple endocrine neoplasia type 2
  (MEN 2), 75, 197, 494
Multiple Risk Factor Intervention
  Trial (MRFIT), 370
multivitamin, 485t
mumps, 504f
muscarinic receptor, 463–464
muscarinic receptor blockade, 401
muscle, 396t, 473
musculoskeletal deformity, 306
musculoskeletal system, 258, 347
myalgia, 341, 344t
mycophenolate, 229t
myocardial infarction (MI). *See
also* non-ST-elevated myocardial
  infarction
    antihypertensive medication, 328

antiplatelet therapy, 355, 362–363, 365*t*
anti-VEGF agent, 444
aspirin, 259, 357
atherosclerotic cardiovascular disease, 339
autonomic neuropathy, 397
β-blocker, 250, 261, 263
cardiovascular outcome trial, 267*t*
clopidogrel, 358–359
clopidogrel/aspirin, 363
empagliflozin, 154
evolocumab, 256
hypertension, 242
lactic acidosis, 85
liraglutide, 195, 264
lixisenatide, 265
niacin/laropiprant, 258
nortriptyline, 386
pioglitazone, 107, 111
prasugrel, 363
repaglinide, 142
rosiglitazone, 106
semaglutide, 196
simvastatin, 257
statin therapy, 346
ticagrelor, 359
vorapaxar, 362
myopia, 496
myositis, 257, 346
myristic acid, 14, 30

N
n-3 fatty acid, 251, 340
nadolol, 326*t*
naltrexone-bupropion SR, 488*t*, 490*t*, 497–499
nasopharyngitis, 182, 344*t*
nateglinide, 56*t*, 71, 138–146, 147*t*
Nateglinide And Valsartan in Impaired Glucose Tolerance Outcomes Research (NAVIGATOR) study, 144
National Average Drug Acquisition Costs (NADAC), 51, 54, 58
National Institute of Diabetes and Digestive and Kidney Diseases (NIDDK), 127

Native American population, 411
nausea
bile acid sequestrant, 228, 345*t*
bromocriptine, 237
bupropion, 464
calcium channel blocker, 324*t*
diabetic gastroparesis, 403
duloxetine, 400
erythromycin, 404
fibric acid derivative, 345*t*
glucagon-like peptide 1 (GLP-1) receptor agonist, 202
HMG-CoA reductase inhibitor, 344*t*
liraglutide, 494
niacin, 345*t*
nicotine replacement therapy, 373, 375
paroxetine, 462
pramlintide, 20, 218
selective serotonin-norepinephrine reuptake inhibitor, 463
varenicline, 378
nebivolol, 326*t*, 331*t*
needle, 3, 32. *See also* injection
nephrologist referral, 288
nephropathy
cardiovascular outcome trial, 268*t*, 293
combination products, 429
combination therapy, 422–423, 428
cost, 411
diabetic retinopathy, 297, 447
goals of treatment, 411–412
medication, 412–421
medication and dosing, 424*t*–427*t*
medication for the management of, **411–438**
monograph, 429–430
nephrotic syndrome, 288, 413
nephrotoxin, 290
neural presynaptic voltage-gated calcium channel, 397
neurocognitive swelling, pain or bruising, 344*t*
neuroendocrine effect, 403
neurogenic bladder, 301
neuroglycopenic symptom, 473

neuroleptic-like malignant syndrome, 237
neuroleptic malignant syndrome (NMS), 486*t*, 490–491
neurological assessment, 304
neuronal cell death, 396
neuronal damage, 395
neuronal sodium, 396
neuropathic pain, 400–401
neuropathy
  anticonvulsant, 397–400
  antidepressant, 400–401
  diabetic-induced, 396*t*
  diagnosis, 301–302
  erectile dysfunction, 404–406
  foot care, 305
  gastroparesis, 402–404
  management, medication for the, **395–410**
  metformin, 49
  monograph, 406–407
  polyneuropathy symptoms, 397*t*
  recommendation, 300
  topical medication, 401–402
  treatment, 302–304
  tricyclic antidepressant, 463
  type 1 diabetes, 395
  type 2 diabetes, 395
neuropsychiatric adverse event, 378–379, 381–382
neurotoxic medication, 301
neutral protamine Hagedorn (NPH) insulin. *See* insulin, NPH
new-onset diabetes, 258, 346
New York Heart Association (NYHA), 72, 107, 109, 113
niacin, 39, 257–258, 345*t*, 346–347, 350*t*, 351
niacinamide, 13, 29
niacin/laropiprant, 258
niacin/lovastatin, 347
nicotine, 370–376
nicotine receptor, 373
nicotine receptor antagonist, 380, 385
nicotine receptor partial agonist, 376
nicotine replacement therapy (NRT)
  adverse events/warnings and precautions, 373

  drug interaction, 373–374
  gum, 375, 388*t*, 389
  inhaler, 375–376, 388*t*, 390
  long-acting, 374–375
  lozenge, 375, 388*t*, 390
  mechanism of action, 373
  nasal spray, 376, 388*t*, 390
  over the counter (OTC), 373
  short-acting, 375–376
  smoking cessation, 372–376
  transdermal patch, 373–375, 388*t*, 390
  transdermal patch/bupropion SR, 387
  transdermal patch/nicotine gum/nasal spray, 389
  transdermal patch/nicotine inhaler, 387
  transdermal patch/nortriptyline, 389
  transdermal patch/second-generation antidepressant, 389
nicotine withdrawal, 383, 387
nifedipine, 89, 172, 247
nisoldipine, 416
nitrate therapy, 405
nitric oxide, 356, 395, 404–405
N-methyl-D-aspartate (NMDA) blockade, 401
nocturnal hypoglycemia, 2, 14–15, 30–32, 54, 474
nonalcoholic fatty liver disease (NAFLD), 86, 106–107, 110–111
nonalcoholic steatohepatitis (NASH), 53*t*, 106, 110–111
nondihydropyridine calcium antagonist (NDCAs), 420–421, 427*t*, 430
nondihydropyridine calcium antagonists/ACE inhibitor, 423
nondihydropyridine calcium channel blocker, 324*t*, 331*t*
non-HDL cholesterol, 346
noninsulin glucose-lowering agent, 3–4, 22, 50, 55*t*–57*t*
non-potassium sparing diuretic, 487*t*, 497

nonproliferative diabetic retinopathy (NPDR), 439–441, 442*t*, 444, 446
nonselective β-blockers, 326*t*
nonstatin LDL-lowering therapy, 341–342
non-ST-elevated myocardial infarction (NSTEMI), 358–359
nonsteroidal anti-inflammatory drugs (NSAIDs), 130, 145, 229*t*, 357–359, 361
nonteratogenic skeletal deformities, 143
noradrenaline reuptake inhibition, 303
noradrenergic receptor system, 385
norepinephrine (NE), 303, 385, 400, 406, 463, 483, 495–497
norepinephrine reuptake inhibitor, 464
norethindrone, 116, 488*t*
normoalbuminuria, 413–414, 420, 446–447
normotension, 413–414, 446–447
nortriptyline, 372, 384–387, 388*t*, 390, 407, 463, 465*t*, 467
Novolog, 13, 28*t*, 29
nuclear imaging, 262
nursing. *See* breast-feeding
nutrition intervention, 127, 251, 291

O

obesity
 cardiovascular risk factor, 355
 combination products, 495–499
 cost, 482
 depression, 460–461
 drug interaction, 485*t*–488*t*
 hypertension, 340
 insulin, 27
 medication for the management of, **482–502**
 monograph, 499
 nephropathy, 411
 nonalcoholic fatty liver disease, 110
 pharmacological management, 483–484, 488, 490–495
 pramlintide, 212
obstructive bowel disorder, 72

occlusive artery disease, 404
octanoic acid breath test, 302
ocular effect, 114
ocular hemorrhage, 444
ocular hypertension, 445, 451
ocular motor disturbance, 362
olanzapine, 467
oligosaccharide, 168
olmesartan, 325*t*, 330*t*, 333, 416, 424*t*, 429
ombitasvir, 90
omega-3 acid ethyl ester, 344*t*, 350
omega-3 carboxylic acid, 344*t*
omega-3 fatty acid, 344*t*, 350
omeprazole, 359
ondansetron, 90
ONTARGET study, 422
ophthalmological exam, 114, 296
ophthalmologist, 296–297
opioid analgesic, 303–304, 374, 485*t*, 498
opioid receptor antagonist, 497
Optimum, 476*t*
optometrist, 296–297
oral antihyperglycemic agent, 38, 80, 156
oral cleft, 496
oral contraceptive, 116, 229*t*, 488*t*, 496
oral glucose-lowering drug, 3–4
oral therapy, 67–74
orlistat, 486*t*, 489*t*, 491–492, 499
orthopedic surgeon, 307
orthostatic blood pressure, 322
orthostatic hypotension, 235, 237, 246, 301, 303–304, 327*t*, 328–329, 384, 396*t*, 463
osteoarthritis, 482
overall survival (OS), 84
overdose, 32, 373, 386, 463, 498
over the counter (OTC), 373
ovulation, 90, 108
oxidative stress, 396
ozempic, 206

P

P2Y12 platelet inhibitor, 359
P2Y12 receptor antagonist, 261

Pacific Islander population, 411
palpitation, 324*t*, 327*t*
Pan, D, 110–111
pancreas, 18, 69, 190, 473, 477
pancreatic α-cell, 20, 176, 212
pancreatic β-cell
  dipeptidyl peptidase-4 (DPP-4)
    inhibitor, 176
  glinide, 138–139
  glucagon-like peptide 1 (GLP-1)
    receptor agonist, 191, 202
  pramlintide, 211
  sulfonylurea, 124
  thiazolidinedione, 106, 108
  type 1 diabetes, 8–9, 20, 26
  valproic acid, 400
pancreatic cancer, 83, 197, 265
pancreatic lipase inhibitor, 491
pancreatitis, 75, 179–180, 182, 196–
  197, 226, 228, 256, 265, 340, 494
panic disorder, 463
panretinal laser photocoagulation
  (PRP), 296, 441, 442*t*, 443–444
panretinal photocoagulation surgery,
  298–299
parathyroid hormone (PTH), 291*t*
paricalcitol, 486*t*
Paris Prospective Study, 370
paritaprevir, 90
Parkinson's disease, 233, 235
paroxetine, 462, 465*t*, 467
pars plana vitrectomy, 449
patch technology, 41
"Pathway for Tobacco Cessation
  Treatment" (American College of
  Cardiology), 371
patiromer, 90
pedal pulse, 305–306
pediatric patient. *See also* children
  α-glucosidase inhibitor, 170
  biguanide, 87
  bile acid sequestrant, 227
  canagliflozin, 158
  dapagliflozin, 159
  dopamine-2 receptor agonist, 236
  empagliflozin, 159
  ertugliflozin, 160
  glinide, 143

glucagon-like peptide 1 (GLP-1)
  receptor agonist, 199
glucagon prescribing information,
  478*t*
  pramlintide, 216–217
  sulfonylurea, 128
  thiazolidinedione, 112
pegaptanib, 441–442, 450*t*, 451
pegvisomant, 89, 487*t*
penicillin, 229*t*
penile prostheses, 304
peptic ulcer disease, 302, 345*t*
percutaneous coronary intervention
  (PCI), 358, 362–363
percutaneous transluminal coronary
  angioplasty, 357*t*
perinatal outcomes, 247
peripheral alpha 1 adrenergic receptor,
  464
peripheral arterial disease (PAD), 241,
  261, 305–307, 339, 355, 358–359,
  362, 364, 365*t*
peripheral dopamine D_2 antagonist,
  403
peripheral edema, 324*t*
peripheral glucose uptake, 76
peripheral nervous system, 373, 473
peripheral polyneuropathy, 396*t*
peroxisome proliferator activated
  receptor alpha (PPAR-α), 345*t*, 448
peroxisome proliferator-activated
  receptor gamma (PPARγ), 72, 104,
  106, 109, 112-113
pertussis, 504*f*, 505, 507
pharmacologic stress
  echocardiography, 262
pharmacologic therapy
  antihyperglycemic drug therapy,
    52*t*–53*t*
  blood pressure, 248
  cardiovascular outcomes trial, 51
  glinide, 138
  hypertension, 322, 329
  hypertriglyceridemia, 256
  sulfonylurea, 124
  type 1 diabetes, **1–7**
  type 2 diabetes, **48–65**
phenformin, 80

phenobarbital, 382, 486*t*
phenol, 15, 32
phenothiazine, 145
phentermine, 483–484, 489*t*, 499
phentermine/topiramate, 487*t*–489*t*, 499
phentermine/topiramate ER, 495–497
phenylalanine, 227
phenylketonuric, 227
phenytoin, 146, 229*t*, 382, 486*t*
pheochromocytoma, 478
phlorizin, 73, 151
phosphodiesterase III, 361
phosphodiesterase inhibitor, 404, 405*t*
phosphodiesterase type 5 inhibitors (PDE5-I), 304, 404–406, 486*t*
phospholipid, 339
photocoagulation, 198, 444
photocoagulation surgery, 298–299
phototoxicity, 324*t*
physical activity
    depression, 460
    hypertension, 247–248, 322
    lipid management, 251, 340
    obesity, 482
    orthostatic hypotension, 303
    type 1 diabetes, 9, 33
    type 2 diabetes, 82
    weight loss, 263
pioglitazone, 56*t*, 72, 97*t*–98*t*, 103–117, 118*t*–119*t*, 120, 134, 155
pitavastatin, 256*t*, 343*t*–344*t*, 348*t*, 350
pituitary insufficiency, 142
PLACID trial, 449
plantar pressure, 306
plant stanol/sterol, 251, 340
plasma lipid level, 340
plasma lipoprotein, 339
PLATO trial, 360
pneumococcal conjugate vaccine (PCV13), 504*f*, 505–507
pneumococcal disease, 506–507
pneumococcal polysaccharide vaccine (PPSV23), 504*f*, 505–507
pneumonia, 506
podiatrist, 307
POINT trial, 363

polycystic ovary syndrome (PCOS), 81–82, 90, 108, 111
polydipsia, 8
polyneuropathy. *See* diabetic polyneuropathy
polyol flux pathway, 395–396
polyphagia, 8
polypharmacy, 246
polyuria, 8
postherpetic neuralgia, 507
postmenopausal women, 107
postprandial glucose (PPG) level
    α-glucosidase inhibitor, 71, 168
    glucagon-like peptide 1 (GLP-1) receptor agonist, 191–193, 203
    insulin, 13, 29, 32, 42
    pramlintide, 211–213, 215–216
    thiazolidinedione, 108
post-vitrectomy patient, 446
potassium
    acute kidney injury, 250
    chronic kidney disease, 287, 290–291
    glinide, 139
    hyperkalemia, 161, 250–251
    hypertension, 248, 329
    hypokalemia, 34, 36
    nephropathy, 422, 428
    sulfonylurea, 124–125
potassium-wasting action, 487*t*
PPARα (alpha), 72, 104
PPARβ/δ (beta/delta), 104
PPAR-γ (peroxisome-proliferator-activated receptor gamma), 72, 104, 106, 109, 112–113
pramipexole, 233
pramlintide, **211–222**
    adverse effects and monitoring, 217–218
    availability, dosing, and administration requirements, 219*t*
    cost, 57*t*
    dosage and administration, 219–220
    drug interaction, 39, 218
    efficacy and safety, 214*t*
    gastroparesis, 304
    hypoglycemia, 215–218
    insulin, 213, 215–216, 218–219

mechanism of action, 212
monograph, 220
pharmacokinetic, 212
pharmacology, 212
special population, 216–217
therapeutic consideration, 215–220
treatment advantages/
    disadvantages, 212–213, 215
type 1 diabetes, 3, 20, 22, 218–220
type 2 diabetes, 219–220
warnings/precautions, 215–216
weight loss, 16, 38
prasugrel, 261, 358, 363, 365t, 366
pravastatin, 229t, 256t, 343t–344t,
    349t, 350
prediabetes, 9t, 82, 225
prednisone, 88
preeclampsia, 247
pregabalin, 116, 300, 302–303, 397,
    398t, 399, 401–402, 407
pregnancy
    α-glucosidase inhibitor, 171
    antihypertensive medication, 246–
        248, 328
    bile acid sequestrant, 227
    bupropion SR, 382
    cilostazol, 361
    clomiphene, 90
    clonidine, 384
    clopidogrel, 359
    diabetic retinopathy, 296–298
    dipeptidyl peptidase-4 (DPP-4)
        inhibitor, 181
    dipyridamole/aspirin, 361
    dopamine-2 receptor agonist, 236
    erythromycin, 404
    GABA analog, 399–400
    glinide, 143
    glucagon, 478–479
    glucagon-like peptide 1 (GLP-1)
        receptor agonist, 199
    hypertension, 243
    insulin, 36
    liraglutide, 494
    lorcaserin, 490
    metformin, 82
    naltrexone/bupropion XR, 498
    nicotine replacement therapy, 373

nortriptyline, 386
oral contraceptive, 488t
orlistat, 492
phentermine, 484
phentermine/topiramate ER, 496
pramlintide, 216
prasugrel, 358
selective serotonin-norepinephrine
    reuptake inhibitor, 400
sodium–glucose cotransporter 2
    (SGLT2) inhibitor, 158–160
statin therapy, 252
sulfonylurea, 128
thiazolidinedione, 108, 110
ticagrelor, 360
tricyclic antidepressant, 401
type 1 diabetes, 1
varenicline, 379
vorapaxar, 362
premenopausal women, 90, 108
priapism, 406, 486t
primary prevention, 339
primary pulmonary hypertension
    (PPH), 484, 490
probenecid, 130, 145, 474
procainamide, 90
progestin, 39
progression-free survival (PFS), 84
prolactin, 236, 491
proliferative diabetic retinopathy
    (PDR), 296–297, 439–444, 448–450
pro-opiomelanocortin (POMC)
    neuron, 488
propafenone, 486t
propranolol, 90, 128, 172, 229t, 326t
proprioceptive impairment, 395
proprotein convertase subtilisin/kexin
    type 9 (PCSK9) inhibitor, 254–255,
    258, 341, 343, 344t, 349t, 351
PROspective pioglitAzone Clinical
    Trial In macroVascular Events
    (PROactive) trial, 107, 109–111, 113
prostacyclin, 356
prostaglandin cyclo-oxygenase-1
    (COX-1), 357
prostaglandin D2 receptor DP1, 346
prostaglandin E, 406
prostate cancer, 84

protamine, 13, 30
protease-activated receptor-1 (PAR-1) antagonist, 362
protease inhibitor, 39
PROTECT (Precose Resolution of Optimal Titration to Enhance Current Therapies), 168
protective sensation, 305
protein, 2, 16, 37, 287, 291, 475–476
protein-bound medication, 401
proteinuria, 108, 413, 421, 423, 428
prothionamide, 89, 487*t*
Protocol S study, 443–444
proton pump inhibitors (PPI), 359
provider-patient communication, 205
proximal tubule epithelial cell, 152
pruritus, 326*t*
pseudophakic eye, 446
psychiatric disorder, 235, 381, 490, 497
psychotherapy, 461–462, 466
puberty, 1
pudendal penile arteries/ arterioles, 404
pulmonary function, 38
pyelonephritis, 157, 161–162

Q
Qsymia, 488*t*
QTc interval prolongation, 462, 473
quinapril, 330*t*
quinidine, 90
quinine, 90
quinolone, 89, 116, 487*t*

R
race, 217, 411, 460
radiological studies, 85
ramipril, 325*t*, 330*t*, 332, 414–415, 422, 424*t*, 429
randomized controlled trial, 244, 245*t*, 254, 258–259, 262–265, 269, 307, 323, 340. *See also under specific trial*
ranibizumab, 296–297, 299, 441–445, 449–451
ranitidine, 90, 172
ranolazine, 90

rapid-acting analogs (RAAs), 12–13, 29
rapid-acting analogs (RAAs) blockade, 415
rapid-acting analogs (RAAs) inhibitor, 417–419
rapid-acting analogs (RAAs) study, 414
rash, 172, 182, 362, 379, 404–405
RASS trial, 446
Ratner, RE, 213, 214*t*
READ2 trial, 449
rebound hypertension, 383
recombinant DNA technology, 11, 26
registered dietitian (RD), 482
regular human insulin (RHI), 11–12, 28–29
rehabilitation specialist, 307
RENAAL trial, 415, 423
renal
    blood flow, 290
    disease, 180, 196, 301, 304, 492
    dysfunction, 69, 72–73, 112, 128, 131, 143, 362
    effect, 74
    failure, 330, 361, 420, 465*t*, 494
    fibrosis, 421
    function, 85, 178, 199, 345*t*, 359, 492
    glucose, 417
    hypertrophy, 411
    injury, 329
    insufficiency, 87, 128, 198, 217, 348*t*, 463
    outcome, 288
    replacement therapy, 155, 295, 417–419
    tubular secretion, 89
renal impairment
    α-glucosidase inhibitor, 171
    alogliptin, 181, 183
    antihypertensive medication, 325*t*, 330*t*–331*t*
    antiplatelet therapy, 360
    atypical antidepressant, 465*t*
    bile acid sequestrant, 228
    bupropion SR, 380
    canagliflozin, 158
    cilostazol, 361
    clopidogrel, 359

dapagliflozin, 159, 418
dipeptidyl peptidase-4 (DPP-4)
    inhibitor, 179
dopamine-2 receptor agonist, 236
duloxetine, 400
empagliflozin, 160
ertugliflozin, 160
exenatide XR, 193
GABA analog, 399
glinide, 143
glucagon-like peptide 1 (GLP-1)
    receptor agonist, 199, 203
insulin, 36–37
linagliptin, 177, 181
liraglutide, 494
lorcaserin, 490–491
metformin, 85
metformin XR, 95*t*
metformin XR/dapagliflozin, 95*t*
metoclopramide, 403
naltrexone/bupropion SR, 498–499
phentermine/topiramate ER, 496
prasugrel, 358
saxagliptin, 178, 181, 183
selective serotonin-norepinephrine
    reuptake inhibitor, 400, 465*t*
selective serotonin reuptake
    inhibitor, 465*t*
semaglutide, 194
sitagliptin, 178, 183
sodium–glucose cotransporter 2
    (SGLT2) inhibitor, 156, 158–160,
    164*t*–165*t*
statin therapy, 348*t*–349*t*
ticagrelor, 360
type 1 diabetes, 199
varenicline, 377
renal-related adverse event, 159–160
renin-angiotensin-aldosterone system,
    330
renin-angiotensin-aldosterone system
    modulator, 156, 161
renin-angiotensin system (RAS)
    inhibitor, 412–417, 421–423, 428–
    429, 446–447
renin-angiotensin system (RAS)
    inhibitor-calcium antagonist, 423

renin inhibitor, 248, 250, 412–413,
    425*t*, 429–430
repaglinide, 56*t*, 71, 94*t*, 138–146, 147*t*
reserpine, 39
resistant hypertension, 250–251,
    328–329
respiratory problems, 482
resting tachycardia, 301
RESTORE study, 449
retina, 439, 441, 448
retinal detachment, 444
retinal neovascularization, 299
retinal photography, 297–298
retinopathy. *See* diabetic retinopathy
retrograde ejaculation, 302
revascularization, 106, 256, 262–263,
    363
reverse cholesterol transport, 339
Reye's syndrome, 260, 357, 361
rhabdomyolysis, 257, 341, 346
rhinitis, 237, 361
rifampicin, 163, 182
rifampin, 116, 145, 358
riomet, 92*t*
Risk Evaluation and Mitigation
    Strategy (REMS), 103
ritodrine, 90
ritonavir, 90, 382
ROADMAP trial, 416
ropinirole, 233
rosiglitazone, 56*t*, 72, 103–117, 118*t*,
    120, 126
Rosiglitazone Evaluated for
    Cardiovascular Outcomes in Oral
    Agents Combination Therapy for
    Type 2 Diabetes (RECORD) trial,
    106–107, 110–111
rosuvastatin, 256*t*, 258, 343*t*–344*t*,
    348*t*, 350
rubella, 504*f*
"rule of 15", 16, 37, 475

S

salicylate, 39, 89, 114, 130, 145, 487*t*
salt, 303
satiety, 20, 75, 211–212, 403

Satiety and Clinical Adiposity—
Liraglutide Evidence in Nondiabetic
and Diabetic Individuals (SCALE)
program, 493
saturated fat, 251, 340
SAVOR-TIMI 53 trial, 179,
266*t*–268*t*, 420
saxagliptin
antihyperglycemic medication with
metformin, 93*t*
cardiovascular outcome trial,
266*t*–268*t*, 269
cost, 56*t*
dipeptidyl peptidase-4 (DPP-4)
inhibitor, 73, 177–183, 184, 185
nephropathy, 420, 426*t*, 430
Saxagliptin Assessment of Vascular
Outcomes Recorded in Patients with
Diabetes Mellitus – Thrombolysis in
Myocardial Infarction 53 (SAVOR-
TIMI 53) study, 269
SCALE Maintenance trial, 493
SCALE Obesity and Prediabetes trial,
493
Scartozzi, Dawn, 70*f*
schizophrenia, 379, 382
sclerosis, 421
seasonal affective disorder (SAD), 464
secondary amines, 401
secondary prevention, 339
second-hand smoke (SHS), 374*f*
sedation, 384, 386, 399, 462–464
sedentary time, 322
seizure, 379–382, 386, 398, 463–464,
472, 485*t*, 496, 498
seizure threshold-lowering drug, 486*t*,
488*t*
selective serotonin-2c (5-HT2C)
receptor agonist, 488*
selective serotonin-norepinephrine
reuptake inhibitors (SNRIs), 398*t*,
400, 461–463, 465*t*, 467
selective serotonin reuptake inhibitors
(SSRIs), 89, 303, 372, 461–462, 465*t*,
467, 487*t*
self-monitoring blood glucose
(SMBG), 54, 203, 216–218, 228, 237,
474, 506

semaglutide
cardiovascular outcome trial, 51,
264–265, 266*t*–268*t*
cost, 57*t*
diabetic retinopathy, 198, 449
glucagon-like peptide 1 (GLP-1)
receptor agonist, 74–75, 190, 192*t*,
193–197, 201*t*
nephropathy, 293, 419, 426*t*, 430
type 2 diabetes, 68*f*
septicemia, 85
SEQUEL randomized clinical trial,
495
serotonergic agent, 486*t*, 490
serotonin, 385, 463
serotonin (5-HT), 400
serotonin-3 receptor (5HT$_3$)
antagonist, 403
serotonin-4 receptor (5HT$_4$) agonist,
403
serotonin 5-HT$_{2C}$ receptor, 488
serotonin modulator, 461, 464, 466*t*,
468
serotonin receptor, 233
serotonin syndrome, 386, 401, 466,
486*t*, 490–491
sertraline, 462, 465*t*
serum creatinine
acute kidney injury, 250, 290
chronic kidney disease, 287, 293
glucagon-like peptide 1 (GLP-1)
receptor agonist, 203
hyperkalemia, 250–251
hypertension, 248, 329, 345*t*
nephropathy, 413, 415, 418–419,
422
serum creatinine kinase level, 341
serum iron, 171
serum lipid control, 296
serum potassium. *See* potassium
serum transaminase, 71, 113, 172
severe hepatic impairment, 360
severe hypoglycemia
cognitive impairment, 472–473
glucagon, 16, 37
glucagon-like peptide 1 (GLP-1)
receptor agonist, 202
insulin, 474

insulin pump therapy, 2
insulin therapy in people with T2D, 76
meglitinide, 130
pramlintide, 20, 213, 214*t*, 215–217
prevention, 475
sulfonylurea, 127, 130
severe nonproliferative diabetic retinopathy, 296
sexual dysfunction, 302, 324*t*, 396*t*, 397, 462–464
shingles, 504*f*
shoe, 305–306
sight-threatening diabetic retinopathy (STDR), 447
sildenafil, 404–407
silent ischemia, 262
Simcor, 347
simvastatin, 254–255, 256*t*, 257, 342–343, 344*t*, 346–347, 349*t*, 350, 360
simvastatin/ezetimibe, 347
simvastatin/niacin, 347
sinus bradycardia, 384
sitagliptin
    antihyperglycemic medication with metformin, 93*t*–94*t*
    cardiovascular outcome trial, 179–180, 266*t*–268*t*, 269
    cost, 56*t*
    dipeptidyl peptidase-4 (DPP-4) inhibitor, 73, 178, 181–183
    dosing recommendation, 184
    metformin and, 185
    nephropathy, 420, 426*t*, 430
skin, 258, 304–306, 347
sleep apnea, 482
sleep disorder, 460, 496
sleep onset, sudden, 235
sleepwalking, 379
SMART goal, 69*f*
smokeless tobacco, 370
smoking. *See also* nicotine replacement therapy; tobacco
    "5 As", 372*t*
    cardiovascular risk factor, 355
    cessation, **370–394**, 464
    cessation, combination therapy for, 387, 388*t*, 389

    cessation, first-line combination therapies, 387
    cessation, first-line medications, 372–382
    cessation, non-nicotine medication, 376
    cessation, second-line combination therapies, 387
    cessation, second-line medication, 372, 383–387
    cigarette, 370, 374*f*
    cost, 60
    diabetes risk factor, 370, 371*t*
    electronic cigarettes (e-cigarettes), 370
    foot care recommendation, 304–305
    hypertension, 322
    monograph, 389–390
    second-hand smoke, 374*f*
    tobacco cessation treatment, 374*f*
Snellen visual acuity, 441
social support system, 460
sodium, 247–248, 291, 322, 329, 417
sodium-channel blockade, 401
sodium–glucose cotransporter 2 (SGLT2) inhibitor, **151–167**
    acute kidney injury, 290
    adverse effects and monitoring, 160–162
    antidiabetic medication, 77*t*
    atherosclerotic cardiovascular disease, 242, 262
    cardiovascular outcomes trial, 263, 266*t*–268*t*, 269, 294
    cardiovascular/renal outcome, 154–155
    chronic kidney disease, 286, 292–293
    combination products, 165
    cost, 56*t*, 74, 156
    dosage and administration, 164*t*–165*t*, 425*t*
    drug interaction, 162–163
    insulin, 38
    mechanism of action, 151–153
    monograph, 165, 430

nephropathy, 417–418, 425*t*, 428, 430
pharmacodynamic, 162–163
pharmacogenomics, 161
pharmacokinetic, 153–154, 163–164
pharmacology, 151–154
renal protection, 155
special population, 158–159
therapeutic consideration, 156–157
treatment advantages/
  disadvantages, 154–156
type 1 diabetes, 4, 21
type 2 diabetes, 48, 50–51, 52*t*–53*t*,
  61, 67, 68*f*, 73–74
warnings/precautions, 156–157
sodium–glucose cotransporter 2
  (SGLT2) inhibitor/DPP-4 inhibitor
  combination, 428
sodium–glucose cotransporter 2
  (SGLT2) inhibitor/RAS inhibitor
  combination, 428
sodium valproate, 399
soliqua, 206
somnambulism, 379
somnolence, 235, 327*t*, 400, 467
sotagliflozin, 4, 73, 153
Special Interest Group on
  Neuropathic Pain of the
  International Association for the
  Study of Pain, 303
spirometry (FEV₁) testing, 60
spironolactone, 247, 325*t*, 331*t*, 332–
  333, 421, 423, 427*t*, 428, 430
stable ischemic heart disease, 364*t*
Standards of Medical Care in Diabetes
  (ADA), 3, 16, 33, 36–37, 82, 224, 234,
  241, 269, 286, 472
staphylococci, 307
statin, 145, 257, 342–343, 344*t*
statin/bile acid sequestrant, 347
statin/fibrate, 257
statin/niacin, 257, 346–347
statin/omega-3 fatty acid, 347
statin therapy, 252–254, 256*t*, 263,
  266*t*, 340–343, 347, 412, 440
ST-elevated myocardial infarction
  (STEMI), 358–359
steroid therapy, 450–451

Stevens-Johnson syndrome, 180, 379
St. John's Wort, 386
stomach pain/cramps, 344*t*–345*t*, 462
stomach ulcer, 357
streptococci, 307
stroke
  antihypertensive medication, 246,
    328
  antiplatelet therapy, 355, 363, 365*t*
  aspirin therapy, 259
  atherosclerotic cardiovascular
    disease, 339
  bromocriptine, 237
  cardiovascular outcome trial, 154,
    179, 244, 263–265, 268*t*
  clopidogrel, 358–359
  clopidogrel/aspirin, 363
  coronary artery disease, 261
  cost, 355
  dipyridamole/aspirin, 360
  evolocumab, 256
  glucagon-like peptide 1 (GLP-1)
    receptor agonist, 195–196
  obesity, 482
  pioglitazone, 111
  prasugrel, 358
  prevention, 356*t*
  rosiglitazone, 106–107
  smoking, 370
  statin/niacin, 257–258
  ticagrelor, 359
  vorapaxar, 362
structural abnormalities, 199, 305
ST-segment elevation myocardial
  infarction (STEMI), 328, 364*t*
studies/trials. *See* randomized
  controlled trial; *under specific trial*
Substance Abuse and Mental Health
  Services Administration (SAMHSA),
  460
substance use/abuse, 460, 484
sudden death, 463
sudomotor dysfunction, 301
suicide/suicidal ideation, 381, 386,
  460, 466, 496, 498
sulfa allergy, 129, 141
sulfonamide, 130, 145
sulfonamide antibiotic, 39

sulfonylurea, **124–137**
  adverse effects and monitoring,
    129–130
  α-glucosidase inhibitor and, 172
  BIDS: bedtime insulin daytime
    sulfonylurea, 132
  bile acid sequestrant and, 225, 229*t*
  bromocriptine and, 234
  combination therapy, 61, 131, 134
  cost, 55*t*
  dosage and administration, 131–
    132, 133*t*
  drug interaction, 130–131
  duration of action, 131
  glinide and, 141
  glucagon and, 130
  glucagon-like peptide 1 (GLP-1)
    receptor agonist, 202
  hypoglycemia, 37, 86, 108, 126–131,
    474, 487*t*
  insulin and, 131
  linagliptin and, 183
  meglitinide and, 131
  monograph, 134
  pharmacokinetic, 132*t*
  pharmacology, 124–126
  rosiglitazone and, 106–107
  saxagliptin and, 181
  special population, 128–129
  therapeutic consideration, 127–134
  treatment advantages/
    disadvantages, 126–127
  type 2 diabetes, 50, 53*t*, 67–71, 77*t*
  warnings/precautions, 127–128
  weight gain, 126, 129–130
surgery/surgical procedure, 86, 304,
  307, 359
SUSTAIN-6 (Trial to Evaluate
  Cardiovascular and Other Long-
  term Outcomes with Semaglutide
  in Subjects With Type 2 Diabetes),
  195*t*, 196, 198, 266*t*–268*t*, 293, 419,
  449
sweat gland, 396*t*
symbyax, 467
sympatholytic, semiselective
  dopamine-2 (D2) receptor agonist,
  233

sympathomimetic agent, 39, 146, 237,
  387
sympathomimetic amine, 483, 495
symptomatic diabetic neuropathy, 300
syncopal migraine, 236
syncope, 237, 250, 325*t*, 406
synthetic ghrelin agonist, 404
syringe, 3, 32
Systolic Blood Pressure Intervention
  Trial (SPRINT), 244, 245*t*, 246

T

tachycardia, 327*t*, 361, 396*t*, 485*t*
tachyphylaxis, 304, 404
tadalafil, 404–407
tamoxifen, 382
Tang, YL, 83
tapentadol, 302–303
tardive dyskinesia, 403
TECOS trial, 179, 266*t*–268*t*, 420
telemedicine program, 296
telmisartan, 330*t*, 416, 422, 424*t*, 429
temperature variation, 11, 27
10-hydroxynortriptyline, 385
teratogen, 496
teratogenicity, 361
tertiary amines, 401
testosterone, 82
tetanus, 504*f*, 505, 507
tetanus, diphtheria, whooping cough
  (pertussis) (Tdap, Td), 504*f*, 505
tetracyclic antidepressant, 463–464
tetracycline, 229*t*
therosclerotic cardiovascular disease,
  261
thiazide, 487*t*
thiazide diuretic, 145, 172, 324*t*, 330*t*
thiazide-like diuretic, 248, 249*t*, 250–
  251, 295, 323, 324*t*, 328, 330*t*, 487*t*
thiazolidinediones (TZDs), **103–123**
  adverse effects and monitoring,
    112–114
  alogliptin, 118*t*
  antihyperglycemic medication with
    metformin, 97*t*
  bladder cancer, 109–110
  cardiac, 109

colesevelam, 225
cost, 56*t*
dosage and administration, 117
drug interaction, 114–116
edema, 109
fracture, 110
heart failure, 269
hematology, 108
hepatic, 109
hypoglycemia, 108
mechanism of action, 104
monograph, 120
neuropathy, 399
nursing, 110
ovulation, 108
pharmacokinetic, 105
pharmacology, 104–108
pioglitazone, 118*t*–119*t*
pioglitazone combination, 118*t*–119*t*
pregnancy, 110
rosiglitazone, 118*t*
special population, 110–112
therapeutic consideration, 108–117
treatment advantages/disadvantages, 105–108
type 1 diabetes, 108
type 2 diabetes, 50, 53*t*, 61, 67–68, 72–73, 77*t*
weight gain, 109, 155
thienopyridine, 358–360
3-hydroxy-3-methylglutaryl coenzyme A reductase (HMG-CoA reductase), 339
threonine, 14, 30
thrombin receptor agonist peptide (TRAP), 362
thrombocytopenia, 129
thrombosis, 355–356, 404
thrombotic cardiovascular event, 362
thromboxane A_2, 261, 356, 360
thyroid C-cell carcinoma, 197
thyroid C-cell tumor, 75, 196, 494
thyroid function, 492
thyroid hormone, 39
Tian, S, 83
ticagrelor, 261, 359–360, 363, 365*t*, 366

ticlopidine, 488*t*
time-domain optical coherence tomography (TD-OCT), 441
tissue catabolism, 1
T_{max}, 153–154, 398
TNF-α (tumor necrosis factor alpha), 104
tobacco, 370, 371*t*–372*t*, 374*f. See also* smoking
tolazamide, 124, 132*t*–133*t*, 134
tolbutamide, 124, 127, 129, 131, 132*t*–133*t*, 134
topical capsaicin, 303
topical medication, 398*t*, 401–402
topiramate, 90, 116, 487*t*–488*t*
torsemide, 326*t*
toxin, 301
trandolapril, 415–416, 447
trandolapril/verapamil SR, 423
transaminase, 257, 346, 350*t*
Transcend, 476*t*
transdermal patch. *See* nicotine replacement therapy
trans fat, 251, 340
transient ischemic attack (TIA), 106–107, 111, 259, 261, 339, 357–358, 360, 362–363, 365*t*
transmembrane G-protein coupled receptor (TGR5), 224
transplantation, 413
trazodone, 464, 466*t*, 468
tremor, 386, 399
Trial Evaluating Cardiovascular Outcomes with Sitagliptin (TECOS), 269
Trial to Evaluate Cardiovascular and Other Long-term Outcomes with Semaglutide in Subjects with Type 2 Diabetes (SUSTAIN-6), 264–265
triamcinolone, 444–445, 450*t*, 451
triamcinolone cream, 375
triamcinolone/laser therapy combination, 445
triamterene, 90, 327*t*, 332
tricyclic, 462
tricyclic antidepressants (TCA)
bupropion SR, 382
depression, 461, 463, 467

diabetic-induced neuropathy, 398*t*
diabetic peripheral neuropathy, 303
dose and dosage adjustment, 465*t*
gastroparesis, 304
hypoglycemia, 486*t*
neuropathy, 400–401
nortriptyline, 384–387
trigeminal neuralgia, 399
triglyceride
  bile acid sequestrant, 225–226, 228,
    345*t*
  bromocriptine, 234
  lipid management, 251–252, 256,
    339–340
  metformin, 81
  orlistat, 492
  pioglitazone, 106
  rosiglitazone, 106
  statin/fibrate, 257, 346
  statin/niacin, 346
  statin/omega-3 fatty acid, 347
  thiazolidinedione, 104
trimethoprim, 90, 116–117
triptan, 386
TRITON-TIMI 38 trial, 363
troglitazone, 103, 109
trospium, 89
Trueplus Glucose, 476*t*
trulicity, 206
tubular secretion, 81
tubuloglomerular feedback, 417
2C8 isoenzyme, 178
2014 U.S. Surgeon General's report,
  370
2018 European Atherosclerosis
  Society Consensus Panel statement,
  258
2018 Heart Disease and Stroke
  Statistics Update, 355
type 1 diabetes (T1D)
  adjunctive drug therapies, 20–21
  α-glucosidase inhibitor, 168
  albuminuria, 290–291, 413–414
  amylin, 211
  antihyperglycemic drug therapy,
    10–17
  antihypertensive therapy, 294–295
  bile acid sequestrant, 225

bromocriptine, 234
cardiovascular risk factor, 355
chronic kidney disease, 286–287,
  292
diabetic ketoacidosis, 157
diabetic kidney disease, 288
diabetic peripheral neuropathy,
  300–302
diabetic retinopathy, 296–298,
  439–440
dipeptidyl peptidase-4 (DPP-4)
  inhibitor, 178, 180
distal symmetric sensorimotor
  polyneuropathy, 395
glinide, 142
glucose-lowering medication, 3
glycemic management, 9–21
hyperglycemia, **8–25**
hypertension, 244, 413–414
hypoglycemia, 1, 472, 474, 477
incretin-based therapy, 21
inhaled human insulin, 58
insulin, 33
insulin dosing, 17–20
insulin secretion, 27
lipid profile, 252
medical nutrition therapy, 482
metformin, 21
mineralocorticoid receptor
  antagonist, 421
monograph, 21–22
natural history of, 9*t*
neuropathy, 395
noninsulin treatment, 3–4
normoalbuminuria, 413–414, 446
normotension, 413–414, 446
pathophysiology, 8
pharmacologic therapy, **1–7**
pramlintide, 213, 215–216, 218–220
pregnancy, 297
recommendation, 1
renin-angiotensin system (RAS)
  inhibitor, 413–414, 446–447
severe hypoglycemia, 76
sodium–glucose cotransporter 2
  (SGLT2) inhibitor, 418
statin therapy, 253–254
statistics, 8

sulfonylurea, 127
thiazolidinedione, 108
vaccine-preventable disease, 503
weight gain, 38
Type 1 Diabetes Through the Life Span
(ADA), 20
type 2 diabetes (T2D), **66–79**
α-glucosidase inhibitor, 168, 171
albuminuria, 290, 414–415
amylin, 211
antihyperglycemic drug therapy,
52*t*–53*t*
antihypertensive therapy, 294–295
atherosclerotic cardiovascular
disease, 252–253, 269, 339
bile acid sequestrant, 225
bromocriptine, 234, 238
cardiovascular outcomes trial, 51,
263
cardiovascular risk factor, 355
chronic kidney disease, 286, 292
colesevelam, 223
combination injectable therapy, 35*f*,
60–61
combination therapy, 50–51, 422–
423, 428
cost, 76
diabetic kidney disease, 288
diabetic peripheral neuropathy,
300–302
diabetic retinopathy, 296–298,
439–440
dipeptidyl peptidase-4 (DPP-4)
inhibitor, 176, 419
distal symmetric polyneuropathy,
396*t*
distal symmetric sensorimotor
polyneuropathy, 395
glinide, **138–150**
glucagon-like peptide 1 (GLP-1)
receptor agonist, 190, 419
glucose-lowering medication, 68*f*,
292–294
histone deacetylase (HDAC)
enzyme, 399
hyperglycemia, 105
hypertension, 244, 414–415
hypertriglyceridemia, 340

initial therapy, 49–50
injectable therapy, 74–76
insulin, 33–34, 75–76
insulin secretion, 27
linagliptin, 419–420
liraglutide, 493
lixisenatide, 419
lorcaserin, 488
major depressive disorder, 460
medical nutrition therapy, 482
medication, choice of, 66–67
mineralocorticoid receptor
antagonist, 421
naltrexone/bupropion XR, 497
neuropathy, 395
normoalbuminuria, 414–416, 419,
447
normotension, 414–416, 447
obesity, 482
oral therapy, 67–74
orlistat, 491
orthostatic hypotension, 329
patient-centered glycemic
management, 48–49, 69*f*
pharmacologic therapy, **48–65**
pramlintide, 20, 213, 215, 219–220
prevention, 82
recommendation, 48–49
regular insulin U-500, 32
renin-angiotensin system (RAS)
inhibitor, 447
semaglutide, 193–194, 419
smoking, 370, 371*t*
sodium–glucose cotransporter 2
(SGLT2) inhibitor, 417–418
statin therapy, 253–254
sulfonylurea, **124–137**
symptomatic hypoglycemia, 474
vaccine-preventable disease, 503
weight gain, 38
tyrosine kinase activity, 75–76

U
UK Prospective Diabetes Study
(UKPDS) risk engine, 262
ulceration, 301, 304–305, 307

United Kingdom Prospective Diabetes
  Study (UKPDS), 82, 127, 130, 440
University Group Diabetes Program,
  127
unstable angina (UA), 358–359
upper limit of normal (ULN), 109
upper respiratory tract infection, 182,
  325t
uric acid, 345t
uridine diphosphate
  glucuronosyltransferase (UGT),
  153–154, 161, 163–164
urinary acidifying agent, 486t
urinary albumin excretion (UAE),
  287–288, 412–416, 418, 421
urinary albumin-to-creatinine ratio
  (UACR), 248, 249t, 250, 286–288,
  293, 295, 323, 328, 414–423, 428
urinary incontinence, 302, 397
urinary oxalate, 492
urinary protein excretion, 423
urinary retention, 386, 396t
urinary sediment, 288
urinary tract infection (UTI), 157, 160
urinary tract symptom, 302
urine creatinine (Cr), 288
urine glucose excretion (UGE), 73,
  151, 153
urogenital infection, 74, 157
urosepsis, 157, 161–162
U.S. Department of Health and
  Human Services, 371, 380, 387
U.S. Food and Drug Administration
  (FDA)
  α-glucosidase inhibitor, 168
  alogliptin, 183
  anti-VEGF agent, 441
  bupropion SR, 380, 382
  cardiovascular outcomes trial,
    263–264, 269
  chronic kidney disease, 294
  clonidine, 383
  colesevelam, 223
  dipeptidyl peptidase-4 (DPP-4)
    inhibitor, 179
  duloxetine, 302, 400
  empagliflozin, 264
  exendin-4, 190

gabapentin, 398
gastroparesis, 304
glinide, 138
glucagon-like peptide 1 (GLP-1)
  receptor agonist, 197, 265
hybrid closed-loop pump system, 2
influenza vaccine, 506
insulin glargine, 14, 30
insulin lispro, 13, 29, 58
liraglutide, 196, 264, 493, 495
lorcaserin, 488
metformin, 49, 82, 292
metoclopramide, 403
nonparenteral glucagon
  preparation, 478
nortriptyline, 384
obesity pharmacotherapy, 483
olmesartan, 416
orlistat, 491
orthostatic hypotension, 304
phentermine/topiramate ER, 495
pioglitazone, 110
pramlintide, 211
pregabalin, 302, 399
ranibizumab, 299
Risk Evaluation and Mitigation
  Strategy (REMS) program, 103
rosiglitazone, 110
semaglutide, 194, 264–265
serotonin norepinephrine reuptake
  inhibitors, 462
smoking cessation, 372–373
sodium–glucose cotransporter 2
  (SGLT2) inhibitor, 21, 151, 265,
  418
sotagliflozin, 4
statin therapy, 258
tapentadol, 303
tri-cyclic antidepressant, 400
varenicline, 376, 378–379
weight loss medication, 38
zoster vaccine, 507

V

vaccination, **503–508**
vacuum device, 304
vagus nerve, 402

valproate, 382, 407
valproic acid, 229*t*, 399–400, 487*t*
valsartan, 330*t*, 332, 415, 421, 424*t*, 429
valvular heart disease, 484, 490–491
vancomycin, 90
vandetanib, 90
VA-NEPHRON D trial, 422
Vanilloid Transient Receptor Potential cation channel (TRPV1), 402
vardenafil, 404–407
varenicline, 372, 388*t*, 390
varenicline (chantix), 376–379
varenicline/bupropion SR, 387
varenicline/nicotine transdermal patch, 387
varicella (Chickenpox), 504*f*
varicella zoster virus, 507
vascular assessment, 305–306
vascular disease, 261, 304
vascular endothelial growth factor (VEGF), 441, 444
vascular endothelial growth factor (VEGF)-binding affinity, 441
vascular endothelial growth factor (VEGF) isoform specificity, 441
vascular mortality, 259, 340, 444
vascular surgery, 304, 307
vasculitis, 301
vasodilation, 327*t*, 405
vegetable, 322
venlafaxine, 303, 398*t*, 400, 462–463, 465*t*, 467
venlafaxine XR, 407, 465*t*
venous thromboembolism, 474
ventricular arrhythmia, 404, 473
verapamil, 90, 331*t*, 333, 415–416, 427*t*, 430, 447
verapamil SR, 324*t*
verapamil/trandolapril, 423, 429
VERTIS trial, 155
very-low-density lipoproteins (VLDL), 339, 345*t*
victoza, 206
vilazodone, 464, 466*t*, 468
viscous fiber, 251, 340
vision issues, 17, 39, 42, 114
vision loss, 296–298, 439–440

visual impairment, 305
vitamin A, 226
vitamin B$_{12}$ deficiency, 48–49, 68–69, 86, 88, 301
vitamin D, 226, 486*t*
vitamin E, 226
vitamin K, 226, 479
vitamin K deficiency-induced hemorrhage, 227
vitamin supplement, fat-soluble, 492
vitreoretinal ophthalmologist specialist, 441
vitreous hemorrhage, 198, 443, 448
voglibose, 168
voltage- dependent sodium channel, 399
voltage-gated sodium channel, 401
volume depletion, 329
volume overload, 291*t*
vomiting, 20, 88, 202, 218, 228, 237, 345*t*, 400, 404, 494
vorapaxar, 362, 365*t*, 366
voriconazole, 145
vortioxetine, 464, 466*t*, 468
Vytorin, 347

W
Wang, JS, 170
warfarin
   bile acid sequestrant, 229*t*
   clopidogrel, 359
   exenatide, 204
   glucagon, 479
   hypoglycemia, 474, 486*t*
   miglitol, 172
   pioglitazone, 117
   repaglinide, 145
   rosiglitazone, 117
   sulfonylurea, 130
   tricyclic antidepressant, 401
   vorapaxar, 362
weight, 3–4, 49, 477, 491
weight gain
   antipsychotic medication, 467
   depression, 460
   duloxetine, 463
   GABA analog, 399

glinide, 144–145
glucose-lowering medication, 68*f*
injectable therapy, 35*f*
insulin, 11, 16, 38, 76
mirtazapine, 464
phentermine, 484
pioglitazone, 108, 111
selective serotonin reuptake
  inhibitors, 462
sulfonylurea, 70, 126, 129–130
thiazolidinedione, 72, 107–109,
  112–113
tricyclic antidepressant, 463
type 2 diabetes, 50
weight loss
  α-glucosidase inhibitor, 169–170
  bupropion, 464
  cardiovascular disease, 263
  dipeptidyl peptidase-4 (DPP-4)
    inhibitor, 184
  gastroparesis, 403
  glucagon-like peptide 1 (GLP-1)
    receptor agonist, 75, 191, 194–
    195, 199
  glucose-lowering medication, 68
  hypertension, 247–248, 322
  hypertriglyceridemia, 256
  lipid management, 251, 340
  liraglutide, 493–495
  naltrexone/bupropion XR, 497–499
  obesity, 482–483
  orlistat, 491–492

phentermine, 483–484
phentermine/topiramate ER,
  495–497
pramlintide, 20, 212–213, 215
sodium–glucose cotransporter 2
  (SGLT2) inhibitor, 74, 155
Wellbutrin, 381
Weyer, C, 213
Whipple triad, 472
white blood cell, 361
white coat hypertension, 243, 250,
  322, 328
Whitehouse, F, 213, 214*t*
whooping cough, 504*f*
withdrawal syndrome, 464, 466

X

XENDOS trial, 491
xerostomia, 327*t*
xultophy, 206

Y

young adult, 381, 386, 466

Z

Zhou, PT, 83
zinc, 15, 32
zoster (shingles), 504*f*, 505
Zyban, 381